HOW TO FIND

THE BEST

METROPOLITAN CHICAGO

DOCTORS

HOW TO FIND THE BEST METROPOLITAN CHICAGO DOCTORS

CASTLE CONNOLLY GUIDE

HOW TO FIND

THE BEST

METROPOLITAN CHICAGO

DOCTORS

All Rights Reserved

Copyright © 1999, by Castle Connolly Medical Ltd.

Library of Congress Catalog Card Number 99-070719

The selection of medical providers for inclusion in this book was based in part on opinions solicited from physicians, nurses, and other health care professionals. The author and publishers cannot assure the accuracy of information provided to them by third parties, since such opinions are necessarily subjective and may be incomplete. The omission from this book of particular health care providers does not mean that such providers are not competent or reputable.

The purpose of this book is educational and informational. It is not intended to replace the advice of your physician or to assist the layman in diagnosing or treating illness, disease, or injury. Following the advice or recommendations set forth in this book is entirely at the reader's own risk. The author and publishers cannot ensure accuracy of, or assume responsibility for, the information in the book as such information is affected by constant change. Liability to any person or organization for any loss or damage caused by errors or omissions in this book is hereby declaimed. Whenever possible, readers should consult their own primary care physician when selecting health care providers, including any selection based upon information contained in this book. In order to protect patient privacy the names of patients cited in anecdotes throughout the book have been omitted.

"The confidence of our readers in our editorial integrity is crucial to the success of the Castle Connolly Guides. Any use of the Castle Connolly name, or of any list or listing (or portion of either) from any Castle Connolly Guide, for advertising or for any commercial purpose, without prior written consent, is strictly prohibited and may result in legal action."

For more information, please contact Castle Connolly Medical Ltd., 150 East 58th St, New York, New York 10155, 212-980-8230. E-mail: CCMedical@aol.com. Web site: http://www.castleconnolly.com, http://www.bestdocs.com

ISBN 1883769-11-6 (paperback)
ISBN 1883769-12-4 (hardcover)

Printed in the United States of America

CASTLE CONNOLLY GUIDE

TABLE OF CONTENTS

SECTION TWO
Directory of Doctors

SECTION THREE

SECTION FOUR

SECTION FIVE

ABOUT THE PUBLISHERS

The mission of Castle Connolly Medical Ltd. is to help individuals and families find the best health care. The company was founded in 1992 by John K. Castle and John J. Connolly, Ed.D.

PUBLISHERS

John K. Castle is the Chairman of Castle Connolly Medical Ltd. He has spent much of the last two decades involved with health care institutions and issues. Mr. Castle served as Chairman of the Board of New York Medical College for eleven years, an institution where he has continued on the Board for more than twenty years.

Mr. Castle has been extensively involved in other health care and voluntary activities as well. He served for five years as a public commissioner on the Joint Commission on Accreditation of Healthcare Organizations (JCAHO), the body which accredits most public and private hospitals throughout the United States. Mr. Castle has also served as a trustee of five different hospitals in the metropolitan New York region and is a director emeritus of the United Hospital Fund as well as a trustee of the Whitehead Institute.

In addition to his health care activities, Mr. Castle has served on many voluntary boards including the Corporation of the Massachusetts Institute of Technology, as well as numerous corporate boards of directors, including the Equitable Life

Assurance Society of the United States. He is chairman of a leading merchant bank and has been chief executive of a major investment bank.

Mr. Castle holds a Bachelor of Science degree from MIT; an MBA with High Distinction from the Harvard Business School, where he was a Baker Scholar; and an honorary doctorate from New York Medical College.

John J. Connolly, Ed.D., is the President and CEO of Castle Connolly Medical Ltd. His experience in health care and education is extensive.

Dr. Connolly served as president of New York Medical College, the state's largest private medical college, for more than ten years. Dr. Connolly is a fellow of the New York Academy of Medicine, a member of the New York Academy of Sciences, a director of the New York Business Group on Health, a member of the President's Council of the United Hospital Fund, and a member of the Executive Committee of Funding First. Dr. Connolly has served as a trustee of two hospitals and as Chairman of the Board of one. He is extensively involved in health care and community activities, and serves on a number of voluntary and corporate boards, including the Board of the American Lyme Disease Foundation, of which he is a founder, the Friends of the National Library of Medicine, and the Board of Advisors of the Whitehead Institute. He has a Bachelor of Science degree from Worcester State College, a Master's degree from the University of Connecticut, and a Doctor of Education degree in College and University Administration from Teacher's College, Columbia University.

MEDICAL ADVISORY BOARD

We are pleased to have associated with Castle Connolly Medical Ltd. a distinguished group of medical leaders who offer invaluable advice and wisdom in our efforts to assist consumers in obtaining the best health care. While the Medical Advisory Board is not involved in the selection of doctors included in this edition of the Castle Connolly Guide, many of them offered suggestions that helped us formulate appropriate selection criteria. We thank each member of the Medical Advisory Board for their valuable contributions.

CASTLE CONNOLLY MEDICAL ADVISORY BOARD

Charles Bechert, M.D.
Director
The Sight Foundation
Fort Lauderdale, FL

Roger Bulger, M.D.
President
Association of Academic Health Centers
Washington, DC

Harry J. Buncke, M.D.
Davies Medical Center
San Francisco, CA

Paul T. Calabresi, M.D.
Professor of Medicine and Medical Science
Chairman Emeritus
Department of Medicine
Brown University
Rhode Island Hospital
Providence, RI

Joseph Cimino, M.D.
Professor and Chairman
Community and Preventive Medicine
New York Medical College
Valhalla, NY

MEDICAL ADVISORY BOARD

Jane Clark, M.D.
Ear, Nose, Throat,
and Hearing Center of Framingham
61 Lincoln St.
Framingham, MA

John C. Duffy, M.D.
Medical Director for Youth Services
Charter Pines Behavioral Health System
Charlotte, NC

J. Richard Gaintner, M.D.
Chief Executive Officer
Shands Health Care
University of Florida
Gainesville, FL

Menard M. Gertler, M.D., D. Sc.
Clinical Professor of Medicine
Cornell University Medical School
New York, NY

Yutaka Kikawa, M.D.
Professor and Chairman
Department of Pathology
University of California Irvine College of Medicine
Irvine, CA

Nicholas F. LaRusso, M.D.
Chairman
Division of Gastroenterology
Mayo Medical School Clinic and Foundation
Rochester, MN

Benedict S. Maniscalco, M.D.
Chief Executive Officer
Access America Medical Care Inc.
Tampa, FL

David Paige, M.D.
Professor
Department of Maternal and Child Health
Johns Hopkins University
Baltimore, MD

Ronald Pion, M.D.
Chairman & CEO
Medical Telecommunications Associates
Los Angeles, CA

James Sammons, M.D.
Haines City, FL

Leon G. Smith, M.D.
Director of Medicine and Chief of Infectious Diseases
St. Michael's Medical Center
Newark, NJ

Ralph Snyderman, M.D.
Chancellor for Health Affairs
Duke University School of Medicine
Durham, NC

FOREWORD

Dear Reader:

Choosing a doctor is one of the most important choices in your life. However, most of us put little effort into this selection. We simply pick a name from a list or get a recommendation from a friend.

Most of us have very little information about our doctors, and/or don't know where to get it. Now with the publication of the *Castle Connolly Guide—How To Find The Best Doctors*, you can learn about doctors' medical school education, residency training, fellowships, board certifications, hospital appointments and much more. The Guide also describes in simple terms what information about each doctor you should ascertain and how to evaluate it. This information gathering is essential for everyone who wants to find a good doctor to truly meet *his or her* health care needs.

FOREWORD

As an administrator and nurse who deals with the problems of health on a daily basis, I know well the importance of getting the best health care. Our center assists medical malpractice victims. The human tragedy we often encounter is heartbreaking.

In many cases, had the patient taken a few minutes to make a modest effort to learn more about their doctor's background, a serious incident may have been avoided.

That is why the *Castle Connolly Guide* is so important to consumers. In this new and rapidly changing health care environment, patients must be well informed. Many do not trust the health care system. They are not confident their HMO, their hospital, or even their doctor, is motivated to protect them and to ensure that they get excellent care.

The *Castle Connolly Guide* is a comprehensive guide chock full of valuable information. It is completely consumer-friendly, giving readers all they need to know to make intelligent, informed choices.

Use it well and in good health!

Sincerely,

Sandra Gainer RN
Associate Director
National Center for Patient Rights

INTRODUCTION

HOW THIS BOOK CAN HELP YOU IMPROVE YOUR HEALTH

A savvy consumer, searching for a car, restaurant, house, or even a spouse, can easily find a guidebook to help. Yet, when it comes to choosing health care providers, the bookshelves are nearly bare.

How To Find The Best Doctors has been written to fill that void. It will guide you in making critical—even lifesaving—choices.

This book has two goals:

- *To provide you with a base of information and a framework of understanding so that you can participate in the important health care choices that will maximize your own health, your family's health, and the quality of your life.*
- *To provide detailed information on approximately 2,000 well-trained, highly competent physicians from which you may confidently choose your personal best doctors for your own health care needs and those of your family.*

INTRODUCTION

Medicine is often described as a combination of art and science. This description holds true for the process of selecting the best medical care. This book describes the "science" of making that selection. It is not magical or even difficult. It is simply a matter of knowing what information you should have and where to find it.

The "art" is what you will bring to the selection process. It is based upon your feelings, your needs, and the chemistry that develops between you and those who provide your health care. *How To Find The Best Doctors: Metropolitan Chicago* will help you prepare for that interaction and guide you in getting the most from it.

Most important, *How To Find The Best Doctors: Metropolitan Chicago* will tell you how to combine the art and science so that you can make the best choices.

HOW TO USE THIS BOOK

This book has been written as a basic, "how to" guide to selecting the best health care. The first section contains important information on how to choose the best doctors. Doctors are the most important providers of health care and whether you are part of an HMO or covered by traditional medical insurance, you want the very best doctor to attend to your health care needs. The second section contains the listings of doctors as well as information on the hospitals invited to participate in the Guide's Hospital Information Program. The third section includes information on Centers of Excellence – special programs and services – offered by a number of the hospitals participating in the Hospital Information Program. The fourth section offers 14 appendices presenting information that may be important and useful. Three indexes complete the book and are a useful tool for finding doctors by name or specialty.

There are three effective ways to use this book:

- *Start at the beginning. This method will give you a broad understanding of the health care field and a clearer perspective of where you fit into it. This method will arm you with information necessary to make informed choices that will help you find the best doctors.*
- *Study the doctor listings. While at least a brief reading of some or all of the introductory chapters is recommended so that, in the end, you will make well-informed choices, it is understandable that you may wish to go straight to the physician listings. The organization of these listings is outlined on pages 101 to 113. You will find guidelines for effectively using the listings on these pages.*
- *You may also wish to begin with the doctor listings. Index I is a listing of special practice interests, Index II is a listing of primary care physicians and Index III is an alphabetical listing, by name, of doctors.*

Each chapter begins with explanations of terms that may be new to you. Reviewing these terms will help you read the section easily.

In preparing this book, we've left little to chance or question. We hope to inspire you to assume that curious and insistent attitude as you make the health care choices that will take you and your family through life.

SECTION ONE

THE DOCTOR OF CHOICE

QUICK TIPS.

1. THE TIME TO ESTABLISH A RELATIONSHIP WITH A DOCTOR IS *WHILE YOU ARE HEALTHY*. THE BEST DOCTOR TO ESTABLISH YOUR RELATIONSHIP WITH IS THE ONE WHO IS MOST LIKELY TO KEEP YOU HEALTHY: A PRIMARY CARE DOCTOR.

2. PRIMARY MEANS FIRST, SO A PRIMARY CARE DOCTOR IS THE FIRST ONE YOU SEE FOR MOST HEALTH PROBLEMS.

3. IT IS DIFFICULT FOR ANY DOCTOR, HOWEVER SKILLED, TO MAKE JUDGEMENTS BASED ON ONLY ONE VISIT OR A SINGLE TEST.

4. YOUR PRIMARY CARE DOCTOR CAN EDUCATE YOU ABOUT THE HOWS AND WHYS OF HEALTH MAINTENANCE AND DISEASE PREVENTION AND FOLLOW UP TO HELP YOU STAY FAITHFUL TO THE COURSE THE TWO OF YOU HAVE AGREED UPON.

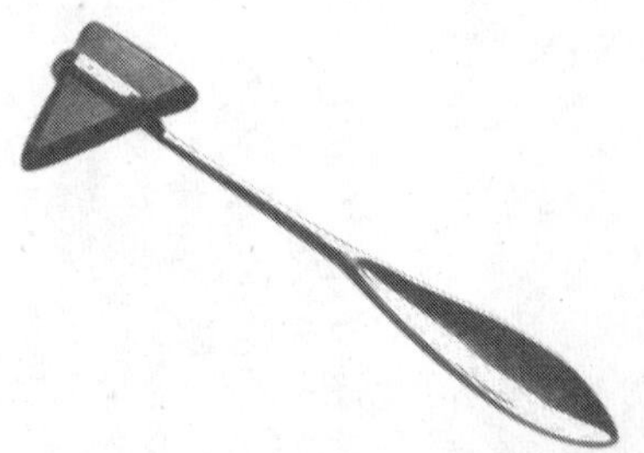

KEY TERMS CHAPTER 1

LUPUS ERYTHEMATOSUS

An autoimmune disorder, also referred to as SLE, or simply lupus. It can cause inflammation and possible damage to a number of vital organs and is commonly marked by joint pain, facial and other rashes, abnormally high antibody levels, and diminished red blood cell levels.

LYME DISEASE

An infectious disease, transmitted through the bite of a deer tick, which may or may not produce a distinctive bull's-eye rash at the site of the tick bite. First identified in Lyme, Connecticut, the infection may also produce other symptoms, including flu-like aches, arthritic joint pain, and, in complicated cases, cardiac abnormalities.

MANAGED CARE

The process of integrating the finance and delivery of health care to control costs and improve quality. A managed care plan typically involves a group of practitioners who "manage" care for a specified population.

OSTEOPATH

A health care professional who has earned a degree in osteopathic medicine, a D.O. Osteopathic Medicine emphasizes massage and bone manipulation while traditional western allopathic medicine emphasizes treatment with drugs and surgery.

PREVENTIVE MEDICINE/CARE

Health services that are aimed at maintaining good health and preventing illness. These services include routine physical examinations, immunizations, certain screening tests such as mammograms or Pap tests, as well as the practice of good health habits.

PRIMARY CARE PHYSICIAN

The first doctor consulted for any health problem, a Primary Care Physician is a specialist who offers basic, including preventive, medical care. It is important to maintain an ongoing relationship with your primary care physician.

SPECIALIST

A physician who practices one or more of the 25 specialties defined by the American Board of Medical Specialties (ABMS). The term is also used to denote a physician's area of practice, such as pediatrics, geriatrics, surgery, etc.

SUBSPECIALIST

A specialist who obtains further training and certification in one or more of the 70 subspecialties approved by the American Board of Medical Specialties.

QUICK TAKES

... Primary care physician. That's a hot term in health care today. Who is this physician? And how do you find one?...

CHAPTER 1

PRIMARY CARE PHYSICIANS

When it comes to choosing a doctor, too many people let the decision slide until they are sick or hurt and need medical attention fast. That's unfortunate if an illness that could have been managed successfully develops to a stage where it becomes difficult to control or cure. It's even more unfortunate if the illness could have been prevented in the first place.

The time to establish a relationship with a doctor is *while you are healthy,* and the best one to establish your relationship with is the one who is most likely to keep you healthy: a primary care doctor.

Primary means first, so a primary care doctor is the first one you see for any health problem. Primary also means basic, so a primary care doctor offers the kind of fundamental care that can keep you healthy.

CHAPTER ONE

YES, YOU DO NEED A DOCTOR WHEN YOU'RE HEALTHY.

Here are four good reasons why you should start your search for a primary care doctor now:

REASON ONE

A primary care doctor can put your medical condition in context. Context is important: this consists of your medical history, current condition as compared with past medical status, and changes in your body and environment over time. It is difficult for any doctor, however skilled, to make judgements based on only one visit or a single test. Conditions well out of normal range are easy to pick up, but extreme variations do not always occur, and a serious illness may develop slowly with only a gradual increase in symptoms. The operative word is continuity: ideally, your medical care should not be interrupted by changes in providers.

REASON TWO

A primary care doctor is better able to treat you as a whole person. Medicine has become very specialized and procedure-oriented, but the human body is not a loose collection of unrelated parts. It is a "whole," with strong interrelationships among all biological systems. Some of the poorest medical care results from people jumping from subspecialist to subspecialist. Despite talent, skill, and training, no specialist knows the patient well enough, or for long enough, to be able to take the whole person into consideration and track the normal patterns of evolution and change. We end up with a specialist for every organ and system instead of a doctor who will care for the whole person.

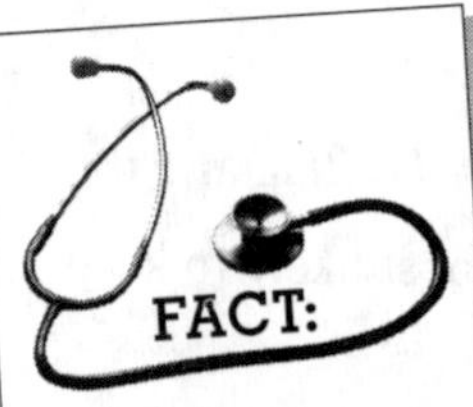

Our health care system does not place enough emphasis on preventing illness; most health care dollars are spent on curative, rather than preventive, medicine.

REASON THREE

A primary care doctor can establish preventive programs. Our health care system does not place enough emphasis on preventing illness; most health care dollars are spent on curative, rather than preventive, medicine. But the status quo is slowly changing, and it is within primary care that the change is most evident. Your primary care doctor can educate you about the hows and whys of health maintenance and disease prevention and follow up to help you stay faithful to the course the two of you have agreed upon. Only an ongoing relationship makes this possible.

REASON FOUR

A primary care doctor can save you money. Managed care advocates, among others, have long deplored the waste inherent in a system in which patients can simply call any specialist any time they have an ache or pain or are not feeling well. Primary care doctors can monitor referrals to specialists, following the patient closely to put together a variety of observations, opinions, and test results in order to treat each person on an individual basis. This improves the quality of care and also controls costs.

A BUSINESSMAN IN HIS LATE FIFTIES, A LONG-TIME COMPETITIVE RUNNER, HAD SURGERY IN ONE OF NEW YORK'S TOP HOSPITALS TO REPAIR A BADLY TORN ACHILLES TENDON. AT HIS FIRST FOLLOW-UP VISIT TO THE ORTHOPEDIC SURGEON, HE WAS ASSURED THAT "EVERYTHING WAS HEALING PERFECTLY," THAT HE HAD NOTHING TO BE CONCERNED ABOUT, AND THAT HE WOULD SOON BE UP AND RUNNING AGAIN. SHORTLY

THEREAFTER, JUST BEFORE A SUMMER CAMPING TRIP, HE DECIDED TO HAVE HIS YEARLY PHYSICAL EXAMINATION. THE PRIMARY CARE DOCTOR EXAMINED THE SITE OF THE SURGERY, PROBING UP AND DOWN THE WHOLE LENGTH OF THE LEG. EXPLAINING THAT HE WAS CONCERNED ABOUT CERTAIN SWELLING AND DISCOLORATION, THE DOCTOR ARRANGED FOR A FURTHER EXAMINATION WITH ULTRASOUND IMAGING. THIS SOPHISTICATED TEST SHOWED THAT A BLOOD CLOT HAD FORMED IN THE UPPER PART OF THE LEG, WHICH COULD HAVE CAUSED SEVERE DISABILITY AND EVEN DEATH HAD IT GOTTEN INTO THE BLOODSTREAM AND TRAVELED TO THE HEART OR BRAIN. IT WAS THE PRIMARY CARE DOCTOR, CAREFULLY CONDUCTING A FULL PHYSICAL EXAM AND WHO KNEW THE PATIENT WELL, WHO DISCOVERED THE POTENTIALLY FATAL CONDITION.

Patients who visit specialists without some guidance from a primary care doctor may choose the wrong specialist based on a general observation and self-diagnosis about the problem or illness they're experiencing. While in some cases the problem may be obvious (for example, an eye injury), in others it may be more subtle. Diseases such as lupus erythematosus and Lyme disease, for example, often have myriad symptoms that are easily misinterpreted by laypersons; in fact, they are often difficult even for doctors to diagnose accurately. While certain problems may require the collaboration of several specialists, it is important to have a primary care doctor navigating the course.

Finally, it is estimated that almost half of all emergency room visits in some areas are for non-emergencies; it's the most expensive place to receive primary care. When people have primary care doctors, they tend to turn to them rather than to hospital emergency departments.

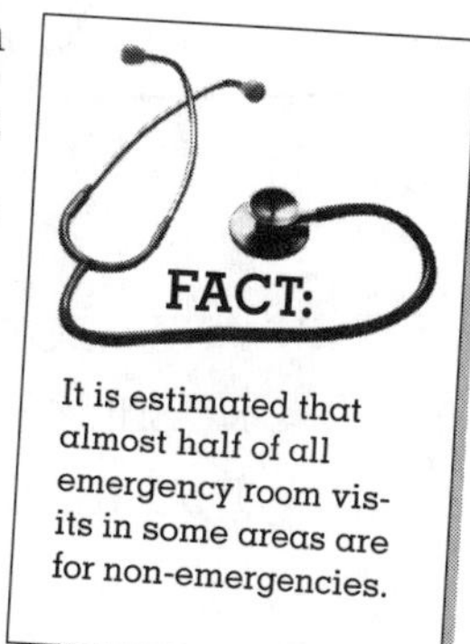

It is estimated that almost half of all emergency room visits in some areas are for non-emergencies.

If you are enrolled in any kind of managed care program, health maintenance organization (HMO) or other, you will almost always be required to select a primary care doctor from its roster. Managed care executives recognize the necessity of a primary care doctor, not only for delivering quality health care, but also for controlling costs.

HOW TO FIND A DOCTOR

Unless you already have a primary care doctor you are satisfied with, you will have to find one. How? Here are five possible avenues to *begin* the process of finding the doctor that best suits your needs. Each has limits, however.

DOCTOR REFERRALS

If you are moving and are leaving a trusted doctor behind, get a recommendation or two before you go. Furthermore, ask in what context and how well your doctor knows the new doctor—they may not have met since medical school.

FRIENDS AND RELATIVES

Always keep in mind that such recommendations are based largely on what may be "simpatico," or a personal affinity. Ask why your friend likes the doctor. It might be because the fees are low or the doctor makes house calls or is warm and sociable—all valid considerations, but certainly not principal determinants. So be

QUICK TIPS.

5. ANY DOCTOR WITH A LICENSE CAN PRACTICE IN ANY SPECIALTY HE/SHE CHOOSES. BOARD CERTIFICATION IS YOUR ASSURANCE THAT THE DOCTOR HAS APPROPRIATE TRAINING FOR THE SPECIALTY.

6. WHEN CONSIDERING RECOMMENDATIONS, USE THE OLD NAVIGATIONAL TECHNIQUE OF TRIANGULATION: FOCUS ON DOCTORS WHOSE NAMES ARE MENTIONED BY THREE OR MORE PEOPLE.

7. HOSPITAL TELEPHONE REFERRAL LINES ARE NOT DESIGNED TO DISTINGUISH AMONG HUNDREDS OF DOCTORS WHO MAY BE MORE OR LESS WELL REGARDED BY OTHER DOCTORS, OR WHO MAY BE BETTER SUITED TO A PARTICULAR CALLER WHEN FACTORS OTHER THAN LOCATION, INSURANCE COVERAGE, AND OFFICE HOURS ARE TAKEN INTO CONSIDERATION.

8. MANY LOCAL MEDICAL SOCIETIES PUBLISH DIRECTORIES, SOME OF WHICH ARE INTENDED PRIMARILY FOR DOCTOR-TO-DOCTOR REFERRALS, WHILE OTHERS ARE DISTRIBUTED TO THE PUBLIC. THEY PROVIDE INFORMATION BUT DO NOT ADDRESS QUALITY.

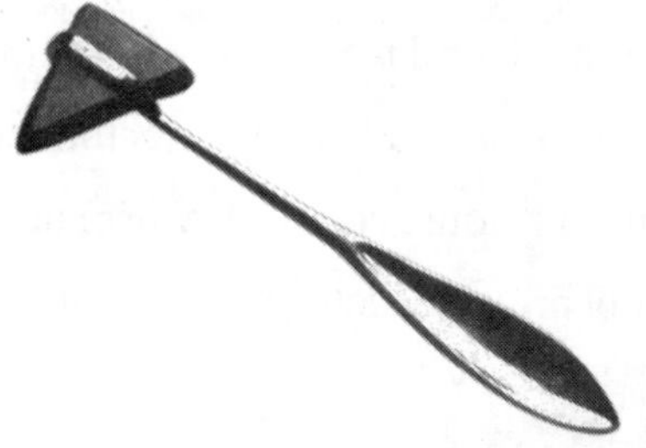

wary of the generalized recommendation that "Dr. Jones is just wonderful." When considering recommendations, use the old navigational technique of triangulation: focus on doctors whose names are mentioned by three or more people.

ONE WOMAN—A LONG-TIME CITY RESIDENT WHO MOVED TO THE SUBURBS TO BE NEAR HER CHILDREN—FOUND OUT THE HARD WAY ABOUT ADVICE WHEN SHE SELECTED A DOCTOR ON THE BASIS OF HER NEIGHBOR'S GLOWING PRAISE. DURING THE INITIAL VISIT, THE PATIENT'S NUMEROUS QUESTIONS ABOUT HER CHRONIC ARTHRITIS CONDITION WENT UNANSWERED WHILE THE DOCTOR MERELY PATTED HER ON THE SHOULDER AND ASSURED HER THAT HE WOULD "TAKE CARE OF EVERYTHING." WHILE THE PATERNALISTIC ATTITUDE MIGHT HAVE SUITED THE NEIGHBOR'S NEEDS, IT FELL FAR SHORT FOR THIS SENIOR PATIENT, WHO WAS USED TO A GOOD GIVE-AND-TAKE WITH HER FORMER INTERNIST. SHE RESUMED HER SEARCH FOR A DOCTOR—THIS TIME WITH THE ADVICE OF HER FORMER DOCTOR, A MORE RELIABLE SOURCE THAN A FRIEND'S RECOMMENDATION.

HOSPITAL REFERRAL SERVICES

Hospital telephone referral lines are not designed to distinguish among hundreds of doctors who may be more or less well regarded by other doctors, or who may be better suited to a particular caller when factors other than location, insurance coverage, and office hours are taken into consideration. It would be impolitic for hospital referral services to rate their members. Their recommendations are based on specialty and geographic proximity, usually by way of a computer that rotates through the lists to "recommend" the next three names in line, and all members of the medical staff are eligible to participate.

MEDICAL SOCIETY DIRECTORIES

Many local medical societies publish directories, some of which are intended primarily for doctor-to-doctor referrals, while others are distributed to the public. These directories usually provide names, addresses, phone numbers, and specialties, and can be useful sources. However, they do not distinguish among doctors in any way. All members of the medical society, usually a countywide organization, are eligible for inclusion. This also applies to the referral lines offered by many medical societies.

ADVERTISING

Responding to advertising is the least effective way to find a doctor. While more and more health professionals now advertise, a practice which is no longer considered unethical, some stigma still remains. Advertising could lead you to a doctor who receives few or no referrals from colleagues and whose orientation to the profession is more entrepreneurial than medical. Most referral lines not sponsored by hospitals charge a fee to doctors who want to be listed. This is simply another form of advertising.

MANY WAYS TO SAY DOCTOR

In this book, the term "doctor" is used to describe only medical doctors who have received a doctor of medicine degree (MD) and osteopaths who have received a doctor of osteopathic medicine degree (DO). Doctors who have been trained in the British system may hold a degree of bachelor of medicine (MB), bachelor of surgery (BS), or bachelor of chirurgia (BCh), which is based on the ancient Greek term that refers to surgery.

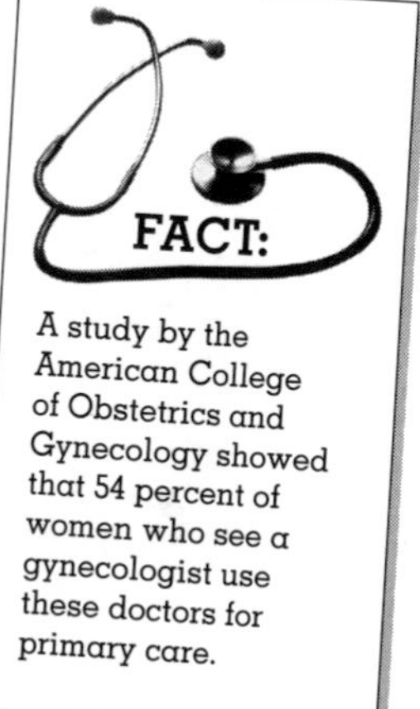

A study by the American College of Obstetrics and Gynecology showed that 54 percent of women who see a gynecologist use these doctors for primary care.

The more formal term for any of these practitioners is "physician." However, most people use the more popular term "doctor," which is the one generally used in this book. Our discussions do not include other kinds of doctors such as dentists, podiatrists, psychologists, or chiropractors, who also deliver health care.

PRIMARY CARE: THE FUNDAMENTAL FOUR

There is not complete agreement in medicine on which specialties are practiced by the group of doctors known as primary care specialists. For the purposes of this book, we have included the following specialties: Internal Medicine; Pediatrics; Family Practice; and Obstetrics and Gynecology. Most adults choose general internists as their primary care doctors, and select pediatricians for their children. There is also a relatively new type of specialist, the family practitioner, who cares for both children and adults. In addition to such generalists, many women also select obstetrician/gynecologists as primary care providers.

- **A GENERAL INTERNIST**, specializing in internal medicine, is trained to treat all internal organs and systems of the body. Many internists are also board certified in a subspecialty, such as cardiology, gastroenterology, or geriatric medicine. Therefore, if you have a history of heart disease, you may wish to select an internist who has additional training in cardiology, but who primarily practices general internal medicine. On the other hand, your primary care doctor may refer you to a cardiologist when necessary, and both may treat you over a period of years. In fact, it is not unusual for a patient with a serious or complex illness to be followed by two or three doctors, with the primary care doctor "quarterbacking" the team.

- **A FAMILY PRACTITIONER** belongs to a relatively new specialty. Such doctors come closest to the general practitioner of the past. They are qualified to treat all family members, including children.

- **A PEDIATRICIAN** is the doctor you would choose for the care of your children. As with doctors in internal medicine, pediatricians often have a subspecialty such as cardiology, rheumatology, or endocrinology.

- **OBSTETRICIANS** and **GYNECOLOGISTS** are the subject of significant debate in terms of their appropriateness as primary care doctors. The American Board of Obstetrics and Gynecology states that these doctors are specialists and are not generally trained for primary care. However, the reality is that many, particularly those who solely practice gynecology, often serve as a woman's primary care doctor. Gynecologists are divided on the issue. One recent study showed that 95 percent of visits to ob-gyns are self-referred and that about 60 percent of visits to these specialists are for diagnostic services and preventive services. Another study, by the American College of Obstetricians and Gynecologists, showed that 54 percent of women who see a gynecologist use these doctors for primary care. Reflecting the reality of current medical practice, we have included these specialists in the primary care category.

QUICK TIPS.

9. RESPONDING TO ADVERTISING IS THE LEAST EFFECTIVE WAY TO FIND A DOCTOR.

10. MANY WOMEN SELECT OBSTETRICIAN/GYNECOLOGISTS AS PRIMARY CARE PROVIDERS.

11. TO CHECK ON A DOCTOR'S (MD) BOARD CERTIFICATION CALL THE AMERICAN BOARD OF MEDICAL SPECIALTIES INFORMATION LINE ESTABLISHED FOR THAT PURPOSE (800) 776-2378 OR CHECK THEIR WEBSITE AT www.abms.org.

12. SINCE MOST PEOPLE WILL OBTAIN ALL, OR CERTAINLY MOST, OF THEIR MEDICAL CARE NEAR WHERE THEY LIVE, IT IS IMPORTANT FOR YOU TO IDENTIFY WHICH DOCTORS ARE AMONG THE BEST IN YOUR OWN COMMUNITY.

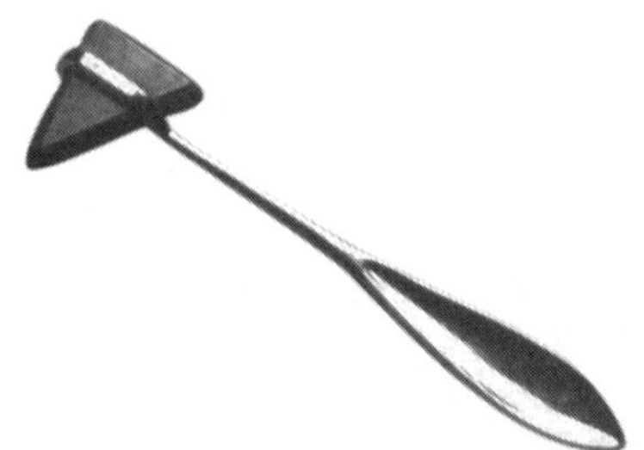

KEY TERMS CHAPTER 2

ACADEMIC MEDICAL CENTER

A large medical complex that centers around a teaching hospital in which diversified residency programs are offered and where the medical school faculty practices full time with fellowship programs and major clinical research activities. Many hospitals call themselves medical centers to indicate a broader range of clinical services even if they do not have teaching programs.

BOARD CERTIFIED

Term signifying that a doctor is qualified for specialization by one of the American Board of Medical Specialties (ABMS) boards. Qualification includes completing an approved residency and passing a rigid exam.

BOARD ELIGIBLE

Term signifying that a doctor has completed an approved residency but has not yet taken the exam given by one of the ABMS recognized boards. The term conveys no official status in the eyes of the ABMS.

CLINICAL

Medical care that involves direct contact with patients.

CREDENTIALING

A process of screening conducted by hospitals by means of which they review the training and licenses of doctors applying to practice on their medical staffs.

INDEMNITY

A form of health insurance coverage that pays for health care but permits the patients to select their provider. Until 1990, indemnity insurance covered most insured people in the United States.

LICENSURE

Official credentials by individual states that permit a doctor to practice medicine in that state. In some states doctors may be licensed with no more than one year of post-graduate training.

RESIDENCY

A training period spent by a graduate of a medical school in a hospital before going into practice. Residents have earned a medical degree and, therefore, are doctors but must complete an approved residency and pass an exam to become board certified.

TERTIARY CARE

Medical services provided by a hospital or medical center that include complex treatments and procedures such as open heart surgery, organ transplants, and burn care.

QUICK TAKES

... You should consider four broad criteria in selecting a primary care doctor: professional preparation; professional reputation; office and practice arrangements; and professional or bedside manner...

CHAPTER 2

WHAT MAKES A DOCTOR "BEST"?

While the overwhelming majority of doctors are competent practitioners, some are less well trained or, for various other reasons, lack a desired level of professional skill or personal characteristics. They have met certain minimum standards, passed the necessary exams, and are licensed, but you would still be better off to avoid them. At the same time, among the many good doctors you could choose from, there will be some who are better for you and your family for a variety of reasons.

Identifying "the best" doctors in a particular specialty is a challenge. There may be some who are generally acknowledged as leaders in a particular field, but that level of national reputation is typically built on appointments to important academic positions, innovative research, or the development of cutting-edge clinical techniques and treatments. Unless you are in need of those techniques and treatments, those doctors may not be the best for you. Since most people will obtain all, or certainly most, of their medical care near where they live, it is important for you to identify which doctors are among the best in your own community.

There are four basic criteria for selecting your own best doctor: Professional preparation; professional reputation; office and practice arrangements; and personal or bedside manner. The first three of these assessments can be made prior to your first visit, which is when you can make your fourth evaluation.

PROFESSIONAL PREPARATION

EDUCATION

Your review of your prospective doctor's education and training should begin with medical school. While you may feel that the institution where someone earned a bachelor's degree could be an indication of the quality of the doctor, most people in the medical field do not believe it plays a major role. A degree from a highly selective undergraduate college or university will help an aspiring doctor gain admission to a medical school, but once there, all students are peers. However, the information on undergraduate colleges, if important to you, is available in the American Board of Medical Specialties' (ABMS) *Compendium of Certified Medical Specialists* and other medical directories.

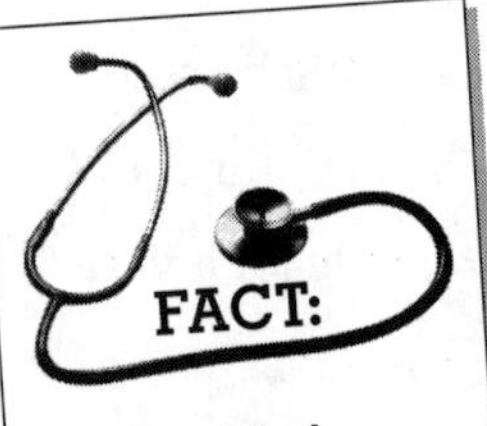

All US medical schools that grant medical degrees (MDs) and osteopathic degrees (DOs) are accredited by a group known as the LCME (Liaison Committee for Medical Education).

American medical schools are highly standardized, at least in terms of minimum quality. All US medical schools that grant medical degrees (MDs) and osteopathic degrees (DOs) are accredited by a group known as the LCME (Liaison Committee for Medical Education). Most are also accredited by the appropriate state agency, if one exists, and by regional accrediting agencies that accredit colleges and universities of all kinds.

Furthermore, US medical schools have universally high standards for admission, including success on the undergraduate level and on the Medical College Admissions Tests (MCATs). Although frequently criticized for being slow to change and for training too many specialists, the system of medical education in the United States has insured high quality in medical practice. One recent positive change is a strong effort in most medical schools to diversify the composition of the student body. While these schools have been less successful in enrolling racial minorities, the number of women in U.S. medical schools has increased to the point that they now make up about 40 percent of most classes. In certain specialties preferred by women medical graduates (pediatrics, for example), it is possible that in coming years the majority of specialists will be female.

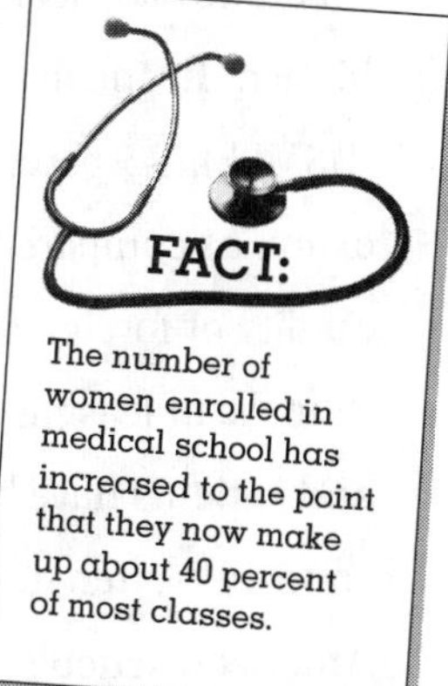

The number of women enrolled in medical school has increased to the point that they now make up about 40 percent of most classes.

Most doctors practicing in the United States are graduates of US medical schools. There are two other groups of doctors in practice who make up a relatively small proportion of the total doctor population. They are: (1) foreign nationals who graduated from foreign schools; and (2) US nationals who graduated from foreign schools (Canadian medical schools are not considered foreign).

FOREIGN MEDICAL GRADUATES

Foreign medical schools vary greatly in quality. Even some of the oldest and finest European schools have become virtually "open door," with huge numbers of unscreened students making teaching and learning difficult. Others are excellent and provided the model for our system of medical education.

The fact that someone graduated from a foreign school does not mean that he or she is a poor doctor. Foreign schools, like US schools, produce good doctors and poor doctors. Foreign medical graduates must pass the same exam taken by US graduates for licensure, but the failure rate for foreign graduates is significantly higher. In the first year of using the new United States Medical Licensing Exam (USMLE), 93 percent of US medical school graduates passed Step II, the clinical exam, as compared with 39 percent of the foreign graduates. It is clear that the quality of foreign schools, if not individual doctors, is not the same as US medical schools, at least as measured by our standards. Nonetheless, many communities and patients have been well served by foreign medical graduates practicing in this country—often in areas where it has been difficult to attract graduates of American schools.

RESIDENCY

Most doctors practicing today have at least three years of postgraduate (following the MD or DO) training in an approved residency program. This is not only an important step in the process of becoming a competent doctor, but it is also a requirement for board (specialty) certification. Most people assume that a prospective doctor needs to complete a three-year residency program to obtain a medical license. This is not true in some states. New York State, for example, requires only one postgraduate year. However, since all approved residencies last at least three years and some, such as those in neurosurgery, general surgery, orthopedic surgery, and urology, may extend for five or more years, it is important to know the details of a doctor's training. Licensure alone is not enough of a basis on which to make a good choice.

Without undertaking extensive and detailed research on every residency program, the best assessment you can make of a doctor's residency program is to see if it took place in a large medical center whose name you recognize. The more prestigious institutions tend to attract the best medical students, sometimes regardless of the quality of the individual residency program. If in doubt about a doctor's training, ask the doctor if the residency completed was in the specialty of the practice. If not, ask why.

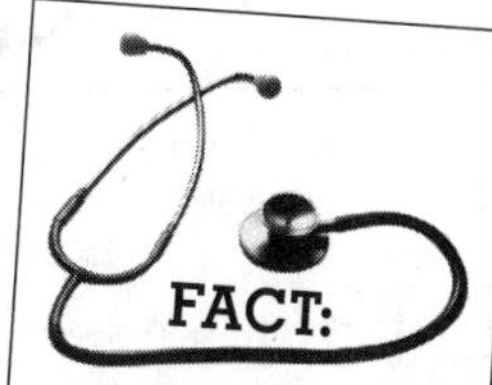

In the first year of using the new United States Medical Licensing Exam (USMLE), 93 percent of US medical school graduates passed Step II, the clinical exam, as compared with 39 percent of the foreign graduates.

It is also important to be certain that a doctor completed a residency that has been approved by the appropriate governing board of the specialty, such as the American Board of Surgery, the American Board of Radiology, or the American Osteopathic Board of Pediatrics. These board groups are listed in Appendices A and B. If you are really concerned about a doctor's training, you should first call the hospital that offered the residency and ask if the residency was approved by the appropriate specialty group. If still in doubt, review the publication *Directory of Graduate Medical Education Programs,* often called the "green book," found in medical school or hospital libraries, which lists all approved residencies.

QUICK TIPS.

13. IF IN DOUBT ABOUT A DOCTOR'S TRAINING, ASK THE DOCTOR IF THE RESIDENCY COMPLETED WAS IN THE SPECIALTY OF THE PRACTICE. IF NOT, ASK WHY.

14. BOARD CERTIFICATION IS THE BEST WAY TO MEASURE COMPETENCE AND TRAINING.

15. THE EASIEST WAY YOU CAN ASSESS THE QUALITY OF A DOCTOR'S RESIDENCY PROGRAM IS TO SEE IF IT TOOK PLACE IN A LARGE MEDICAL CENTER WHOSE NAME YOU RECOGNIZE.

16. IF A DOCTOR DOES NOT HAVE ADMITTING PRIVILEGES OR IS NOT ON THE ATTENDING STAFF OF A HOSPITAL, YOU MAY WISH TO CONSIDER CHOOSING ANOTHER DOCTOR.

17. THERE ARE MANY EXCELLENT, WELL-TRAINED DOCTORS AT COMMUNITY HOSPITALS AND THEY SHOULD BE AS CAREFULLY EVALUATED AND CONSIDERED IN YOUR SEARCH AS A DOCTOR IN A LARGE INSTITUTION.

BOARD CERTIFICATION

With an MD or DO degree and a license, an individual may practice any kind of medicine—with or without additional special training. For example, doctors with a license but no special training may call themselves radiologists or pediatricians. This is why board certification is such an important factor. Twenty-five specialties are recognized by the American Board of Medical Specialties (ABMS). Eighteen boards certify in 106 specialties under the aegis of the American Osteopathic Association (AOA). Doctors who have qualified for such specialization are called board certified; they have completed an approved residency and passed the board's exam. (See Appendix A for an approved ABMS list; see Appendix B for the AOA list; see Appendix C for a description of each specialty and subspecialty.) While many doctors who are not board certified do call themselves specialists, board certification is the best standard by which to measure competence and training.

You can be confident that doctors who are board certified have at a minimum the proper training in their specialty and have demonstrated their proficiency through supervision and testing. While there are many non-board certified doctors who are highly competent, it is more difficult to assess the level of their training. Board certification alone does not guarantee competence, but it is a standard that reflects successful completion of an appropriate training program.

BOARD ELIGIBILITY

There are doctors without board certification who are highly competent, including many who have been more recently trained and are waiting to take the boards. They are sometimes described as "board eligible," a common term that is, however, frowned upon by the ABMS. Board eligible means that the doctor has completed an approved residency and is qualified to sit for the board exams, which may be given only infrequently. Most of the specialty boards permit unlimited attempts to pass the exam. Only the American Board of Internal Medicine (ABIM) continues to use and recognize the term board eligible. The other boards neither use the term, nor sanction its use. The description board eligible should not be viewed as a real qualification, especially if a doctor has been out of medical school long enough to have taken the certification exams. To the boards, a doctor is either board certified or not. In some cases, doctors who have failed the exams twice continue to call themselves board eligible. In osteopathic medicine, the board eligible status is recognized only for the first six years after completion of a residency.

In addition to the ABMS- and AOA-approved list of specialties and subspecialties, there is a wide variety of other doctors, and groups of doctors, who may call themselves specialists. There are, at present, at least 100 such groups called self-designated medical specialties. They range from doctors who are working to create a recognized body of knowledge and subspecialty training to less formal groups interested in a particular approach to the practice of medicine. These groups may or may not have standards for membership. There is no way of determining the true extent of their members' training, and they are not recognized by the ABMS or the AOA. While you should be cautious of doctors who claim they are specialists in these areas, many do have advanced training, and the groups at least offer a listing of people interested in a particular approach to medical care. Rely on board certification to assure yourself of basic competence, and use membership in one of these groups to indicate strong interest and possible additional training in a particular aspect of medicine. A list of these self-designated medical specialties may be found in Appendix D.

FELLOWSHIPS

The purpose of a fellowship is to provide advanced training in the clinical techniques and research of a particular subspecialty. In the US there are a variety of fellowship programs available to doctors, and they fall into two broad categories: approved and unapproved. Approved fellowships are those that are approved by the appropriate medical specialty board (e.g., the American Board of Radiology) and that lead to a subspecialty certificate. Fellowship programs that are not approved are often in the same areas of training as those that are, but they do not lead to a subspecialty certificate. Unfortunately, all too often, unapproved fellowships exist only to provide relatively inexpensive labor for the research and/or patient care activities of a clinical department in a medical school or hospital. In such cases, the learning that takes place is secondary and may be a good deal less than in an approved fellowship. On the other hand, any fellowship is better than none at all, and some unapproved fellowships have that status for a valid reason, which should not reflect negatively on the program. For example, the fellowship may have been recently created, with approval being sought. To check that a fellowship is an approved one, call the hospital where the training took place or the medical board for that specialty.

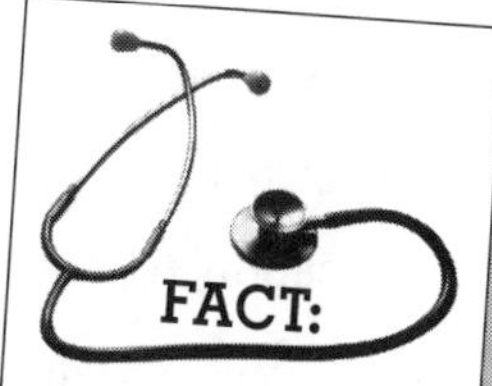

Many states typically require a minimum number of continuing medical education (CME) credits for a doctor to maintain a medical license. Twenty-eight states require 150 CME credits over a three-year period. Osteopathic doctors are required to take 150 hours of CME credits within three years to maintain certification.

RECERTIFICATION

A relatively new focus of the specialty boards is the area of recertification. Until recently, board certification lasted for an unlimited time period. Now, almost all the boards have put time limits on the certification period. For example, in internal medicine, it is 10 years; in family practice, six, and under some circumstances, seven years; in anesthesiology there is no defined time period. In osteopathic medicine, most of the boards need to set a recertification period within 10 years. Many have done so already. These more stringent standards reflect an increasing emphasis, by both the

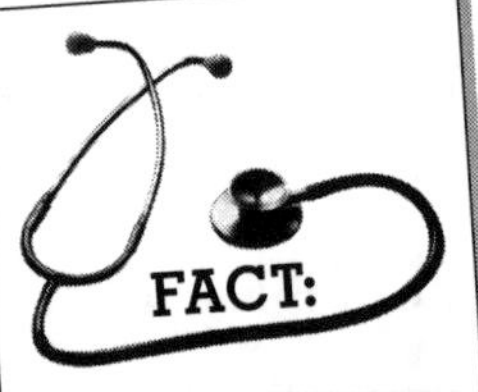

In a consumer survey conducted by Towers Perrin, the management consulting firm, the chief criterion by which the respondents selected doctors was reputation. This was the most important factor for those enrolled in either managed care or indemnity plans.

medical boards and state agencies responsible for licensing doctors, on recertification.

Since the policies of the boards vary widely, it is good procedure to ask a doctor if certification was awarded and when. If the date was seven to ten years ago, ask if he/she has been recertified. Unfortunately, many boards permit "grandfathering," whereby already certified doctors do not have to be recertified, and recertification demands apply only to newly certified doctors. Appendix A contains a list of the names and addresses of the boards and the certification period for each board specialty. Even if recertification is not required, it is good professional practice for doctors to undertake the process. It assures you, the patient, that they are attempting to stay current.

Many states have a continuing medical education requirement for doctors. These states typically require a minimum number of continuing medical education (CME) credits for a doctor to maintain a medical license. Twenty-eight states require 150 CME credits over a three-year period. Osteopathic doctors are required to take 150 hours of CME credits within three years to maintain certification.

PROFESSIONAL REPUTATION

There are doctors who meet every professional standard on paper, but who are simply not good doctors. In all probability the medical community has ascertained that and, while the individual may still practice medicine, his or her reputation will reflect that collective assessment. There are also doctors who are outstanding leaders in their fields because of research or professional activities, but who are not particularly strong or perhaps even active in patient care. It is important to distinguish that kind of professional reputation from a reputation as a competent, caring doctor in delivering patient care. In a consumer survey conducted by Towers Perrin, the management consulting firm, the chief criterion by which the respondents selected doctors was reputation. This was the most important factor for those enrolled in either managed care or indemnity plans.

HOSPITAL APPOINTMENT

Most doctors are on the medical staff of one or more hospitals and are known as attendings; some are not. If a doctor does not have admitting privileges or is not on the attending staff of a hospital, you may wish to consider choosing another doctor. It can be very difficult to ascertain whether the lack of hospital appointment is for a good reason or not. For example, it is understandable that some doctors who are raising families or heading toward retirement choose not to meet the demands (meetings, committees, etc.) of being an attending. However, if you need care in a hospital, the lack of such an appointment means that another doctor will have to oversee that care. In some specialties such as dermatology and psychiatry, doctors may conduct their entire practice in the office, and a hospital appointment is not as essential, or as good a criterion for assessment, as in other specialties.

While mistakes are made, most hospitals are quite careful about admissions to their medical staffs. The best hospitals are highly selective, so a degree of screening (or "credentialing") has been done for you. In other words, the best doctors practice at the best hospitals. Since caring for a patient in the hospital is also often a team effort involving a number of specialists, the reputation of the hospital where the doctor admits patients carries special weight. Hospital medical staffs also review their colleagues to authorize them to perform specific procedures. In addition, they typically reappoint their medical staffs—and review them—every two or three years. In effect, this is an additional screening to protect patients. It is especially true of hospitals that have what are known as closed staffs, where it is impossible to obtain admitting privileges unless there is a vacancy that the administration and medical staff deem necessary to fill. If you are having some type of surgical procedure and are concerned about the doctor's skill or experience with it, it may be worthwhile to call the medical affairs office at the doctor's hospital to see if he or she is authorized to perform that procedure in the hospital.

The reasons for a hospital's selectivity are easy to understand: no hospital, excellent or not, wishes to expose itself to liability, and every hospital wants to have the best reputation possible in order to attract patients. Obviously, the quality of the medical staff is immensely important in creating that reputation. Unfortunately, some hospitals are less diligent when a major group practice of doctors, all of whom have previously been affiliated with the institution, adds new members. In such cases, the hospital may almost automatically grant privileges without conducting the same intensive review given to individual doctors who are not members of a group practice. Also, some hospitals are less selective in granting privileges when beds are empty than when beds are full.

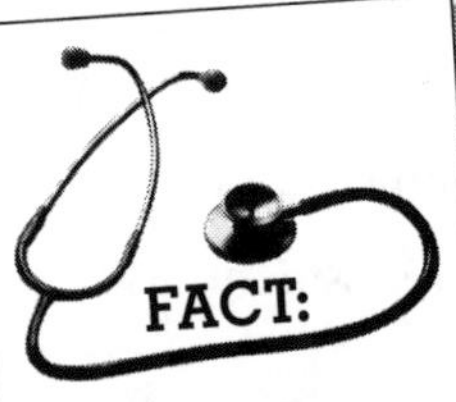

Few hospitals permit doctors to practice in them unless they carry malpractice insurance. This not only protects the hospital, but the patient as well.

A last and very important reason why a hospital appointment is an essential requirement in your choice of a doctor is that many states permit doctors to practice *without* malpractice insurance. If you are injured as a result of the doctor's poor care, you could be without recourse. However, few hospitals permit doctors to practice in them unless they carry malpractice insurance. This not only protects the hospital, but the patient as well.

Many people believe that they should choose a doctor with an appointment at a major medical center as opposed to a community hospital. This assumption is incorrect on two counts. For one thing, there are many excellent, well-trained doctors at community hospitals and they should be as carefully evaluated and considered in your search as a doctor in a large institution. What's more, the term "medical center" has less significance today than it did years ago when the term was used to describe only the major university hospitals of medical schools. A true medical center is a teaching hospital which offers multiple residency programs and where the medical school faculty practices full-time with fellowship programs and major clinical research activities as an integral part of the teaching of medical students. These large centers are also involved in tertiary care, offering services such as organ transplants, burn care, and cardiovascular surgery.

Today many community hospitals have added the term medical center to their name. They do this to indicate that they, too, offer advanced and sophisticated medical programs, as well as to compete with the academic medical centers for patients. With academic medical centers turning out many well-trained specialists and subspecialists who establish practices in nearby communities and then want to continue the highly specialized techniques they have learned, many community hospitals have initiated tertiary care programs of their own, further blurring the distinction between medical centers and hospitals.

In any case, most of our health care today is delivered *outside* of the hospital. Those who are hospitalized for acute illness (e.g., surgery, serious infection) will find that community hospitals and their staffs are well-suited to the task.

When extremely difficult and complex problems develop, or when tertiary care is needed, many communities have excellent academic medical centers. Of course, they offer primary care as well, especially to those who live nearby. This illustrates the point, once again, that medical care is a local issue.

QUICK TIPS.

18. DOCTORS WHO ARE FULL-TIME ACADEMICIANS MAY BE IN THE FOREFRONT OF NEW TECHNIQUES AND RESEARCH, BUT THEY ARE NOT NECESSARILY BETTER DOCTORS.

19. THE BEST CARE IS PROVIDED BY A COMBINATION OF PRIMARY CARE DOCTORS AND OTHER SPECIALISTS AND SUBSPECIALISTS.

20. DO NOT HESITATE TO ASK HOW FREQUENTLY YOUR DOCTOR HAS PERFORMED A PROCEDURE AND WITH WHAT DEGREE OF SUCCESS. PRACTICE MAY NOT LEAD TO PERFECTION, BUT IT IMPROVES SKILLS AND ENHANCES THE PROBABILITY OF SUCCESS.

21. CHECK THE DATE OF GRADUATION FROM MEDICAL SCHOOL OR COMPLETION OF RESIDENCY IF YOU WANT TO KNOW PRECISELY HOW LONG A DOCTOR HAS BEEN IN PRACTICE.

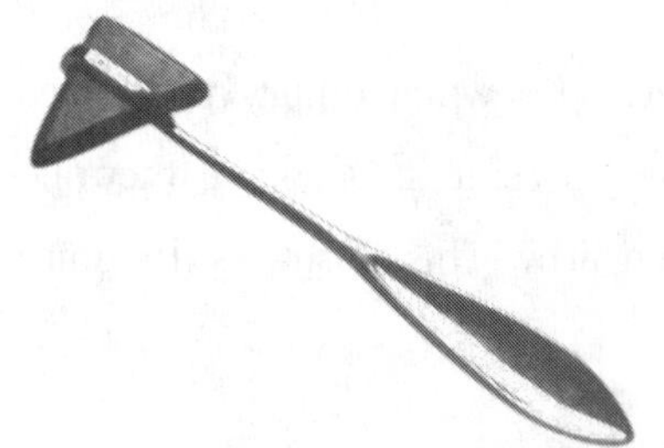

MEDICAL SCHOOL FACULTY APPOINTMENT

Many doctors have appointments on the faculties of medical schools. There is a range of categories from "straight" appointments—meaning full-time appointment as professor, associate professor, assistant professor, or instructor—to clinical ranks that may reflect lesser degrees of involvement in teaching or research. If someone carries what is known as a straight academic rank (i.e., professor of surgery, without clinical in the title), this usually means that the individual is engaged full-time in medical school research and/or teaching activities. The title professor of clinical surgery usually describes a doctor who has a full-time appointment in a medical school, but who puts a greater emphasis on clinical practice (patient care) than on research or teaching. The title clinical professor of surgery usually specifies a part-time or adjunct appointment and less direct involvement in medical school activities.

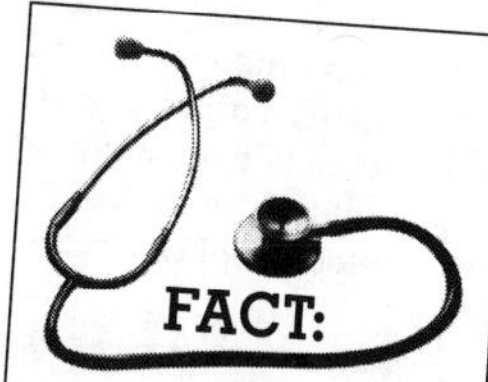

The newest approaches and techniques in medicine, for the most part, are explored and developed by medical school faculties in their laboratories and clinical practice settings.

Doctors who are full-time academicians may be in the forefront of new techniques and research, but they are not necessarily better doctors. Nonetheless, you would be assured that they have the support of other faculty, residents, and medical students.

When you are seeking a subspecialist, a doctor's relationship to a medical school becomes more meaningful since medical school faculties tend to be made up of subspecialists. You are less likely to find large numbers of general or primary care practitioners engaged full-time on a medical school faculty. The newest approaches and techniques in medicine, for the most part, are explored and developed by medical school faculties in their laboratories and clinical practice settings. This is where they practice their subspecialties, as well as teach and perform research. Such leading specialists are not necessarily better doctors than com-

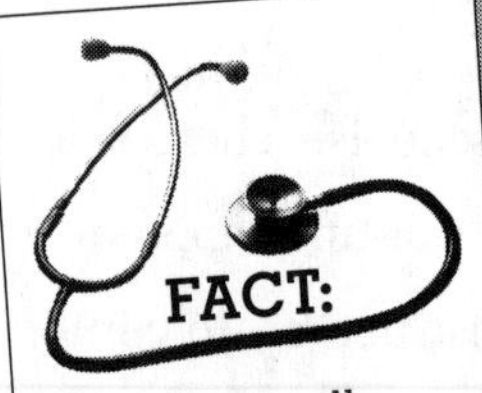

A consumer poll conducted for the Robert Wood Johnson Foundation identified office location as one of the two most important factors in the selection of a doctor.

munity doctors—they are trained to provide a *different* kind of medical care. The best care is provided by a combination of primary care doctors and other specialists and subspecialists.

MEDICAL SOCIETY MEMBERSHIP

Most medical society memberships sound very prestigious and some are; however, there are many societies that are not selective and which virtually any doctor can join. In addition, membership in many of the more prestigious societies is based on research and publication, or on leadership in the field, and may have little to do with direct patient care. While it is clearly an honor to be invited to join these groups, membership may be less than helpful in discerning whether a doctor can meet your needs.

Board certified doctors are referred to as Diplomates of the Board. Some of the colleges of medical specialties (e.g., the American College of Radiology; the American College of Surgeons) have multiple levels of recognition. The first is basic membership and the second, more prestigious and difficult to obtain, is status as a Fellow. Fellowship status in the colleges is meaningful and is based on experience, professional achievement, and recognition by one's peers, including extensive experience in patient care. It should be viewed as a significant professional qualification.

EXPERIENCE

Experience is difficult to assess. Obviously, in most cases, an older doctor has more experience; on the other hand, a younger doctor has been more recently immersed in residency, the challenge of medical school, or even a fellowship, and may be the most up-to-date. If a doctor is board certified, you may assume that assures at least a minimal amount of experience, but it could be as little as a year.

So check the date of graduation from medical school or completion of residency if you want to know precisely how long a doctor has been in practice.

The one type of experience you should specifically want to know about is that dealing with any special procedure, particularly a surgical one, that has recently been developed and introduced into practice. For example, many doctors using a new surgical technique for removing gallbladders—laparoscopic cholecystectomy—experienced a high percentage of problems because they were not properly trained. This prompted new standards to be issued by the American College of Surgeons to make sure doctors using this new approach would be adequately trained. Do not hesitate to ask how frequently your doctor has performed a procedure and with what degree of success. Practice may not lead to perfection, but it improves skills and enhances the probability of success.

OFFICE AND PRACTICE ARRANGEMENTS

Although clearly not as important as training or reputation, office and practice arrangements are usually of great significance to patients. Practice arrangements include office hours, office location, billing procedures, and office testing among the many factors that result in how well the office is run.

Many years ago most doctors practiced independently in private offices. They were called solo practitioners and usually had agreements with other doctors to respond to their patients' calls when they were unavailable. In recent decades, most doctors have entered group practices; indeed, this is becoming the most common way for young doctors to begin to practice. Two or more doctors in the same specialty, or in different specialties (a multi-specialty group), share offices and staff to lower their costs of operations. They also cover for each other on rotation for weekends, evenings, and vacations. As a patient you may prefer one of

QUICK TIPS.

22. IF YOU DON'T THINK YOU WILL BE SATISFIED HAVING YOUR OFFICE VISIT AND EXAMINATION CONDUCTED BY ANYONE BUT THE DOCTOR, YOU SHOULD DETERMINE UP FRONT HOW MANY MIDLEVEL PROVIDERS ARE ON STAFF AND HOW EXTENSIVE THEIR RESPONSIBILITIES ARE.

23. THE SITE OF THE OFFICE CAN BE VERY IMPORTANT IN CHOOSING A DOCTOR YOU MAY VISIT ON A REGULAR BASIS. IF THE LOCATION IS INCONVENIENT, YOU MAY BE DISCOURAGED FROM MAKING NEEDED VISITS.

24. YOU SHOULD DISCUSS ANY CHRONIC PROBLEMS WHEN FIRST ESTABLISHING A RELATIONSHIP WITH A DOCTOR. IN FACT, YOU MAY WANT TO FIND A DOCTOR WITH SPECIAL INTEREST OR TRAINING IN THAT PROBLEM.

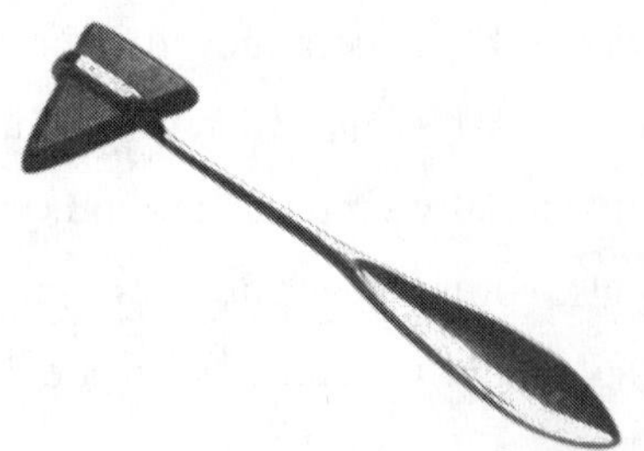

the following: a solo practitioner who is covered occasionally; a group where you usually, but not always, see the same doctor; or a multi-specialty group where, if a consultation or referral is necessary, the specialist is at the same location. The choice is really one of personal preference.

There are other factors relating to practice arrangements that may or may not be important to an individual choosing a doctor. One is the location of the office. A consumer poll conducted for the Robert Wood Johnson Foundation identified office location as one of the two most important factors in the selection of a doctor (the other was a recommendation by a relative or friend). Actually, the site of the office can be very important in choosing a doctor you may visit on a regular basis. If the location is inconvenient, you may be discouraged from making needed visits.

FACT:

According to an article in the professional journal *Family Practice Management*, these "midlevel providers," as they are called, "can handle 80 to 90 percent of the problems that occasion office visits."

Another important factor concerns the use of nurse practitioners and physician's assistants in the office. Licensed nurse practitioners are advanced practice nurses in primary care. They have additional training beyond the basic requirements for nursing licensure, usually a master's degree or special certificate. They perform a broad range of nursing functions as well as functions that, historically, have been performed by doctors, including assessing and diagnosing, conducting physical examinations, ordering diagnostic tests, implementing treatment plans and monitoring patient status. Physician's assistants are licensed to provide medical care in many states. Unlike nurses, they may practice only under a doctor's direction and supervision. According to an article in the professional journal *Family Practice Management*, these "midlevel providers," as they are called, "can handle 80 to 90 percent of the problems that occasion office visits." These providers have become more of a presence in health care in recent years, especially in medical groups and HMOs. If you don't think you will be satisfied having your office visit and examination conducted by anyone but the doctor, you should determine up front how many midlevel providers are on staff and how extensive their responsibilities are.

NARROWING THE CHOICE

Here are 10 additional questions that will guide you in assessing the practice patterns or arrangements of a doctor to see if they meet your needs. If there are other items not listed that are important to you, add them to the list before you make your initial appointment. You should try to obtain as much of the information as possible from the staff.

- *Are you currently accepting new patients and, if so, is a referral required?*
- *On average, how long does a patient have to wait for an appointment?*
- *Are you open on weekends? In the evening?*
- *If lab work and X-rays are performed in the office what are the qualifications of the people doing the test?*
- *Is full payment, deductibles or co-payments required at the time of the appointment?*
- *Do you accept my insurance plan? Medicare? Medicaid? Worker's Compensation? No-fault insurance?*
- *Do you accept credit cards and, if so, which do you accept?*
- *Do you accept patient phone calls?*
- *Will you care for patients in their homes?*
- *Is your office handicapped-accessible?*

If you have a chronic illness or disease, there may be certain additional aspects of a doctor's practice that could be particularly important to you. You should discuss any chronic problems when first establishing a relationship with a doctor. In fact, you may want to find a doctor with special interest or training in that problem.

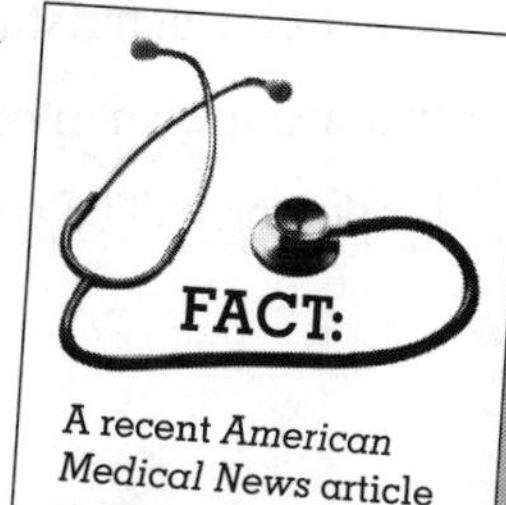

A recent *American Medical News* article suggested that 43 percent of internal medicine specialists and 65 percent of family practice specialists made one or more house calls a year.

House calls also continue to be important to some people. Yes, some doctors still do make house calls! In fact, a recent *American Medical News* article suggested that 43 percent of internal medicine specialists and 65 percent of family practice specialists made one or more house calls a year. However, it is important to point out that house calls have declined not because doctors are lazy or arrogant, but because of technology, liability risks, and time pressures. Important diagnostic equipment often cannot be carried around in a doctor's little black bag and is only available in the office or hospital. Also, the time required to visit one patient at home markedly reduces the time available to see other patients.

PERSONAL OR BEDSIDE MANNER

To many patients, once they have determined that a doctor is competent, the doctor's professional manner—also known as bedside manner—is the most important part of their choice. The Towers Perrin report cited earlier indicated that after reputation, communications skill was the most important factor sought in doctors. Patients want sensitive and caring doctors who listen carefully and demonstrate their concern. Studies show that such doctors are sued less often than others!

What characteristics make up a doctor's personal manner? The four described below may, when considered together, give you a clear idea of whether a particular doctor will be your personal "best."

- **Listening. Professional manner includes the doctor's willingness to listen to patients, be supportive and understanding, explain procedures, and exhibit concern and respect. These skills are expressed at the bedside, in the office, or in any setting where there is doctor/patient contact. Listening is also a valuable diagnostic tool. Unfortunately, these skills often have not been taught well in medical schools, and the lack of them forms the primary basis for complaints from patients. However, there is a growing emphasis on these vital interpersonal and communications skills in medical schools today, and with good reason. They are critically important to most patients.**

- **Cultural sensitivity. Some patients may prefer doctors who speak their language or are familiar with their cultural background. The term "culturally competent physician" is a relatively new one describing doctors who have the skills and attitudes to deal with minority cultures.**

- **Ethical, religious, and philosophical views. Religion, or at least views on issues such as abortion, utilization of life-sustaining measures, natural childbirth, breast-feeding, and other matters can also be important. It is perfectly appropriate to ask doctors questions about sensitive issues.**

- **Decision-making procedures. Years ago patients took the words of the doctor as law, not to be questioned, or perhaps even discussed. That is not the case today. Consumers are better informed about health issues and may want to be actively involved in the decision-making affecting their health. Some patients do not feel this way and are comfortable accepting a doctor's diagnosis or course of treatment without question. Some doctors—in diminishing numbers, thankfully—feel uncomfortable with patients who want everything explained to them or want to be involved in decision-making. Consider how you feel about this issue and discuss it with your doctor to be certain you are on compatible wavelengths.**

Of course, what ultimately makes a doctor "best" are the results, the "outcomes," of care. Unfortunately, there is relatively little information available to consumers on the outcomes of physicians and hospitals. Some states, New York for example, have produced studies on outcomes for cardiac surgery. Also, some HMOs are talking about producing report cards for doctors. Generally, however, consumers will have difficulty finding outcome studies for individual doctors.

QUICK TIPS.

25. ALWAYS OBTAIN COPIES OF ALL MEDICAL RECORDS AND TESTS FOR YOUR FILES.

26. WHEN SELECTING A DOCTOR, ESPECIALLY A PRIMARY CARE DOCTOR, IT IS APPROPRIATE TO REQUEST AN INTERVIEW TO GET ACQUAINTED.

27. GOOD DOCTORS LISTEN, GOOD PATIENTS TALK.

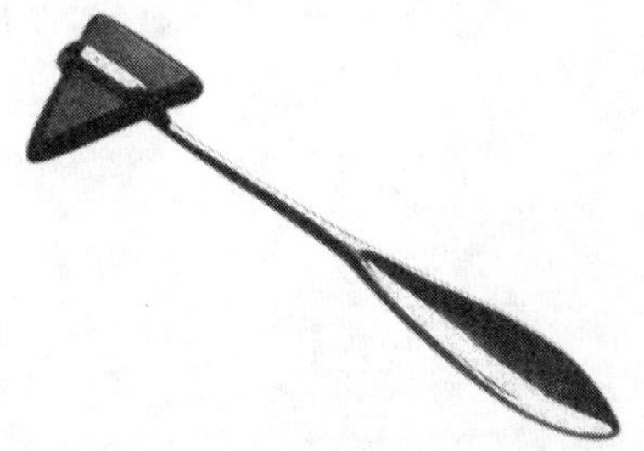

KEY TERMS CHAPTER 3

AMERICAN MEDICAL ASSOCIATION

A partnership of physicians and their professional associations dedicated to promoting the art and science of medicine and the betterment of public health through establishing and promoting ethical, educational, and clinical standards for the medical profession. It represents the interests of physicians on the national level.

BASELINE TESTS

A series of basic, routine medical tests—such as electrocardiogram, complete blood count, blood pressure measurement, weight measurement, and chest X-ray—that are usually completed by a physician upon a patient's initial visit in order to provide a standard for comparison during subsequent health examinations.

GENERIC DRUGS

Prescription medications that have been marketed by one company under a proprietary or brand name and which may be sold, after the original exclusive 17-year patent expires, under a generic name or the name assigned to it during early stage of development. Most generic drugs are less expensive than proprietary versions and are just as effective except in cases when, because of different manufacturing processes, they are not bioequivalent or handled by the body in an identical manner.

THIRD PARTY PAYER

An organization such as indemnity insurance company or managed care organization that provides individual and group health insurance, or a governmental department which assumes responsibility for the payment of an individual's health care, either directly to the health care provider or by means of reimbursement to the individual (medicare and medicaid are such government programs).

QUICK TAKES

...The best doctor-patient relationship is based on a two-way dialogue. Be open and honest and seek a doctor who is the same...

CHAPTER 3

YOU AND YOUR DOCTOR: A TEAM

Trust and respect between doctors and patients have reached a low point in modern American society. A recent poll of consumers sponsored by the American Medical Association (AMA) concluded that approximately 70 percent of those who responded agreed with the statement that "people are beginning to lose faith in their doctors." (Despite concerns about doctors in general, much research has shown patients tend to rate their own doctors well.)

Trust between doctors and patients has declined for many reasons, including unrealistic expectations on the part of some patients and the patronizing attitudes of some doctors, which clash with the higher education level and medical sophistication of many patients. This has been further complicated by changing financial arrangements, particularly those involving the government and third-party payers, and the perception that some doctors seem to be motivated not by

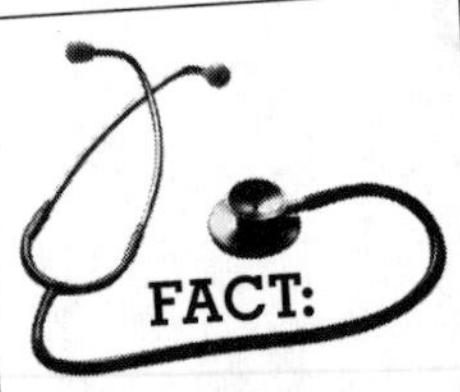

A recent poll of consumers sponsored by the American Medical Association (AMA) concluded that approximately 70 percent of those who responded agreed with the statement that "people are beginning to lose faith in their doctors," and that 69 percent of the respondents agreed that doctors "are too interested in making money."

the values of the Hippocratic Oath (See Appendix E), but by those of the marketplace. The AMA poll cited earlier found that 69 percent of the respondents agreed that doctors "are too interested in making money." Perhaps a significant factor in creating this atmosphere is that in many cases the relationship between doctor and patient now has another dimension, the managed care organization. Another significant contributor is the huge amount of paperwork required from doctors. Generated by quality-assurance efforts, regulation, complex billing, and managed care procedures, this burden reduces the time doctors are able to spend with patients.

Given the formidable obstacles, it might seem impossible to find a primary care doctor who is well suited to your needs. If you have carefully read the preceding chapters, your work is half done. What remains is to find that special individual who fits the criteria.

THE INITIAL INTERVIEW

When selecting a doctor, especially a primary care doctor, it is appropriate to request an exploratory interview. Frequently, doctors will engage in such brief interviews at no charge or at a reduced fee or by telephone. It is preferable to find out about a doctor's credentials, office hours, and billing procedures from the staff beforehand so you don't waste time asking about basic facts. This leaves time to ask the doctor questions that will allow you to determine what kind of relationship could develop. It is interesting that many parents will insist on interviewing a pediatrician for their child but wouldn't think of interviewing a physician for themselves.

ASK THE RIGHT QUESTIONS

The most important aspect of this session is to see if you can develop a positive doctor/patient relationship. Are you comfortable with the doctor's manner, style, and general personality? Do you feel a strong sense of trust in the doctor? Here are five questions to ask the doctor plus two questions to ask yourself that may lead you closer to a selection.

- *What is your experience in treating __________ (if you are seeking care for a particular illness or condition)?*
- *Are you open to treatments and therapies that do not rely heavily on medication?*
- *What preventive programs do you suggest for someone of my age, sex, and health status?*
- *How do you feel about involving patients in decision-making?*
- *What are your views on__________(ethical and moral issues of importance to you as a patient)?*

Even when the doctor is responding to your questions, you should ask yourself:

- *Is the doctor paying attention to me and really considering my questions or do the impersonal, "stock" answers indicate that the doctor's thoughts are elsewhere?*
- *Does this doctor speak about good health and prevention with the personal knowledge of someone who seems to practice it?*

If your prospective doctor seems to measure up to your standards, get the relationship off to a good start by making an appointment for a complete check-up. During this appointment, you will have an opportunity to share your medical and family history, and baseline tests will be performed to serve as a standard in the years ahead.

ONE WOMAN, IMBUED WITH HER NEW "TAKE CHARGE" ROLE IN HER HEALTH CARE, CARRIED THE INTERVIEWING PROCESS TO THE LIMIT WHEN SHE VISITED MORE THAN 20 DOCTORS FOR EXPLORATORY INTERVIEWS IN THE COURSE OF A SINGLE YEAR. EACH TIME THERE WAS SOME LITTLE PROBLEM: THE DOCTOR WAS BEHIND SCHEDULE, THE DOCTOR WAS VERY BRUSQUE, THE DOCTOR DISCUSSED EVERYTHING IN COMPLICATED MEDICAL LANGUAGE, EVEN ONE INSTANCE WHEN SHE CONCLUDED THAT THE DOCTOR WAS JUST TOO YOUNG. NOT ONLY WAS SHE IMPOSING ON THE PROFESSIONALISM OF THE DOCTORS WHO CONDUCTED THE INTERVIEWS WITH HER, BUT SHE WAS ACTUALLY NEGLECTING HER HEALTH CARE; DURING THAT YEAR, SHE NEVER HAD A SINGLE MEDICAL EXAMINATION. IF A SERIOUS HEALTH PROBLEM HAD BEEN IN THE DEVELOPING STAGES, A YEAR WOULD HAVE BEEN TOO LONG TO GO WITHOUT MEDICAL TREATMENT.

TALKING WITH YOUR DOCTOR

After you have selected your doctor, your first appointment should include an extensive medical history. Your doctor should spend time with you, ask questions, and listen to your responses carefully.

Medical students are often told, "Listen to your patients. They'll tell you what's wrong with them." This conveys an important lesson not only for doctors, but for patients: *Good doctors listen, good patients talk.*

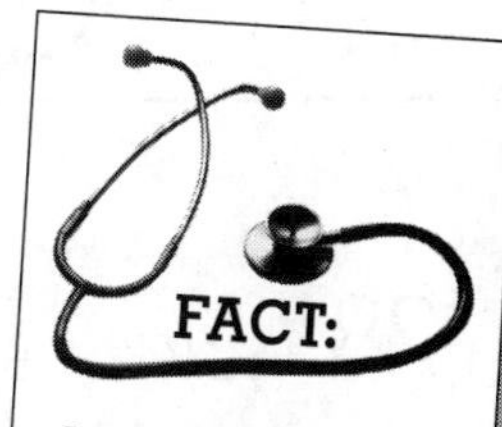

Analysis of doctor/patient conversations has revealed that many patients wait until the end of a conversation, even until they are saying goodbye, to tell their doctors what is really bothering them.

Analysis of doctor/patient conversations has revealed that many patients wait until the end of a conversation, even until they are saying goodbye, to tell their doctors what is really bothering them. This is just a small example of the dynamics of doctor/patient relationships. It is also a good example of a waste of valuable time—the doctor's and the patient's. One reason doctors need to be trained to be good listeners is that they frequently must ascertain what is troubling the patient not by what is said directly, but by what is said indirectly, not at all, or through body language and other signs. However, it is always easier, less time-consuming, and certainly more effective if a patient can describe problems completely and accurately.

Before you even see a doctor, you should prepare thoroughly. You should have a complete record of your medical history, including a record of X-rays and any other diagnostic tests, as well as blood workups. You need information about childhood diseases, chronic conditions, hospitalizations, past and present medications, doses, and drug reactions, if any, and, if possible, something about the health history of your parents and even their siblings. Except for the last item, these are available to patients from their previous doctors or hospitals. That is why it is useful to obtain copies of all medical records and tests for your own files. Not only will this save you time and effort, but it may avoid additional testing and expense. Your doctor will also ask many seemingly personal questions about your work, education, sex life, and even drug and alcohol use. These are all part of a complete medical history and will help your doctor understand you better.

If you have a particular problem or concern, describe all your symptoms. Try not to minimize or exaggerate and, most of all, don't deny.

QUICK TIPS.

28. ALWAYS BRING A PAD AND PENCIL WITH YOU TO MEDICAL APPOINTMENTS. WHEN THE DOCTOR GIVES YOU INSTRUCTIONS, TAKE NOTES.

29. *THE PHYSICIAN'S DESK REFERENCE*, COMMONLY KNOWN AS THE PDR, IS AVAILABLE IN MOST LIBRARIES AND IS AN EXCELLENT RESOURCE FOR LEARNING MORE ABOUT MEDICATIONS. (THE PDR WEB PAGE IS AT http://www.pdr.net)

30. DO NOT HESITATE TO ASK YOUR PHARMACIST ABOUT SIDE EFFECTS, GENERIC SUBSTITUTIONS, AND OTHER QUESTIONS RELATED TO YOUR MEDICATIONS.

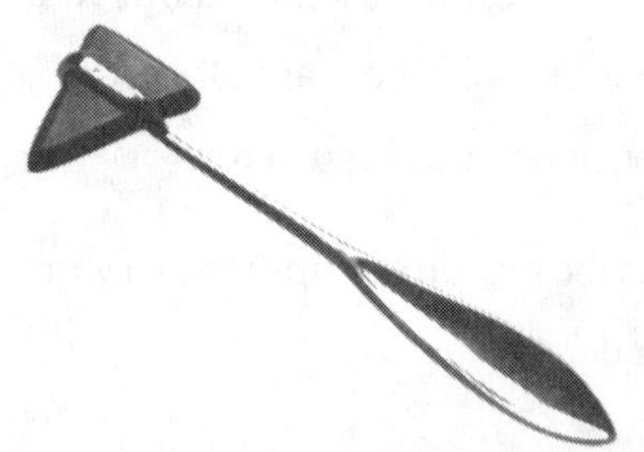

AN EXECUTIVE OF A LARGE COMPUTER SOFTWARE FIRM ASSURED HIS DOCTOR THAT HE WAS "FEELING FIT," CHOOSING NOT TO MENTION THE SOMETIMES SEVERE PAIN IN HIS SCROTUM. SIX MONTHS LATER THE PAIN HAD WORSENED TO THE DEGREE THAT IT DEMANDED ATTENTION. UNFORTUNATELY, THE DIAGNOSIS WAS ADVANCED TESTICULAR CANCER.

If you have questions to ask your doctor, make a list. Always bring a pad and pencil with you to medical appointments. When the doctor gives you instructions, take notes or ask the doctor to write them down for you. If a prescription is written, ask about doses, side effects, efficacy, and alternative medications, as well as generic substitutes. The *Physician's Desk Reference*, commonly known as the PDR, is available in most libraries and is an excellent resource for learning more about medications. There is also a PDR Web page on the Internet at http://www.pdr.net. You can also get a great deal of information on medications from another health professional, your pharmacist. Do not hesitate to ask your pharmacist about side effects, generic substitutions, and other questions related to your medications. However, if the information you receive conflicts with that given by your doctor, consult with the doctor and follow his or her directions.

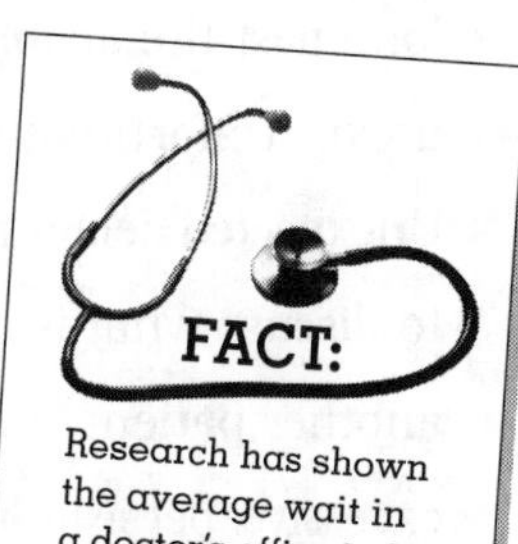

Research has shown the average wait in a doctor's office is 20 minutes. However, the doctor who spends extra time with another patient probably is the doctor you want for yourself.

CHAPTER THREE

A MATTER OF TIME

Patients want and expect doctors who listen, express concern, explain conditions and procedures in a clear and understandable manner, discuss medications and their effects and side effects thoroughly, return calls, are available when needed and, perhaps most important, spend sufficient time with them. With increasing demands on their time, many doctors are left with an uneasy feeling of "running to stay in place." The end result may be a tendency, unintended for the most part, to rush through a patient visit. This situation contributes to the erosion of the doctor-patient relationship.

Also contributing to this problem is pervasive lateness on the part of doctors. Patients frequently complain that they spend hours in a doctor's waiting room, long past the appointed hour (research has shown the average wait is 20 minutes). Unfortunately, the duration of a patient visit is not always predictable. Unexpected delays may occur if the diagnosis is complicated or if a patient needs to discuss what is on his or her mind. The doctor who spends extra time with another patient is probably the doctor you want for yourself. If the lateness is excessive, persistent, and without apparent good reason, discuss it with your doctor and, if it is interfering with your relationship, consider changing doctors.

AFTER A DELAY OF TWO HOURS IN HIS DOCTOR'S OFFICE, ONE PATIENT, A SELF-EMPLOYED MARKETING CONSULTANT, MADE SURE THAT IT WOULD NEVER HAPPEN AGAIN. DID HE HAVE A SHOWDOWN WITH THE DOCTOR? DID HE DECIDE NEVER TO RETURN? NOT AT ALL. HE SIMPLY MADE IT A POINT TO CALL THE DOCTOR'S OFFICE

TWO HOURS BEFORE HIS SCHEDULED APPOINTMENT TO SEE HOW THE SCHEDULE WAS RUNNING. HE THEN ADJUSTED HIS OWN SCHEDULE TO COINCIDE WITH THE DOCTOR'S.

QUICK TIPS.

31. THE MORE COMPLEX AND DIFFICULT THE PROBLEM, THE MORE IMPORTANT REPUTATION IS. IN FACT, YOU MIGHT WELL NARROW YOUR FOCUS TO DOCTORS ON THE STAFFS OF CERTAIN MEDICAL CENTERS NOTED FOR EXCELLENCE WITH SPECIFIC PROBLEMS.

32. DOCTORS TYPICALLY REFER PATIENTS TO DOCTORS ON THE STAFFS OF THE SAME HOSPITALS WHERE THEY PRACTICE.

33. IN MANY CASES, INSURANCE COMPANIES WILL PAY FOR SECOND OPINIONS, BUT CHECK AHEAD OF TIME TO MAKE SURE YOUR INSURANCE PLAN DOES COVER THEM.

34. IF YOU ARE NOT COMFORTABLE WITH YOUR PRIMARY CARE DOCTOR'S REFERRAL, ASK FOR A NUMBER OF OPTIONS. IF NECESSARY, YOU MAY CONSIDER GOING "OUT OF NETWORK" EVEN IF YOU HAVE TO PAY SOME OR ALL OF THE FEE.

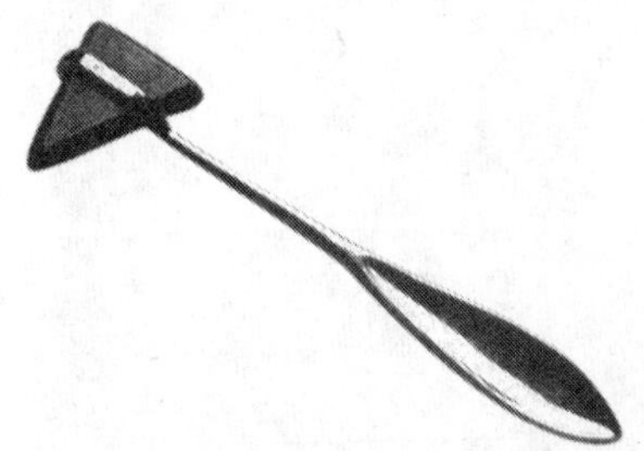

KEY TERMS CHAPTER 4

ALTERNATIVE THERAPY

Non-traditional forms of health care—including acupuncture, homeopathy, naturopathy, massage, reflexology, biofeedback, hypnotherapy, herbology, therapeutic touch, and prayer—that are often based on ancient healing methods and have not been tested in a conventional scientific manner.

CLINICAL TRIAL

An experimental trial of a new drug or therapy in a selected group of human volunteers who suffer from the condition for which the experimental drug or treatment is to be used.

DOUBLE BLIND STUDY

One form of a clinical trial in which two groups of volunteers—one group receiving the real drug or treatment and the other receiving a placebo or dummy—are followed for a specific period of time by researchers who do not know themselves who is receiving which therapy.

PROTOCOL

A rigid set of rules set up for a clinical trial by the Food and Drug Administration (FDA) which must be followed strictly by all researchers and volunteers participating in the trial.

QUICK TAKES

...The old adage, two heads are better than one, often applies in health care, too. Expanded options include referrals, second opinions, alternative therapies, and clinical trials...

CHAPTER 4

STRENGTHENING YOUR TEAM

WHEN YOU NEED A SPECIALIST

For the most part, selecting a specialist is similar to choosing a primary care doctor. There is one major difference, however; typically you will be referred to a specialist by your primary care doctor. Suggesting a consultation does not show a weakness on the part of the doctor. On the contrary, the real weakness lies in a reluctance to suggest consultations when advisable. Your primary care doctor will receive a written report from any consultation or referral. You should get a copy as well.

Ask your doctor why this particular specialist is being recommended. Find out about the specialist's training and experience. If your doctor has sent many patients to the same doctor for the same treatment, you should find out how successful the treatment was and if the patients were satisfied. You might also ask if the specialist would be the one selected for your doctor's personal care. You should feel comfortable about seeing the specialist and, if you are not, ask for another recommendation or you may want to find a different one on your own.

Frequently, patients do seek out specialists on their own. If you are attempting to find a specialist or subspecialist without the guidance of your primary care doctor, use the various kinds of selection procedures described in Chapters one, two and three. However, even greater emphasis should be placed on board certification in the relevant specialty. If you are trying to find someone to care for a very specific problem, make certain that the individual is well trained in that area. You may check to see if a doctor is board certified by calling the American Board of Medical Specialties at (800) 776-2378 or visit their website at www.abms.org.

You will also want to know if the specialist you select is well respected. The more complex and difficult the problem, the more important reputation is. In fact, you might well narrow your focus to doctors on the staffs of certain medical centers noted for excellence with specific problems. There are a number of books and magazine articles such as the annual *U.S News and World Report* issue on America's best hospitals, that offer views on the best medical centers for specific problems.

Last, make certain your doctor and the specialist communicate easily about your case. If you should have a problem with a specialist, or if you are not pleased with the care given, let your primary care doctor know about it right away.

EASY ACCESS TO SPECIALISTS AND SUBSPECIALISTS, ESPECIALLY IN LARGE METROPOLITAN AREAS, PRESENTS CERTAIN PROBLEMS IN COORDINATION THAT A PATIENT SHOULD BE AWARE OF. THIS DIFFICULTY IS PROBABLY EPITOMIZED BY ONE WOMAN WHO WAS TREATED BY A

DERMATOLOGIST, AN OPHTHALMOLOGIST, A RHEUMATOLOGIST, A PSYCHIATRIST, AND AN ALLERGIST, ALL OF WHOM HAD OFFICE SPACE IN HER VERY LARGE APARTMENT COMPLEX ON MANHATTAN'S UPPER WEST SIDE LEASED PRIMARILY TO DOCTORS, THUS ELIMINATING HER NEED TO TRAVEL ANYWHERE, OR, IN FACT, EVEN TO PUT ON HER COAT. FORTUNATELY, ALL WERE QUITE COMPETENT AND HAD ALL THE NECESSARY QUALIFICATIONS. UNFORTUNATELY, EACH WAS AFFILIATED WITH A DIFFERENT MEDICAL CENTER, WHICH MADE COORDINATING HER CARE WITH HER PRIMARY CARE DOCTOR VERY COMPLEX.

Doctors typically refer patients to doctors on the staffs of the same hospitals where they practice. There are good and poor reasons for this:

WHY DOCTORS USUALLY REFER TO DOCTORS IN THE SAME HOSPITALS

Good

- **They know the doctors better.**
- **They continue to be involved in the case.**
- **Coordination of multiple specialists may be easier.**

Poor

- **It is easier.**
- **They will get referrals back.**

- **It reduces the chances of losing the patient.**
- **It may help build social or professional relationships.**
- **The hospital may pressure doctors to refer within the institution.**

In today's managed care environment doctor referrals are usually restricted to other doctors in the managed care organization's network. Sometimes the referring doctor may not even be familiar with the other doctor's qualifications. If you are not comfortable with your primary care doctor's referral, ask for a number of options. If necessary, you may consider going "out of network" even if you have to pay some or all of the fee.

SECOND OPINIONS

Second opinions are a valuable medical tool, too infrequently used in many instances, overused in others. Clearly, you do not want to get another doctor's opinion on every ailment or problem, but there are definitely times you should seek out a second opinion:

- **Before major surgery.**
- **When the diagnosis is serious or life-threatening.**
- **If a rare disease is diagnosed.**
- **If the diagnosis is uncertain.**
- **If you think the number of tests or procedures recommended is excessive.**

- **If a test result has serious implications—a positive pap smear for example—have the test redone immediately before taking further action.**
- **If the treatment suggested is risky or expensive.**
- **If you are uncomfortable with the prescribed diagnosis and treatment.**
- **If a course of treatment is not working.**
- **If you question your doctor's competence.**
- **If your insurance company requires it.**

Most doctors will be supportive if you request a second opinion, and many will recommend it. In many cases, insurance companies will pay for second opinions, but check ahead of time to make sure your insurance plan does cover them. In an HMO, you may have to be more assertive because one way HMOs control costs is by limiting second opinions. This is especially true if you want an opinion outside the plan's network.

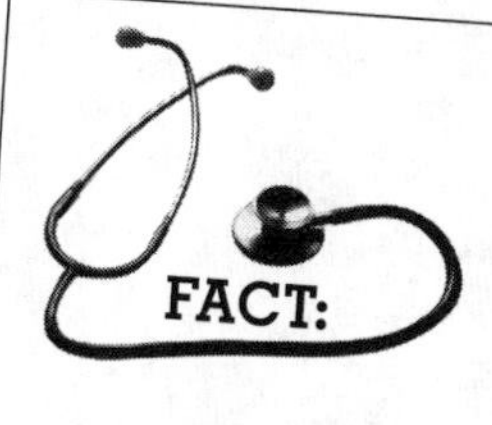

Total out-of-pocket expenditures for alternative and complimentary medicine approach $30 billion annually, estimated David Eisenberg and colleagues at the Harvard/Beth Israel Center for Alternative Medicine Research.

Often, the opinion of a second doctor will affirm the opinion of the first, but the reassurance may be worth the time and extra cost. On the other hand, if the second opinion differs from the first, you have two remaining alternatives: seek the opinion of a third doctor, or educate yourself as much as possible by talking with both doctors and reading up on the problem, and trusting your instincts about which diagnosis is correct.

QUICK TIPS.

35. IN MANY CASES, INSURANCE COMPANIES WILL PAY FOR SECOND OPINIONS, BUT CHECK AHEAD OF TIME TO MAKE SURE YOUR INSURANCE PLAN DOES COVER THEM.

36. ONE WAY HMOS CONTROL COSTS IS BY LIMITING SECOND OPINIONS.

37. DOCTORS MAY HAVE DIFFERENT SOLUTIONS TO THE SAME PROBLEM—AND ANY ONE OR MORE COULD WORK.

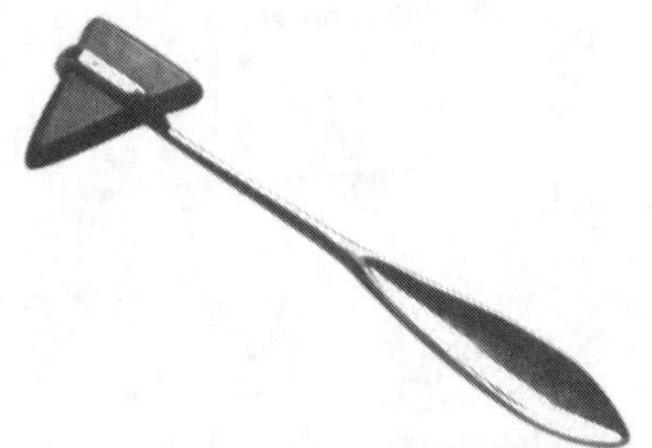

If the diagnosis is the same but the recommended treatments differ, remember that doctors may have different solutions to the same problem—and any one or more could work. For example, an orthopedic surgeon may recommend surgery to correct a knee injury while a physiatrist (a doctor certified in physical medicine and rehabilitation) may recommend rehabilitation. One might work better than the other or they could both work equally well. The choice may be based on your preference. Remember, however, that surgical solutions can rarely be reversed. It usually is best to try a non-surgical solution first if possible.

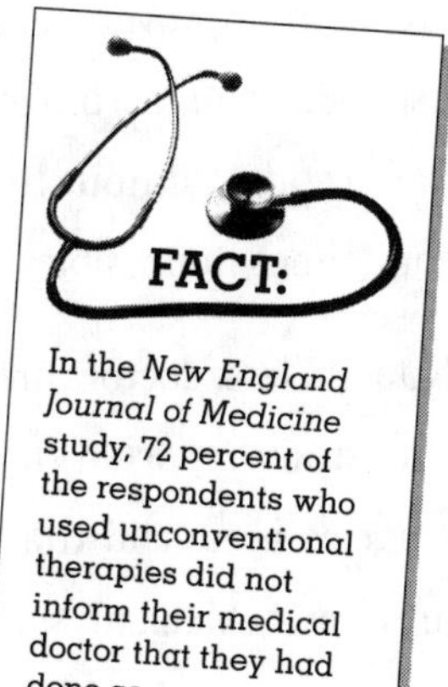

In the *New England Journal of Medicine* study, 72 percent of the respondents who used unconventional therapies did not inform their medical doctor that they had done so.

ALTERNATIVE MEDICINE: EXPLORING YOUR OPTIONS

A recent study conducted by the University of Florida estimated that 86% of households in the US use some sort of alternative therapies. Total out-of-pocket expenditures for alternative and complimentary medicine approach $30 billion annually, estimated David Eisenberg, M.D. and colleagues at the Harvard/Beth Israel Center for Alternative Medicine Research. They further point out that total visits to complimentary/alternative providers numbered 629 million in 1997 as compared to 386 million visits to primary care physicians.

One of the reasons conventional medical therapies are conventional is that most have been proven to be effective in a rigorous scientific manner. Many alternative therapies have not been tested under accepted scientific conditions. You should always consider the possibility that alternative therapies, since they are often unproven, may do more harm than good. The alternative approaches in use today range from legitimate searches for new therapies to outright quackery and fraud. Without the guidance of the scientific and medical community, it is sometimes impossible for doctors, let alone consumers, to tell the difference.

Nonetheless, doctors are becoming more open to the use of alternative approaches. One study reported that about 30 percent of the doctors questioned in the Los Angeles area said that they were open to alternative practices in one form or another. Medical scientists are also indicating a new interest in studying approaches to health that may complement the strengths of Western medicine. Some of the therapies being explored include mind-body medicine, hypnotherapy, biofeedback, chiropractic, vital energy, metabolic therapy, naturopathy, homeopathy, therapeutic touch, acupuncture, prayer, and the use of herbs.

In a *New England Journal of Medicine* study, 72 percent of the respondents who used unconventional therapies did not inform their medical doctor that they had done so. That is unfortunate, because such treatments could be greatly enhanced with the support and advice of a primary care doctor. More worrisome is the great danger that some people may seek alternative treatments in lieu of, rather than as a supplement to, more conventional and proven medical therapies. A classic and tragic example of this was the surge of patients who traveled to Mexico to seek a "magic bullet" cure for cancer promised by the drug Laetrile (made from apricot pits). There was no magic; indeed, patients lost money, hope, and, in some cases, the opportunity for timely use of proven treatment. If you do explore alternative therapies, be certain to let your doctor know about it. Some may be harmful, especially if you are undergoing another treatment under your doctor's direction.

To learn more about alternative medicine contact the National Center for Complementary and Alternative Medicine Clearing House (see Appendix K). To locate a source of reliable information on the practice you are considering, see Appendix K.

HOW TO USE ALTERNATIVE/ COMPLEMENTARY MEDICINE WISELY AND WELL

- **Try to learn everything you can about the particular therapy you are interested in. Your local library may have materials on alternative medicine. Many consumer magazines feature articles on alternative medicine, and the librarian should be able to direct you to these publications.**
- **Discuss your plans with your doctor. You might gain some insight into the therapy in terms of its possible risks. Furthermore, if you are currently under medical treatment, you should make certain that the two approaches will not conflict in some way.**
- **If you start an alternative therapy and it does not appear to be providing relief, or worse, seems to be worsening the condition, contact your doctor immediately.**

CLINICAL TRIALS: SHOULD YOU PARTICIPATE?

Each year, more than half a million Americans, some of them sick, but even more of them healthy, volunteer to take part in experimental trials of new drugs and therapies. Before drugs, vaccines, biological agents, and medical devices are made available for general use by doctors and their patients, they must go through extensive testing on animals and humans. The latter are called "clinical trials." There is probably at least one in process at some medical center for almost any serious disease.

On the plus side, a clinical trial offers the opportunity for prompt use of a drug or other treatment that seems promising, and comes with the bonus of regular and thorough medical examinations at no cost to you (some trials even make allowances for participants' travel and other expenses). Moreover, patients are encouraged to discuss all of their experiences regarding the trial. You will probably learn more about your condition and, therefore, feel more in control, which can have a very positive effect. On the downside, you may be giving up standard treatment for something that may or may not be better. There is even the possibility that you will not get a drug at all, because most trials are conducted by the double-blind method, in which half of the participants get the drug and half get a placebo, or "dummy" medicine. Even the doctors conducting the trials do not know who is getting which.

WHAT TO KNOW BEFORE YOU GET INVOLVED

If you are considering participating in a clinical trial, you will want to know:

- **Who is the sponsor? Look for a federal government, major health organization, drug company, or university-sponsored trial.**
- **Do any impartial authorities monitor the trial? Every hospital conducting research has an institutional review board (IRB) consisting of medical professionals and community leaders to approve**

that hospital's participation. There are also data and safety monitoring boards that oversee trials.

- **What is the financial relationship, if any, between the doctor, hospital and the company or agency sponsoring the trial?**
- **Will there be pain or discomfort? Will diagnostic tests be involved? Get detailed answers to these concerns before you sign any form.**
- **How often will I be examined? This depends on the guidelines of the trial (called the protocol). You should make every effort to keep your appointments.**
- **Does my own doctor get a record of my participation in the trial? Routine health information is sent to your doctor, but details relevant to a "blinded" trial are not disclosed until the trial is over.**
- **Is the drug in this trial approved for treatment of any other disorder? If the answer is yes, you then know that the drug has a prior safety record.**
- **After the study has ended, if I have responded well to the drug, will I be able to continue using it, even before it is approved?**
- **Can I drop out?**

If you are interested in participating in a clinical trial, make your desire known to your doctor, who can track down openings in trials being conducted by medical centers, private foundations, drug companies, physician groups and the federal government.

QUICK TIPS.

38. SURGICAL SOLUTIONS CAN RARELY BE REVERSED. IT USUALLY IS BEST TO TRY A NON-SURGICAL SOLUTION FIRST, IF POSSIBLE.

39. YOU SHOULD ALWAYS CONSIDER THE POSSIBILITY THAT ALTERNATIVE THERAPIES, SIMPLY BECAUSE THEY ARE UNPROVEN, MAY DO MORE HARM THAN GOOD.

40. IF YOU DO EXPLORE ALTERNATIVE THERAPIES, BE CERTAIN TO LET YOUR DOCTOR KNOW ABOUT IT. SOME MAY BE HARMFUL, ESPECIALLY IF YOU ARE UNDERGOING ANOTHER TREATMENT UNDER YOUR DOCTOR'S DIRECTION.

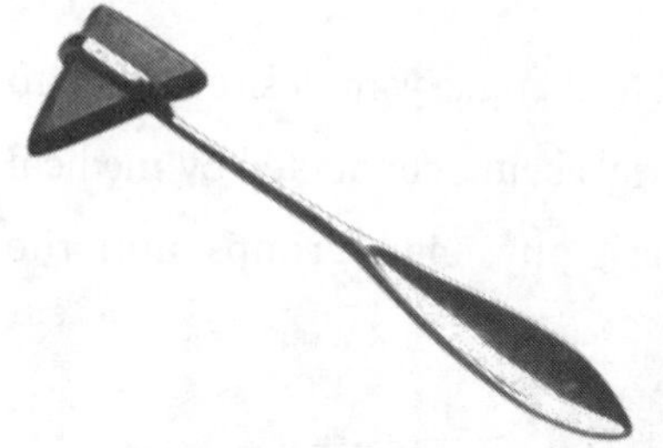

KEY TERMS CHAPTER 5

NATIONAL PRACTITIONER DATA BANK

A computerized listing, created in 1986 by an Act of Congress, to track health professionals who are disciplined for unprofessional behavior and to deter them from simply moving their practices from one state to another.

PUBLIC CITIZEN'S HEALTH RESEARCH GROUP

A Washington, D.C. based consumer advocacy group that has been publicly critical of many medical practices that the group considers detrimental to public health care.

QUICK TAKES

...There's a big difference between doctor-hopping and changing doctors for a good reason. Most failed doctor-patient relationships can be attributed to some common complaints but sometimes it is a matter of self-defense...

CHAPTER 5

CHANGING YOUR DOCTOR

Obviously, at times there are good reasons for changing doctors. Some are very simple and straightforward, such as a doctor's retirement, illness, or death, your own relocation, or a change in your health plan. About 40 percent of people enrolling in managed care plans have to change their doctor to one who is affiliated with the plan.

An onset of a chronic condition may also prompt a change to a different medical specialist, such as a rheumatologist or cardiologist, if a condition needs to be managed by a specialist other than a primary care doctor.

If you have continuing symptoms that your doctor has been unable to diagnose or if, after a diagnosis, your problems continue to linger without improvement, you should at least consider getting a second opinion and, depending on that opinion, possibly changing doctors. Doctors often have different approaches to the same problem. A different doctor may offer a different perspective and, perhaps, a solution.

You might also change doctors in order to find one who includes alternative medicine in the treatment or to find one who can help you enroll in a clinical trial.

People who have hostile feelings toward organized medicine tend to change doctors frequently; their complaints then become a self-fulfilling prophecy. They don't get continuous, quality care because it's impossible for anyone to deliver it. On the other hand, negative feelings may be prompted by unfortunate encounters with incompetent doctors or by the patronizing or otherwise inappropriate attitudes expressed by some doctors toward patients. Patients on the receiving end of such a relationship should continue their search for a doctor who better meets their needs.

EIGHT REASONS TO SAY GOODBYE

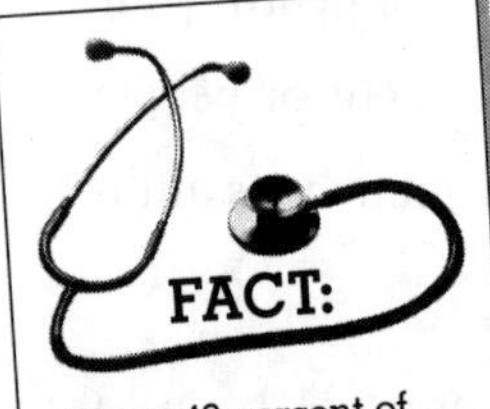

About 40 percent of people enrolling in managed care plans have to change their doctor to one who is affiliated with the plan.

Here are the eight most common complaints about "doctors I don't go to anymore."

POOR BEDSIDE MANNER

Good medical care is more than diagnosis and treatment; it's also an attitude on the part of the doctor that sparks a sense of trust in the patient. Being under the care of a doctor who is impersonal, abrupt, bored, arrogant, condescending, or sarcastic, may in the end be counterproductive.

The doctor's aloofness could have a more serious explanation: substance abuse or psychological impairment, which according to a recent American Medical

Association report affects 30,000 to 40,000 physicians. Mood swings and detachment are signs to watch for.

TOO VAGUE AND EVASIVE

A doctor who dismisses problems with "it's nothing to worry about," or "let me take care of it," or who uses medical jargon isn't interested in having you as a partner in your health care. The effect of this evasiveness can be anger, fear, and confusion, leading to failure to follow directions and failure of treatment.

NEVER ON SCHEDULE

Medical emergencies can make appointment scheduling an inexact science, but when snafus become chronic, it's a sign of trouble. An explanation can ease the frustration, but make-up time should not be at your expense.

COULDN'T DIAGNOSE THE PROBLEM

Some conditions can't be diagnosed on-the-spot. Others aren't attributable to one specific cause. That doesn't excuse an incomplete workup, however, which may leave you with a condition that could have been treated earlier.

ORDERED TOO MANY TESTS

Sophisticated technology is available and doctors tend to use it, although some testing may not be necessary. The number of tests performed for diagnosis seems to be reduced in patient-doctor relationships where communication is strong.

DISCOURAGED SECOND OPINIONS

A doctor who dissuades you from talking to another doctor may perceive it as questioning his or her professional abilities.

DIDN'T PROTECT MY MEDICAL PRIVACY

No patient should have to discuss the reason for a visit, payment, or payment problems within earshot of other patients or staff.

Medical records can be requested by and turned over to insurance companies, lawyers, employers, and others without your consent, but you can certainly see them, too, to make sure they contain the proper information. In 23 states and the District of Columbia the law grants patients access to medical records from doctors and hospital records; in other states, a doctor may let you see them anyway.

UNPLEASANT OFFICE STAFF

Repeated incidents such as rudeness over the telephone, a brusque physician's assistant, or being kept waiting in an examining room for a long time before the doctor shows up are all annoying indications that a staff could do better.

The staff takes its cues from the chief. A doctor who doesn't demand the highest level of performance from a staff may be sending a message about his or her own laxity in diagnosis and treatment.

SHOULD YOU SWITCH?

If your doctor fits these important factors in a doctor-patient relationship, it may be time to consider finding a new doctor. But before you decide to part company with your doctor, ask yourself if you've been a responsible patient. Often problems arise when patients don't reveal their full medical history, or if they forget to alert their doctor about other drugs they are taking. A doctor-patient relationship is like a marriage—both sides have to work to make it successful.

If you're sure the problem isn't on your side, however, confront your doctor with your grievances. Or if it's easier for you, you may want to write them in a letter. Expressing your dissatisfaction may open the communication lines between you and your doctor. You might even end up in a better relationship with your present doctor. Sometimes doctors aren't aware that they are in the midst of a deteriorating relationship until a patient wants to leave.

But if you are still unhappy with your doctor and you've decided a change is necessary, you can make a clean break by simply going to another doctor. Keep in mind, however, that your most important concern should be continuity of care. So, unless the situation is intolerable or the doctor is impaired, stay with your current doctor until you have found another one that you like.

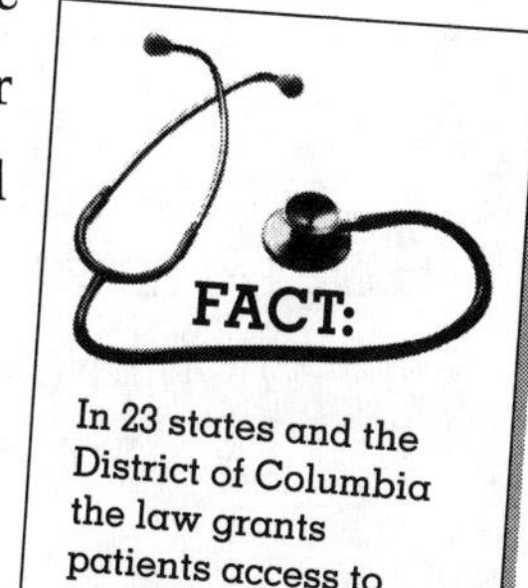

In 23 states and the District of Columbia the law grants patients access to medical records held by physicians; in other states, a doctor may let you see them anyway.

Generally, medical records are kept by your doctor until you have found a new one. You will then have to sign a release with your new doctor approving the transfer of all your medical records to the new office. These records cannot be withheld for any reason, even if you have not yet paid your last bill.

Finally, don't feel embarrassed or guilty if you decide to change doctors. Remember, good quality medical care is your right!

IN ONE CASE INVOLVING A WOMAN IN HER MID-THIRTIES, THE DOCTOR-PATIENT RELATIONSHIP WAS SEVERED OVER WHAT WAS BASICALLY A CONFLICT IN PERSONALITIES: THE WOMAN WISHED TO HAVE MORE CONTROL OVER HER HEALTH CARE, AND THE DOCTOR WAS RELUCTANT TO GIVE IT. THE IMPASSE WAS REACHED

QUICK TIPS.

41. BEFORE YOU DECIDE TO PART COMPANY WITH YOUR DOCTOR, ASK YOURSELF IF YOU'VE BEEN A RESPONSIBLE PATIENT.

42. A DOCTOR-PATIENT RELATIONSHIP IS LIKE A MARRIAGE—BOTH SIDES HAVE TO WORK TO MAKE IT SUCCESSFUL.

43. EXPRESSING YOUR DISSATISFACTION MAY OPEN THE COMMUNICATION LINES BETWEEN YOU AND YOUR DOCTOR. YOU MIGHT EVEN END UP IN A BETTER RELATIONSHIP WITH YOUR PRESENT DOCTOR.

44. UNLESS THE SITUATION IS INTOLERABLE OR THE DOCTOR IS IMPAIRED, STAY WITH YOUR CURRENT DOCTOR UNTIL YOU HAVE FOUND ANOTHER ONE THAT YOU LIKE.

45. WHEN CHANGING DOCTORS YOU MAY HAVE TO SIGN A RELEASE WITH YOUR NEW DOCTOR APPROVING THE TRANSFER OF ALL YOUR MEDICAL RECORDS TO THE NEW OFFICE. THESE RECORDS CANNOT BE WITHHELD FOR ANY REASON, EVEN IF YOU HAVE NOT YET PAID YOUR LAST BILL.

BEFORE THE TWO COULD ATTEMPT ANY KIND OF A COMPROMISE, AND THE WOMAN WENT OFF IN SEARCH OF A DOCTOR WHO WOULD BETTER SUIT HER PERSONAL NEEDS. A YEAR LATER, AFTER A FRUITLESS SEARCH FOR A DOCTOR WHOSE MEDICAL EXPERTISE SHE RESPECTED, SHE RETURNED TO HER ORIGINAL DOCTOR.

SELF DEFENSE: AVOIDING QUESTIONABLE DOCTORS

In addition to finding good doctors, you also want to be able to identify and avoid doctors who have a history of professional problems. One way to do this is to make certain a doctor has not been disciplined by your state or, in fact, any state. You can call the appropriate state agency (listed in Appendix G) or check names in the book *16,638 Questionable Doctors*, published by the Public Citizens' Health Research Group. This book lists the names of doctors who have been disciplined by states or by the federal government. The disciplinary actions were taken for a variety of reasons, including overprescribing or misprescribing medications, criminal convictions, alcohol or drug abuse, and patient sexual abuse.

You may also visit the Castle Connolly Medical Ltd. website (www.castleconnolly.com) which links directly to the website (www.docboard.org) which lists disciplined doctors. You may also link to the American Medical Association (AMA, www.ama-assn.org) and American Board of Medical Specialities (ABMS, www.abms.org) websites for biographical information, including board certification, on doctors (see Appendix K).

The Public Citizens' Health Research Group, which publishes a report on the number of physicians disciplined in each state, believes that many states are not aggressive enough in monitoring doctors. They have been leading the call for public access to the National Practitioner Data Bank. The Data Bank was created in 1986 by an Act of Congress in order to track professionals who are disciplined for unprofessional behavior and to deter them from simply moving their practices from one state to another. The Data Bank became operational in 1990 and contains a record of adverse actions such as license removal, loss of clinical privileges, and professional society membership actions taken against doctors and other licensed health professionals, such as dentists. It contains the names of over 170,000 health practitioners who have either a licensing action or malpractice judgement or settlement against them. There is strong pressure from some medical groups either to do away with the Data Bank or to place even stricter controls on access. They support their position with examples of errors in the handling of sensitive information. It is unlikely that Congress would permit the elimination of the Data Bank, however. In fact, it is possible that at some time in the future, access may be made more available to the public. However, at the present time there is no public access to this information.

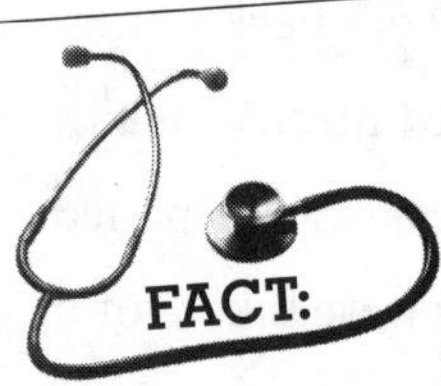

The National Practitioner Data Bank contains the names of over 170,000 health practitioners who have either a licensing action or malpractice judgement or settlement against them. You can write directly to the National Practitioner Data Bank if you wish more information.

A data service used by lawyers to check on a doctor's or hospital's malpractice history is LEXIS/NEXIS, the computerized legal information service. Some libraries will do a LEXIS/NEXIS search for a fee, usually over $65.00. Public access to the listing of malpractice payments is one issue on which doctors are very sensitive, and rightfully so. Many malpractice payments are made by insurance companies over the objections of doctors because the insurers feel it's cheaper to settle than to fight. Yet doctors who feel they are blameless contend that these settlements reflect negatively on them. Also, since so many specialists, such as those in obstetrics and gynecology, are subject to more frequent lawsuits because of the nature of their practice, doctors are concerned about how patients will interpret a malpractice settlement.

People who believe they have a problem with a doctor, whether in regard to fees, treatment, or ethics, may contact the appropriate local medical society in the county in which the doctor practices, or the state medical society. State health departments are also places consumers may turn to for assistance or information on disciplinary actions taken against doctors. The health department, typically, will only divulge that an action has been taken but will not give you any specific information about it (See Appendix G for phone numbers and addresses).

Changing your doctor should not be considered a setback in your search for the best doctor to meet your needs. As you may have come to understand throughout preceding chapters in this book, the personal and treatment styles doctors bring to their practices vary greatly. What is important for you, as a patient, to realize is that these subtle and immeasurable characteristics can be as important as clinical skills. There is, in fact, substantial empirical and anecdotal evidence demonstrating that confidence in the healer and the healing process plays a major role in many cures. Your main objective is to find the therapy—in combination with the professional who is providing the therapy—that works best for you.

QUICK TIPS.

46. A DATA SERVICE USED BY LAWYERS TO CHECK ON A DOCTOR'S OR HOSPITAL'S MALPRACTICE HISTORY IS LEXIS/NEXIS, THE COMPUTERIZED LEGAL INFORMATION SERVICE. LEXIS WILL DO A SEARCH AND ISSUE A REPORT ON ANY MALPRACTICE AWARDS OR SETTLEMENTS ORDERED BY A COURT.

47. STATE HEALTH DEPARTMENTS ARE ALSO PLACES CONSUMERS MAY TURN TO FOR ASSISTANCE OR INFORMATION ON DISCIPLINARY ACTIONS TAKEN AGAINST DOCTORS.

48. THERE IS SUBSTANTIAL EMPIRICAL AND ANECDOTAL EVIDENCE DEMONSTRATING THAT CONFIDENCE IN THE HEALER AND THE HEALING PROCESS PLAYS A MAJOR ROLE IN MANY CURES.

49. PEOPLE WHO BELIEVE THEY HAVE A PROBLEM WITH A DOCTOR, WHETHER IN REGARD TO FEES, TREATMENT, OR ETHICS, MAY CONTACT THE APPROPRIATE LOCAL MEDICAL SOCIETY IN THE COUNTY IN WHICH THE DOCTOR PRACTICES, OR THE STATE MEDICAL SOCIETY.

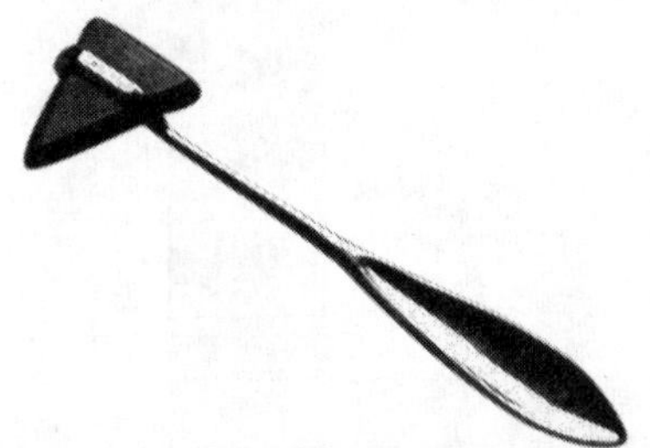

KEY TERMS CHAPTER 6

CAPITATION

A method of payment to physicians and other health care providers whereby a fixed amount of money is allotted for each patient served.

EPO

An Exclusive Provider Organization is similar to a PPO except the patients must use only providers in the EPO.

GROUP MODEL HMO

A model of an HMO in which the HMO contracts with large multi-specialty groups of doctors to provide care, usually from a number of central locations.

HEALTH MAINTENANCE ORGANIZATION (HMO)

One type of managed care organization that provides for a wide range of comprehensive health care services for its members in return for a fixed, predetermined fee. The care is provided by a network or group of physicians affiliated with the organization and possibly other health care professionals.

IPA

An Independent Practice Association is one model of health maintenance organization (HMO) in which the organization contracts with individual doctors, or groups of doctors, to provide care for the enrolled patients in the doctors' own offices.

PHO

A Physician Hospital Organization is an organization of a hospital and its physicians that may contract with managed care organizations (MCO) or may become licensed as a MCO itself.

PPO

A Preferred Provider Organization is a managed care model that offers health care provided by a group of doctors and/or hospitals that have negotiated discounted rates, either capitated or fee-for-service, for enrollees while continuing to provide care for other patients. Patients typically pay less if they use the PPO provider.

PSO

A Provider Service Organization, sometimes called a provider service network (PSN), is a group of doctors that are organized to provide care to a large number of patients, typically under contract to managed care organizations.

STAFF MODEL HMO

A managed care model where the HMO employs the doctors, usually on salary. Care is provided out of a number of centralized locations.

QUICK TAKES

... The rules are different but they are not difficult to play by. The first step is to sort out the alphabet soup of models. The model of HMO usually determines how your care will be delivered and often your satisfaction with it...

CHAPTER 6

CHOOSING A DOCTOR IN AN HMO

At one time only doctors looking for new patients joined HMOs. Today, there is a new reality. Almost *all* doctors—over 80 percent—participate in some kind of managed care arrangement. So it is likely that you will find the best for your own care if you know how to work the system.

When managed care achieves a significant market penetration and begins to control the flow of large numbers of patients, more doctors sign on. Also, many hospitals encourage their doctors to sign on with as many different plans as possible in order to insure that the hospital does not lose any potential patients. Managed care now enrolls more than one out of every three people in the country, and over 80% of workers who get health insurance through their employer are in some form of managed care. A doctor who has not joined a managed health plan provider network could have few patients!

The main factor to focus on in assessing an HMO is its resources, primarily doctors and hospitals. First, is there an ample selection of primary care doctors near where you live and work? Second, are the doctors well qualified? This can be answered by following the approach outlined in this book for finding the best doctors. When choosing doctors, it is usually a good idea to call their offices to confirm they are still affiliated with the particular plan. Doctors frequently change affiliations with managed care plans. Also, it is a good idea to check on the procedure for using the doctor listed.

HMOs may list hundreds of doctors but not all of them are necessarily accessible to all members. A large HMO, for example, may restrict the number of specialists that primary care doctors can refer to for various reasons, including location, hospital capacity, and general resource allocation. So although you may see the name of an ophthalmologist, gynecologist, or other specialist you want to use, and indeed that doctor may be affiliated with the HMO, it does not necessarily follow that your primary care doctor is free to refer you to them. Those specialists may see HMO patients only on a certain basis—for specific procedures, for example, or in a certain geographic region—and then possibly only after a rigorous screening process. These possibilities illustrate the varying styles of operation you will find in managed care plans.

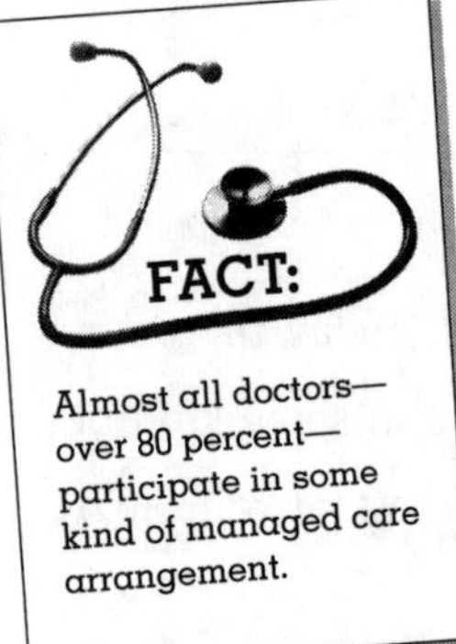
FACT:
Almost all doctors—over 80 percent—participate in some kind of managed care arrangement.

Doctors in HMOs are bound by the same professional ethics that guide all doctors. However, there is a major difference: In an HMO, the plan is responsible for providing you with care as well as with a doctor. If your doctor leaves the plan, you don't follow him or her. The plan provides a new doctor for you.

SELECTING DOCTORS IN AN HMO

Selecting a doctor in an HMO can be a greater challenge than selecting one when you have indemnity insurance that leaves you free to select a doctor without the restrictions of the plan. Obviously, in an HMO arrangement you need to select a doctor who belongs to that plan. Studies have shown that about 40 percent of enrollees in managed care plans have to choose a new doctor when they join. However, even in a plan of small size, you will usually have the option of choosing among a number of primary care doctors as well as other specialists and subspecialists. In doing so, utilize the same criteria you would apply to selecting a doctor in a fee-for-service practice.

The first doctor you select in an HMO plan is your primary care doctor. Typically, you will be sent a list with little information other than the doctor's name, specialty, and address. *Find out more about those doctors you may be considering.* Use the process described earlier in this book. If you make a selection and are not satisfied, request a change. Ask about the procedure for changing doctors before you join the plan.

When you need a specialist, it is your primary care doctor who will refer you, as in traditional indemnity plans. But, unlike indemnity plans in which you can find a specialist on your own if you choose, in managed care plans you must be referred to see a specialist. Again, your choices will be limited in selecting specialists, but be assertive. Ask for a choice of doctors and ask why your primary care doctor recommends a particular specialist. One disadvantage to the IPA model and the network referral process is that primary care doctors can end up making referrals to specialists and/or subspecialists they do not know. This may result in poor communication between the primary care doctor and the specialist, which is not in the patient's best interest. If you are not satisfied with the choices offered, ask to go outside the plan. Choice of providers outside a plan is built into certain managed care plans and is permitted in many others under certain conditions.

However, if you do not have a choice, or if the choices are not ones with which you agree, consider going outside the HMO. Although you are likely to have to pay more, it may be worth it if you get a correct diagnosis and appropriate treatment for your problem. In some cases, the HMO will agree to pay at least a consultation fee if you feel strongly that you need to discuss your problem with another doctor outside the HMO network. After the consultation, if you still feel the need for a different doctor, at least your choice will be based on more complete information.

One of the most popular plans offered by HMOs permits going outside of the network of doctors and hospitals—but at an added cost. The point of service, or POS plan, one of the fastest growing offerings of many HMOs, permits the HMO member to use doctors, hospitals, and other services that are not part of the HMO network. Typically, the member will pay an additional fee for this choice—for example, 20 percent or 30 percent of the cost—whereas if the member stays "in-network" the HMO will pay all or close to all of the cost.

When leaving the network of a POS, however, patients should find out exactly how much it will cost to do so. Some HMOs will pay a percentage of "appropriate and prevailing fees" while others will pay a percentage of their own fee schedule, which is usually lower.

HMO MODELS

Although a large alphabet soup of HMO models has appeared since the big move toward managed care began in the late 1980s, and we now have PPOs, PSOs, and EPOs, two models are most important to the health care consumer. One is the staff or group model where patients visit their doctors in a single, or perhaps in a few, locations and where all the doctors and most, if not all, diagnostic and treatment facilities are located. The second is the independent practice association or IPA model where doctors see patients in their private offices. Organizations such as PPOs, EPOs and PSOs tend to be organized on the IPA model.

Whether a group/staff model or an IPA, all HMOs require a primary care physician and all have certain protocols, usually involving referral by the primary care physician, to access a specialist.

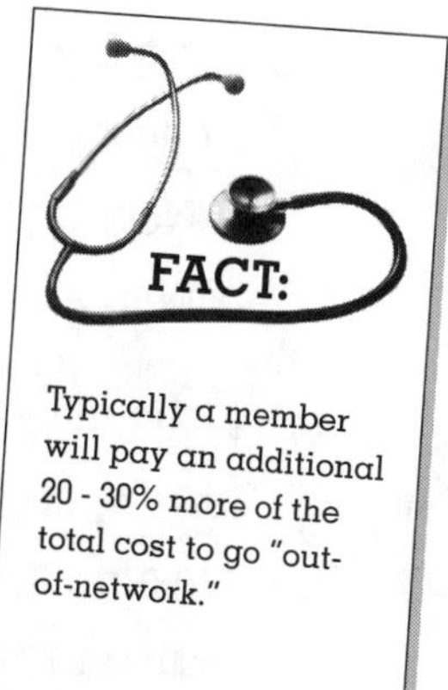

Typically a member will pay an additional 20 - 30% more of the total cost to go "out-of-network."

DOCTOR COMPENSATION

There is virtually no difference in the types of doctors who practice in the two HMO models and each should be evaluated in terms of benefits to the individual patient. There is, however, a separate matter of how doctors in HMOs are compensated, and this issue has become a major concern to both patients and doctors.

HMOs compensate doctors in a number of ways. Doctors who are employed by staff model HMOs are usually on salary, perhaps with a quality bonus based on patient satisfaction. In group model HMOs the physician group has a contract with the HMO and the doctors are employed by the group, usually on salary and, again, often with a quality bonus.

QUICK TIPS.

50. THE MAIN FACTOR TO FOCUS ON IN ASSESSING AN HMO IS ITS RESOURCES, PRIMARILY DOCTORS AND HOSPITALS.

51. HMOS MAY LIST HUNDREDS OF DOCTORS BUT NOT ALL OF THEM ARE NECESSARILY ACCESSIBLE TO ALL MEMBERS.

52. WHEN YOU NEED A SPECIALIST, IT IS YOUR PRIMARY CARE DOCTOR WHO WILL REFER YOU, AS IN TRADITIONAL INDEMNITY PLANS. BUT, UNLIKE INDEMNITY PLANS IN WHICH YOU CAN FIND A SPECIALIST ON YOUR OWN IF YOU CHOOSE, IN MANAGED CARE PLANS YOU TYPICALLY MUST BE REFERRED TO SEE A SPECIALIST.

53. WHEN LEAVING THE NETWORK IN A POS PLAN PATIENTS SHOULD FIND OUT EXACTLY HOW MUCH IT WILL COST TO DO SO.

54. WHEN CHOOSING DOCTORS, IT IS USUALLY A GOOD IDEA TO CALL THEIR OFFICES TO CONFIRM THAT THEY ARE STILL AFFILIATED WITH THE PARTICULAR PLAN.

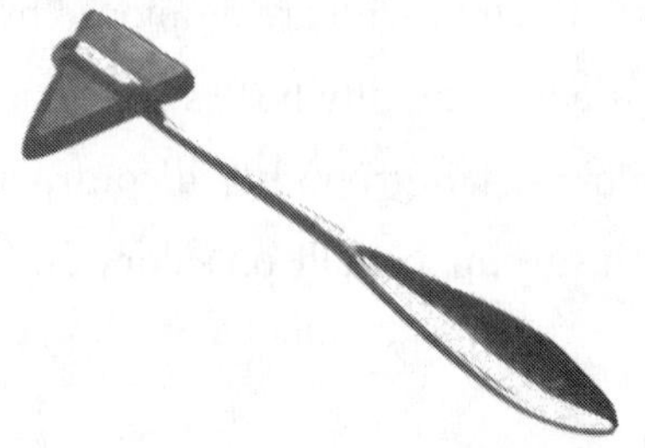

In the IPA model HMOs, or in PPOs, EPOs, PSOs and other types of managed care organizations the doctors are usually paid in one of two ways. In the past, the predominant payment method was a negotiated fee schedule, typically designed at some discount to the doctor's normal fee. Doctors simply traded the promise of higher volume for a reduced fee. Today, a major method of payment in an IPA is capitation. While this is fast becoming the most common method of payment in IPAs it is also the one generating the most controversy.

Under a capitated or capitation system doctors are paid a set amount per month or per year to provide care to a patient during that time period. So, for example, a primary care physician may be paid $15 per member per month.

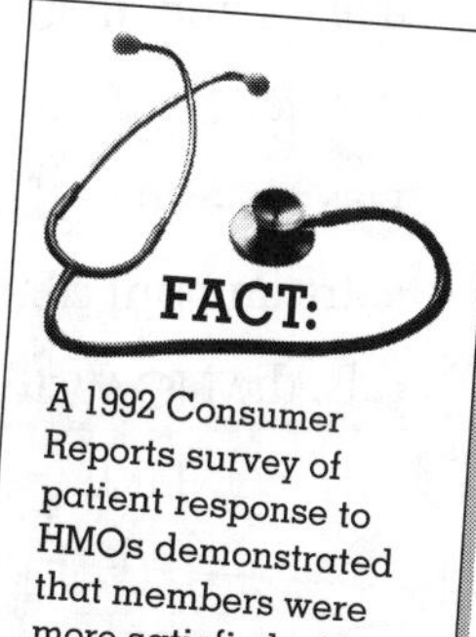

A 1992 Consumer Reports survey of patient response to HMOs demonstrated that members were more satisfied with plans that paid their doctor on a fee basis than they were with those that paid on a capitated, or per person, basis.

HMOs have moved toward capitation as a method of payment because they found that discounted fee-for-service payment methods did not reduce costs as much as had been hoped, if at all. To make up for discounted fees of 20 percent, for instance, some doctors simply scheduled 20 percent more patient visits so that their incomes would not decrease. Doctors openly comment that discounted fees translate to discounted time with patients!

Capitation has helped to control costs. However, it also has introduced a number of important ethical issues for doctors, other health care providers, and for patients. Many are troubled by the notion that a doctor could be placed in a situation that appears to promise rewards for *not* providing care. It is generally recognized that under a fee-for-service system doctors have an incentive to provide more care, even if it is not necessary, because they are paid by the amount of care they deliver. But the reverse is not accepted in such a benign fashion: the concept of a doctor being rewarded to provide *less* care is of major concern to many people, including many doctors.

Another technique involved in payment systems utilized by managed care companies is called "withholds" or "set-asides." This method is also used to motivate doctors to control costs and, as in capitation, raises similar ethical concerns. Under this method, for example, a group of pediatricians is contracted to care for 1,000 children. That contract is based on a budget of $15,000 a month. A certain amount of that budget, say 20 percent, is reserved for referrals to subspecialists and another 20 percent is set aside or withheld. If the group of doctors uses fewer subspecialist referrals than budgeted they receive the 20 percent that was set aside. If they use more subspecialist referrals than were budgeted the extra amount comes out of the set-aside. The more set-aside that is used for referrals, the less doctors will be able to receive from it.

A great deal of controversy has ensued over these payment mechanisms. Some states, in fact, are legislating to prohibit or restrict these practices. Individual "horror stories" of patients who have been denied appropriate care, such as not being referred to a subspecialist in a timely manner, have been used to demonstrate the issue in human terms.

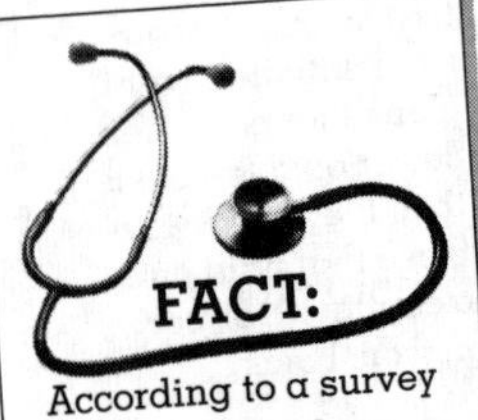

According to a survey conducted by the American Medical Association, just over a third (210,811) of physicians in this country are now members of group practices, and, in 1995, those practices numbered 19,788, an increase of 361 percent since 1965.

Some studies demonstrate that when physician-run health plans are paid by capitation and are in control they reduce costs more substantially than other plans. Some doctors strongly support capitation. They believe it makes them, rather than managers, responsible for allocating resources and making medical decisions.

And, despite the outcry, most of the studies of HMO patients versus non-HMO patients demonstrate no differences in their health status.

In fact, there is a substantial body of research suggesting that HMO members receive more in the way of preventive services than do non-HMO populations.

If method of payment is an issue of concern to you, it may be wise to ask your doctor about the method of compensation in the HMO in which you are enrolled. If you believe the method would work against you as a patient you should discuss it with your doctor and ask if and how it influences the manner of care for patients. If you are not satisfied by the answer you may want to change doctors or, better yet, change HMOs, if possible.

While the wisest course of action is to ask about this issue before joining an HMO, rather than after you have become a member, most HMO members have not done this. If you believe you are not recieving appropriate care because of an HMO policy, you can contact your state health insurance department (see Appendix G).

In response to patient and physician concerns about payment policies, groups of doctors in various parts of the country have formed organizations to receive and investigate complaints against HMOs. You can contact them with any grievances you have about your HMO (see Physicians Who Care, Appendix K).

QUICK TIPS.

55. IF YOU BELIEVE YOU ARE NOT RECEIVING APPROPRIATE CARE BECAUSE OF AN HMO POLICY YOU CAN CONTACT YOUR STATE HEALTH OR INSURANCE DEPARTMENT.

56. TYPICALLY, YOU WILL BE SENT A LIST WITH LITTLE INFORMATION OTHER THAN THE DOCTOR'S NAME, SPECIALTY, AND ADDRESS. FIND OUT MORE ABOUT THOSE DOCTORS YOU MAY BE CONSIDERING.

57. IN SOME CASES, AN HMO WILL AGREE TO PAY AT LEAST A CONSULTATION FEE IF YOU FEEL STRONGLY THAT YOU NEED TO DISCUSS YOUR PROBLEM WITH ANOTHER DOCTOR OUTSIDE THE HMO NETWORK.

58. IF METHOD OF HMO PAYMENT TO PHYSICIANS IS AN ISSUE OF CONCERN TO YOU, IT MAY BE WISE TO ASK YOUR DOCTOR ABOUT THE METHOD OF COMPENSATION IN THE HMO IN WHICH YOU ARE ENROLLED.

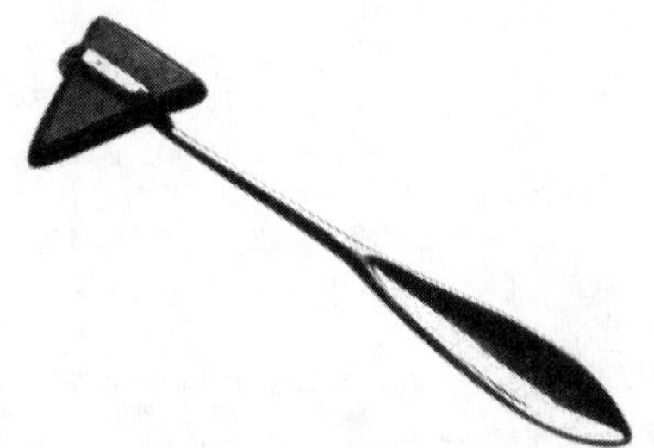

HOW DOCTORS AND PATIENTS FEEL ABOUT MANAGED CARE

People enrolled in HMOs tend to like them. However, most doctors do not like managed care—and understandably so! Managed care organizations negotiate deep discounts in fees for doctors. There is no reason doctors should prefer this process, but when managed care controls so many patients there is little choice but to join managed care and negotiate.

Managed care organizations also require doctors to do a substantial amount of paper work and to follow policies and procedures that control costs and monitor quality. All of this creates a level of business management most doctors resent.

At least a portion of these negative attitudes toward managed care can be ascribed to differences in the organization of medical practices in different parts of the country.

The northeast, south, and southwest regions have been the slowest to accept managed care because doctors generally resisted it more strongly than those in other parts of the country. Doctors in large group practices, which are more common in the far west and midwest than in the east, adapted to managed care more readily. In the northeast, where doctors practice solo or in small groups, the change has been greater and the adjustment more difficult.

Most doctors have adapted and learned to practice successfully in this new medical environment. According to a survey conducted by the American Medical Association, just over a third (210,811) of physicians in this country are now members of group practices. In 1995 group practices numbered 19,788, an increase of 361 percent since 1965. From 1991 to 1995, the number of groups increased by 16.4 percent and the number of group physicians by 14.3 percent.

The survey shows that, in an environment that is organizationally complex, medical groups have changed how they are organized legally, with partnerships declining to 13.8 percent and professional corporations increasing to 77.9 percent. In the latter group, control of decision making remains largely in physician hands. This ability to retain decision making power has dramatically altered physicians' attitudes towards managed care.

FACT:

Most studies have shown that enrollees in HMOs use about the same amount of health care resources at about the same rate as people not enrolled in HMOs, with the exception of hospital days, which HMOs reduce by about 30 percent.

The view of patients and the public, however, is decidedly more positive about managed care.

A study sponsored by the Medstat Group, J.D. Power and Associates and the New England Medical Center reported that in 20 markets across the United States, HMOs recieved more top scores than PPOs and fee-for-service plans.

The study asked plan members to assess their health plans on choice of providers, physician care, premiums and deductibles and access to care. HMOs topped fee-for-service and point-of-service plans in over half the markets.

One of the findings uncovered in a Louis Harris Associates poll of consumers was that the majority surveyed, 59 percent, believed the trend toward managed care was a good thing as compared to 28 percent who viewed it as a bad thing. Also, 48 percent as compared to 39 percent believed managed care would improve quality, and 59 percent versus 30 percent believed it would help contain the costs of care. Of note was that the response of those people in communities with a high penetration by managed care tended to be the most positive!

There are many studies that have examined the quality of care and the satisfaction of patients in managed care settings. Most show that members of HMOs and other managed care organizations are at least as satisfied or more satisfied with their care than people covered by indemnity insurance. Some studies have shown indemnity-covered people more satisfied, particularly when it relates to choice of doctors. In fact, the issue of greatest concern to HMO enrollees is usually access, particularly to specialists. Advocates of either view can point to studies to support managed care or to criticize it. The key may lay in the studies that have demonstrated that when individuals have a choice, and select a managed care plan, they tend to be more satisfied than those who have no choice.

In terms of quality the conclusion is similar. While critics may contend that the care delivered by managed care organizations is not adequate, and a study of Medicaid patients is frequently cited to support this view, the overwhelming majority of studies demonstrate no difference in the health status and quality of care of those people covered by managed care plans or by indemnity insurance.

The variability in the results of all of the studies on quality and satisfaction in managed care reinforces the important premise that as there are good doctors and poor doctors there are good HMOs and poor HMOs. It is important for consumers to know how to discern the difference and to put some effort, however modest, into finding the best.

POINTS TO REMEMBER

- **To summarize, there is basically no difference in quality between doctors in HMOs and those in private practice. You can find excellent doctors if you're a member of an HMO and you can find poor ones, just as you can find excellent and poor doctors if you carry indemnity insurance. The key is making sure that you find the best available for your own needs and the needs of your family.**

Some simple guidelines to remember:

- Review the credentials and training of *any* doctor who cares for you.
- Make certain a doctor you select is taking new patients and the waiting period for an appointment is not unreasonable
- Be sure the HMO has a sufficient number of specialists and subspecialists you may need to see and that they are of high quality. For example, if you have diabetes, you will want to make sure that the HMC has endocrinologists on staff or as part of its network. If you have coronary heart disease, you will want to make sure that the HMO has first rate cardiologists and an arrangement with an outstanding center where the doctors perform invasive and non-invasive diagnostic techniques and which has a good record for open heart surgery.
- Determine beforehand the HMO's policy for patient referral to subspecialists, especially whether you will have a choice and how it may be exercised.
- Inquire about the rules for changing doctors in the HMO if you are not satisfied with your initial choice. You will want to know not only the procedure but how often such change is allowed.
- Ask about your options to go out of network

and what your additional percentage of payment will be if you exercise this option. In determining what percentage the HMO pays, try to find out whether their payment is based on the HMO fee scale or "usual and customary" fees.

- Ask your doctor about the HMO's compensation system. You want to be sure that the system for paying your doctor will not have a negative influence on your care.

QUICK TIPS.

59. IF YOU BELIEVE YOU ARE NOT RECEIVING APPROPRIATE CARE BECAUSE OF AN HMO POLICY YOU CAN CONTACT YOUR STATE HEALTH OR INSURANCE DEPARTMENT.

60. PEOPLE IN COMMUNITIES WITH A HIGH PENETRATION BY MANAGED CARE TENDED TO BE THE MOST POSITIVE ABOUT IT.

61. THE ISSUE OF GREATEST CONCERN TO HMO ENROLLEES IS USUALLY ACCESS, PARTICULARLY TO SPECIALISTS.

62. THE VARIABILITY IN THE RESULTS OF ALL OF THE STUDIES ON QUALITY AND SATISFACTION IN MANAGED CARE REINFORCES THE IMPORTANT PREMISE THAT AS THERE ARE GOOD DOCTORS AND POOR DOCTORS THERE ARE GOOD HMOS AND POOR HMOS.

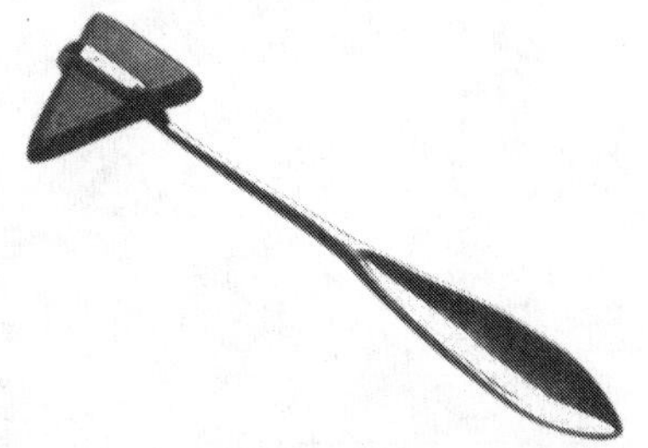

SECTION TWO

DIRECTORY OF DOCTORS

INCLUDES HOSPITAL INFORMATION PROGRAM

DIRECTORY OF DOCTORS

SECTION TWO

HOW TO USE THE DIRECTORY OF DOCTORS

This first edition of the Castle Connolly Guide, *How to Find the Best Doctors: Metropolitan Chicago*, contains vital information on approximately 2,000 of the finest doctors in the region. Nominated by their peers, these doctors have met exacting criteria established by the Castle Connolly Medical Ltd. research staff. The result of the intensive screening process is a rigorously selected and outstanding group of doctors representing less than ten percent in the region, each one chosen for excellence in patient care.

WHY THIS BOOK IS YOUR BEST GUIDE

How to Find the Best Doctors is unique in a number of ways. The first edition of the Guide, published in 1994, was the first selective directory of doctors who practice in the New York metropolitan region. Our decision to publish regional guides, rather than a countrywide directory of the best medical specialists was based on the simple and widely proven fact that most people, unless motivated by an extremely unusual health problem, will seek health care as close to home as possible. Health care consumers in the Chicago metropolitan region are very fortunate in the abundance of doctors—approximately 22,000—who practice in the area. On the other hand, making a selection of one out of such a multitude can be a daunting task; it's hard even to know where to start. With *How to Find the Best Doctors: Metropolitan Chicago* in hand, you are already well on your way to finding the very best doctor for your individual needs and the needs of your family members.

With the profusion of outstanding academic medical centers, tertiary care teaching hospitals, and fine community hospitals in the region, virtually any medical procedure or treatment can be found close to home. By virtue of this fact, it would be a simple matter to compile a book identifying the outstanding leaders in medical research and academic medicine in the region. Although many of these doctors are included in the listings, their names are to be found among the many excellent and caring doctors who deliver outstanding patient care in every community in the area. The goal—first and foremost—is to help you find the best doctors to meet your health care needs where you live and work. Again, a good reason why the Castle Connolly Guide is exceptional.

Further, the Castle Connolly Guide is different from most other listings of doctors in its selection process. Our selection is predicated on an extensive nomination procedure and a set of exacting standards which each doctor nominated was required to meet. To you, this means that the basis for inclusion of every one of the doctors in the listings was twofold: respect of their peers and medical excellence.

HOW CASTLE CONNOLLY SELECTED 2,000 OF THE BEST DOCTORS

How to Find the Best Doctors: Metropolitan Chicago is the result of a meticulous search process that consumed six months. To begin the selection process, Castle Connolly Medical Ltd. randomly selected 16,000 board certified doctors from over 22,000 doctors who practice in Cook, Du Page, Kane, Lake, McHenry, and Will counties.

A nomination form was mailed to each of the 16,000 doctors asking them to share with us the names of the best among their peers. We made it clear in this initial survey that we were not looking for the leaders in academic medicine and research, but rather *excellence in patient care.* Respondents were asked to nominate excellent, caring physicians "to whom you would send members of your own family." In addition, Castle Connolly Medical Ltd. invited 3,000 nurses, who were also randomly selected from registered nurses in the region, and more than 741 health care professionals in major medical centers and hospitals in the region, to participate in the nomination process. These health care professionals included hospital executives, vice presidents of medical affairs, directors of clinical services, nursing vice presidents, and leading specialists and subspecialists. Following the extensive mail survey, follow-up telephone calls were made to the same group of health care leaders and to leading specialists to gather further nominations and to validate all nominations.

This process garnered nominations of over 5,400 different doctors. Using this pool of names, the Castle Connolly Medical Ltd. research staff set to work to validate and confirm the nominations. After thousands of personal telephone calls to trusted health care professionals in the region, as well as extensive review of the professional credentials of the nominated doctors, the research staff whittled down the initial list to a final selection of approximately 2,000 doctors. These doctors were notified of their nomination and each was asked to complete a professional information form. Medical credentials were verified and accompanying information checked whenever possible. These data forms became the basis for the information in the directory.

HOW *YOU* CAN SELECT THE BEST DOCTORS

How can you begin to make a choice from such a compilation of names? There is, in fact, a basic, step-by-step process which varies somewhat depending on what your individual needs are as you approach the list. Here are the possibilities:

ONE: IF YOU ARE LOOKING FOR A DOCTOR IN A PARTICULAR COUNTY

The key: Physicians listed in the following pages are organized under the county where their office is located so that you can go directly to the section listing doctors in your county of residence.

Key fact: Like most health care consumers, you probably receive your health care locally. If you think about it, you usually have been treated by doctors close to where you live and in community hospitals. If necessary, you may be referred to regional specialists and nearby medical centers.

TWO: IF YOU ARE LOOKING FOR A PRIMARY CARE PHYSICIAN—A GENERALIST

The key: The doctors who practice predominantly primary care, in the specialties of internal medicine, family practice, pediatrics, and obstetrics/gynecology, are designated by the notation **PCP** in the listing.

Key fact: Every board certified physician is a specialist. The term "having boards" signifies that a physician has completed an approved residency in a given specialty and has passed a rigorous examination given by that particular board. Therefore, doctors who practice primary care—internists, family practitioners, pediatricians, and Ob/Gyns—are specialists in their respective fields, just as are urologists, otolaryngologists, and radiologists. They are the specialists in primary care. Index II lists primary care specialists.

THREE: IF YOU ARE LOOKING FOR A PHYSICIAN IN A PARTICULAR SPECIALTY

The Key: Each entry contains the specialty practiced by the doctor and, in most cases, the year of *initial* board certification.

Key Fact: Many physicians specialize in fields of medicine that are not primary care. These specialists have completed an approved residency in a given specialty and have passed a rigorous exam given by that specialty board. For example, some physicians are board certified in psychiatry, surgery, allergy and immunology, or dermatology.

Many doctors choose to specialize further. They choose an additional training program called a fellowship and upon completion of the program, they are required to take another exam in order to be certified as a subspecialist. An example of such subspecialization is an internist (initially board certified in internal medicine), who subspecializes in nephrology or cardiology. This doctor would be termed "double boarded" and would very likely practice nephrology or cardiology rather than internal medicine as a primary care physician.

FOUR: IF YOU ARE LOOKING FOR A DOCTOR WITH EXPERTISE IN A PARTICULAR DISEASE OR TECHNIQUE

The Key: Particular skills and interests of the doctors are found under the heading Special Practice Interest.

Key Fact: A physician may have a special practice interest in a particular field of medicine without actually being board certified in that area. Special practice interests should not be confused with a board certified medical specialty. For example, cosmetic surgery is not an American Board of Medical Specialties recognized specialty, but it may constitute a major practice activity for many plastic surgeons. Certain doctors may develop a reputation as "specialists" in AIDS, diabetes or arthroscopic surgery. None of these are recognized medical specialties, yet they are indications of a doctor's expertise in a disease or medical or surgical procedure which may be helpful if you have the disease or need the procedure.

Many doctors who have a strong interest in, or consider themselves "specializing in," a particular health problem or medical technique form special interest groups referred to as "self-designated medical specialties." These groups are often confused with recognized medical specialties, which they are not. Some of the groups would like to be recognized by the ABMS and may even work toward that goal. For example, adolescent medicine was a special interest and self-designated specialty that is now an ABMS recognized subspecialty.

Choosing a doctor with a special practice interest is an additional step to be considered after you have already narrowed your choices to particular specialists and/or subspecialists. Index I lists the special practice interests of the doctors in this book. Self-designated medical specialties are listed in Appendix D.

FIVE: IF YOU ARE LOOKING FOR A DOCTOR BY NAME

The Key: Index III lists the doctors in alphabetical order. This alphabetical listing will indicate the page on which information on the doctor's credentials can be found.

Key Fact: Most people start their search for a doctor through recommendation by family and friends. As a savvy health care consumer you realize that such recommendations are often based on personal "chemistry" and may be made by someone who actually knows very little about doctors or health care. Therefore, you will want to check the credentials of any recommended doctor and follow the additional recommendations we have outlined in Sections One and Two.

SIX: IF YOU ARE LOOKING FOR A DOCTOR AFFILIATED WITH YOUR HMO OR PPO

The Key: Each doctor's listing includes the first five health plans listed by the doctor and a (+) if the doctor belongs to more than five.

Key Fact: Most doctors have relationships with at least one managed care organization. Some doctors, in fact, listed 20 or more affiliations on their response form. In the listing, the HMO, PPO or other health plan is abbreviated; you will find the full names of the major health plans with which doctors in this book are affiliated in Appendix N.

Since doctors' relationships with health plans change frequently and since we could not list all the managed care affiliations of the doctors, you should call the doctor's office to verify the information before you make an appointment.

SEVEN: IF YOU WANT DETAILED INFORMATION ON A PARTICULAR DOCTOR

The Key: Each doctor's listing includes a substantial amount of information about the doctor.

Key Fact: Wise choices in health care are made by consumers who have gathered as much information as possible about a particular doctor. If a professional information form was not returned by a doctor in time for inclusion in the book, our research staff verified certain major points of information (name, address, telephone, hospital affiliation, and specialty) from public sources and we have included this limited information. Even if a doctor's full credentials are included in this book, it is possible that, since the time of publication, the doctor has moved his or her offices, changed telephone numbers, joined new medical groups, resigned from or joined hospital staffs, and, especially, changed relationships with HMOs and PPOs. Nonetheless, you can, in most cases, track down the doctor by using the following sources:

- **Doctor's office—call the office number listed in the directory and ask for a new number.**
- **Hospitals—call the hospital listed in the directory and ask for help in locating a particular doctor.**
- **HMO or PPO—call the HMO or PPO listed and ask for further help.**
- **County Medical Societies—all county medical numbers are listed in Appendix H.**
- **State Medical Society—all state medical society numbers are listed in Appendix H.**
- **State Health Department—all state health**

department numbers are listed in Appendix G.

- **American Board of Medical Specialties—a complete listing of ABMS Specialty Boards is found in Appendix A.**
- **American Osteopathic Association—a complete listing of AOA Specialty Boards is found in Appendix B.**

CONCLUSION

You are now ready to work with our directory of approximately 2,000 of the finest doctors in the Metropolitan Chicago area. Although you may be well-informed as a result of reading Sections One and Two of this book, it is possible that choosing the doctor will seem to be a complex endeavor. The tendency might be to try to get the job done as quickly as possible by picking a doctor based solely on the convenience of the office's location. To do so would be a big mistake. You want the best health care. You deserve it. A little effort will help you get the best.

There are many excellent doctors in the region not listed in this book. You can identify them by using the process we have described in Sections One and Two, or, if a doctor in this book is unable to meet your needs, ask about others whom that doctor regards highly.

We believe that this book will educate and enlighten you throughout its pages and that it will prove its value in the end—when you decide on the doctor with whom you plan to have a lasting relationship "in sickness and in health."

A. MEDICAL SPECIALTIES AND SUBSPECIALTIES

The following medical specialties and subspecialties are indicated by their abbreviations in the doctors' listings. Only those specialties and subspecialties for which we solicited nominations are included; therefore, certain specialties and subspecialties do not appear. For example, space medicine and emergency medicine have been omitted. In the case of the former specialty, it is not one that most people would have an occasion to use. In the case of the latter specialty, it is one that is most often assigned rather than selected by patients.

For a brief description of each specialty and subspecialty refer to Appendix C. Also, please note that specialties are indicated in bold and subspecialties in regular typeface. The four primary care specialties are in capital letters and bold italic. This list has been created for use in the Castle Connolly Guide to make it easy for you to find doctors in a given specialty or subspecialty. To review the official American Board of Medical Specialties (ABMS) organization of specialties, refer to Appendix A.

MEDICAL SPECIALTIES AND SUBSPECIALTIES

SPECIALTY & SUBSPECIALTY	ABBREVIATION
Addiction Psychiatry	AdP
Adolescent Medicine	AM
Allergy & Immunology	A&I
Anesthesiology	Anes
Cardiac Electrophysiology (Clinical)	CE
Cardiology (Cardiovascular Disease)	Cv
Child & Adolescent Psychiatry	ChAP
Child Neurology	ChiN
Colon & Rectal Surgery	CRS
Critical Care Medicine	CCM
Dermatology	D
Diagnostic Radiology	DR
Endocrinology, Diabetes & Metabolism	EDM
FAMILY PRACTICE	FP
Forensic Psychiatry	FPsy
Gastroenterology	Ge
Geriatric Medicine	Ger
Geriatric Psychiatry	GerPsy
Gynecologic Oncology*	GO
Hand Surgery	HS
Hematology	Hem
Infectious Disease	Inf

MEDICAL SPECIALTIES AND SUBSPECIALTIES

SPECIALTY & SUBSPECIALTY	ABBREVIATION
INTERNAL MEDICINE	IM
Maternal & Fetal Medicine	MF
Medical Genetics	MG
Medical Oncology*	Onc
Neonatal-Perinatal Medicine	NP
Nephrology	Nep
Neurological Surgery	NS
Neurology	N
Neuroradiology	NRad
Nuclear Medicine	NuM
Nuclear Radiology	NR
OBSTETRICS & GYNECOLOGY	ObG
Occupational Medicine	OM
Ophthalmology	Oph
Orthopaedic Surgery	OrS
Otolaryngology	Oto
Pain Management	PM
Pediatric Allergy & Immunology	PA&I
Pediatric Cardiology	PCd
Pediatric Critical Care Medicine	PCCM
Pediatric Emergency Medicine	PEM
Pediatric Endocrinology	PEn
Pediatric Gastroenterology	PGe
Pediatric Hematology–Oncology*	PHO
Pediatric Infectious Disease	PInf
Pediatric Nephrology	PNep
Pediatric Otolaryngology	POto
Pediatric Pulmonology	PPul
Pediatric Radiology	PR
Pediatric Rheumatology	PRhu
Pediatric Sports Medicine	PSpMed
Pediatric Surgery	PS
PEDIATRICS (GENERAL)	Ped
Physical Medicine & Rehabilitation	PMR
Plastic Surgery	PlS
Preventive Medicine	PrM
Psychiatry	Psyc
Public Health & General Preventive Medicine	PHGPM
Pulmonary Disease	Pul
Radiation Oncology*	RadRO
Radiology	Rad
Reproductive Endocrinology	RE
Rheumatology	Rhu
Spinal Cord Injury Medicine	SCI
Sports Medicine	SM
Surgery	S
Surgical Critical Care	SCC
Thoracic Surgery (includes open heart surgery)	TS
Urology	U
Vascular & Interventional Radiology	VIR
Vascular Surgery (General)	GVS

Specialties are indicated in bold-type face. Capital letters indicate Primary Care Specialties. Subspecialties are listed in non-bold type. Listings indicate if a doctor is certified in a subspecialty but predominately practices primary care medicine.

*Oncologists deal with Cancer

B. GUIDE TO SYMBOLS

- Handicapped accessible
- Open weekends
- Evening office hours
- Calls by phone
- Referral required
- Accepting new patients
- Require payment of deductibles & co-payment at appointment
- Accept Medicare
- Accept Medicaid
- Accept no fault insurance
- Accept Credit cards

Languages Spoken

Language	LangAbbr	Language	LangAbbr
African	Afr	Japanese	Jpn
Afrikaans	Afk	Kannada	Kan
Albanian	Alb	Kasamini	Kas
Amharic	Amh	Khmer	Khm
Arabic	Ar	Korean	Kor
Armenian	Arm	Laotian	Lao
Ashanti	Ash	Latvian	Lat
Basque	Bsq	Lebanese	Leb
Bengali	Bng	Lithuanian	Lth
Bulgarian	Bul	Malaysian	Mly
Burmese	Brm	Mandarin	Man
Byelorussian	Blr	Marathi	Mar
Cambodian	Cam	Norwegian	Nwg
Cantonese	Can	Pakistani	Pak
Catalan	Cat	Patois	Pat
Ceylonese	Cey	Persian	Per
Chinese	Chi	Philipino	Fil
Creole	Cre	Polish	Pol
Croatian	Crt	Portugese	Prt
Czech	Czc	Punjabi	Pun
Danish	Dan	Romanian	Rom
Dutch	Dut	Russian	Rus
East Indian	EIn	Serbian	Srb
Estonian	Est	Serbo-Croatian	SCr
Farsi	Frs	Signing	Sgn
Filipino	Fil	Sindhi	Sin
Finnish	Fin	Sinhalese	Shl
Flemish	Flm	Slovak	Slv
French	Fr	Spanish	Sp
Gaelic	Gae	Swahili	Swa
German	Ger	Swedish	Swd
Greek	Grk	Tagalog	Tag
Gujarati	Guj	Taiwanese	Twn
Hebrew	Heb	Tamil	Tam
Hindi	Hin	Telugy	Tel
Hungarian/Magyar	Hun	Thai	Thai
Icelandic	Ice	Turkish	Trk
Ilocano	Ilo	Ukrainian	Ukr
Indonesian	Ind	Urdu	Ur
Italian	Itl	Uzbeki	Uzb
		Vietnamese	Vn
		Yiddish	Yd

C. SAMPLE LISTING

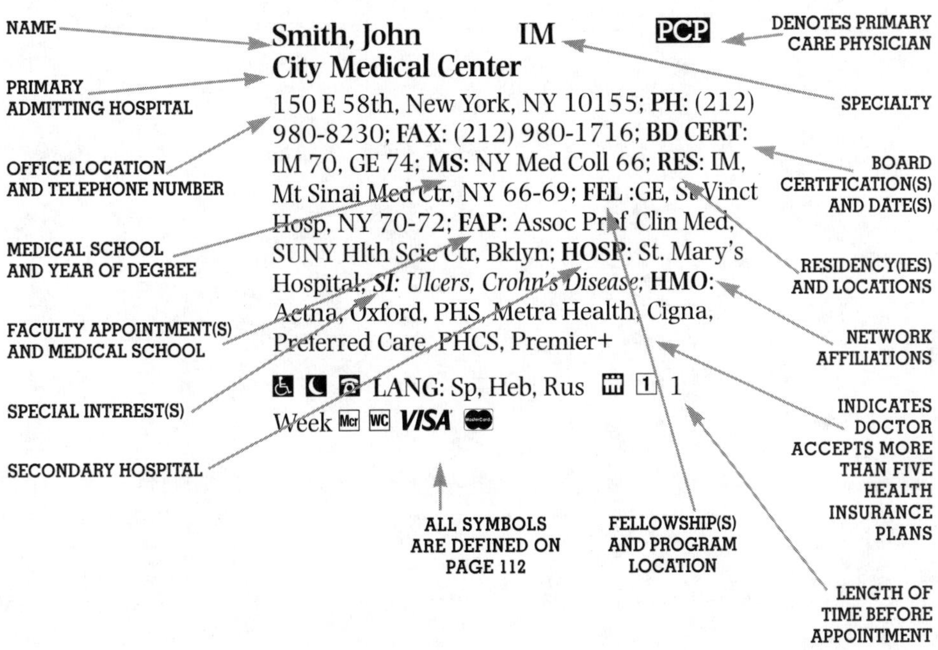

In our listings of the professional information on doctors, we have abbreviated medical schools, hospitals and managed care affiliations. The abbreviations are designed to be self-explanatory, but if you need assistance, refer to the following appendices: Medical Schools, Appendix L; Hospitals, Appendix M; and HMOs, Appendix N.

Note on Special Interest(s):
These are not medical specialties as described in Appendix C, but the areas of expertise or practice interests indicated by the doctor.

The information reported in each doctor's listing is, for the most part, provided by the doctor or his/her office staff. Castle Connolly attempts to verify the data through other sources but cannot guarantee that in all cases all data have been so verified or are accurate. All such information is subject to change from time to time due to changes in physician practices.

HOSPITAL INFORMATION PROGRAM

THE HOSPITAL INFORMATION PROGRAM

Castle Connolly Medical Ltd. has received many requests from book buyers to provide information on hospitals. There are over 100 acute care and specialty hospitals in the Metropolitan Chicago area, many of which have extraordinary capabilities for superior patient care.

Therefore, in order to respond to these requests, we have invited a select group of outstanding hospitals to profile their services in the Castle Connolly Guide through the medium of paid advertorials. These selected hospitals were invited to sponsor the Hospital Information pages you will see in the Guide which are organized into three groupings: Major Medical Centers; Hospital Networks; and Regional Medical Centers and Community Hospitals. This partnership with the participating hospitals is totally separate from the physician selection process which is based upon a totally independent review system.

The Major Medical Centers and Hospital Networks will be found on pages 118 to 134 prior to the listings of doctors. The Regional Medical Centers and Community Hospitals will be found at the beginning of each county section. The information presented will give you an overview of many of the programs and services offered by these hospitals, as well as vital information related to their accreditation and sponsorship. Also included in each hospital profile is the hospital's physican referral number, should you wish to ask the hospitals for recommendations of physicians not listed in the Castle Connolly Guide.

The "Centers of Excellence" section is also in response to requests by our readers. Not only are many people searching for the best doctors and hospitals to meet their needs, they also want to know which hospitals have special programs or services focusing on a particular illness or health need. The "Centers of Excellence" section describes those special programs offered by the hospitals that are participating in the Hospital Information section of the Castle Connolly Guide. They reflect the depth of commitment to these special health care needs by the hospitals. Typically, the hospitals have recruited physicians, nurses and other staff with special interests and training and provided the attention and financial support necessary to develop these special programs. We believe you will find this information helpful in your search for the best health care — from both physicians and hospitals — for you and your family.

We are pleased to have these distinguished institutions as partners in our effort to provide you with useful information to help you meet your health care needs.

MAJOR MEDICAL CENTERS

The following pages contain vital information on four of the region's Major Medical Centers. A Major Medical Center is an acute care hospital with tertiary care services, residency programs, a major affiliation with a medical school and clinical research programs. A major medical center draws its patients from a broad geographic region, even nationally and internationally and, in many instances, is the center of a network or consortium of hospitals.

The Chicago metropolitan region is nationally and internationally known for its major medical centers and their excellent programs and services. Some of the nation's leading academic centers are in this region and, in addition to superior patient care and cutting edge patient research, they produce thousands of talented, well trained physicians and other health professionals each year. Castle Connolly Medical Ltd. has invited a number of major medical centers in the region to sponsor the profiles and information that follows.

Major Medical Centers

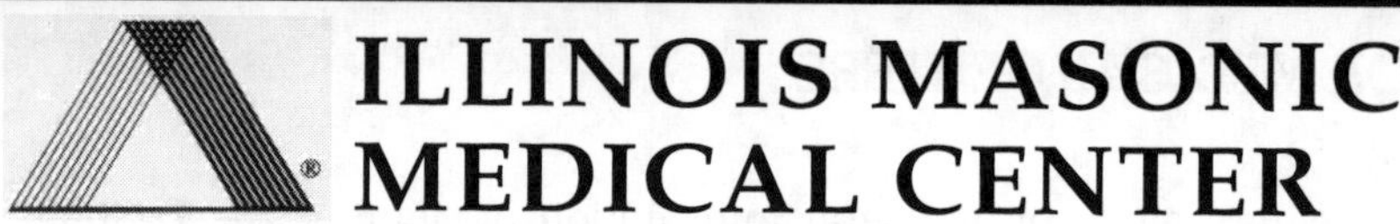

ILLINOIS MASONIC MEDICAL CENTER

836 WEST WELLINGTON AVENUE
CHICAGO, ILLINOIS 60657
PHONE (773) 975-1600

WEB SITE: HTTP://WWW.IMMC.ORG

Sponsorship	Voluntary Not-for-Profit
Beds	801 (Licensed)
Accreditation	Joint Commission on Accreditation of Healthcare Organizations All 14 graduate medical education programs fully accredited

GENERAL DESCRIPTION

Illinois Masonic Medical Center (IMMC) is located on the north side of Chicago, a diverse community of ethnic groups, ages, economic classes and lifestyles. It was here that the Masons of Illinois founded IMMC in 1921. Today, the Medical Center consists of a 507-bed teaching hospital; a 294-bed skilled care facility serving older adults in need of medical attention, long-term care or rehabilitative services; and a health network of services featuring nine primary care centers located on the north and northwest sides of Chicago. The mission of IMMC is to improve the health of its patients and the community it serves. It accomplishes this mission through the efforts of 1,000 physicians, 200 doctors in post-graduate training, 3,300 employees and 500 volunteers.

EDUCATION PROGRAMS

Illinois Masonic Medical Center is the primary teaching affiliate of Rush-Presbyterian-St. Luke's Medical Center and Rush University. Almost 200 residency and fellowship positions are offered annually to new doctors in the fields of pathology, internal medicine, dentistry, primary care, family medicine, anesthesiology, obstetrics/gynecology, radiology and podiatry. IMMC also participates in affiliated residency programs in surgery, pathology and emergency medicine with the University of Illinois College of Medicine. It has its own cardiology and electrophysiology fellowship programs and participates in an affiliated gastroenterology fellowship program. IMMC is the primary teaching hospital for Scholl College of Podiatric Medicine, the nation's first and largest podiatric school. Illinois Masonic is also affiliated with Midwestern University Chicago College of Osteopathic Medicine in both graduate and undergraduate training.

CENTERS OF EXCELLENCE

Cancer Care

The Angelo P. Creticos, M.D. Cancer Center offers an interdisciplinary approach to the diagnosis and treatment of cancer, allowing patients to take advantage of the latest techniques in surgery, chemotherapy and radiation therapy. The Center provides blood disorder and hematology services, screening and detection programs, and enrollment in local, regional and national clinical trials. A special four-part breast assessment includes a physician's exam, mammogram, risk assessment and self-exam instruction. Psychology support services by a dedicated psycho-oncologist are provided to patients and families.

Cardiac Care Cardiac specialists provide a full range of services for diagnosing and treating patients with cardiovascular disease, including diagnostic tests, traditional treatments and innovative investigational therapies, as well as patient and family support programs. The newly remodeled cardiac catheterization/electrophysiology facility offers the latest equipment for diagnosing and clearing blocked blood vessels and evaluating and treating patients with arrhythmias. Program includes comprehensive approach to patients with complex arrhythmias, cardiovascular surgery, and a full range of noninvasive cardiology options.

Emergency Care One of four Level I Trauma Centers in Chicago, IMMC provides immediate assessment and care for severely injured patients. The Emergency Department features 17 exam rooms, and a state-of-the-art trauma suite to provide medical care more quickly and with greater privacy. The newest digital x-ray equipment and a complete laboratory reduce waiting time by as much as one hour. Specially equipped and staffed rooms speed treatment of the most common emergency ailments, like the eye-ear-throat diagnostic treatment area. There is a separate treatment area for children. In addition, IMMC is a resource hospital for clinical training of paramedics, both public and private.

HIV/AIDS Care IMMC had the first designated AIDS unit in Chicago, and today remains the only designated inpatient unit on the north side. A cadre of more than 80 healthcare professionals in both inpatient and outpatient settings help people with HIV/AIDS live healthier, more fulfilling lives. Among these professionals is an internal medicine health practice specializing in this area. Services include research, infusion, transfusion, dietary, podiatry, pharmacy and wellness activities. More than 60 patients are enrolled in multiple HIV clinical research trials at IMMC.

Women's Care In 1982, IMMC responded to the growing need for alternative and specialized care for women by opening Women's Health Resources, the first such program in the country. This program provides comprehensive care for women, by women. This includes providing complete physical examinations, obstetric/gynecological care, family planning, nutritional assessments, mid-life women's services and counseling. In addition, IMMC offers a full range of reproductive health services, including the Alternative Birthing Center, the first such center in the Midwest (1978); a Level III Perinatal Facility, which treats low birth weight and high risk babies; an Antenatal Resource Center, providing comprehensive antepartum care for both mother and fetus; an Assisted Reproductive Technology Center, to assist couples who are experiencing infertility problems but do not respond to traditional methods of treatment; and one of the largest and most experienced Certified Nurse Midwifery programs in Chicago.

Other Specialties Among IMMC's other nationally recognized programs are: the Pediatric Developmental Center, which provides complete diagnostic work-ups and evaluation services to children when developmental problems are suspected; the IMMC Eye Center, which offers advanced medical, laser and surgical techniques for both adults and children; and the Special Patient Dental Care Program, which treats developmentally disabled adults and children.

Physician Referral Call (773) 296-7091 if you are looking for a primary care or specialist physician at IMMC.

LOYOLA UNIVERSITY HEALTH SYSTEM

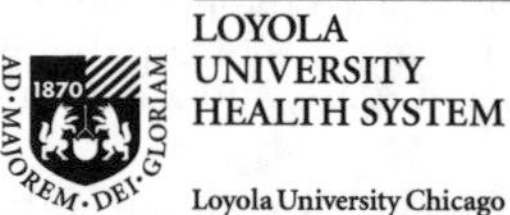

2160 SOUTH FIRST AVENUE
MAYWOOD, IL 60153
(888) LUHS-888
WEB SITE: WWW.LUHS.ORG

Sponsorship	**Voluntary Not-for-Profit**
Beds	**541 (includes 18 psychiatric; 21 burn; 24 rehabilitation; 30 obstetrics; 32 pediatrics; 50 neonatal; 113 ICU; 253 medical/surgical.)**
Accreditation	**Joint Commission on Accreditation of Healthcare Organizations (JCAHO), Quality Management Network member, American College of Surgeons (Level I Trauma Program), American Burn Association (Burn Center),**

WHO WE ARE

Loyola University Health System (LUHS) is an academic integrated health delivery system, owned by Loyola University Chicago, designed to meet all of an individual's lifelong health needs, from primary care to transplants, from clinic and hospital care to home health services.

Loyola University Medical Center is a component of LUHS and resides on a 73-acre campus in Maywood, Ill. It is one of the nation's leading academic medical centers, and is comprised of a Burn Center, the Cardinal Bernardin Cancer Center, a Cardiovascular Institute, the Foster G. McGaw Hospital, the Ronald McDonald Children's Hospital of Loyola, the Mulcahy Outpatient Center, an Oral Health Center, the Russo Surgical Pavilion, a Level 1 Trauma Center and the Loyola University Chicago Stritch School of Medicine, one of only four Jesuit medical schools in the country.

LUHS sends its world class medical expertise into the community through 14 off-campus Primary Care Centers and two Ambulatory Surgical Centers located throughout the DuPage and western Cook counties. LUHS also has partnered with the Rehabilitation Institute of Chicago to offer a full continuum of high-quality rehabilitative care to adult and pediatric patients disabled due to multiple trauma, burns, stroke or amputation, as well as those with congenital deformities or disorders or diseases such as arthritis. To improve the long-term acute care provided to ventilator-dependent patients, LUHS joined Rush-Presbyterian-St. Luke's Medical Center and MacNeal Health Network in the ownership of RML Specialty Hospital. In addition, LUHS operates a mobile clinic for the Ronald McDonald Children's Hospital of Loyola, a 40-foot doctor's office on wheels that serves underprivileged children in nearby communities.

CLINICAL SERVICES

Burn Center	One of only three state-designated burn centers in metropolitan Chicago and the only center in the Midwest with accreditation from both the American College of Surgeons and the American Burn Association. Its 21-bed Burn Center is the largest in Illinois and treats more than 350 burn patients a year from a four-state area. Home to one of only 24 specialized hyperbaric oxygen chambers in the nation, used to speed the healing of burn center and cancer center patients.

Cardinal Bernardin Cancer Center	The only free-standing facility in Illinois that combines cancer research, diagnosis, treatment and prevention under one roof. Recognized nationally for its pioneering cancer research and treatment programs using stem cell and bone marrow transplantation, chemotherapy, biologic response modifiers, surgery and radiation therapy. Supported by a National Cancer Institute Cancer Center Planning Grant for cancer research and treatment, and is a center selected for conducting research on the development of new cancer-fighting drugs. Established the nation's first day hospital for bone marrow transplant recipients. Provides many unique multispecialty cancer services including breast, GI, lung, head and neck, neuro-oncology, melanoma and genetic counseling.
Cardiovascular Institute (CV Institute)	More than 460 people have received a heart transplant at Loyola since 1984, and the CV Institute's expertise has created a patient survival rate that exceeds the national average. Physicians at the CV Institute have performed more minimally invasive heart procedures than anyone else in Illinois. In addition, Loyola's Heart Failure Center offers one of the widest ranges of conventional and leading edge treatments to keep patients with failing hearts alive, including specialized devices and investigative drugs not yet available elsewhere.
Level I Trauma Center	The first trauma center in Illinois to gain Level 1 Trauma Center status and be certified by the American College of Surgeons. LIFESTAR, the LUMC helicopter and ground transport system, stands guard 24-hours a day to transport critically ill or injured patients to Loyola from as far away as 150 miles.
Neurosciences	Specializing in the treatment of pediatric and adult disorders and diseases of the nervous system, brain, pituitary gland, spinal cord, and cranial and spinal nerves. One of only a few medical centers in the nation that can perform a new catheter-based procedure to treat cerebral aneurysms. In addition, patients with Alzheimer's, myasthenia gravis, multiple sclerosis or Parkinson's disease benefit from the latest research and medications, as well as gain access to the most sophisticated diagnostic equipment available.
Orthopaedics & Rehabilitation	Diagnoses and treats a wide spectrum of musculoskeletal conditions for both adult and pediatric patients, including hand, spinal and sports related injuries. Specialists in the treatment of congenital pediatric diseases such as Spina Bifida and scoliosis, and congenital malformations such as clubfeet. With the Rehabilitation Institute of Chicago, created RIC&LOYOLA, A Partnership in Rehabilitation, to provide acute, subacute and outpatient rehabilitative care.
Ronald McDonald Children's Hospital of Loyola (RMCH)	Chicago suburbs' only comprehensive pediatric emergency room and pediatric trauma program. Recognized by the National Association of Children's Hospitals and Related Institutions (NACHRI) for its breadth of pediatric services and child care expertise. Home to the state's largest neonatal intensive care unit. Consistently achieves Illinois' best survival rates for low-birthweight babies and is among the top three programs in the U.S.
Transplantation	Offers one of the most complete solid organ transplantation programs in the country. Operates one of the largest programs in Illinois for heart, lung and bone marrow transplantation. Specializes in kidney, heart-lung and liver transplantation.
Women's Health Services	Offers continuum of care for women from pre-pregnancy through menopause, specializing in cardiovascular disease in women, high-risk pregnancies, intrauterine surgery, gynecological care, hormone replacement therapy and nutritional assessment. Comprehensive Breast Care Center offers full array of diagnostic and screening programs for a variety of breast diseases. Midwifery services offer alternative delivery care for low-risk mothers.
Physician Referral	Loyola believes patients receive the best care when they and their doctor have access to world class specialty physicians. To make a referral, call (888) LUHS-888, 24-hours a day. © 1999, Loyola University Health System

RUSH-PRESBYTERIAN-ST. LUKE'S MEDICAL CENTER

RUSH

Rush System for Health

1653 W. CONGRESS PARKWAY
CHICAGO, IL 60612
PHONE (312) 942-5000

Sponsorship	**Private, Not-for-Profit**
Beds	**963**
Accreditation	**Joint Commission on Accreditation of Healthcare Organizations, Commission for Accreditation of Rehabilitation Facilities**

A TRADITION OF LEADERSHIP

For more than 160 years, Rush-Presbyterian-St. Luke's Medical Center has been recognized as a leader in patient care, teaching and research. Located minutes from the Loop on Chicago's near West Side, Rush is the largest private hospital in Illinois and home to one of the first medical schools in the Midwest. The Medical Center campus includes:

- Presbyterian-St. Luke's Hospital, an 832-bed tertiary care hospital with a medical staff of more than 1,200 physicians and scientists
- Rush Children's Hospital, which includes intensive care and intermediate care units for critically ill children
- The Johnston R. Bowman Health Center for the Elderly, a 131-bed, skilled-nursing facility for rehabilitation and geriatric care
- Rush University, with colleges in medicine, nursing, the allied health sciences, basic sciences and health care administration

The Medical Center also includes the Rush Institutes — comprehensive, multidisciplinary centers that offer primary health care services, along with leading-edge diagnostic techniques and treatments for a variety of problems, including **arthritis** and **orthopedic problems**, **cancer**, **heart disease**, **mental illness**, **diseases associated with aging** and **neurological disorders**.

The Institutes bring together patient care and research to address major health problems facing Chicago and the nation. Physicians not only conduct research on the latest treatments for disease, they see complex and rare illnesses not seen at other hospitals. Rush fosters a unique collaborative environment in which physicians and laboratory scientists work together to advance medical knowledge and improve patient care. Rush researchers received $50.4 million in outside funding in 1998, and are conducting more than 1,100 research studies.

Rush-Presbyterian-St. Luke's Medical Center is the heart of the Rush System for Health, an integrated health care system designed to serve 3 million people in the Chicago area. The Rush System for Health has a number of affiliated hospitals in Illinois, including:

- Holy Family Medical Center in Des Plaines
- Illinois Masonic Medical Center in Chicago
- Oak Park Hospital
- Riverside HealthCare in Kankakee
- Rush-Copley Medical Center in Aurora
- Rush North Shore Medical Center in Skokie

The Rush System for Health also offers a variety of outpatient and other services, including occupational health, executive health, behavioral health, home care and hospice.

CENTERS OF EXCELLENCE

Arthritis and Orthopedics	The **Rush Arthritis and Orthopedics Institute** offers comprehensive research, diagnosis and treatment for osteo- and rheumatoid arthritis, back pain, spine surgery, foot and ankle problems, hand and elbow disorders, sports medicine and bone cancer. Doctors at Rush pioneered joint replacement techniques and are internationally recognized for their work. Researchers are developing innovative new treatments for all forms of arthritis, as well as for spinal disorders, such as scoliosis.
Brain & Nervous System	Physicians at the **Rush Neuroscience Institute** are studying innovative surgical and pharmaceutical treatments for people with epilepsy, Parkinson's disease, multiple sclerosis, Tourette's syndrome, stroke, Alzheimer's disease; neuromuscular disorders, such as muscular dystrophy, Lou Gehrig's disease (ALS) and myasthenia gravis. In addition, the Rush Alzheimer's Disease Center is one of the nation's largest programs providing diagnostic services for people with signs and symptoms of dementia.
Cancer	The **Rush Cancer Institute** offers multidisciplinary centers for patients with breast cancer; leukemia and lymphoma; chest, head and neck cancers; bone and soft tissue cancers; bone marrow cancers, including multiple myeloma; prostate cancer; skin cancer; cervical, uterine, ovarian and related cancers; and brain tumors. (For more information, see Rush in the Centers of Excellence section.)
Heart Care	The **Rush Heart Institute** is ranked among the country's top medical centers for heart disease prevention, treatment and research. Rush doctors offer leading edge therapies for a variety of complex conditions. (For more information, see Rush in the Centers of Excellence section.)
Mental Health	The **Institute for Mental Well-Being at Rush** is internationally known for helping people with depression and manic-depression who have not been helped by standard treatments. The Institute is a leader in testing new drugs, for depression and other conditions, that are more effective with fewer side effects. The Institute also provides comprehensive care for children and adults with obsessive-compulsive disorder; panic disorder; anxiety disorder; schizophrenia; and alcohol and drug abuse. The Institute is a leader in the study and prevention of suicide.
Older Adult Care	The **Rush Institute for Healthy Aging** offers medical, psychiatric and rehabilitative care for people over age 55. (For more information, see Rush in the Centers of Excellence section.)
Pediatrics	The **Rush Children's Hospital** provides compassionate, state-of-the-art care to children and adolescents. Many of the physicians are internationally recognized for their research efforts to improve care for patients with asthma, cystic fibrosis, sickle cell anemia and infectious diseases, such as congenital toxoplasmosis and Group B strep. Programs to treat childhood cancers and congenital heart disorders draw patients from throughout the Midwest. All programs provide comprehensive, multidisciplinary care.
Women's Health	At Rush, physicians and researchers work in concert to develop innovative new treatments for women's most important health concerns, including **osteoporosis, heart disease** and other conditions that occur with greater frequency after menopause. In addition, doctors are studying new ways to treat infertility, sexual problems and urogynecological problems, such as incontinence.

Rush on Call Physician Referral Service

(888) 352-RUSH or on the Web at www.rush.edu

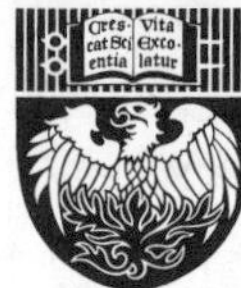

The University of Chicago Hospitals & Health System

5841 S. Maryland Avenue • For general information: (773) 702-1000
Chicago, IL 60637-1470 • Web address: www.uchospitals.edu

Sponsorship	**Private. Not-for-profit**
Beds	**890**
Accreditation	**Joint Commission on Accreditation of Healthcare Organizations**

AT THE FOREFRONT OF MEDICINE

We have been at the forefront of medicine for decades — delivering extraordinary care to patients who come from the Chicago area, as well as from all parts of the world. According to *U.S. News and World Report's* ranking of America's best hospitals, the University of Chicago Hospitals rank 12th in the nation and first in Illinois. We were named best in Illinois in nine specialty areas: cancer, cardiology/cardiac surgery, endocrinology, gastroenterology, geriatrics, neurology/neurosurgery, otolaryngology, pulmonary medicine, and rheumatology.

Our mission is to provide superior health care in a compassionate manner, ever mindful of each patient's dignity and individuality. To accomplish our mission, we call upon the skills and expertise of all our medical professionals, who work together to advance biomedical innovation, serve the health needs of the community, and further the knowledge of medical students, physicians, and others dedicated to caring.

WORLD-RENOWNED UNIVERSITY OF CHICAGO PHYSICIANS

All patients are encouraged to establish an ongoing relationship with a personal University of Chicago physician. Should the need arise, this physician will collaborate with or refer to any one of over 400 U of C board-certified specialists, many of whom are world leaders in their areas of expertise. Our faculty physicians see patients at the main Hospitals' campus, as well as at several other locations in the Chicago area. At the main campus, adult inpatient care is provided at Bernard Mitchell Hospital and Chicago Lying-in Hospital.

THE CENTER FOR ADVANCED MEDICINE

The Duchossois Center for Advanced Medicine is home to nearly all specialty clinics of the University of Chicago Hospitals, along with an unparalleled range of outpatient diagnostic and treatment services. The Center for Advanced Medicine is designed with the patient's best interests in mind. Physician offices are conveniently located next to related diagnostic and treatment suites, enabling patients to receive care for all related medical conditions within the same area of the building.

At the Center, patients have access to significant advances in medical treatment. Our physicians bring to its outpatient setting all of the knowledge and resources of the University of Chicago: virtually every clinical trial available and more research funded by the National Institutes of Health than any other place in the state.

There is simply no other outpatient facility in the five-state area where so many internationally-renowned medical specialists care for patients in such an integrated and seamless fashion.

THE UNIVERSITY OF CHICAGO CHILDREN'S HOSPITAL

Staffed by more than 100 faculty physicians, the University of Chicago Children's Hospital is dedicated to helping children with medical problems ranging from the routine to the complex. Our pediatricians provide advanced therapies in virtually all clinical areas, including allergy, arthritis, asthma, cancer, cardiology, child development, diabetes, ear/nose/throat, emergency medicine, gastroenterology, genetics, gynecology, infectious disease, neonatology, neurology, orthopaedics, psychiatry, and surgery.

Critically ill or injured children are cared for in the state-of-the-art Frankel Pediatric Intensive Care Unit. In addition, a 53-bassinet neonatal intensive care unit provides premature and critically ill infants with the most advanced medical care and life support systems. The pediatric liver transplantation program is one of the largest in the country and was the first living-donor program in the world. The University of Chicago Children's Hospital offers every available form of therapy, both conventional and investigational, for a child afflicted with cancer.

OTHER OUTSTANDING PROGRAMS

Cancer. The University of Chicago Hospitals' cancer program ranks ninth in the nation and first in Illinois, according to *U.S. News and World Report.* Designated by the National Cancer Institute as a Comprehensive Cancer Center, the University of Chicago Hospitals are currently working with more than $30 million in cancer research grants — more funding than any other hospital in the state.

Cardiology/Cardiac Services. The University of Chicago Hospitals' cardiac center ranks 14th in the nation and first in Illinois, according to *U.S. News and World Report.* Our team of cardiologists and cardiac surgeons have two goals: to provide state-of-the-art, high quality care to all patients, and to develop new therapies that will improve the health and prolong the lives of our patients with cardiovascular disease.

Women's Programs. The University of Chicago Hospitals provide health care for women during every stage of life. Our physicians and nurse practitioners specialize in assisting women through the reproductive years and menopause. Specialized services, such as our new Breast Center, help women who experience chronic or serious health problems.

Geriatrics. The University of Chicago Hospitals' geriatrics program ranks 12th in the nation and first in Illinois, according to *U.S. News and World Report.* The University of Chicago Hospitals have one of the nation's largest groups of physicians who are fellowship-trained and board-certified in geriatric medicine. Special areas of focus include arthritis, orthopaedics, and the care of dementias, Alzheimer's disease, and memory disorders.

WEISS MEMORIAL HOSPITAL AND OTHER OFF-CAMPUS LOCATIONS

Off-campus, care is provided at Louis A. Weiss Memorial Hospital, a 225-bed hospital on Chicago's North Side, and through a network of more than 30 physician offices located throughout Chicago, Chicago's suburbs, and northwest Indiana.

Physician Referral — Call 1-888-UCH-0200 for help in choosing a physician suitable to your needs. Visit our web site: www.uchospitals.edu

HOSPITAL NETWORKS

Hospital Networks are alliances of a number of hospitals. The networks are typically led by a Major Medical Center and may include Regional Medical Centers & Community Hospitals. Several networks are under common ownership; others are strong affiliations between hospitals that may share joint marketing purchasing and medical programs.

Hospital Networks

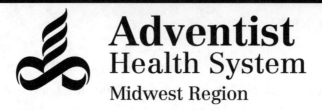

Adventist Health System
Midwest Region

120 N. OAK STREET, HINSDALE, IL 60521; PHONE (630) 856-9000
WWW.AHSMIDWEST.ORG

Sponsorship	**Non-profit. A member of Adventist Health System.**
Beds	**952 licensed beds**
Accreditation	**JCAHO, CARF**

GENERAL DESCRIPTION:

Hinsdale Hospital is the flagship of the Midwest Region. Other facilities include GlenOaks Hospital (Glendale Heights), La Grange Memorial Hospital (La Grange), Chippewa Valley Hospital (Durand, WI), Bolingbrook Medical Center, Hinsdale Surgical Center, Health Care at Home, St. Thomas Hospice, and primary care physician group practices, Adventist Health Partners.

The hospital's community outreach program offers education support classes, screenings, behavior modification programs, health fairs, lectures to the community.

MISSION:

A Christian health-care leader committed to a partnering with physicians and community to provide whole-person care and promote wellness.

HINSDALE HOSPITAL

For nearly 100 years, Hinsdale Hospital has been providing compassionate, quality care to residents of the western suburbs of Chicago. The 404-bed facility is widely known for its comprehensive diagnostic and treatment programs. Centers of excellence include the Opler Cancer Center, Rooney Heart Institute, Level II Trauma Center, Birck Family Women's and Children's Center, Paulson Rehab Network, Orthopedic and Spine Center, Sleep Center and Behavioral Health Services, including the New Day Center substance abuse program. The only teaching hospital in DuPage County, Hinsdale Hospital is the site of the Hinsdale Family Practice Residency program, a three-year postgraduate program that provides training to physicians specializing in family practice medicine.

GLENOAKS HOSPITAL

In a caring, homelike environment, GlenOaks Hospital provides residents of the western suburbs a full range of health care services. These include the Special Additions Birth Centre, a Level II Trauma Center, occupational health services, outpatient rehabilitation services, outpatient surgery, a full range of diagnostic services including cardiology, sleep lab and radiology, and the most comprehensive behavioral medicine program in the area. With 186 beds, GlenOaks is dedicated to serving its community's needs.

LA GRANGE MEMORIAL HOSPITAL

The hospital is known for its Level II Trauma Center, Family Maternity Center, cancer services, cardiovascular services, rehabilitation services, geriatric assessment program, Transitional Care Pavilion, McCormick -Alexander Pain Management Center and a Family Practice Residency Program. A network of Family Medical Centers provides comprehensive primary care to patients at convenient locations throughout the western suburbs.

BOLINGBROOK MEDICAL CENTER

With extensive outpatient services and physician offices, Bolingbrook is one of the largest and most comprehensive outpatient centers in Illinois. Due to its superb Emergency Services Department, it recently became the first outpatient facility in Illinois designated to receive emergency ambulance services.

CHIPPEWA VALLEY HOSPITAL

Chippewa Valley Hospital and Oak View Care Center have proven that high quality health care can be provided to small population areas. The hospital's 88-bed inpatient facility, with the combination of acute and long-term care beds, serves the broad needs of the community, while its outpatient services have set new standards in preventive care.

HINSDALE SURGICAL CENTER

This outpatient surgery center has been providing high quality surgical services to the community for nearly 25 years. Its 120 member medical staff provides surgical services in a variety of specialty areas including gynecology, orthopedics, ophthalmology, otolaryngology, podiatry, cosmetic and plastic surgery, and general surgery.

HEALTH CARE AT HOME

Health Care at Home continues the healing process with home care services for patients in Cook, DuPage, Will and Kane Counties. A wide array of medical and wellness services are provided by registered nurses, mental health nurses, physical and occupational therapists, speech-language therapists, social workers, and home health aides. Private duty nursing services are provided through Health Care at Home, Plus. Health Care at Home also serves communities in Michigan and Wisconsin.

ST. THOMAS HOSPICE

Caring for the terminally ill in their own homes, St. Thomas Hospice provides an interdisciplinary team of experts who assist those with limited life expectancy by providing skilled medical care, pain management, and a full complement of holistic services. Emphasis is placed on human dignity and the preservation of the quality and sanctity of life.

ADVENTIST HEALTH PARTNERS

Adventist Health Partners is a physician group practice specializing in pediatrics, family medicine and internal medicine. It is affiliated with Hinsdale Hospital, GlenOaks Hospital, and Bolingbrook Medical Center. Practice sites are conveniently located throughout the western suburbs.

Physician Referral — Please call (630) 856-7500 for a physician referral (weekdays 8 a.m. - 5 p.m.).

ADVOCATE HEALTH CARE

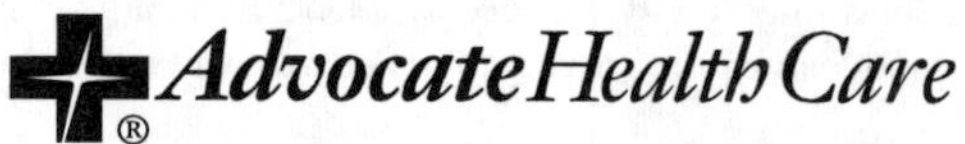

2025 WINSOR DRIVE
OAK BROOK, ILLINOIS 60523
1-800-3-ADVOCATE (1-800-323-8622)

Sponsorship Voluntary Not-for-Profit
Evangelical Lutheran Church in America and the United Church of Christ

Advocate Health Care brings together nearly 4,000 physicians, eight respected local hospitals, health centers and physician practices across the six-county Chicago area to provide you with close-to-home access to quality health programs and services. While we're recognized as one of the top 10 health care systems in the country, we always try to listen to you — our customers — on a one-to-one basis.

Our toll-free customer service center — HealthAdvisor — can help you obtain medical information you need on doctors, health-related topics or seminars. Just dial 1-800-3-ADVOCATE (1-800-323-8622). We're also on the World Wide Web. You can meet our doctors, read health articles and learn more about our system. Check us out on-line at www.advocatehealth.com.

ADVOCATE: WE'RE HIGHLY RESPECTED HOSPITALS AND MEDICAL GROUPS
Each year, Advocate's hospitals and physicians treat more than 1 million Chicago-area residents. From large teaching institutions to smaller community hospitals and outpatient centers, Advocate is listening and responding to your needs.

Advocate Health Centers, Chicago Est: 1998
This multi-specialty, physician-led medical group offers preventive care programs and 150 physicians at 13 convenient, city and suburban locations. Formerly Humana Health Centers, these friendly practices are now open to numerous health plans.

Advocate Medical Group Est: 1980
With more than 250 physicians at multiple locations throughout the northwest metropolitan area, Advocate Medical Group offers a wide array of primary care physicians and services. There also are advanced physician and diagnostic services in 46 specialty areas. Advocate Medical Group is affiliated with Lutheran General Hospital, recognized as one of the Top 100 Hospitals in the country.

Bethany Hospital, Chicago Est : 1920
Bethany Hospital, on Chicago's West Side, works closely with community groups, social service agencies, schools and churches to improve the quality of life for area residents through innovative asthma programs, a comprehensive emergency department and neighborhood health centers.

Christ Hospital and Medical Center, Oak Lawn Est: 1961
Christ Hospital is renowned for its expert care in cardiovascular services, pediatrics, women's and infant's services, oncology, rehabilitation services, psychiatry and substance abuse. This major medical center and teaching hospital has the highest level designation for trauma and

perinatal care. Hope Children's Hospital, on the Christ Hospital campus, brings state-of-the-art pediatric services to Chicago's south suburbs.

Dreyer Medical Clinic Est. 1922
With over 100 board-certified physicians representing 27 specialties, and 39 allied health professionals, Dreyer serves the residents of the greater Fox Valley area at a dozen convenient satellite sites located in Aurora, Batavia, St. Charles, Oswego, Yorkville, Plainfield and Hinckley.

Field Medical Group, Chicago Est. 1939
Field Medical Group is an organization of 45 primary care physicians and specialists who provide comprehensive health care services to Chicago's north and northwest sides.

Good Samaritan Hospital, Downers Grove Est: 1976
Good Samaritan hospital offers the highest level of trauma care and excels in the delivery of cardiac care, oncology, mental health services, outpatient testing and therapies, and women's and children's services. The hospital's special care nursery provides the highest level of care for newborns in DuPage County. A health and wellness center will open in 1999.

Good Shepherd Hospital, Barrington Est: 1979
Good Shepherd hospital provides a warm and confident combination of personal care and medical expertise. Good Shepherd is a trauma center and provides care for critically ill and underweight newborns. It also is recognized for its oncology, orthopedics, surgical, rehabilitative and women's services.

Lutheran General Hospital, Park Ridge Est: 1898
Named as one of the top 100 hospitals in the country as well as one of the nation's most preferred hospitals by consumers, Lutheran General provides the highest level of trauma and perinatal care. This academic medical center is a recognized leader in cardiology, cancer services, critical care, mental health and addiction, obstetrics, pediatrics, rehabilitation services and women's health care.

Ravenswood Hospital Medical Center, Chicago Est: 1907
Ravenswood Hospital is an acute care teaching hospital that offers family-centered birthing, day surgery, skilled nursing, cardiac, hospice, pediatrics, psychiatric, rehabilitation and oncology services, and a comprehensive 24-hour emergency department. Ravenswood also has extensive outpatient care programs.

South Suburban Hospital, Hazel Crest Est: 1946
South Suburban is a community-based, full-service hospital committed to providing comprehensive inpatient, outpatient and diagnostic services to Chicago's southern suburbs. It offers an on-site skilled nursing facility, a Family Birth Center with 16 single-room maternity suites and a state-of-the-art emergency department.

Trinity Hospital, Chicago Est: 1895
Trinity Hospital serves the health care needs of Chicago's South Side. The hospital features a full range of inpatient and outpatient services, including renovated pediatric and birthing units. Trinity also operates a School of Respiratory Care and School of Radiologic Technology.

For more information about our doctors and services, call 1-800-3-ADVOCATE (1-800-323-8622)

NORTHWESTERN
HEALTHCARE

Northwestern Healthcare is dedicated to providing superior quality and the most cost-effective medical care available. Comprised of affiliated physicians, academic medical centers and community-based hospitals, we are the largest integrated health delivery system in the metropolitan Chicago area.

Our comprehensive geographic coverage links more than 4,500 physicians, nine hospitals and 50 satellite facilities. By bringing together the individual strengths of eight locally integrated delivery systems and using nationally recognized procedures and research, Northwestern Healthcare provides convenient access to superior health care services delivered in a caring and compassionate manner. Our members include:

CHILDREN'S MEMORIAL MEDICAL CENTER

The #1 specialty pediatric care provider in the Midwest, Children's has locations and affiliated pediatricians throughout the Chicago Metropolitan area. Offering all specialty and subspecialty services and comprehensive treatment in secondary and tertiary care and rehabilitative care, Children's breadth and depth of pediatric services is unsurpassed in the area. Children's is a Level I pediatric trauma center of the state of Illinois.

EVANSTON NORTHWESTERN HEALTHCARE

Comprised of Evanston and Glenbrook Hospitals, ENH Medical Group, ENH Home Services and ENH Research Institute. The hospitals, which offer a complete range of specialty and subspecialty care, have been ranked among the "Top 100 Hospitals" and "Top 15 Major Teaching Hospitals" in the nation for the past five years.

HIGHLAND PARK HOSPITAL

A leader in health care delivery for Lake and northern Cook Counties with more than 50 areas of clinical specialization. Areas of excellence include comprehensive cancer and cardiac care, advanced surgical capabilities, dedicated Breast Center, nationally renowned Fertility program, enhanced pediatric care, LDRP Family Birthing Center, Osteoporosis Prevention and Research Centers, and Highland Park Hospital Health & Fitness Center in Buffalo Grove.

INGALLS HEALTH SYSTEM

Comprised of Ingalls Memorial Hospital, three community-based treatment centers, a physician-hospital organization, home care subsidiary, diagnostic center, physician practice management company and an outpatient rehab center. The Wellness Center works in cooperation with the local park district to bring health care services out into the community.

NORTHWEST COMMUNITY HEALTHCARE

Comprised of Northwest Community Hospital, the Continuing Care Center, Day Surgery Center, the Wellness Center, three 24-hour Treatment Centers and Home Healthcare. The Hospital's new North Pavilion offers a convenient outpatient center, as well as medically advanced services for surgical and critical care needs. Summer 1999 will mark the opening of a newly expanded and renovated emergency department which ranks among the ten busiest in the Chicago area.

NORTHWESTERN MEMORIAL HOSPITAL

NMH is the primary teaching hospital for Northwestern University Medical School and is consistently ranked one of the nation's leading hospitals. And year after year, the people of Chicago rank us their most preferred hospital and their choice for best quality, best physicians, best nurses and most personalized care, as measured by the National Research Corporation. In Spring 1999 we opened our state-of-the-art replacement hospital, which will set new standards in health care for decades to come.

SILVER CROSS HOSPITAL

Located in Joliet with a network of eight health care centers, a full range of services is provided to Will, Grundy and Cook Counties including a center for diabetes, and specialists from Children's Memorial, the Chicago Institute of Neurosurgery and Neuroresearch and Northwestern's Lurie Cancer Center. The newly added pavilion features diagnostic services, inpatient/outpatient surgical suites and a 14-station dialysis unit.

SWEDISH COVENANT HOSPITAL

Services include family practice, OB/maternity, occupational health, cancer treatment, on-site extended care nursing facility, home health and a comprehensive pain management clinic. The hospital also operates the Galter LifeCenter which has been recognized as one of the top five hospital-based health and wellness centers in the country.

MEMBER INSTITUTIONS

Children's Memorial Medical Center
705 West Fullerton
Chicago, IL 60614

Physician Referral: (800) KIDS-DOC

Evanston Northwestern Healthcare
1301 Central Street
Evanston, IL 60201

Physician Referral and Health Information:
(847) 570-5020

Highland Park Hospital
718 Glenview Avenue
Highland Park, IL 60035

Physician Referral: (847) 432-1161

Ingalls Health System
One Ingalls Drive
Harvey, IL 60426

Physician Referral: (800) 221-2199

Northwest Community Healthcare
800 West Central Road
Arlington Heights, IL 60005

Physician Referral: (847) 618-3463

Northwestern Memorial Hospital
251 East Huron Street
Chicago, IL 60611

Physician Referral: (312) 926-8400

Silver Cross Hospital and Medical Centers
1200 Maple Road
Joliet, IL 60432

Physician Referral: (800) 934-6937

Swedish Covenant Hospital
5145 North California Avenue
Chicago, IL 60625

Physician Referral: (773) 989-3838

980 North Michigan Avenue
Suite 1500
Chicago, IL 60611
Northwestern Healthcare is also affiliated with
Northwestern University Medical School

REGIONAL MEDICAL CENTERS AND COMMUNITY HOSPITALS

The Chicago metropolitan region is fortunate to have a large number of truly excellent regional medical centers and community hospitals. Many of these institutions offer sophisticated services that in years past were offered only at academic medical centers. However, with advancements in medical technology, regional medical centers and community hospitals have access to the equipment, and by virtue of the medical schools and teaching hospitals in the region, the well-trained physicians and staff, to offer these programs.

Regional medical centers and community hospitals range in size from the small (100 beds) to the very large (800 beds) but they share a common theme: a primary focus on patient care.

We have invited a selected number of excellent community hospitals to provide readers of the Castle Connolly Guide with information on their institutions and services by sponsoring the following profiles.

THE STATE OF ILLINOIS

DOCTOR LISTINGS

Information on hospitals in Illinois may be found as follows:

COOK COUNTY

ALEXIAN BROTHERS MEDICAL CENTER

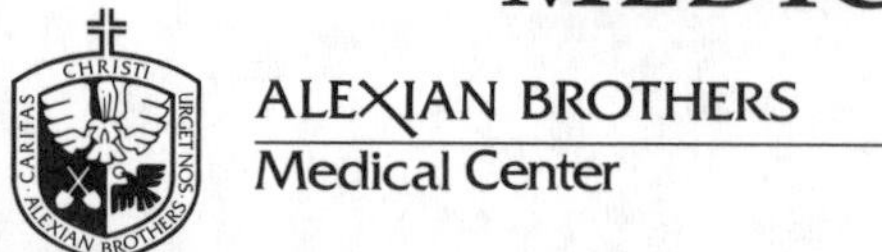

800 Biesterfield Road
Elk Grove Village, IL 60007
Phone: (847) 437-5500
Fax: (847) 981-3580
website: www.alexian.org

Sponsorship	**A not for profit hospital and trauma center; member of the Alexian Brothers Health System, a national Healthcare system sponsored by the Immaculate Conception Province of the Congregation of the Alexian Brothers**
Beds	**473**
Accreditation	**Joint Commission on the Accreditation of Healthcare Organizations; American Sleep Disorders Association Accreditation**

MISSION

The mission of Alexian Brothers Medical Center is to serve the health care needs of the community with a constant striving for the highest quality care, innovative and responsible use of resources, and an abiding regard for the individual. The health care provided at the Medical Center is the outward sign of the Alexian Brothers' enduring vision, holistic perspective, and sensitivity to the dignity of every person, advantaged and disadvantaged. It is care illuminated by the teachings of Christ and His church. The Medical Center delivers health care in partnership with those who would share our ministry. Only with and through the community can we fully and faithfully serve those who come from the community to find healing and blessing.

MEDICAL/DENTAL STAFF

Over 700 physicians representing more than 50 medical and dental specialties who provide care through multidisciplinary teams.

SPECIALTIES

Cardiology	Complete continuum of care from advanced diagnostics and state-of-the-art treatment to rehabilitation and home health care.
Oncology	Full spectrum of advanced care including the latest assessment and treatment tools combined with emotional and spiritual support.
Obstetrics	Advanced medical technology combined with a comfortable, home-like environment that offers patients flexibility in the delivery process.
Surgery	Technologically advanced surgical suites offering Day Surgery, laser and minimally invasive surgery and home health follow up.
Rehabilitation	Together with the Rehabilitation Institute of Chicago, ABMC offers an intensive, acute rehabilitation program in inpatient and outpatient settings to address a variety of physical disabilities.

COMMUNITY BASED PROGRAMS

Alexian Brothers Home Health; Community Health Alliance; Community Family Health Center, Mount Prospect, IL; Catholic Charities Physician Referral Service; Parish Nurse Program; Community Outreach Health Services.

For more information about services and physicians, please call HealthSource at 888-394-9400.

CHILDREN'S MEMORIAL MEDICAL CENTER

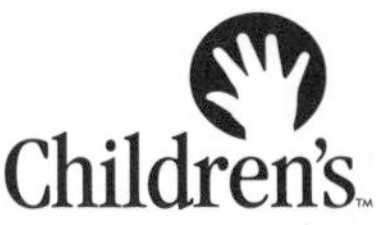

2300 CHILDREN'S PLAZA
AT LINCOLN AND FULLERTON AVES.
CHICAGO, IL 60614
PHONE (773) 880-4000
FAX (773) 880-3068

Sponsorship	Not-for-Profit, a member of Northwestern Healthcare, affiliated with Northwestern University Medical School
Beds	265
Accreditation	Joint Commission on Accreditation of Healthcare Organizations, American College of Surgeons, American College of Radiology, Accreditation Council for Graduate Medical Education (ACGME), College of American Pathologists, Foundation for the Accreditation of Hematopoietic Cell Therapy (FAHCT)

A TRUSTED NAME

Children's has been a trusted name for families since 1882. Children's remains the only hospital in the Chicago area dedicated to caring only for kids. Our commitment to children is unique and drives us to be the leader in patient care, medical education, pediatric research and child advocacy. In a recent survey by U.S. News & World Report, Children's was named the #1 children's hospital in the Midwest. Children's consistently ranks in the top 10 in the nation and #1 in the Chicago area. Children's is nationally recognized for its dedication and caring for all children and families who seek our help.

Children's breadth and depth of service is unsurpassed in the Chicago area. Children's offers every pediatric specialty and subspecialty. All services are specially designed to meet the unique needs of children. Our specialties include Pediatric Cardiology and Cardio-Thoracic Surgery, Pediatric Hematology and Oncology, Pediatric Neurology and Neurosurgery, Pediatric Organ and Stem Cell Transplantation, Neonatology and all others.

AFFILIATED WITH NORTHWESTERN UNIVERSITY MEDICAL SCHOOL

The full-time physicians and surgeons at Children's are board-certified and hold faculty positions at Northwestern University Medical School. Children's exclusive teaching relationship with NUMS means a multifaceted approach toward patient care as well as expertise in the latest developments in pediatric specialty medicine.

CHILDREN'S® IS ACCESSIBLE TO ALL FAMILIES

Children's is truly a network of care, comprised of a freestanding pediatric hospital, suburban inpatient facility, convenient suburban outpatient center, a home health service and a broad network of referring physicians - ensuring that Children's care is always near.

Children's pediatric specialists are available in Chicago and throughout the suburbs in:

Arlington Heights	Harvey	Joliet	Tinley Park
Glenview	Highland Park	LaGrange	Westchester

Physician Referral	To make an appointment with a Children's specialist, or to get help finding a Children's-affiliated pediatrician near you call 1.800.KIDS DOC. Parents can also call 1.800 KIDS DOC to learn more about free community lectures given in their area or to learn more about Children's free automated resource for parents, the Parent Advice Line.

CHRIST HOSPITAL AND MEDICAL CENTER

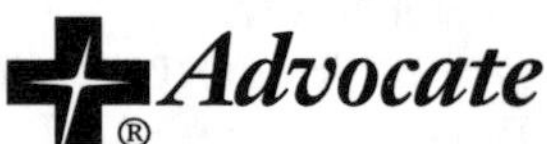

CHRIST HOSPITAL AND MEDICAL CENTER
HOPE CHILDREN'S HOSPITAL
4440 WEST 95TH STREET
OAK LAWN, ILLINOIS 60453
708-425-8000

Sponsorship:	Voluntary, not-for-profit
Beds:	Christ Hospital 754 licensed beds; Hope Children's Hospital 60 licensed beds, including 15 pediatric intensive care unit beds
Accreditation:	Joint Commission on Accreditation of Healthcare Organizations, named one of the nation's Top 100 Hospitals

Christ Hospital and Medical Center is the largest private hospital in Illinois, based on admissions. It is one of the region's leading providers of care in pediatrics, cardiology, women and infant's services, cancer, trauma and emergency services, physical rehabilitation, and mental health and addictions.

Hope Children's Hospital is widely respected for its superior capabilities in pediatric cardiology, oncology, critical care, perinatology, neonatology, neurology, gastroenterology and rehabilitation and development. More than 5,000 pediatric inpatients are treated annually, and approximately 65,000 outpatient visits made.

Christ Hospital and Medical Center is a member of Advocate Health Care, a non-profit organization of Chicagoland hospitals, health centers, and physician practices. To learn more, visit our web site at www.advocatehealth.com.

A Leading Cardiac Center	As the largest provider of cardiovascular services in northern Illinois, Christ Hospital offers a full spectrum of advanced diagnostic, treatment and rehabilitative services. The hospital performs more than 1,000 adult and 450 pediatric open heart surgeries each year. Christ Hospital also leads the region in heart disease prevention and the management of congestive heart failure. The hospital's Heart Institute for Children is a regional center of excellence in the care of newborns and children with heart disease.
Comprehensive Cancer Care	The staff at Christ Hospital and Medical Center treats more than 1,200 patients diagnosed with cancer each year. Christ Hospital's approach to treatment is guided by the standards of the National Cancer Institute. The program's strength has earned the designation of Comprehensive Cancer Care Center, granted by the Commission on Cancer for the American College of Surgeons.
Emergency Medical Care	Christ Hospital is a state-designated Level I trauma center, allowing the hospital to provide the most sophisticated level of emergency medical care and expertise for trauma patients. The hospital's emergency department treats more than 60,000 patients each year, including the highest volume of trauma patients in the state.
Rehabilitation Services	Christ Hospital boasts the state's most broadly accredited hospital-based physical rehabilitation program. Accredited services include spinal cord injury, traumatic brain injury and comprehensive inpatient rehabilitation, vocational evaluation, work adjustment and job placement.
Physician Referral	Christ Hospital and Medical Center's physician referral line at 1-800-3-ADVOCATE (1-800-323-8622) provides easy access to information about physicians and services at the hospital, general health information and information about health education programs, screenings and support groups. English- and Spanish-speaking health representatives are available.

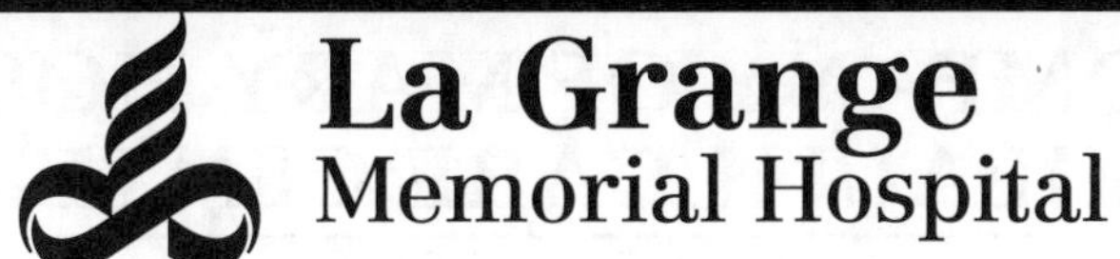

A Member of Adventist Health System

5101 S. Willow Springs Road, La Grange, IL 60525; PHONE: (708) 352-1200
www.ahsmidwest.org

Sponsorship	Non-profit. A member of Adventist Health System Midwest Region.
Beds	274 licensed beds
Accreditation	JCAHO, CARF

General Description:

La Grange Memorial Hospital has been a leader in offering a comprehensive range of modern medical services including: complete inpatient and outpatient diagnostics, therapeutic and rehabilitative cardiology services; a comprehensive oncology program affiliated with a Chicago-based academic medical center and other specialty services that cater to the community; and a Community Family Practice Center, staffed by a group of physicians on staff at La Grange Memorial Hospital and in the Family Practice Residency Program.

The hospital's community outreach program offers education support classes, screenings, behavior modification programs, health fairs, and lectures to the community.

Mission:

A Christian health-care leader committed to a partnering with physicians and community to provide whole-person care and promote wellness.

Family Maternity Center

The Family Maternity Program is a comprehensive program dedicated to nurturing and informing the parents and ensuring the most comfortable and memorable experience for mother and newborn. Services include LDR birthing rooms, family suites for extra privacy, childbirth education classes and a Special Delivery Club which provides exclusive amenities to its expectant mothers.

Convenient Primary Care

The hospital operates six Family Medical Centers which provide a full range of high quality primary and ambulatory care services from pediatrics to geriatric patients. These centers are conveniently located throughout the western suburbs and are staffed by primary care physicians.

List of Services:

Air Ambulance
Cardiology
Emergency Department - Level II Trauma
Enterology/Endoscopy
Geriatric Services
Hematology
Intermediate Nursing Beds
Laparoscopic Surgery
Lithotripsy
Medical Intensive Care Unit
Nephrology
Nutritional Services
Neonatal Intensive Care
Obstetrics/Gynecology
Occupational Medicine
Oncology Services
Ophthalmology
Orthopedics
Outpatient Surgery
Pain Center
Pastoral Care
Pediatrics
Physical Therapy
Psychiatry
Pulmonary Medicine
Radiology
Rehabilitation Services
Research Programs
Residency Program
Skilled Nursing Beds
Speech Therapy
Sports Medicine Center
Sub-Acute Care
Teaching Program
Transitional Care Unit
Urology
Women's Services

Physician Referral — Please call (630) 856-7500 for a physician referral (weekdays 8 a.m. - 5 p.m.).

LITTLE COMPANY OF MARY HOSPITAL AND HEALTH CARE CENTERS

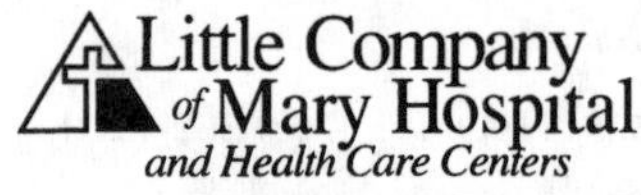

2800 W. 95th Street
Evergreen Park, Illinois 60805
708-422-6200

Sponsorship	Not-for-profit
Beds	492 beds
Physicians	81.5% Board Certified
Accreditation	American Association of Blood Banks, American College of Surgeons Commission on Cancer-Oncology Programs, College of American Pathologists, Joint Commission on Accreditation of Healthcare Organizations

General Description
Little Company of Mary Hospital and Health Care Centers was founded in 1930 by the Sisters of the Little Company of Mary. With a fully accredited hospital, two urgent care centers, a physicians' pavilion, home health equipment center, two health education centers in local malls, and a home based services program, Little Company continues its tradition of providing quality health care with a compassionate touch on Chicago's southwest side. The hospital offers a wide range of medical, surgical, pediatric, obstetrical, gynecological, and psychiatric services.

Medical Staff
Over 500 physicians with outstanding reputations in their respective fields support Little Company of Mary Hospital.

Pioneering Medicine
Little Company of Mary, which has always devoted itself to providing quality care, was the site of the world's first human organ transplant in 1950. The successful kidney transplant extended the life of 44-year-old Ruth Tucker, and has been the basis for thousands of other transplants performed around the world annually.

Special Programs

Cancer Center:	A leading center for cancer diagnosis and treatment, the specially accredited Cancer Center promotes cancer prevention within the community with free and reduced-fee screenings. Recent affiliation with the Medical Oncology Group of the University of Chicago Hospitals promises to bring the best in cancer care to the Southwest Side.
Orthopedic Center:	For full-service care of bones and joints, the Little Company Orthopedic Center's dedicated physician and nursing staff offers a multidisciplinary approach to care. Services include physical therapy, nutrition counseling, social work, home care, and pastoral care.
Breast Health Center:	This home-like, private environment provides professional breast exams, mammograms and instruction for self-evaluation. The Little Company Breast Health Center is dedicated to early detection, diagnostic services and treatment consultation.
Osteoporosis Center:	A state-of-the-art detection system enables our Osteoporosis Center specialists to identify bone thinning in its earliest stages so that treatment options can begin before problems develop.
Physical Therapy Center:	Little Company's Monsignor Thomas S. Obrycki Physical Therapy Center offers the very latest in treatment and services -- from underwater treadmills to an unweighting system to provide the best in physical and occupational therapy.

Physician Match	Little Company offers a physician referral service to help your family find a doctor to satisfy your health care needs. Call 708/423-3070 for more information.

LUTHERAN GENERAL HOSPITAL

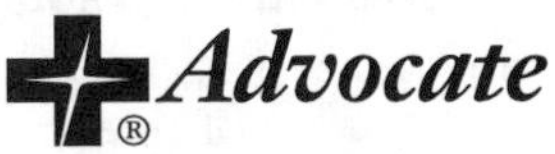

1775 DEMPSTER STREET
PARK RIDGE, ILLINOIS 60068
847-723-2210

Sponsorship:	Voluntary, not-for-profit
Beds:	608 licensed beds, including 150 bed children's hospital
Accreditation:	Joint Commission on Accreditation of Healthcare Organizations, American College of Surgeons, American College of Radiology, American College of Pathologists, American College of Radiology, American Association of Blood Banks, Illinois State Medical Society, Commission on Accreditation of Rehabilitation Facilities

Lutheran General Hospital is a teaching, research and referral hospital; a level I Trauma Center for both adult and pediatric care; and a Level III Perinatal Center, the highest designation. A leader in cancer services, orthopedic services, pediatric services, cardiology, women's health, trauma care and mental health and addiction programs, Lutheran General has been selected as one of the nation's top 100 hospitals and top 15 major teaching hospitals according to the "100 Top Hospitals: Benchmarks for Success" study. It was also ranked #1 in quality of care in 1998 in a "Chicago's Top Hospitals" survey.

Lutheran General Hospital's medical staff consists of more than 1,075 physicians representing over 65 specialties. The medical staff includes over 570 Primary Care Physicians.

Lutheran General Hospital is a member of Advocate Health Care, a non-profit organization of Chicagoland hospitals, health centers and physician practices. To learn more, see page (#) or visit our web site at advocatehealth.com.

Lutheran General Children's Hospital	Lutheran General Children's Hospital is one of the largest and most comprehensive children's hospitals in Illinois with over 185 pediatricians and pediatric subspecialists that provide primary and tertiary care in every major subspecialty. For more information see our page in the Center of Excellence section under Pediatrics.
Cancer Care Center	Lutheran General Cancer Care Center is the most comprehensive center in the northwest suburban corridor providing a multidisciplinary approach to prevention, evaluation, diagnosis, treatment, follow-up and cancer research studies. For more information see our page in the Center of Excellence section under Cancer.
Cardiovascular Services	Lutheran General Hospital is a recognized leader in cardiology services, with 42 board-certified or board-eligible cardiologists, and 3 three cardiac surgeons. The hospital houses 3 three state-of-the-art catheterization labs and two operating rooms dedicated to cardiac surgery around the clock . An entire range of the latest technology is offered: Electrophysiology for adults and pediatrics, Noninvasive Cardiac Testing, Pacing and Monitoring, Cardiac Rehabilitation, Adult and Pediatric Cardiac Catheterization and Cardiac Nuclear Imaging.
Women's Health	Lutheran General Hospital offers a Women's Health and Resource Center, a Breast Center, Continence Center, Osteoporosis Screening, a Women's Cancer Care Program and a Women's Research and Education Program.
Physician Referral	Call 1-800-3-ADVOCATE (1-800-323-8622) for easy access to information on hospital services, general health topics, physician referrals, education programs and support groups. Spanish-speaking health representatives are available.

COOK COUNTY

Specialties are indicated in bold-type face. Capital letters indicate Primary Care Specialties. Subspecialties are listed in non-bold type. Listings indicate if a doctor is certified in a subspecialty but predominately practices primary care medicine.

*Oncologists deal with Cancer

ALLERGY & IMMUNOLOGY

Aaronson, Donald W (MD) **A&I**
Resurrection Med Ctr
Aaronson Asthma & Allergy Ltd, 7447 W Talcott Ave Ste 422; Chicago, IL 60631; (773) 775-2600; **BDCERT:** A&I 75; **MS:** Univ IL Coll Med 61; **RES:** IM, Hines VA Hosp, Chicago, IL 62-65; **FEL:** A&I, Northwestern Mem Hosp, Chicago, IL 65-66; **FAP:** Assoc Clin Prof U Chicago-Pritzker Sch Med; **HOSP:** Lutheran Gen Hosp
Mcr Mcd 1 Week

Detjen, Paul (MD) **A&I**
Evanston Hosp
Kenilworth Medical Assoc, 534 Green Bay Rd; Kenilworth, IL 60043; (847) 256-5505; **BDCERT:** A&I 93; IM 89; **MS:** Washington U, St Louis 84; **RES:** IM, Northwestern Mem Hosp, Chicago, IL 86-88; Northwestern Mem Hosp, Chicago, IL 88-89; **FEL:** A&I, Northwestern Mem Hosp, Chicago, IL 89-91; **HOSP:** Glenbrook Hosp; ***SI:** Asthma; Allergies*; **HMO:** Guardian, PHCS, United Healthcare, Prudential +
Mcr Mcd 2-4 Weeks VISA

Goldberg, Salmon (MD) **A&I**
Good Shepherd Hosp
Chudwin & Goldberg, 500 Skokie Blvd Ste 140; Northbrook, IL 60062; (847) 272-4296; **BDCERT:** A&I 75; Ped 70; **MS:** Israel 61; **RES:** Path, Jewish Hosp, Cincinnati, OH 67; Ped, U IL Med Ctr, Chicago, IL 67-69; **FEL:** A&I, U Chicago Hosp, Chicago, IL 69-71; **HOSP:** Highland Park Hosp; **HMO:** Aetna Hlth Plan, Blue Choice, Californiacare, CIGNA, Healthamerica

Grammer III, Leslie C (MD) **A&I**
Northwestern Mem Hosp
Northwestern U Med Sch, 303 E Chicago Ave; Chicago, IL 60611; (312) 908-8171; **BDCERT:** A&I 81; IM 79; **MS:** Northwestern U 76; **RES:** A&I, Northwestern Mem Hosp, Chicago, IL 77-79; IM, Northwestern Mem Hosp, Chicago, IL 79-91; **FAP:** Prof Med Northwestern U

Grant, Evalyn N (MD) **A&I**
Rush-Presbyterian-St Luke's Med Ctr
(see page 122)
1725 W Harrison St Ste 207; Chicago, IL 60612; (312) 942-6296; **BDCERT:** Ped 89; A&I 95; **MS:** Rush Med Coll 86; ***SI:** Asthma; Sinusitis*
Mcr Mcd 2-4 Weeks

Greenberger, Paul (MD) **A&I**
Northwestern Mem Hosp
303 E Chicago Ave Ste 3705; Chicago, IL 60611; (312) 908-8171; **BDCERT:** IM 76; A&I 79; **MS:** Ind U Sch Med 73; **RES:** IM, Jewish Hosp, St Louis, MO 74-76; **FEL:** A&I, Northwestern Mem Hosp, Chicago, IL 76-78

Langiewicz, Janusz (MD) **A&I**
Resurrection Med Ctr
Allergy Center, 3933 N Cicero Ave; Chicago, IL 60641; (773) 777-4522; **BDCERT:** A&I 97; Ped 97; **MS:** Poland 72; **RES:** IM, Univ Hosp, Bialystok, Poland 73-76; Ped, Graduate Med Edu Inc, Lansing, MI 84-87; **FEL:** A&I, Samter Inst Allergy & Clin Immunol, Chicago, IL 87-89; **HOSP:** Illinois Masonic Med Ctr; ***SI:** Asthma; Hives*; **HMO:** Aetna Hlth Plan, Blue Cross & Blue Shield, Prudential, Masonicare +
LANG: Pol; Mcr NFI Immediately VISA

Lisberg, Edward E (MD) **A&I**
West Suburban Hosp Med Ctr
Asthma and Allergy Center of Chicago S C, 7420 Central Ste 2020; River Forest, IL 60305; (708) 366-9300; **BDCERT:** A&I 89; IM 85; **MS:** Rush Med Coll 82; **RES:** IM, Rush Presbyterian-St Luke's Med Ctr, Chicago, IL 82-85; **FEL:** A&I, Nat Jewish Med Ctr, Denver, CO 86-87; A&I, Rush Presbyterian-St Luke's Med Ctr, Chicago, IL 82-88; **FAP:** Assoc Prof Rush Med Coll; ***SI:** Asthma; Allergy/Sinus Disease*

McGrath, Kris (MD) **A&I**
St Joseph Hosp-Chicago
500 N Michigan Ave Ste 1640; Chicago, IL 60611; (312) 222-9500; **BDCERT:** A&I 85; IM 82; **MS:** U Iowa Coll Med 79; **RES:** A&I, Northwestern Mem Hosp, Chicago, IL 80-82; **FEL:** A&I, Northwestern Mem Hosp, Chicago, IL 82-84; **FAP:** Assoc Prof of Clin Med Northwestern U; **HOSP:** Northwestern Mem Hosp; ***SI:** Asthma; Allergies*; **HMO:** Blue Cross & Blue Shield, Aetna Hlth Plan, Prudential
LANG: Sp; Mcr Mcd 2-4 Weeks

Melam, Howard (MD) **A&I**
Lutheran Gen Hosp (see page 143)
Advanced Allergists, 455 S Roselle Rd Ste 206; Schaumburg, IL 60193; (847) 298-5151; **BDCERT:** A&I 74; Ped 70; **MS:** Northwestern U 65

Pollock, James (MD) **A&I**
Evanston Hosp
3633 W Lake Ave Ste 412; Glenview, IL 60025; (847) 998-6229; **BDCERT:** A&I 75; Ped 73; **MS:** Med Coll Wisc 68; **HOSP:** Glen Oaks Hosp and Med Ctr; **HMO:** Aetna Hlth Plan, Blue Cross & Blue Shield, CIGNA, Humana Health Plan, Metlife

Rosenberg, Michael (MD) **A&I**
Resurrection Med Ctr
Advanced Allergists Ltd, 241 Golf Mill Ctr; Niles, IL 60714; (847) 298-5151; **BDCERT:** A&I 79; IM 78; **MS:** Northwestern U 70; **RES:** IM, Northwestern Mem Hosp, Chicago, IL 71-73; **FEL:** A&I, Northwestern Mem Hosp, Chicago, IL 75-77; **FAP:** Asst Clin Prof Med Univ IL Coll Med; **HMO:** Aetna Hlth Plan, Blue Cross & Blue Shield, Chicago HMO, CIGNA, Principal Health Care

ANESTHESIOLOGY

Abreu, Jose (MD) **Anes**
South Suburban Hosp
South Suburban Hosp, 17800 S Kedzie Ave; Hazel Crest, IL 60429; (708) 799-8000; **BDCERT:** Anes 71; **MS:** Dominican Republic 60; **RES:** S, Ottawa General Hosp, Ottawa, Canada 63-64; Anes, St Joseph Med Ctr-Joliet, Joliet, IL 64-66; **FEL:** Anes, Mass Eye & Ear Infirmary, Boston, MA 66-67

Albrecht, Ronald (MD) **Anes**
Univ of Illinois at Chicago Med Ctr
1740 W Taylor St Ste 3200; Chicago, IL 60612; (312) 996-4020; **BDCERT:** Anes 67; **MS:** Univ IL Coll Med 61; **RES:** Anes, U IL Med Ctr, Chicago, IL 62-64; **FEL:** Anes, Nat Inst Health, Bethesda, MD 64-66; **FAP:** Prof Anes Univ IL Coll Med; **HOSP:** Michael Reese Hosp & Med Ctr

Ampel, Leon Louis (MD) **Anes**
Evanston Hosp
Evanston Hospital, 2650 Ridge Ave; Glenview, IL 60201; (847) 657-5812; **BDCERT:** Anes 76; **MS:** Univ Mo-Columbia Sch Med 62; **RES:** Evanston Hosp, Evanston, IL 65-67; **FAP:** Asst Prof Anes Northwestern U

Aronson, Solomon (MD) **Anes**
U Chicago Hosp **(see page 124)**
Univ of Chicago - Dept of Anes/Critical Care, 5841 S Maryland Ave; Chicago, IL 60637; (773) 702-0017; **BDCERT:** Anes 88; **MS:** Med Coll Wisc 83; **RES:** Anes, U TX Med Branch Hosp, Galveston, TX 85-86; **FEL:** Cv/Anes, Texas Heart Inst, Houston, TX 87; **FAP:** Assoc Prof Anes U Chicago-Pritzker Sch Med

Baughman, Verna (MD) **Anes**
Univ of Illinois at Chicago Med Ctr
Univ of IL at Chicago - Dept Anes, 1740 W Taylor St M/C515; Chicago, IL 60612; (312) 996-4020; **BDCERT:** Anes 86; **MS:** Loyola U-Stritch Sch Med, Maywood 81; **RES:** Anes, Michael Reese Hosp Med Ctr, Chicago, IL 81-84; **FEL:** Anes, Michael Reese Hosp Med Ctr, Chicago, IL 84-85; **FAP:** Assoc Prof Univ IL Coll Med; **HOSP:** Michael Reese Hosp & Med Ctr; ***SI:*** *Neurosurgical Anesthesia*
Mcr Mcd NFI A Few Days
VISA

Benzon, Honorio (MD) **Anes**
Northwestern Mem Hosp
Northwestern Mem Hospital, 303 E Superior St Rm 360; Chicago, IL 60611; (312) 908-2500; **BDCERT:** Anes 95; PM 93; **MS:** Philippines 71; **RES:** Anes, U of Cincinnati, Cincinnati, OH 73-75; Northwestern Mem Hosp, Chicago, IL 75-76; **FEL:** NPh, Brigham & Women's Hosp, Boston, MA 85-86; **FAP:** Prof PM Northwestern U; ***SI:*** *Pain Management; Regional Nerve Blocks*; **HMO:** Blue Cross & Blue Shield, Aetna Hlth Plan, HealthStar, United +
LANG: Fil; Mcr Mcd 2-4 Weeks VISA

Berkowitz, Richard A (MD) **Anes**
Univ of Illinois at Chicago Med Ctr
University of Illinois Department Of Anesthesiology, 1740 W Taylor St Ste 3200; Chicago, IL 60612; (312) 996-4020; **BDCERT:** Anes 90; Ped 87; **MS:** Univ IL Coll Med 83; **RES:** Ped A&I, Michael Reese Hosp Med Ctr, Chicago, IL 84-86; Anes, Michael Reese Hosp Med Ctr, Chicago, IL 86-88; **FAP:** Clin Prof Anes Univ IL Coll Med; **HOSP:** Michael Reese Hosp & Med Ctr; ***SI:*** *Pediatric Anesthesiology; Pediatric Critical Care*
Mcr Mcd Immediately

Blasco, Thomas (MD) **Anes**
Lutheran Gen Hosp **(see page 143)**
Lutheran General Hospital, 1775 Dempster St; Park Ridge, IL 60068; (847) 696-5524; **BDCERT:** Anes 86; **MS:** Loyola U-Stritch Sch Med, Maywood 78

Boarden, Wilfred (MD) **Anes**
Christ Hosp & Med Ctr **(see page 140)**
4440 W 95th St; Oak Lawn, IL 60453; (708) 346-5745; **BDCERT:** Anes 89; **MS:** Univ IL Coll Med 81; **RES:** Anes, Michael Reese Hosp Med Ctr, Chicago, IL 82-84; **FEL:** Cv, Michael Reese Hosp Med Ctr, Chicago, IL 84-85; **FAP:** Asst Clin Prof Univ IL Coll Med

Brey, Steven (MD) **Anes**
Alexian Brothers Med Ctr
(see page 138)
Alexian Bros Med Ctr, 800 Biesterfield Rd; Elk Grove Village, IL 60007; (847) 437-5500; **BDCERT:** Anes 95; **MS:** Med Coll Wisc 88; **RES:** Anes, Loyola U Med Ctr, Maywood, IL 90-93

Brown, Douglas V (MD) **Anes**
Rush-Presbyterian-St Luke's Med Ctr
(see page 122)
Rush Presbyterian St Luke's Medical, 1653 W Congress Pkwy; Chicago, IL 60612; (312) 942-6504; **BDCERT:** Anes 94; **MS:** U Chicago-Pritzker Sch Med 89; **RES:** Johns Hopkins Hosp, Baltimore, MD 90-93; **FAP:** Assoc Prof Rush Med Coll; ***SI:*** *Cardiac Anesthesia; Thoracic Anesthesia*; **HMO:** +

Childers, Sara Jean (MD) **Anes**
Columbus Hosp
Columbus Hosp, 2520 N Lakeview; Chicago, IL 60614; (773) 883-7952; **BDCERT:** Anes 88; **MS:** Univ Ky Coll Med 81; **RES:** S, Northwestern Mem Hosp, Chicago, IL 81-83; Anes, Northwestern Mem Hosp, Chicago, IL 83-85; **FEL:** Ped Anes, Children's Mem Med Ctr, Chicago, IL 85-86; **FAP:** Asst Prof Northwestern U; ***SI:*** *Pain Management*
LANG: Sp;

Davis-Fourte, Felicia (MD) **Anes**
Cook Cty Hosp
1835 W Harrison; Chicago, IL 60612; (312) 633-6167; **BDCERT:** Anes 96; **MS:** Howard U 83; **RES:** Anes, Cook Cty Hosp, Chicago, IL 86-87; **FEL:** Ped Anes, Cook Cty Hosp, Chicago, IL 88; Northwestern Mem Hosp, Chicago, IL 88

Desai, Kirtiben P (MD) **Anes**
Victory Mem Hosp
Dept of Anesthesiology, 1324 N Sheridan Rd; Chicago, IL 60641; (847) 360-4212; **BDCERT:** Anes 94; **MS:** Ind U Sch Med 75; **RES:** Anes, U IL Med Ctr, Chicago, IL 80-81; **FEL:** Cv & ObG, U IL Med Ctr, Chicago, IL 83

Fermin, Ramone E (MD) **Anes**
Bethany Hosp
Bethany Hosp, 3435 W Van Buren St; Chicago, IL 60624; (773) 947-7560; **BDCERT:** Anes 94; **MS:** Philippines 79; **RES:** Cook Co Hosp, Chicago, IL 83-85

Gelfand, Richard (MD) **Anes**
Evanston Hosp
Evanston Hosp, 2650 Ridge Ave; Evanston, IL 60201; (847) 570-2760; **BDCERT:** Anes 84; **MS:** Univ IL Coll Med 76; **RES:** Anes, Northwestern Mem Hosp, Chicago, IL 80-82; **FEL:** ObG, Northwestern Mem Hosp, Chicago, IL 82-83; **FAP:** Assoc Clin Prof Northwestern U

Greene, Scott (MD) **Anes**
Northwestern Mem Hosp
710 N Fairbanks Ct Ste 6210; Chicago, IL 60611; (312) 908-5149; **BDCERT:** Anes 83; **MS:** Northwestern U 78; **RES:** Anes, Northwestern Mem Hosp, Chicago, IL 79-81; **FEL:** CCM, Northwestern Mem Hosp, Chicago, IL 81-82; **FAP:** Asst Clin Prof Anes Northwestern U; **HMO:** Aetna Hlth Plan, Blue Cross & Blue Shield, Chicago HMO, CIGNA, Healthplus

Hahn, June (MD) **Anes**
Lutheran Gen Hosp **(see page 143)**
1775 Dempster St; Park Ridge, IL 60068; (847) 696-7003; **BDCERT:** Anes 78; **MS:** South Korea 69; **RES:** Anes, Johns Hopkins Hosp, Baltimore, MD 72-74; UCLA Med Ctr, Los Angeles, CA -96; **HOSP:** Christ Hosp & Med Ctr; ***SI:*** *Back Pain*; **HMO:** +
LANG: Kor; SA SU Mcr NFI
A Few Days

Hall, Steven (MD) **Anes**
Children's Mem Med Ctr **(see page 139)**
Children's Memorial Med Ctr, 2300 Children's Plaza; Chicago, IL 60614; (773) 880-4414; **BDCERT:** Anes 78; **MS:** Northwestern U 74; **RES:** Anes, Northwestern Mem Hosp, Chicago, IL 75-77; Hosp For Sick Children, Toronto, Canada 78; **FEL:** Ped Anes, Children's Mem Med Ctr, Chicago, IL 77; **HOSP:** Glenbrook Hosp; ***SI:*** *Pediatric Anesthesia; Pediatric Pain Management*; **HMO:** Aetna Hlth Plan, Blue Choice, CIGNA PPO, Principal Health Care
LANG: Dut, Fr, Sp, Pol, Grk; Mcd
Immediately ***VISA***

Ivankovich, Anthony (MD) **Anes**
Rush-Presbyterian-St Luke's Med Ctr
(see page 122)
Ste 740 Jelke, 1653 W Congress Pkwy; Chicago, IL 60612; (312) 942-6504; **BDCERT:** Anes 71; **MS:** Yugoslavia 63; **RES:** U Chicago Hosp, Chicago, IL 67-69; **FAP:** Prof Rush Med Coll; ***SI:*** *Pain Management*; **HMO:** Aetna Hlth Plan, Blue Cross & Blue Shield, Californiacare, CIGNA, Maxicare Health Plan

Jellish, Walter Scott (MD & PhD) **Anes**
Loyola U Med Ctr **(see page 120)**
Loyla University Physicans Fnd, 2160 S 1st Ave Ste 3116; Maywood, IL 60153; (708) 821-6450; **BDCERT:** Anes 92; **MS:** Rush Med Coll 86; **RES:** Anes, Barnes Hosp, St Louis, MO 87-90; **FEL:** Neuro Anes, Barnes Hosp, St Louis, MO 90-91; **FAP:** Assoc Prof Loyola U-Stritch Sch Med, Maywood; ***SI:*** *Anesthesia For Neurosurgery; Skull Base Surgery*
LANG: Sp, Pol, Rus; Mcr Mcd NFI
4+ Weeks

Klowden, Arthur (MD) **Anes**
Illinois Masonic Med Ctr
(see page 118)
M Ramez Salem & Assoc SC, 836 W Wellington Ave Ste 4815; Chicago, IL 60657; (773) 296-5211; **BDCERT:** Anes 75; **MS:** Univ IL Coll Med 66; **RES:** IM, Michael Reese Hosp Med Ctr, Chicago, IL 66-67; Anes, U IL Med Ctr, Chicago, IL 67-69; **FAP:** Asst Prof Anes Rush Med Coll; **HOSP:** Shriners Hosp for Children; ***SI:*** *Pediatric Anesthesiology*; **HMO:** Blue Cross & Blue Shield, Chicago HMO, Metlife, Prudential

Koht, Antoun (MD) Anes
Christ Hosp & Med Ctr (see page 140)
Midwest Anesthesiologist, 4440 W 95th St; Oak Lawn, IL 60453; (708) 346-5745; **BDCERT:** Anes 79; **MS:** Syria 72; **RES:** Anes, Northwestern Mem Hosp, Chicago, IL 75-77; **FEL:** CCM, Northwestern Mem Hosp, Chicago, IL 77-78; **FAP:** Asst Clin Prof Anes Northwestern U; **HMO:** Blue Cross & Blue Shield, Chicago HMO, Health Options

Lipov, Eugene G (MD) Anes
Alexian Brothers Med Ctr
(see page 138)
Poplar Creek Surg Ctr, 1800 McDonough Rd; Hoffman Estates, IL 60192; (847) 742-7272; **BDCERT:** Anes 91; PM 94; **MS:** Northwestern U 84; **RES:** Anes, U IL Med Ctr, Chicago, IL 87-89; Anes, U IL Med Ctr, Chicago, IL 89-90; **FAP:** Asst Prof Rush Med Coll

Marymont, Jesse (MD) Anes
Evanston Hosp
E and H Medical Group, 2650 Ridge Ave; Evanston, IL 60201; (847) 570-2760; **BDCERT:** Anes 87; **MS:** St Louis U 83; **RES:** Anes, Northwestern Mem Hosp, Chicago, IL 84-86; **FEL:** Cv, Northwestern Mem Hosp, Chicago, IL 86-87; **FAP:** Assoc Clin Instr Anes Northwestern U

Mc Laughlin, Desmond (MD) Anes
Lutheran Gen Hosp (see page 143)
1775 Dempster St; Park Ridge, IL 60068; (847) 696-8365; **BDCERT:** Anes 64; **MS:** Ireland 54; **RES:** St Joseph Med Ctr-Joliet, Joliet, IL 59-61; **FAP:** Assoc Clin Prof U Chicago-Pritzker Sch Med

McGee, John (MD) Anes
Evanston Hosp
2650 Ridge Ave; Evanston, IL 60201; (847) 570-2760; **BDCERT:** Anes 75; **MS:** Northwestern U 70; **RES:** Anes, Evanston Hosp, Evanston, IL 71-74; **FAP:** Asst Clin Prof Anes Northwestern U

Miller, Paul E. (MD) Anes
Christ Hosp & Med Ctr (see page 140)
4440 W 95th St; Oak Lawn, IL 60453; (708) 425-8000; **BDCERT:** Anes 88; **MS:** Univ IL Coll Med 83; **RES:** Anes, Michael Reese Hosp Med Ctr, Chicago, IL 84-85; **FAP:** Instr Rush Med Coll; **HMO:** +

Molloy Jr, Robert E (MD) Anes
Northwestern Mem Hosp
Northwestern Mem Hosp - Anesthesiology, Superior St & Fairbanks Ct; Chicago, IL 60611; (312) 908-8254; **BDCERT:** Anes 78; PM 93; **MS:** Northwestern U 74
2-4 Weeks

Moss, Jonathan (MD) Anes
U Chicago Hosp (see page 124)
Anesthesia & Criticl Care Dept, 5841 S Maryland Box 4028; Chicago, IL 60637; (773) 702-6700; **BDCERT:** Anes 79; **MS:** Duke U 74; **RES:** Mass Gen Hosp, Boston, MA 74-76; **FAP:** Prof CCM (Anes) U Chicago-Pritzker Sch Med

Murthy, Vemuri (MD) Anes
West Suburban Hosp Med Ctr
Chairman, Dept of Anesthesia, West Suburban Hospital; Oak Park, IL 60302; (630) 383-6200; **BDCERT:** Anes 87; **MS:** India 74; **RES:** Anes, Rush Presbyterian-St Luke's Med Ctr, Chicago, IL 80-83; ***SI:*** *Pain Management*
VISA

Overton, Margaret Eileen (MD) Anes
Lutheran Gen Hosp (see page 143)
Lutheran General Hospital, 1775 Dempster St; Park Ridge, IL 60068; (847) 723-2210; **BDCERT:** Anes 89; **MS:** Northwestern U 83; **RES:** Anes, Northwestern U, Chicago, IL 83-86; **FEL:** Cv, Northwestern U, Chicago, IL 86-87

Parnass, Samuel (MD) Anes
Rush North Shore Med Ctr
Univ Anesthesiologists SC, 9600 Gross Point Rd; Skokie, IL 60076; (847) 933-6909; **BDCERT:** Anes 88; IM 85; **MS:** Israel 82; **RES:** IM, Michael Reese Hosp Med Ctr, Chicago, IL 83-85; Anes, Michael Reese Hosp Med Ctr, Chicago, IL 85-87; **FEL:** Anes, Rush Presbyterian-St Luke's Med Ctr, Chicago, IL 87; **FAP:** Assoc Prof Anes Rush Med Coll

Porter, Gregory Anthony (MD) Anes
Alexian Brothers Med Ctr
(see page 138)
800 Biesterfield Rd; Elk Grove Village, IL 60007; (847) 437-5500; **BDCERT:** Anes 87; **MS:** Southern IL U 79; **RES:** S, Metro-Five/IL Masonic MC, Chicago, IL 79-80; Anes, IL Masonic Med Ctr, Chicago, IL 80-82

Reddy, Chandra (MD) Anes
Holy Family Med Ctr
100 North River Rd; Des Plaines, IL 60016; (847) 297-7246; **BDCERT:** Anes 93; PM 94; **MS:** India 62; **RES:** Anes, Northwestern Mem Hosp, Chicago, IL 72-73; Anes, Youngstown Hospital 70-72; **FAP:** Asst Prof Anes Univ IL Coll Med; ***SI:*** *Pain Management*

Rodenas, Jesus (MD) **Anes**
St Mary's of Nazareth Hosp Ctr
St Mary's of Nazareth Hospital Ctr - Chief of Anes, 2233 W Division; Chicago, IL 60622; (312) 770-2413; **BDCERT:** Anes 75; **MS:** Philippines 55; **RES:** Cook Cty Hosp, Chicago, IL 69-72

Roth, Andrew G (MD) **Anes**
Children's Mem Med Ctr **(see page 139)**
Children's Memorial Hosp, 2300 Children's Plaza; Chicago, IL 60614; (312) 880-4000; **BDCERT:** Anes 81; **MS:** Ind U Sch Med 76; **RES:** Anes, Northwestern Mem Hosp, Chicago, IL 77-79; **FEL:** Ped Anes, Children's Mem Med Ctr, Chicago, IL 79-80; **FAP:** Asst Prof Anes Northwestern U

Roth, David (MD) **Anes**
Little Company of Mary Hosp & Hlth Care Ctrs **(see page 142)**
2800 W 95th St; Evergreen Park, IL 60805; (708) 229-5300; **BDCERT:** Anes 87; **MS:** U Chicago-Pritzker Sch Med 82; **RES:** Anes, U Chicago Hosp, Chicago, IL 83-85; ***SI:*** *Chronic Pain Treatment*; **HMO:** Humana Health Plan, Advocate
LANG: Sp;
Immediately

Rothenberg, David (MD) **Anes**
Rush-Presbyterian-St Luke's Med Ctr
(see page 122)
Rush Presbyterian-Anesthesia, 1653 W Congress Pkwy; Chicago, IL 60612; (312) 942-6504; **BDCERT:** Anes 88; IM 85; **MS:** Univ IL Coll Med 81; **RES:** IM, Michael Reese Hosp Med Ctr, Chicago, IL 81-84; Anes, Michael Reese Hosp Med Ctr, Chicago, IL 85-87; **FEL:** CCM, Rush Presbyterian-St Luke's Med Ctr, Chicago, IL 87-88; **FAP:** Assoc Prof Anes Rush Med Coll; ***SI:*** *Intensive Care Medicine*

Schanbacher, Paul (MD) **Anes**
Resurrection Med Ctr
7345 W Talcott Ave; Chicago, IL 60631; (773) 792-5162; **BDCERT:** Anes 94; **MS:** Creighton U 84; **RES:** Anes, Illinois Masonic Med Ctr, Chicago, IL 90-93; **FEL:** Anes, Children's Mem Med Ctr, Chicago, IL 93-94; ***SI:*** *Pediatric Anesthesia; Pain Management*; **HMO:** Health One, Rush Prudential, BC/BS PPO
LANG: Pol, Sp, Itl;
1 Week VISA

Schulte, Edward (DO) **Anes**
St Alexius Med Ctr
Medical Center Anesthesia Ltd, 1555 Barrington Rd; Hoffman Estates, IL 60194; (847) 490-6932; **BDCERT:** Anes 75; **MS:** Chicago Coll Osteo Med 69; **RES:** Northwestern Mem Hosp, Chicago, IL 71-74

Shapiro, Barry (MD) **Anes**
Northwestern Mem Hosp
Northwestern Hospital, 303 E Superior St Ste 360; Chicago, IL 60611; (312) 908-2280; **BDCERT:** Anes 70; CCM 87; **MS:** U Mich Med Sch 63; **RES:** U Mich Med Ctr, Ann Arbor, MI 64-66; **FAP:** Chrmn Anes Northwestern U

Slogoff, Stephen (MD) **Anes**
Loyola U Med Ctr **(see page 120)**
Loyola University Medical Center, 2160 S First Ave; Maywood, IL 60153; (708) 216-4016; **BDCERT:** Anes 93; **MS:** Jefferson Med Coll 67; **RES:** Anes, Thomas Jefferson U Hosp, Philadelphia, PA 68-71; **FAP:** Prof Anes Loyola U-Stritch Sch Med, Maywood; **HOSP:** VA Med Ctr; ***SI:*** *Cardiac Anesthesiology*; **HMO:** Blue Cross, Aetna-US Healthcare, Champus, Medicare
Immediately VISA

Srinivasan, Chida (MD) **Anes**
Little Company of Mary Hosp & Hlth Care Ctrs **(see page 142)**
2800 W 95th St; Evergreen Park, IL 60805; (708) 229-5300; **BDCERT:** Anes 81; **MS:** India 72; ***SI:*** *Pain Management*

Stephenson, Richard E (MD) **Anes**
Trinity Hosp
SE Anesthesia Consul - Trinity Hosp, 2320 E 93rd St; Chicago, IL 60617; (773) 933-3895; **BDCERT:** Anes 91; **MS:** Univ IL Coll Med 86; **RES:** Anes, U IL Med Ctr, Chicago, IL 87-89; **FEL:** Cv & Anes, U IL Med Ctr, Chicago, IL 89-90; **FAP:** Chrmn Anes U Hlth Sci/Chicago Med Sch; ***SI:*** *Postoperative Pain Control; Acute Pain Control*; **HMO:** +
LANG: Ger;
A Few Days

Terna, Paul (MD) **Anes**
Alexian Brothers Med Ctr
(see page 138)
800 Biesterfield Road; Elk Grove Village, IL 60007; (847) 437-5500; **BDCERT:** Anes 89; **MS:** Loyola U-Stritch Sch Med, Maywood 84; **RES:** Anes, Loyola U Med Ctr, Maywood, IL 85-87

Tobin, Michael (MD) **Anes**
Children's Mem Med Ctr **(see page 139)**
Children's Memorial Hospital, 2300 N Children's Plz Ste 69; Chicago, IL 60614; (773) 880-4414; **BDCERT:** Ped 99; Anes 93; **MS:** Rush Med Coll 86; **HMO:** Aetna Hlth Plan, Blue Cross & Blue Shield, Chicago HMO, CIGNA, Humana Health Plan

Tuman, Kenneth (MD) **Anes**
Rush-Presbyterian-St Luke's Med Ctr
(see page 122)
Rush Presbyterian-St Lukes, 1653 W Congress Pkwy; Chicago, IL 60612; (312) 942-6504; **BDCERT:** Anes 85; CCM 87; **MS:** U Chicago-Pritzker Sch Med 80; **RES:** S, U IL Med Ctr, Chicago, IL 81-82; Anes, Northwestern Mem Hosp, Chicago, IL 82-84; **FEL:** Cv/Anes, Rush Presbyterian-St Luke's Med Ctr, Chicago, IL 84-85; **FAP:** Prof/VChrmn Anes Rush Med Coll
VISA

Vender, Jeffrey (MD) Anes
Evanston Hosp
Evanston Hosp, 2650 Ridge Ave; Evanston, IL 60201; (847) 570-2760; **BDCERT:** Anes 79; CCM 87; **MS:** Northwestern U 75; **FAP:** Prof Anes Northwestern U; ***SI:*** *Respiratory Failure; Cardiac Anesthesia*; **HMO:** +
Immediately

Watt, Cathleen M (MD) Anes
Columbus Hosp
Columbus Hospital-Dept of Anesthesiology, 2520 N Lakeview Ave; Chicago, IL 60614; (773) 883-7300; **BDCERT:** Anes 89; IM 85; **MS:** U Iowa Coll Med 82

Winnie, Alon (MD) Anes
Cook Cty Hosp
Cook County Hosptial, 1835 W Harrison St; Chicago, IL 60612; (312) 633-3360; **BDCERT:** Anes 67; PM 93; **MS:** Northwestern U 58; **RES:** Cook Cty Hosp, Chicago, IL 60-63; **FAP:** Prof Anes Univ IL Coll Med

CARDIOLOGY (CARDIOVASCULAR DISEASE)

Akhter, Iqbal (MD) Cv
Edgewater Med Ctr
Prevention & Treatment Ctr, 3551 N Central Ave; Chicago, IL 60634; (773) 545-9770; **BDCERT:** IM 96; **MS:** India 63

Albert, Brian (MD) Cv
Northwest Comm Hlthcare
Northwest Heart Specialists, 1632 W Central Rd; Arlington Hts, IL 60005; (847) 253-8050; **BDCERT:** Cv 87; **MS:** Univ IL Coll Med 84; **RES:** IM, U IL Med Ctr, Chicago, IL 84-87; **FEL:** Cv, Rush Presbyterian-St Luke's Med Ctr, Chicago, IL 87-89; ***SI:*** *Echocardiography; Coronary Artery Disease*; **HMO:** Blue Cross & Blue Shield, Aetna Hlth Plan, PHCS, Prudential, UHC +
1 Week VISA

Balesteri, Anthony (MD) Cv
Resurrection Med Ctr
Talcott Internal Medicine Ltd, 7447 W Talcott Ave Ste 262; Chicago, IL 60631; (773) 775-1900; **BDCERT:** Cv 75; **MS:** Loyola U-Stritch Sch Med, Maywood 70; **RES:** IM, Cook Cty Hosp, Chicago, IL 71-72; IM, Loyola U Med Ctr, Maywood, IL 72-73; **FEL:** Cv, Loyola U Med Ctr, Maywood, IL 73-75; **FAP:** Asst Clin Prof Loyola U-Stritch Sch Med, Maywood

Bernstein, Ira (MD) Cv
Evanston Hosp
800 Oak St Ste 109; Winnetka, IL 60093; (847) 446-2300; **BDCERT:** Cv 71; IM 67; **MS:** Northwestern U 60; **RES:** IM, Cook Cty Hosp, Chicago, IL 61; Cv, Cook Cty Hosp, Chicago, IL 63-67; **FAP:** Asst Prof of Clin Med Northwestern U

Bonow, Robert O (MD) Cv
Northwestern Mem Hosp
Northwestern Medical Faculty, 250 E Superior St Ste 521; Chicago, IL 60611; (312) 908-1052; **BDCERT:** Cv 81; IM 76; **MS:** Univ Penn 73; **RES:** IM, Hosp of U Penn, Philadelphia, PA 74-76; **FEL:** Cv, Nat Heart Inst, Bethesda, MD 76-79; **FAP:** Prof Cv Northwestern U; **HOSP:** VA Hlthcare Systems-Lakeside; ***SI:*** *Coronary Artery Disease; Valvular Heart Disease*
LANG: Sp, Pol; 1 Week VISA

Briller, Joan (MD) Cv
Univ of Illinois at Chicago Med Ctr
University of Illinois at Chicago Medical Center, 840 S Wood St Ste 787; Chicago, IL 60612; (312) 996-9342; **BDCERT:** IM 84; Cv 89; **MS:** U Conn Sch Med 81; **RES:** IM, Northwestern Mem Hosp, Chicago, IL 81-84; **FEL:** Cv, U Chicago Hosp, Chicago, IL 86-88; **FAP:** Asst Prof Med Loyola U-Stritch Sch Med, Maywood; ***SI:*** *Echocardiography Stress Testing; Women & Heart Disease*
LANG: Fr; 1 Week VISA

Calvin, James E (MD) Cv
Rush-Presbyterian-St Luke's Med Ctr
(see page 122)
University Cardiologists, 1725 W Harrison St Ste 1159; Chicago, IL 60612; (312) 942-5020; **BDCERT:** IM 81; Cv 83; **MS:** Dalhousie U 75; **RES:** CCM, U West Ontario, London, Canada 78-79; Cv, U Ottawa, Ottawa, Ontario 80-81; **FEL:** Cv, UC San Francisco Med Ctr, San Francisco, CA 81-83

Camba, Noel (MD) Cv
St James Hosp & Hlth Ctrs
333 Dixie Hwy; Chicago Heights, IL 60411; (708) 709-6331; **BDCERT:** IM 91; Cv 95; **MS:** Univ IL Coll Med 86; **RES:** IM, Louis A Weiss Hosp, Chicago, IL 86-89; **FEL:** Cv, Chicago Med Sch, Chicago, IL 89-92; Cv, Norhtwestern U, Chicago, IL 92-93; **HOSP:** Ingalls Mem Hosp; ***SI:*** *Angioplasty*; **HMO:** +
2-4 Weeks

Campo, Adalberto (MD) Cv
Norwegian-American Hosp
1431 N Western Ave Ste 506; Chicago, IL 60622; (773) 327-8000; **BDCERT:** IM 86; **MS:** Mexico 79; **RES:** IM, Cook Cty Hosp, Chicago, IL 82-84; **FEL:** Cv, Cook Cty Hosp, Chicago, IL 84-86

Chiu, Y Christopher (MD) Cv
Illinois Masonic Med Ctr
(see page 118)
3000 N Halsted Ave Ste 701; Chicago, IL 60657; (773) 296-3888; **BDCERT:** IM 84; Cv 87; **MS:** Harvard Med Sch 81; **RES:** IM, U Chicago Hosp, Chicago, IL 81-82; IM, Univ of Chicago, Chicago, IL 82-84; **FEL:** Cv, U Chicago Hosp, Chicago, IL 84-87; Cv, Intervent - U Chicago Hosp, Chicago, IL 87-88; ***SI:*** *Invasive Procedures*; **HMO:** +
LANG: Chi, Sp; 2-4 Weeks VISA

Co, Richard (MD) Cv
Holy Family Med Ctr
1400 EastGolf Rd Ste 117; Des Plaines, IL 60016; (847) 297-9922; **BDCERT:** IM 69; Cv 72; **MS:** Philippines 63; **RES:** Mount Sinai Med Ctr, New York, NY 64-66; **FEL:** Cv, St Barnabas Med Ctr, Livingston, NJ 67-68

Cooke, David (MD) Cv
Lutheran Gen Hosp **(see page 143)**
Advocate Medical Group, 1875 Dempster; Park Ridge, IL 60068; (847) 698-3600; **BDCERT:** Cv 81; CCM 89; **MS:** Univ IL Coll Med 76

Dahodwala, Mohamed (MD) Cv
St Anthony Hosp
Cardiac Associates, 6441 S Pulaski Rd Ste 100; Chicago, IL 60629; (773) 284-1234; **BDCERT:** IM 84; Cv 87; **MS:** India 80; **RES:** Grant Hosp, Chicago, IL 82-84; **FEL:** Cv, Mount Sinai Hosp Med Ctr, Chicago, IL 84-85; **HOSP:** Holy Cross Hosp

Davidson, Charles J (MD) Cv
Northwestern Mem Hosp
Northwestern Memorial Hosp, 710 Fairbanks Ct Olson 4220; Chicago, IL 60611; (312) 908-5421; **BDCERT:** Cv 89; IM 85; **MS:** U Conn Sch Med 82; **RES:** IM, Northwestern Mem Hosp, Chicago, IL 82-85; **FEL:** Cv, Duke U Med Ctr, Durham, NC 85-88; **FAP:** Assoc Prof Med Northwestern U; ***SI:*** *Interventional Cardiology*
LANG: Sp;

Davison, Richard (MD) Cv
Northwestern Mem Hosp
Northwestern Univ Medical School, 250 E Superior St; Chicago, IL 60611; (312) 908-2745; **BDCERT:** Cv 74; IM 80; **MS:** Argentina 63; **RES:** IM, Passavant Meml Hosp, Chicago, IL 66-69; **FEL:** Cv, Veteran's Admin Hosp, Chicago, IL 69-71; **FAP:** Assoc Prof Med Northwestern U
LANG: Sp; 4+ Weeks

Dixon, Donald (MD) Cv
Macneal Mem Hosp
Macneal Cardiology Group, 3231 Euclid Ave Ste 201; Berwyn, IL 60402; (708) 783-2055; **BDCERT:** Cv 77; IM 76; **MS:** Univ IL Coll Med 70; **RES:** IM, Evanston Hosp, Evanston, IL 73-75; **FEL:** Cv, Loyola U Med Ctr, Maywood, IL 75-77

Feldman, Ted (MD) Cv
U Chicago Hosp **(see page 124)**
University of Chicago Hospital, 5841 S Maryland Ave M567; Chicago, IL 60637; (773) 702-9461; **BDCERT:** IM 81; Cv 85; **MS:** Ind U Sch Med 78; **RES:** IM, Rush Presbyterian-St Luke's Med Ctr, Chicago, IL 78-82; **FEL:** Cv, U Chicago Hosp, Chicago, IL 82-85; **FAP:** Prof Med U Chicago-Pritzker Sch Med; ***SI:*** *Angioplasty; Heart Valve Disease*
A Few Days

Fisher, Raymond (MD) Cv
Resurrection Med Ctr
North Shore Cardiology Cnslnts, 800 Austin East Tower Ste 363; Evanston, IL 60202; (847) 869-3003; **BDCERT:** IM 80; Cv 89; **MS:** Loyola U-Stritch Sch Med, Maywood 76; **RES:** IM, St Francis Hosp of Evanston, Evanston, IL 77-79; **HOSP:** St Francis Hosp; ***SI:*** *Non-invasive Testing; Carotid Doppler Studies*; **HMO:** United Healthcare, Humana Health Plan, Bc/BS, Rush Prudential +
LANG: Tag, Kor, Sp;

Fishman, David (MD) Cv
Resurrection Med Ctr
5600 W Addison St Ste 505; Chicago, IL 60634; (773) 282-3311; **BDCERT:** Cv 77; CCM 89; **MS:** Univ IL Coll Med 70; **RES:** IM, U IL Med Ctr, Chicago, IL 73-75; **FEL:** Cv, Loyola U Med Ctr, Maywood, IL 75-77; **HOSP:** Our Lady Of the Resurrection Med Ctr; **HMO:** Accord, United Healthcare, AARP +
LANG: Sp, Pol;
1 Week

Gaiha, Vishnu (MD) Cv
St Francis Hosp of Evanston
800 Austin St Ste 602; Evanston, IL 60202; (847) 491-1977; **BDCERT:** IM 80; Cv 77; **MS:** India 68; **RES:** IM, Northwestern Mem Hosp, Chicago, IL 70-72; **FEL:** Cv, U Mich Med Ctr, Ann Arbor, MI 72-74; **HOSP:** Swedish Covenant Hosp; ***SI:*** *Balloon Angioplasty; Stents Heart Angiograms*; **HMO:** Aetna Hlth Plan, Blue Cross, Californiacare, CIGNA, United Healthcare +
LANG: Hin;
A Few Days VISA

Gill, Sukhjit (MD) Cv
Grant Hosp
2266 N Lincoln Ave Fl 3; Chicago, IL 60614; (773) 327-8008; **BDCERT:** IM 75; Cv 77; **MS:** India 65; **RES:** IM, Cook Cty Hosp, Chicago, IL 73-75; **FEL:** Cv, Cook Cty Hosp, Chicago, IL 75-77

Golbus, Glenn (MD) Cv
Good Shepherd Hosp
Northwest Cardiology, 1575 Barrington Rd Ste 215; Hoffman Estates, IL 60194; (847) 882-8448; **BDCERT:** Cv 77; **MS:** Loyola U-Stritch Sch Med, Maywood 72; **RES:** St Louis U Hosp, St Louis, MO 75-77; **FEL:** Cv, Loyola U Med Ctr, Maywood, IL 77-79; **HOSP:** St Alexius Med Ctr; **HMO:** Blue Cross & Blue Shield, United Healthcare, PHCS, One Health Plan
A Few Days VISA

Greenland, Philip (MD) Cv
Northwestern Mem Hosp
Northwestern Medical Faculty Inc, 680 N Lake Shore Dr Ste 1102; Chicago, IL 60611; (312) 908-7914; **BDCERT:** IM 77; Cv 81; **MS:** U Rochester 74; **RES:** IM, Univ of Rochester Med Ctr, Rochester, NY 74-78; **FEL:** Cv, U MN Med Ctr, Minneapolis, MN 78-80; **FAP:** Professor PrM Northwestern U; ***SI:*** *Heart Disease Prevention; Cardiac Rehabilitation*
2-4 Weeks

Greenspahn, Bruce (MD) Cv
Lutheran Gen Hosp **(see page 143)**
Cardiology Specialists Ltd, 1875 Dempster St Ste 555; Park Ridge, IL 60068; (847) 698-5500; **BDCERT:** Cv 78; **MS:** Univ IL Coll Med 75; **RES:** IM, U IL Med Ctr, Chicago, IL 76-78; **FEL:** Cv, U Chicago Hosp, Chicago, IL 79-81; **HMO:** Aetna Hlth Plan, Blue Cross & Blue Shield, Californiacare, CIGNA, Compare Health Service
2-4 Weeks

Hale, David (MD) Cv
Alexian Brothers Med Ctr
(see page 138)
810 Biesterfield Rd Ste 206; Elk Grove Village, IL 60007; (847) 981-3680; **BDCERT:** Cv 75; IM 74; **MS:** Loyola U-Stritch Sch Med, Maywood 71; **RES:** IM, Loyola U Med Ctr, Maywood, IL 72-73; **FEL:** Cv, Loyola U Med Ctr, Maywood, IL 73-75; **FAP:** Prof of Clin Med Loyola U-Stritch Sch Med, Maywood; **HOSP:** Glen Oaks Hosp and Med Ctr
LANG: Pol; 2-4 Weeks VISA

Hueter, David C (MD) Cv
Evanston Hosp
ENH Medical Group Cardiology, 2650 Ridge Ave Burch 300; Evanston, IL 60201; (847) 570-2250; **BDCERT:** Cv 75; IM 74; **MS:** Stanford U 69; **RES:** IM, Mass Gen Hosp, Boston, MA 72-73; **FEL:** Cv, Mass Gen Hosp, Boston, MA 73-75; **FAP:** Asst Prof Cv Northwestern U; ***SI:*** *Cardiac Pacemaker; Cardiology-Invasive*; **HMO:** Aetna Hlth Plan, Blue Cross & Blue Shield, Chicago HMO, Humana Health Plan, Travelers

Hussein, Jaafar (MD) Cv
Grant Hosp
2202 N Lincoln Ave; Chicago, IL 60614; (773) 871-5353; **BDCERT:** IM 70; Cv 74; **MS:** Iraq 59; **RES:** Cook Cty Hosp, Chicago, IL 69-70; Chicago VA Rsrch Hospital, Chicago, IL 70-71; **FEL:** Cv, Cook Cty Hosp, Chicago, IL 68

Ivanovic, Lou (MD) Cv
West Suburban Hosp Med Ctr
Millman Ltd, 7411 Lake St Ste 2110; River Forest, IL 60305; (630) 573-5871; **BDCERT:** Cv 91; IM 89; **MS:** Yugoslavia 83; **RES:** West Suburban Hosp Med Ctr, Oak Park, IL 85-89; **FEL:** U IL Med Ctr, Chicago, IL 89

Jain, Bhagwan (MD) Cv
Thorek Hosp & Med Ctr
850 W Irving Park Rd; Chicago, IL 60613; (773) 975-6772; **BDCERT:** IM 78; Cv 79; **MS:** India 68; **RES:** Mount Sinai Hosp Med Ctr, Chicago, IL 75-76; Edgewater Med Ctr, Chicago, IL 76-77; **FEL:** Cv, Cook Cty Hosp, Chicago, IL 77-79; ***SI:*** *Cardiac Catheterization*
A Few Days

Johnson, Maryl (MD) Cv
Northwestern Mem Hosp
250 E Superior St Ste 512; Chicago, IL 60611; (312) 908-4052; **BDCERT:** Cv 83; IM 81; **MS:** U Iowa Coll Med 77; **RES:** IM, U IA Hosp, Iowa City, IA 78-81; **FEL:** Cv, U IA Hosp, Iowa City, IA 79-82; **FAP:** Assoc Prof Med Northwestern U; **HMO:** Blue Cross & Blue Shield, Chicago HMO, Rush Health Plans

Jones, Paul (MD) Cv
Mercy Hosp & Med Ctr
Mercy Hospital, 2525 S Michigan Ave; Chicago, IL 60616; (312) 567-2380; **BDCERT:** Cv 93; IM 89; **MS:** Univ IL Coll Med 86; **RES:** IM, Mercy Hosp & Med Ctr, Chicago, IL 86-89; **FAP:** Asst Prof Rush Med Coll; **HOSP:** Rush-Presbyterian-St Luke's Med Ctr

Kadish, Alan (MD) Cv
Northwestern Mem Hosp
250 E Superior St Ste 250; Chicago, IL 60611; (312) 908-4753; **BDCERT:** CE 92; Cv 85; **MS:** Albert Einstein Coll Med 80; **RES:** IM, Brigham & Women's Hosp, Boston, MA 80-83; **FEL:** Cv, Hosp of U Penn, Philadelphia, PA 83-86; CE, Hosp of U Penn, Philadelphia, PA 86-87; **FAP:** Prof Med Northwestern U; ***SI:*** *Cardiac Arrhythmia; Pacemakers*

Khadra, Suhail (MD) Cv
Cook Cty Hosp
Division of Cardiology, 1835 W Harrison Ste 2258; Chicago, IL 60612; (312) 633-3296; **BDCERT:** IM 85; Cv 87; **MS:** Syria 79; **RES:** IM, Cook Cty Hosp, Chicago, IL 81-84; **FEL:** Cv, Cook Cty Hosp, Chicago, IL 84-87; ***SI:*** *Coronary Artery Diseases; Interventional Cardiology*; **HMO:** Blue Cross & Blue Shield, Humana Health Plan, Aetna Hlth Plan, Compass +
LANG: Ar, Sp, Pol; A Few Days

Koenigsberg, David (MD) Cv
Columbus Hosp
Lake Shore Cardiology Group, 2515 N Clark St Ste 905; Chicago, IL 60614; (773) 975-6640; **BDCERT:** Cv 81; IM 78; **MS:** Loyola U-Stritch Sch Med, Maywood 75; **RES:** IM, Loyola, Maywood, IL 76-78; **FEL:** Northwestern Cardiology, Chicago, IL 78-80; **HOSP:** Evanston Hosp; ***SI:*** *Angiograms; Stent Placement*

Krause, Philip (MD) Cv
Rush North Shore Med Ctr
150 N River Rd Ste 220; Des Plaines, IL 60016; (847) 296-4888; **BDCERT:** Cv 95; IM 92; **MS:** U Hlth Sci/Chicago Med Sch 87; **RES:** IM, Rush Presbyterian-St Luke's Med Ctr, Chicago, IL 88-90; **FEL:** Cv, Rush Presbyterian-St Luke's Med Ctr, Chicago, IL 90-93; Rush Presbyterian-St Luke's Med Ctr, Chicago, IL 93-94; **FAP:** Asst Prof Med Rush Med Coll; **HOSP:** Holy Family Med Ctr

Guide to symbols and abbreviations can be found on pages 110-113.

Lalmalani, Gopal (MD) Cv
Holy Cross Hosp
Midwest Cardiac Ctr, 2340 S Highland Ave; Lombard, IL 60148; (630) 792-0900; **BDCERT:** IM 76; Cv 79; **MS:** India 72; **RES:** IM, Michael Reese Hosp Med Ctr, Chicago, IL 74-76; **FEL:** Cv, Michael Reese Hosp Med Ctr, Chicago, IL 76-78; **FAP:** Asst Clin Prof U Chicago-Pritzker Sch Med; ***SI:*** *Echocardiography*

Lewis, Gregory (MD) Cv
La Grange Mem Hosp **(see page 141)**
West Suburban Cardiologists, 5201 Willow Springs Rd; La Grange, IL 60525; (708) 482-3215; **BDCERT:** Cv 91; IM 88; **MS:** Vanderbilt U Sch Med 85; **RES:** IM, U Chicago Hosp, Chicago, IL; **FEL:** Cv, U Chicago Hosp, Chicago, IL; **HOSP:** Hinsdale Hosp; ***SI:*** *Cardiac Arrhythmias; Pacemakers*; **HMO:** Blue Cross, Humana Health Plan, United Healthcare +
Mcr Mcd NFI Immediately VISA

Lipinski, Casimir (MD) Cv
Resurrection Med Ctr
Talcott Internal Medicine Ltd, 7447 W Talcott Ave Ste 207; Chicago, IL 60631; (773) 775-1900; **BDCERT:** Cv 87; IM 83; **MS:** Loyola U-Stritch Sch Med, Maywood 79; **RES:** IM, Hines VA Hosp, Chicago, IL 79-82; **FEL:** Cv, Northwestern Mem Hosp, Chicago, IL 82-84; **HMO:** Blue Cross & Blue Shield

Messer, Joseph V. (MD) Cv
Rush-Presbyterian-St Luke's Med Ctr **(see page 122)**
Associates In Cardiology Ltd, 1725 W Harrison St Ste 1138; Chicago, IL 60612; (312) 243-6800; **BDCERT:** IM 72; **MS:** Harvard Med Sch 56; **RES:** IM, Peter Bent Brigham Hosp, Boston, MA 57-58; IM, Peter Brent Brigham Hosp, Boston, MA 60-61; **FEL:** Cv, Brigham & Women's Hosp, Boston, MA 58-60; **FAP:** Prof Med Rush Med Coll; **HMO:** Aetna Hlth Plan, Chicago HMO, Choicecare, HealthNet, Healthpartners
Mcr

Miller, Albert (MD) Cv
Northwestern Mem Hosp
Clinical Cardiology Group Ltd, 676 N Saint Clair St Ste 1930; Chicago, IL 60611; (312) 642-2502; **BDCERT:** Cv 56; **MS:** Northwestern U 45; **RES:** IM, VA Hosp, Hines, IL; IM, Michael Reese Hosp Med Ctr, Chicago, IL; **FEL:** Cv, Michael Reese Hosp Med Ctr, Chicago, IL; **FAP:** Prof Northwestern U; ***SI:*** *Coronary Heart Disease; Hypertension*; **HMO:** Blue Cross & Blue Shield +
LANG: Sp, Itl; Mcr NFI 1 Week
VISA

Miller, Scott (MD) Cv
Lutheran Gen Hosp **(see page 143)**
Cardiology Specialists Ltd, 1875 Dempster St Ste 555; Park Ridge, IL 60068; (847) 698-5500; **BDCERT:** IM 81; Cv 85; **MS:** Univ IL Coll Med 78; ***SI:*** *Cardiac Electrophysiology*; **HMO:** Aetna Hlth Plan, Blue Choice, CIGNA, Compare Health Service

Millman, William (MD) Cv
Oak Park Hosp
O'Donoghue, Millman & Ivanovic, 7411 Lake St Ste 1210; River Forest, IL 60305; (708) 573-5871; **BDCERT:** IM 75; Cv 77; **MS:** Univ IL Coll Med 72; **RES:** IM, Med Coll WI, Milwaukee, WI 72-75; **FEL:** Cv, Med Coll WI, Milwaukee, WI 75-77; **FAP:** Asst Prof Loyola U-Stritch Sch Med, Maywood; **HOSP:** West Suburban Hosp Med Ctr; ***SI:*** *Interventional Cardiology*; **HMO:** +
Mcr Mcd NFI A Few Days

Mukherjee, Ashish (MD) Cv
St Anthony Hosp
Heart Specialist-Sawyer Med Ctr, 3232 W 55th St; Chicago, IL 60632; (773) 471-3600; **BDCERT:** IM 84; Cv 87; **MS:** India 79; **RES:** IM, Illinois Masonic Med Ctr, Chicago, IL 81-83; **FEL:** Cv, Illinois Masonic Med Ctr, Chicago, IL 83-85; **HOSP:** Holy Cross Hosp; ***SI:*** *Chest Pain; Rheumatology*

Nemickas, Rimgaudas (MD) Cv
Illinois Masonic Med Ctr **(see page 118)**
Cardiac Diagnosis Ltd, 3000 N Halsted St Ste 703; Chicago, IL 60657; (773) 296-3600; **BDCERT:** Cv 69; **MS:** Loyola U-Stritch Sch Med, Maywood 61; **RES:** IM, U IL Med Ctr, Chicago, IL 66-67; **FEL:** Cv, Cook Cty Hosp, Chicago, IL 62-63; **FAP:** Clin Prof Med Loyola U-Stritch Sch Med, Maywood; **HOSP:** Holy Cross Hosp; ***SI:*** *Coronary & Valvular Disease; Clinical Cardiology*

Quigg, Rebecca Jayne (MD) Cv
Northwestern Mem Hosp
Northwestern U, 250 E Superior St Ste 512; Chicago, IL 60611; (312) 908-4052; **BDCERT:** Cv 89; IM 83; **MS:** Penn State U-Hershey Med Ctr 80; **RES:** IM, Geo Wash U Med Ctr, Washington, DC 80-83; **FEL:** Cv, Boston Med Ctr, Boston, MA 84-86; ***SI:*** *Heart Failure; Cardiac Transplantation*; **HMO:** +
Mcr Mcd 1 Week

Quinn, Thomas (MD) Cv
Little Company of Mary Hosp & Hlth Care Ctrs **(see page 142)**
Cardiovascular Consultants, 2850 W 95th St Ste 301; Evergreen Park, IL 60805; (708) 425-7272; **BDCERT:** IM 82; Cv 85; **MS:** Loyola U-Stritch Sch Med, Maywood 79; **RES:** IM, U Hawaii, Honolulu, HI 80-82; **FEL:** Cv, Rush Presbyterian-St Luke's Med Ctr, Chicago, IL 82-84

Rich, Stuart (MD) Cv
Rush-Presbyterian-St Luke's Med Ctr **(see page 122)**
Center for Pulmonary Heart Disease, 1725 W Harrison St Ste 202; Chicago, IL 60612; (312) 563-2169; **BDCERT:** Cv 81; IM 78; **MS:** Loyola U-Stritch Sch Med, Maywood 74; **RES:** IM, Jewish Hosp of St Louis, St Louis, MO 76-78; **FEL:** Cv, U Chicago Hosp, Chicago, IL 78-80; **FAP:** Prof Med Rush Med Coll; ***SI:*** *Heart Scan*
LANG: Sp; 2-4 Weeks

Rosenbush, Stuart (MD) Cv
Rush-Presbyterian-St Luke's Med Ctr **(see page 122)**
Associates In Cardiology Ltd, 1725 W Harrison St Ste 1138; Chicago, IL 60612; (312) 243-6800; **BDCERT:** Cv 81; IM 79; **MS:** Univ IL Coll Med 76; **RES:** IM, Michael Reese Hosp Med Ctr, Chicago, IL 77-79; **FEL:** Cv, Rush Presby-St Luke's Med Ctr, Chicago, IL 79-81; **FAP:** Asst Prof Rush Med Coll; **HMO:** Blue Cross & Blue Shield, Chicago HMO, Rush Health Plans
Mcr

Rowan, Daniel (DO) Cv
Christ Hosp & Med Ctr **(see page 140)**
Cardiovascular Consultants, 2850 W 95th St Ste 301; Evergreen Park, IL 60805; (708) 425-7272; **BDCERT:** IM 89; Cv 91; **MS:** Chicago Coll Osteo Med 86; **RES:** IM, Mercy Hosp & Med Ctr, Chicago, IL 86-89; **FEL:** CCM (Anes), Rush Presby-St Luke's Med Ctr, Chicago, IL 91-92; IntvnCd, Rush Presby-St Luke's Med Ctr, Chicago, IL 92-93; **FAP:** Assoc Dir Rush Med Coll

Salinger, Michael H (MD) Cv
Evanston Hosp
2650 Ridge Ave; Evanston, IL 60201; (708) 570-2250; **BDCERT:** Cv 85; CCM 87; **MS:** Loyola U-Stritch Sch Med, Maywood 79; **RES:** IM, Evanston Hosp, Evanston, IL 80-82; Cv, Northwestern Mem Hosp, Chicago, IL 82-84; **FEL:** CCM, Northwestern Mem Hosp, Chicago, IL 84-85; Interventional Cv, Cleveland Clinic Hosp, Cleveland, OH 85-86; **FAP:** Assoc Prof Cv Northwestern U; ***SI:*** *Angioplasty/Stents; Heart Transplant*; **HMO:** Blue Cross & Blue Shield, Humana Health Plan, CIGNA +
SA SU Mcr Mcd 2-4 Weeks VISA

Scanlon, Patrick (MD) Cv
Loyola U Med Ctr **(see page 120)**
2160 S 1st Ave; Maywood, IL 60153; (708) 327-2858; **BDCERT:** IM 68; Cv 73; **MS:** Loyola U-Stritch Sch Med, Maywood 62; **FEL:** IM, Cleveland Clinic Hosp, Cleveland, OH 65-66; Cv, Cleveland Clinic Hosp, Cleveland, OH 68-70; **FAP:** Prof Loyola U-Stritch Sch Med, Maywood; ***SI:*** *Cardiac Catheterization*; **HMO:** +
Mcr Mcd 1 Week VISA

Schreiber, Ronald (MD) Cv
Loyola U Med Ctr **(see page 120)**
2160 S 1st Ave; Maywood, IL 60153; (708) 327-2747; **BDCERT:** IM 74; Cv 77; **MS:** Loyola U-Stritch Sch Med, Maywood 71; **RES:** IM, Mercy Hosp Med Ctr, San Diego, CA 71-73; IM, Med Coll WI, Milwaukee, WI 73-74; **FEL:** Cv, Loyola U Med Ctr, Maywood, IL 74-76; **FAP:** Assoc Prof of Clin Med Loyola U-Stritch Sch Med, Maywood
Mcr NFI 1 Week

Sethi, Manjeet (MD) Cv
Northwest Comm Hlthcare
Northwest Cardio-Vascular, 1100 W Central Rd Ste 301; Arlington Hts, IL 60005; (847) 392-7810; **BDCERT:** Cv 79; IM 77; **MS:** India 71; **RES:** IM, St Francis Hosp of Evanston, Evanston, IL 75-77; **FEL:** Cv, St Francis Hosp of Evanston, Evanston, IL 77-78; **HMO:** Blue Cross & Blue Shield, Healthcare America
Mcr Mcd VISA

Shah, Shirish (MD) Cv
Our Lady Of the Resurrection Med Ctr
5511 1/2 W Montrose Ave; Chicago, IL 60641; (773) 283-8444; **BDCERT:** IM 79; Cv 80; **MS:** India 74; **RES:** IM, VA Hosp, Hines, IL 76-78; **FEL:** Cv, Michael Reese Hosp Med Ctr, Chicago, IL 78-80; **HOSP:** Resurrection Med Ctr; ***SI:*** *Balloon Angioplasty; Coronary Stent Insertion*; **HMO:** Blue Cross, United Healthcare +
SA SU Mcr Mcd NFI

Silverman, Irwin (MD) Cv
Evanston Hosp
1713 Central St; Evanston, IL 60201; (847) 869-1499; **BDCERT:** Cv 87; CCM 91; **MS:** U Hlth Sci/Chicago Med Sch 77; **RES:** IM, Evanston Hosp, Evanston, IL 78-81; **FEL:** Cv, Northwestern Mem Hosp, Chicago, IL 81-83; **FAP:** Assoc Prof of Clin Med Northwestern U; **HOSP:** Glenbrook Hosp
Mcr Mcd A Few Days

Stone, Neil (MD) Cv
Northwestern Mem Hosp
Associates in Internal Medicine, 211 E Chicago Ave Ste 930; Chicago, IL 60611; (312) 944-6677; **BDCERT:** IM 74; Cv 75; **MS:** Northwestern U 68; **RES:** IM, Brigham & Women's Hosp, Boston, MA 68-70; IM, Northwestern Mem Hosp, Chicago, IL 73-74; **FEL:** Cv, Nat Heart Inst, Bethesda, MD 70-73; Cv, Northwestern Mem Hosp, Chicago, IL 74; **FAP:** Professor IM Northwestern U; ***SI:*** *Cholesterol Disorders; Coronary Artery Disease*

Talano, James (MD) Cv
Northwestern Mem Hosp
250 E Superior St Ste 585; Chicago, IL 60611; (312) 908-4687; **BDCERT:** IM 73; Cv 74; **MS:** Loyola U-Stritch Sch Med, Maywood 65; **RES:** IM, Georgetown U Hosp, Washington, DC 66-67; IM, Georgetown U Hosp, Washington, DC 67-68; **FEL:** Cv, Tufts U, Boston, MA 68-69; Cv, Georgetown U, Washington, DC 69-71; **FAP:** Prof Med Northwestern U

Upton, Mark (MD) Cv
Northwestern Mem Hosp
233 E Erie St Ste 412; Chicago, IL 60611; (312) 573-1322; **BDCERT:** IM 78; **MS:** McGill U 73; **RES:** Mary Hitchcock Mem Hosp, Hanover, NH; **FEL:** Cv, Duke Eye Ctr, Durham, NC 77-80; **FAP:** Asst Prof Med Northwestern U; **HMO:** Aetna Hlth Plan, Blue Choice, Californiacare, Chicago HMO, CIGNA
Mcr

Guide to symbols and abbreviations can be found on pages 110-113.

Wilber, David (MD) Cv
U Chicago Hosp (see page 124)
U Chicago Electrophysiology Group, 5758 S Maryland Ave Ste 5734; Chicago, IL 60637; (773) 702-5988; **BDCERT:** Cv 85; CE 92; **MS:** Northwestern U 77; **RES:** IM, Northwestern Mem Hosp, Chicago, IL 77-80; **FEL:** Cv, U Mich Med Ctr, Ann Arbor, MI 82-84; CE, Mass Gen Hosp, Boston, MA 84; **FAP:** Professor CE U Chicago-Pritzker Sch Med; **HOSP:** Alexian Brothers Med Ctr; ***SI:** Cardiac Electrophysiology; Defibrillators*
LANG: Sp, Pol; A Few Days VISA

Wilner, Gary (MD) Cv
Evanston Hosp
Evanston Northwestern Healthcare - Gary N. Wilner, 2650 Ridge Ave; Evanston, IL 60201; (847) 570-2063; **BDCERT:** Cv 77; IM 75; **MS:** U Md Sch Med 67; **RES:** IM, U MD Hosp, Baltimore, MD 67-70; **FEL:** Cv, NY Hosp-Cornell Med Ctr, New York, NY 70-72; **FAP:** Asst Prof Cv Northwestern U; **HOSP:** Glenbrook Hosp; ***SI:** Congenital Heart Disease in Adults; Cardiovascular Wellness*
1 Week

Yellen, Steven (MD) Cv
St Mary's of Nazareth Hosp Ctr
1431 N Western Ave Ste 112; Chicago, IL 60622; (773) 342-1119; **BDCERT:** IM 78; Cv 81; **MS:** U Hlth Sci/Chicago Med Sch 75

CHILD & ADOLESCENT PSYCHIATRY

Crawford, Karen (MD) ChAP
Christ Hosp & Med Ctr (see page 140)
Damen Wells Center, 1947 W 95th St; Chicago, IL 60643; (773) 779-1610; **BDCERT:** ChAP 85; Psyc 82; **MS:** Univ IL Coll Med 75; **RES:** Psyc, U IL Med Ctr, Chicago, IL 76-78; Ped, U IL Med Ctr, Chicago, IL 75; **FEL:** ChAP, Inst Juvenile Rsch, Chicago, IL 78-80

D'Agostino, Anthony M (MD) ChAP
Alexian Brothers Med Ctr
(see page 138)
25 E Schaumburg Rd Ste 101; Schaumburg, IL 60194; (847) 352-4540; **BDCERT:** Psyc 71; ChAP 74; **MS:** Univ IL Coll Med 65; **RES:** ChAP, U Wisc Hosp, Madison, WI 71-72; ChAP, UCLA Med Ctr, Los Angeles, CA 68-69; **FEL:** Psyc, U IL Med Ctr, Chicago, IL 66-68; **FAP:** Asst Prof Psyc Loyola U-Stritch Sch Med, Maywood; **HMO:** United Healthcare, CIGNA, Blue Cross +
2-4 Weeks

Dulcan, Mina K (MD) ChAP
Children's Mem Med Ctr (see page 139)
Children's Memorial Hosp-Dept Psyc 10, 2300 Children's Plaza; Chicago, IL 60614; (773) 880-4811; **BDCERT:** ChAP 79; Psyc 78; **MS:** Penn State U-Hershey Med Ctr 74; **RES:** ChAP, U of Pittsburgh Med Ctr, Pittsburgh, PA 74-78; Psyc, U of Pittsburgh Med Ctr, Pittsburgh, PA 74-77; **FAP:** Prof Psyc Northwestern U; **HOSP:** Northwestern Mem Hosp; ***SI:** Attention Deficit Disorder; Hyperactivity Disorder*

Hanus, Steven (MD) ChAP
Evanston Hosp
2530 Ridge Ave Ste 203; Evanston, IL 60201; (847) 864-3444; **BDCERT:** Psyc 84; **MS:** Northwestern U 77; **RES:** ChAP, U IL Med Ctr, Chicago, IL 78-80; Psyc, Northwestern Mem Hosp, Chicago, IL 80-82

Nierman, Peter (MD) ChAP
Illinois Office of Mental Health, 203 N Wabash St 10th Floor; Chicago, IL 60601; (312) 814-4770; **BDCERT:** ChAP 97; Psyc 95; **MS:** U Hlth Sci/Chicago Med Sch 88; **RES:** Psyc, U Chicago Hosp, Chicago, IL 89-91; **FEL:** ChAP, U Chicago Hosp, Chicago, IL 91-93; **FAP:** Asst Prof Univ IL Coll Med; ***SI:** Young Adults; Adolescence*
1 Week

Pierce, Karen (MD) ChAP
Rush-Presbyterian-St Luke's Med Ctr
(see page 122)
2634 N Dayton St; Chicago, IL 60614; (773) 525-1218; **BDCERT:** Psyc 84; ChAP 85; **MS:** Univ IL Coll Med 78; **RES:** U Mich Med Ctr, Ann Arbor, MI 79-83; **FEL:** ChAP, U Mich Med Ctr, Ann Arbor, MI 81-83; **FAP:** Asst Prof Rush Med Coll

Poznanski, Elva (MD) ChAP
Rush-Presbyterian-St Luke's Med Ctr
(see page 122)
Elva Poznanski & Assoc Ltd, 1725 W Harrison St Ste 956; Chicago, IL 60612; (312) 942-8022; **BDCERT:** Psyc 64; **MS:** Canada 57; **RES:** ChAP, Lafayette Clin, Detroit, MI 60-62; Psyc, Lafayette Clin, Detroit, MI 58-60; **FAP:** Prof Rush Med Coll

Sandage, Scott (DO) ChAP
Lutheran Gen Hosp (see page 143)
Child & Adolescent Psych Svc, 8816 W Dempster St; Niles, IL 60714; (847) 723-8626; **BDCERT:** Psyc 85; ChAP 88; **MS:** Univ Osteo Med & Hlth Sci 78; **RES:** Psyc, Med Coll WI, Milwaukee, WI 79-81; **FEL:** ChAP, Med Coll WI, Milwaukee, WI 81-82; ChAP, Children's Mem Med Ctr, Chicago, IL 82-83

Taylor-Crawford, Karen (MD) ChAP
Christ Hosp & Med Ctr (see page 140)
1947 W 95th St; Chicago, IL 60643; (773) 298-2054; **BDCERT:** ChAP 85; Psyc 82; **MS:** Univ IL Coll Med 75; **RES:** Ped, U IL Med Ctr, Chicago, IL 75-76; Psyc, U IL Med Ctr, Chicago, IL 76-78; **FEL:** ChAP, Inst Juvenile Rsch, Chicago, IL 78-80
4+ Weeks

CHILD NEUROLOGY

Egel, Robert Terrell (MD) **ChiN**
Christ Hosp & Med Ctr **(see page 140)**
Christ & Hope Children's Hosp, 4440 W 95th St; Oak Lawn, IL 60453; (708) 346-5445; **BDCERT:** ChiN 79; Ped 77; **MS:** U Hlth Sci/Chicago Med Sch 71; **RES:** Ped, Children's Mem Med Ctr, Chicago, IL 72-73; ChiN, KY Med Ctr, Lexington, KY 73-76; **FAP:** Clin Prof N Univ IL Coll Med; ***SI:*** *Pediatric Neurology*; **HMO:** Blue Cross & Blue Shield, Humana Health Plan, Rush Health Plans

Huttenlocher, Peter (MD) **ChiN**
U Chicago Hosp **(see page 124)**
University-Chicago Hlth Systms, PO Box Mc3055; Chicago, IL 60637; (773) 702-6487; **BDCERT:** Ped 65; N 67; **MS:** Harvard Med Sch 57; **RES:** Ped, Children's Mem Med Ctr, Chicago, IL 60-61; **FEL:** N, Mass Gen Hosp, Boston, MA 61-64; **FAP:** Prof Path U Chicago-Pritzker Sch Med; ***SI:*** *Epilepsy; Tuberous Sclerosis*

Pasternak, Joseph F (MD) **ChiN**
Evanston Hosp
2650 Ridge Ave; Evanston, IL 60201; (847) 570-2577; **BDCERT:** N 81; Ped 80; **MS:** Washington U, St Louis 75; **RES:** Ped, St Louis Childrens Hosp, St Louis, MO 75-76; Washington U, St Louis, MO 76-79; **FAP:** Assoc Prof Northwestern U

CLINICAL GENETICS

Pergament, Eugene (MD) **CG**
Northwestern Mem Hosp
344 W Willow St D; Chicago, IL 60614; (773) 908-7441; **BDCERT:** CG 82; **MS:** U Chicago-Pritzker Sch Med 70; **RES:** Ped, U Chicago Hosp, Chicago, IL 72; **FAP:** Prof Northwestern U

COLON & RECTAL SURGERY

Abcarian, Herand (MD) **CRS**
Univ of Illinois at Chicago Med Ctr
675 W North Ave Fl 1; Melrose Park, IL 60160; (708) 450-5075; **BDCERT:** CRS 72; S 72; **MS:** Iran 65; **RES:** S, Cook Cty Hosp, Chicago, IL 66-71; CRS, Cook Cty Hosp, Chicago, IL 71-72; **FAP:** Prof Univ IL Coll Med; ***SI:*** *Colon and Rectal Cancer; Crohn's & Ulcerative Colitis*
LANG: Sp, Frs, Arm, Fr; Immediately

Bartizal, John (MD) **CRS**
Loyola U Med Ctr **(see page 120)**
3722 S Harlem Ave Ste 204; Riverside, IL 60546; (708) 863-1691; **BDCERT:** CRS 72; S 72; **MS:** U Hlth Sci/Chicago Med Sch 65; **RES:** CRS, Cook Cty Hosp, Chicago, IL 70-71; S, Cook Cty Hosp, Chicago, IL 66-70; **FEL:** Cook Cty Hosp, Chicago, IL 65-66; **FAP:** Assoc Clin Prof Loyola U-Stritch Sch Med, Maywood; **HOSP:** Macneal Mem Hosp; ***SI:*** *Hemorrhoids-Rectal Bleeding; Colon Cancer*; **HMO:** Aetna Hlth Plan, Blue Cross & Blue Shield, Chicago HMO, Travelers +
1 Week VISA

Hambrick, Ernestine (MD) **CRS**
Michael Reese Hosp & Med Ctr
30 N Michigan Ave Ste 1118; Chicago, IL 60602; (312) 782-4828; **BDCERT:** CRS 73; S 73; **MS:** Univ IL Coll Med 67; **RES:** S, Cook Cty Hosp, Chicago, IL 68-72; **FEL:** CRS, Cook Cty Hosp, Chicago, IL 72-73; **FAP:** Asst Clin Prof S Univ IL Coll Med

Saclarides, Theodore John (MD) **CRS**
Rush-Presbyterian-St Luke's Med Ctr **(see page 122)**
University Surgeons, 1725 W Harrison St Ste 810; Chicago, IL 60612; (312) 942-6543; **BDCERT:** CRS 89; S 96; **MS:** U Miami Sch Med 82; **RES:** S, Rush Presbyterian-St Luke's Med Ctr, Chicago, IL 82-87; **FEL:** CRS, Mayo Clinic, Rochester, MN 87-88; **FAP:** Assoc Prof Rush Med Coll; **HMO:** +
A Few Days

Weisman, Robert (MD) **CRS**
Lutheran Gen Hosp **(see page 143)**
1875 Dempster Ste 280; Park Ridge, IL 60068; (847) 318-9071; **BDCERT:** S 88; CRS 88; **MS:** U Hlth Sci/Chicago Med Sch 81; **RES:** S, Michael Reese Hosp Med Ctr, Chicago, IL 81-86; **FEL:** CRS, Cook Cty Hosp, Chicago, IL 86-87; **FAP:** Asst Clin Prof S Univ IL Coll Med; **HOSP:** Gottlieb Mem Hosp; ***SI:*** *Colon Rectal Cancer; Anorectal Disease*; **HMO:** Highland Park IPA
Immediately VISA

CRITICAL CARE MEDICINE

Hong, Dennis (MD) **CCM**
Univ of Illinois at Chicago Med Ctr
840 S Wood St; Chicago, IL 60612; (312) 996-8039; **BDCERT:** CCM 95; Pul 92; **MS:** U Hlth Sci/Chicago Med Sch 87; **RES:** Evanston Hosp, Evanston, IL 88-89; **FEL:** U IL Med Ctr, Chicago, IL 90-93; **FAP:** Asst Clin Prof Med Univ IL Coll Med
A Few Days VISA

Guide to symbols and abbreviations can be found on pages 110-113.

Luger, Gerald (MD) CCM
Gottlieb Mem Hosp
Pulmonary Medicine Assoc, 675 W North Ave Ste 212; Melrose Park, IL 60160; (708) 450-4557; **BDCERT:** CCM 96; IM 80; **MS:** Albert Einstein Coll Med 76; **RES:** IM, Boston Med Ctr, Boston, MA 77-80; **FEL:** Georgetown U Hosp, Washington, DC 80-82

Parrillo, Joseph E (MD) CCM
Rush-Presbyterian-St Luke's Med Ctr
(see page 122)
University Cardiologists, 1653 W Harrison St Ste 1159; Chicago, IL 60612; (312) 942-2998; **BDCERT:** CCM 95; A&I 77; **MS:** Cornell U 72; **RES:** A&I, Nat Inst Health, Bethesda, MD 74-77; IM, NY Hosp-Cornell Med Ctr, New York, NY 77-78; **FEL:** Cv, Mass Gen Hosp, Boston, MA 78-80; **FAP:** Dir CCM Rush Med Coll

Schmidt, Greg (MD) CCM
U Chicago Hosp **(see page 124)**
Section Of Pulmonary/Critical Care, 5841 S Maryland Avenue MC6026; Chicago, IL 60637; (773) 702-9660; **BDCERT:** IM 85; CCM 97; **MS:** U Chicago-Pritzker Sch Med 81; **RES:** IM, U Chicago Hosp, Chicago, IL 81-84; **FEL:** CCM, U Chicago Hosp, Chicago, IL 84-86; **FAP:** Professor CCM U Chicago-Pritzker Sch Med; ***SI:*** *Respiratory Failure; Pulmonary Embolism*
LANG: Sp, Ger; Mcr Mcd 2-4 Weeks

DERMATOLOGY

Caro, William (MD) D
Northwestern Mem Hosp
676 N Saint Clair St Ste 1840; Chicago, IL 60611; (312) 266-7180; **BDCERT:** D 66; **MS:** Univ IL Coll Med 59; **RES:** D, Hosp of U Penn, Philadelphia, PA 61-62; D, Hosp of U Penn, Philadelphia, PA 64-66; **FAP:** Prof of Clin D Northwestern U

Craig, Nona (MD) D
Evanston Hosp
1220 Meadow Rd Ste 210; Northbrook, IL 60062; (847) 559-0090; **BDCERT:** D 94; IM 90; **MS:** Northwestern U 87; **RES:** IM, Evanston Hosp, Evanston, IL 90-91; **FEL:** D, Northwestern Mem Hosp, Chicago, IL 91-94; **FAP:** Clin Instr Northwestern U
Mcr VISA

Feinberg, James (MD) D
Univ of Illinois at Chicago Med Ctr
University of Illinois at Chicago Medical Center-Dept of Dermatology, 1740 W Taylor St; Chicago, IL 60612; (312) 996-1193; **BDCERT:** D 86; **MS:** Univ IL Coll Med 74; **RES:** D, U IL Med Ctr, Chicago, IL 81-84; **FAP:** Assoc Prof D Univ IL Coll Med; **HOSP:** St Mary's of Nazareth Hosp Ctr

Fretzin, David (MD) D
Michael Reese Hosp & Med Ctr
Robin & Fretzin, 41 S Prospect Ave Ste 205; Park Ridge, IL 60068; (847) 823-1960; **BDCERT:** D 67; **MS:** U Iowa Coll Med 60; **RES:** IM, VA Hosp Hines, Hines, IL 63-64; D, U IL Med Ctr, Chicago, IL 64-67; **FEL:** AFIP, Washington, DC 67-68; **FAP:** Prof Path Univ IL Coll Med; **HMO:** Humana Health Plan

Gendleman, Mark (MD) D
Evanston Hosp
1220 Meadow Rd Ste 210; Northbrook, IL 60062; (847) 559-1502; **BDCERT:** D 76; **MS:** Northwestern U 71; **RES:** D, Northwestern Mem Hosp, Chicago, IL 72-75; **FAP:** Asst Clin Prof Northwestern U; **HOSP:** Glenbrook Hosp; ***SI:*** *Dermatological Manifestations of Systemic Disease*
SA SU Mcr 2-4 Weeks

Glazer, Scott (MD) D
Northwest Comm Hlthcare
Glazer & Clark, 1430 N Arlington Hghts Rd Ste 213; Arlington Hts, IL 60004; (847) 255-9150; **BDCERT:** D 82; **MS:** Northwestern U 78; **RES:** Northwestern Mem Hosp, Chicago, IL 78-82; **HMO:** Aetna Hlth Plan, Blue Cross & Blue Shield, Californiacare, Choicecare, Humana Health Plan

Hoag, J M (MD) D
Central DuPage Hosp
Fahey Medical Ctr, 581 E Golf Rd; Des Plaines, IL 60016; (847) 297-2240; **BDCERT:** D 95; Ped 89; **MS:** Univ IL Coll Med 85; **RES:** Ped, U Chicago Hosp, Chicago, IL 85-88; **FEL:** HO, U Chicago Hosp, Chicago, IL 89-90

Keane, John (MD) D
Christ Hosp & Med Ctr **(see page 140)**
Dermatology Center Assoc, 4647 W 103rd St Ste 2E; Oak Lawn, IL 60453; (708) 636-2840; **BDCERT:** D 77; DP 78; **MS:** Loyola U-Stritch Sch Med, Maywood 72; **RES:** IM, Milwaukee City Hosp, Milwaukee, WI 73-74; D, Rush Presbyterian-St Luke's Med Ctr, Chicago, IL 75-77; **FEL:** DP, U Chicago Hosp, Chicago, IL 77-78; **HOSP:** Little Company of Mary Hosp & Hlth Care Ctrs

Keuer, Edward J. (MD) D
Loyola U Med Ctr **(see page 120)**
1 S 260 Summit Rd; Oak Book Terrace, IL 60181; (630) 953-1190; **BDCERT:** D 79; Ped 79; **MS:** Loyola U-Stritch Sch Med, Maywood 74; **RES:** Ped, Illinois Masonic Med Ctr, Chicago, IL 75-76; D, Illinois Masonic Med Ctr, Chicago, IL 76-79; **FEL:** Ped D, Illinois Masonic Med Ctr, Chicago, IL 78-79; ***SI:*** *Pediatric Dermatology*; **HMO:** Blue Cross & Blue Shield, Affordable Hlth Plan
LANG: Sp; SA SU Mcr Immediately VISA

Kozeny, Keith (MD) D
Northwest Comm Hlthcare
Glazer & Clark, 1430 N Arlington Hghts Rd Ste 213; Arlington Hts, IL 60004; (847) 255-9150; **BDCERT:** D 86; **MS:** Loyola U-Stritch Sch Med, Maywood 82; **RES:** D, Cleveland Clinic Hosp, Cleveland, OH 83-86

La Voo, Elizabeth (MD) D
Columbus Hosp
467 W Deming Pl Ste 916; Chicago, IL 60614; (773) 327-3711; **BDCERT:** IM 79; D 81; **MS:** Northwestern U 76; **RES:** D, Northwestern Mem Hosp, Chicago, IL 76-79; IM, Northwestern Mem Hosp, Chicago, IL 78-81; ***SI:*** *Skin Cancer*; **HMO:** Humana Health Plan, Family Med Net, Blue Cross & Blue Shield
LANG: Sp; VISA

Levit, Fred (MD) D
Northwestern Mem Hosp
233 E Erie St Ste 307; Chicago, IL 60611; (312) 337-1611; **BDCERT:** D 62; **MS:** U Hlth Sci/Chicago Med Sch 53; **RES:** D, VA Rsch Hosp, Chicago, IL 56-57; D, Northwestern Mem Hosp, Chicago, IL 56-59; ***SI:*** *Fevers of Unknown Origin*

Levitt, Leonard (MD) D
Rush-Presbyterian-St Luke's Med Ctr
(see page 122)
6201 N California Ave Ste 104; Chicago, IL 60659; (773) 743-8936; **BDCERT:** IM 78; D 80; **MS:** Rush Med Coll 74; **RES:** IM, Rush Presbyterian-St Luke's Med Ctr, Chicago, IL 76-77; D, Rush Presbyterian-St Luke's Med Ctr, Chicago, IL 78-80; **FAP:** Asst Prof Rush Med Coll; **HOSP:** Edgewater Med Ctr; **HMO:** Blue Cross & Blue Shield

Liebovitz, Susan (MD) D
St Alexius Med Ctr
Northwest Dermatology, 2500 W Higgins Rd Ste 1040; Hoffman Estates, IL 60195; (847) 884-8096; **BDCERT:** D 81; **MS:** Northwestern U 76; **RES:** IM, Northwestern Mem Hosp, Chicago, IL 76-78; D, Northwestern Mem Hosp, Chicago, IL 78-81; ***SI:*** *Psoriasis; Skin Cancer*; **HMO:** Blue Cross & Blue Shield, HealthStar, Preferred Care +
2-4 Weeks VISA

Mandrea, Eugene (MD) D
Christ Hosp & Med Ctr **(see page 140)**
4700 W 95th St Ste 101; Oak Lawn, IL 60453; (708) 425-0669; **BDCERT:** D 64; **MS:** France 58; **RES:** Temple U Hosp, Philadelphia, PA 61-63; Cincinnati Gen Hosp, Cincinnati, OH 60-61

Morgan, Nathaniel (MD) D
11157 S Halsted St; Chicago, IL 60628; (773) 568-5800; **BDCERT:** D 78; **MS:** Univ IL Coll Med 74; **RES:** D, Illinois Masonic Med Ctr, Chicago, IL 75-78; **FEL:** U Chicago Hosp, Chicago, IL 78-79; **FAP:** Asst Clin Prof D U Chicago-Pritzker Sch Med

Paller, Amy Susan (MD) D
Children's Mem Med Ctr **(see page 139)**
Chlidren's Memorial Hosp, 2300 Children's Plaza Ste 107; Chicago, IL 60614; (773) 880-4698; **BDCERT:** Ped 82; D 83; **MS:** Stanford U 78; **RES:** Ped A&I, Children's Mem Med Ctr, Chicago, IL 79-81; D, Northwestern Mem Hosp, Chicago, IL 81-83; **FEL:** U NC Hosp, Chapel Hill, NC 83-84; **FAP:** Prof Ped Northwestern U; ***SI:*** *Pediatric Dermatology*

Robinson, June (MD) D
Loyola U Med Ctr **(see page 120)**
Loyola U Chicago, 2160 S First Ave; Maywood, IL 60153; (312) 908-8106; **BDCERT:** D 78; **MS:** U Md Sch Med 74; **RES:** IM, Greater Baltimore Med Ctr, Baltimore, MD 74-75; D, Dartmouth Hitchcock Med Ctr, Lebanon, NH 75-78; **FEL:** Chemo S, Bellevue Hosp Ctr, New York, NY 78-79; **FAP:** Prof Med Loyola U-Stritch Sch Med, Maywood; ***SI:*** *Skin Cancers*; **HMO:** +
1 Week

Shaw, James C (MD) D
Louis A Weiss Mem Hosp
Dermatology Office, 5841 S Maryland Ave MC 5067; Chicago, IL 60637; (773) 702-6559; **BDCERT:** D 85; **MS:** Boston U 78; **RES:** IM, Good Samaritan H & M Ctr, Portland, OR 80-81; D, Oregon Health Sci U Hosp, Portland, OR 82-85; ***SI:*** *Acne; Melanoma*; **HMO:** +
2-4 Weeks

Spero, Neal (MD) D
St Francis Hosp
Neal A Spero & Assoc, 2348 W Irving Park Rd Ste 110; Chicago, IL 60618; (773) 583-0200; **BDCERT:** D 66; **MS:** Univ IL Coll Med 61; **RES:** D, Northwest Comm Hlthcare, Arlington Heights, IL 62-65; **FAP:** Instr D Northwestern U; **HMO:** Aetna Hlth Plan, Blue Choice, Blue Cross & Blue Shield, Chicago HMO, Humana Health Plan

Wise, Ronald (MD) D
Illinois Masonic Med Ctr
(see page 118)
30 N Michigan Ave Ste 1301; Chicago, IL 60602; (312) 332-7303; **BDCERT:** D 79; **MS:** Univ IL Coll Med 74; **RES:** D, Rush Presbyterian-St Luke's Med Ctr, Chicago, IL 75-78; **FAP:** Asst Prof Rush Med Coll; **HOSP:** St Joseph Hosp-Chicago; **HMO:** UHC, Blue Cross & Blue Shield, HealthStar, HMO of IL +
LANG: Sp; 2-4 Weeks VISA

Woodley, David T (MD) D
Northwestern Mem Hosp
Northwestern Medical Faculty, 222 E Superior St Ste 300; Chicago, IL 60611; (312) 908-8106; **BDCERT:** D 82; IM 76; **MS:** Univ Mo-Columbia Sch Med 73; **RES:** D, U NC Hosp, Chapel Hill, NC 76-78; IM, U NE Med Ctr, Omaha, NE 74-76; **FEL:** D, Univ of Paris, Paris, France 78-80; **FAP:** Chrmn Northwestern U; **HMO:** Blue Cross & Blue Shield, CIGNA, Bay State Health Plan

DIAGNOSTIC RADIOLOGY

(See also Radiology)

Berlin, Leonard (MD) DR
Rush North Shore Med Ctr
Rush North Shore MC - Rad Dept, 9600 Gross Point Rd; Skokie, IL 60076; (847) 793-6111; **BDCERT:** DR 64; **MS:** Univ IL Coll Med 59; **RES:** U IL Med Ctr, Chicago, IL 60-63; **FAP:** Prof Rush Med Coll; ***SI:*** *Open MRI CT Mammography Scans*; **HMO:** Rush Prudential, Aetna Hlth Plan, Humana Health Plan, Blue Cross +

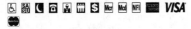

Bernstein, Joel R (MD) DR
Evanston Hosp
2650 Ridge Ave; Evanston, IL 60201; (847) 652-1865; **BDCERT:** DR 75; **MS:** Univ IL Coll Med 71; **RES:** DR, U Chicago Hosp, Chicago, IL 72-75; **FAP:** Assoc Prof Northwestern U; **HOSP:** Glenbrook Hosp; ***SI:*** *Mammography-Breast Imaging; Breast Needle Biopsy*

A Few Days VISA

Bresler, Michael E. (MD) DR
Macneal Mem Hosp
3249 S Oak Park Ave; Berwyn, IL 60402; (708) 783-9100; **BDCERT:** DR 93; **MS:** U Chicago-Pritzker Sch Med 88; **RES:** Northwestern Mem Hosp, Chicago, IL 93; Loyola U Med Ctr, Maywood, IL 89-93; **HMO:** +

Immediately VISA

Bronner, Abraham Jay (MD) DR
Ingalls Mem Hosp
One Ingalls Dr; Harvey, IL 60426; (708) 333-2300; **BDCERT:** DR 83; **MS:** Johns Hopkins U 80; **RES:** DR, Johns Hopkins Hospital, Baltimore, MD 80-83; ***SI:*** *Neuroradiology; MRI*; **HMO:** +

LANG: Fr; Immediately VISA

Cavallino, Robert (MD) DR
Illinois Masonic Med Ctr
(see page 118)
IL Masonic Med Ctr-Dept of Radiology, 836 W Wellington Ave; Chicago, IL 60657; (773) 883-0911; **BDCERT:** DR 68; **MS:** Tufts U 59; **RES:** Rad, NY Hosp-Cornell Med Ctr, New York, NY 64-67; **FAP:** Prof Rad Rush Med Coll; ***SI:*** *Muscular-Skeletal Imaging*; **HMO:** Aetna Hlth Plan, Blue Cross & Blue Shield, Californiacare, HealthNet, Humana Health Plan

Cuasay, Nestor (MD) DR
Roseland Comm Hosp
45 W 111th St; Chicago, IL 60628; (773) 995-3000; **BDCERT:** DR 78; **MS:** Philippines 69; **RES:** DR, Cook Cty Hosp, Chicago, IL 73-75; ***SI:*** *CT Scans; Ultrasound*

LANG: Sp, Fil;

Demos, Terrence (MD) DR
Loyola U Med Ctr (see page 120)
Loyola University Medical Center, 2160 S 1st Ave; Maywood, IL 60153; (708) 216-8625; **BDCERT:** DR 72; **MS:** Univ IL Coll Med 63; **RES:** U WI Sch Med, Milwaukee, MI 66-71; **FAP:** Prof Rad Loyola U-Stritch Sch Med, Maywood

Donaldson, James S (MD) DR
Children's Mem Med Ctr (see page 139)
2300 Children's Plaza; Chicago, IL 60614; (773) 880-4000; **BDCERT:** DR 83; PR 94; **MS:** Loma Linda U 78; **RES:** Rad, Loma Linda U Med Ctr, Loma Linda, CA 80-83; **FEL:** PR, Chldns Hosp, Los Angeles, CA 80-83

Enzmann, Dieter (MD) DR
Northwestern Mem Hosp
222 E Superior St Ste 140; Chicago, IL 60611; (312) 503-5103; **BDCERT:** DR 77; N 96; **MS:** Stanford U 73

Fuld, Irving (MD) DR
Little Company of Mary Hosp & Hlth Care Ctrs (see page 142)
3513 River Falls Dr; Northbrook, IL 60062; (708) 229-5651; **BDCERT:** DR 82; **MS:** Med Coll Wisc 78; **RES:** Rad, Albert Einstein Med Ctr, Bronx, NY 79-82; **FEL:** CT/US/MRI, Northwestern Mem Hosp, Chicago, IL 82-83

Immediately

Ghahremani, Gary (MD) DR
Evanston Hosp
2650 Ridge Ave; Evanston, IL 60201; (847) 570-2552; **BDCERT:** DR 72; **MS:** Germany 65; **RES:** DR, U Chicago Hosp, Chicago, IL 68-72; **FAP:** Prof Rad Northwestern U; ***SI:*** *Gastrointestinal Radiology; Abdominal Imaging*; **HMO:** Aetna Hlth Plan, Blue Cross & Blue Shield, Californiacare, Humana Health Plan, CIGNA +

LANG: Ger, Frs;
A Few Days VISA

Gore, Richard M (MD) DR
Evanston Hosp
Evanston Hospital-Dept Radiology, 2650 Ridge Ave; Evanston, IL 60201; (847) 570-2475; **BDCERT:** DR 81; **MS:** Northwestern U 77; **RES:** RadRO, Northwestern Mem Hosp, Chicago, IL 77-81; Moffit Hosp-UCSF, San Francisco, CA 81-82; **FAP:** Prof Rad Northwestern U; **HMO:** +
1 Week

Grant, Thomas H (DO) DR
Louis A Weiss Mem Hosp
Radiology Dept, Louis A Weiss Mem Hosp, 4646 N Marine Drive; Chicago, IL 60640; (773) 564-5148; **BDCERT:** DR 75; **MS:** Chicago Coll Osteo Med 70; **RES:** Michael Reese Hosp Med Ctr, Chicago, IL 71-74

Hansen, Jack (MD) DR
Holy Family Med Ctr
Des Plaines Radiologists, 1455 E Golf Rd Ste 212; Des Plaines, IL 60016; (847) 296-4220; **BDCERT:** DR 75; **MS:** Univ IL Coll Med 69; **RES:** Rush Presbyterian-St Luke's Med Ctr, Chicago, IL 72-75
Mcr Mcd

Heiser, William (MD) DR
St Joseph Hosp-Chicago
1955 N Maud Ave; Chicago, IL 60614; (773) 665-3240; **BDCERT:** Rad 70; **MS:** Northwestern U 63; **RES:** Rad, Chicago Wesley Mem Hosp, Chicago, IL 64-67; **FAP:** Instr Northwestern U; **HOSP:** Columbus Hosp; ***SI:*** *Mammography; Ultrasound*; **HMO:** Aetna Hlth Plan, Blue Cross & Blue Shield, Californiacare, CIGNA, Humana Health Plan
SA SU Mcr Mcd NFI Immediately
VISA

Lawson, Thomas (MD) DR
Loyola U Med Ctr (see page 120)
Loyola U-Stritch Sch Med, 2160 S First Ave; Maywood, IL 60153; (708) 216-5221; **BDCERT:** DR 70; **MS:** U Mich Med Sch 65; **RES:** UC San Francisco Med Ctr, San Francisco, CA 66-70; **FAP:** Prof & Chrmn Rad Loyola U-Stritch Sch Med, Maywood; ***SI:*** *Body Imaging; CT Ultrasound*; **HMO:** +
Mcr

Mafee, Mahmood (MD) DR
Univ of Illinois at Chicago Med Ctr
Univ Illinois Med Ctr, 1740 W Taylor St Ste 931; Chicago, IL 60612; (312) 996-0234; **BDCERT:** Rad 76; **MS:** Iran 69; **RES:** Rad, Albert Einstein Med Ctr, Bronx, NY 73-74; Rad, U IL Med Ctr, Chicago, IL 74-76; **FEL:** Neuroradiology, U IL Med Ctr, Chicago, IL 76-77; **FAP:** Prof Univ IL Coll Med; ***SI:*** *Eye Diseases; Ear Diseases*; **HMO:** HMO Illinois
LANG: Frs; SA SU Mcr Mcd A Few Days
VISA

Marinberg, Boris (MD) DR
St Anthony Hosp
St Anthony Hospital, 2875 W 19th St; Chicago, IL 60623; (773) 521-1710; **BDCERT:** Rad 86; **MS:** Russia 70; **RES:** DR, Michael Reese Hosp Med Ctr, Chicago, IL 78-81

Matalon, Terrence (MD) DR
Rush-Presbyterian-St Luke's Med Ctr (see page 122)
Diagnostic Radiology Dept Rush-Presby-St Lukes Hosp, 1653 W Congress Pkwy; Chicago, IL 60612; (312) 942-5781; **BDCERT:** DR 81; VIR 94; **MS:** Boston U 77; **RES:** DR, Northwestern Mem Hosp, Chicago, IL; **FEL:** Northwestern Mem Hosp, Chicago, IL 81-82; **FAP:** Assoc Prof Rad Rush Med Coll

Merrill, Timothy (MD) DR
La Grange Mem Hosp (see page 141)
Suburban Radiologists SC, PO Box 415; Western Springs, IL 60558; (708) 579-1616; **BDCERT:** Rad 74; **MS:** Univ Penn 66; **RES:** IM, Rush Presbyterian-St Luke's Med Ctr, Chicago, IL 67-68; DR, Rush Presbyterian-St Luke's Med Ctr, Chicago, IL 71-74

Miller, Frank (MD) DR
Northwestern Mem Hosp
Northwestern Mem Hospital-Dept of Radiology, Superior St and Fairbanks Ct; Chicago, IL 60611; (312) 908-2000; **BDCERT:** DR 93; **MS:** Northwestern U 88; **RES:** DR, Northwestern Mem Hosp, Chicago, IL 89-93; **FEL:** MRI, Brigham & Women's Hosp, Boston, MA 93-94; Ge, Hosp of U Penn, Philadelphia, PA 94; **FAP:** Asst Prof Rad Northwestern U

Rattner, Zachary (MD) DR
Evanston Hosp
Department of Radiology, 2650 Ridge Ave; Evanston, IL 60201; (847) 570-2265; **BDCERT:** DR 90; VIR 96; **MS:** Temple U 85; **RES:** Rad, Yale-New Haven Hosp, New Haven, CT 86-89; **FEL:** NuM, Johns Hopkins U, Baltimore, MD 89; VIR, Yale Med Sch, New Haven, CT 93-94; **FAP:** Asst Prof Northwestern U; **HMO:** Blue Cross & Blue Shield, Humana Health Plan

Guide to symbols and abbreviations can be found on pages 110-113.

Sacy, George (MD) DR
Good Samaritan Hosp (see page 274)
6910 S Madison; Willow Brook, IL 60521; (630) 275-1152; **BDCERT:** Rad 81; NRad 95; **MS:** Syria 74

Wasserman, David (MD) DR
Grant Hosp
Radiology Assoc, 550 W Webster Ave; Chicago, IL 60614; (773) 883-3895; **BDCERT:** DR 75; **MS:** Loyola U-Stritch Sch Med, Maywood 70; **RES:** DR, Loyola U Med Ctr, Maywood, IL 71-74; Loyola U Med Ctr, Maywood, IL; **HMO:** +
Immediately
VISA

ENDOCRINOLOGY, DIABETES & METABOLISM

Baba, Walten (MD) EDM
Swedish Covenant Hosp
Swedish Covenant Med Ed Ctr, 5145 N California Ave; Chicago, IL 60625; (773) 989-3808; **BDCERT:** IM 78; FP 95; **MS:** Iraq 59; **RES:** EDM, U Toronto Hosp, Toronto, Canada 70-72; **FEL:** U Sheffield, Sheffield, England 64-67; **FAP:** Assoc Prof U Chicago-Pritzker Sch Med

Baldwin, David (MD) EDM
Rush-Presbyterian-St Luke's Med Ctr (see page 122)
1725 W Harrison St Ste 250; Chicago, IL 60612; (312) 942-6163; **BDCERT:** IM 84; EDM 87; **MS:** Rush Med Coll 81; **RES:** Brigham & Women's Hosp, Boston, MA 81-82; Brigham & Women's Hosp, Boston, MA 82-84; **FEL:** EDM, U Chicago Hosp, Chicago, IL 84-86; **FAP:** Asst Prof Med Rush Med Coll; ***SI:*** *Diabetes*; **HMO:** HMO, Blue Cross & Blue Shield +
LANG: Sp; 2-4 Weeks
VISA

Berlinger, Frederick (MD) EDM
St Alexius Med Ctr
1575 Barrington Rd Ste 330; Hoffman Estates, IL 60194; (847) 490-9393; **BDCERT:** IM 87; **MS:** U Hlth Sci/Chicago Med Sch 63; **RES:** IM, Montefiore Med Ctr, Bronx, NY 64-65; IM, Bellevue Hosp Ctr, New York, NY 65-66; **FEL:** EDM, U Mich Med Ctr, Ann Arbor, MI 66-68; **FAP:** Prof of Clin Med Univ IL Coll Med; **HMO:** Aetna Hlth Plan, Blue Cross & Blue Shield, Californiacare, Metlife, Principal Health Care

Charnogursky, Gerald (MD) EDM
Macneal Mem Hosp
MacNeal Diabetes Ctr, 3722 Harlem Ave Ste 204; Riverside, IL 60546; (708) 442-0044; **BDCERT:** IM 82; EDM 87; **MS:** Univ Penn 79; **RES:** IM, Univ Hosp SUNY Syracuse, Syracuse, NY 79-82; **FEL:** EDM, Univ Hosp SUNY Syracuse, Syracuse, NY 84-86; **FAP:** Asst Clin Prof Loyola U-Stritch Sch Med, Maywood; ***SI:*** *Diabetes Mellitus; Thyroid Diseases*; **HMO:** Aetna Hlth Plan, Blue Cross & Blue Shield, United Healthcare, Humana Health Plan, Maxicare Health Plan +
2-4 Weeks

De Bustros, Andree C (MD) EDM
Christ Hosp & Med Ctr (see page 140)
Christ Hospital & Medical Center, 4440 W 95th St; Oak Lawn, IL 60453; (708) 346-4274; **BDCERT:** EDM 87; IM 85; **MS:** Lebanon 80; **RES:** EDM, Johns Hopkins Hosp, Baltimore, MD 81-84; IM, Johns Hopkins Hosp, Baltimore, MD 84-85; **FEL:** IM, American U Hosp, Beirut, Lebanon 80-81; **FAP:** Assoc Clin Prof Univ IL Coll Med; ***SI:*** *Diabetes; Thyroid*
A Few Days

De Groot, Leslie (MD) EDM
U Chicago Hosp (see page 124)
University-Chicago Medical Ctr - Mail Code 3090, 5841 S Maryland Ave; Chicago, IL 60637; (773) 702-1470; **BDCERT:** IM 60; **MS:** Columbia P&S 52; **RES:** IM, Columbia-Presbyterian Med Ctr, New York, NY 52-54; IM, Mass Gen Hosp, Boston, MA 57; **FEL:** EDM, Mass Gen Hosp, Boston, MA 57-59; **FAP:** Prof Med U Chicago-Pritzker Sch Med; ***SI:*** *Thyroid Disease*; **HMO:** Blue Cross & Blue Shield, Prudential
2-4 Weeks VISA

Dwarakanathan, Arcot A (MD) EDM
St James Hosp & Hlth Ctrs
St James Diabetes Ctr, 30 E 15th St Ste 314; Chicago Heights, IL 60411; (708) 709-2010; **BDCERT:** IM 74; EDM 77; **MS:** India 67; **RES:** VA Hosp -UCLA, Sepulveda, CA 72-73; IM, Ill Masonic Med Ctr, Chicago, IL 73-74; **FEL:** EDM, Cook Cty Hosp, Chicago, IL 74-75; **FAP:** Asst Prof Rush Med Coll; ***SI:*** *Thyroid; Osteoporosis*

Emanuele, Mary Ann (MD) EDM
Loyola U Med Ctr (see page 120)
2160 S 1st Ave Ste 117N; Maywood, IL 60153; (708) 216-0406; **BDCERT:** EDM 83; IM 78; **MS:** Loyola U-Stritch Sch Med, Maywood 75; **RES:** IM, Northwestern Mem Hosp, Chicago, IL 75-76; IM, Univ of Hawaii, Honolulu, HI 76-78; **FEL:** Loyola U Med Ctr, Maywood, IL 78-80; **FAP:** Prof Med Loyola U-Stritch Sch Med, Maywood; ***SI:*** *Diabetes Mellitus; Thyroid Disease*

Emanuele, Nicholas (MD) EDM
Loyola U Med Ctr (see page 120)
2160 S 1st Ave Bldg 117 Rm 25; Maywood, IL 60153; (708) 216-9218; **BDCERT:** IM 75; EDM 79; **MS:** Northwestern U 71; **RES:** IM, Cook Cty Hosp, Chicago, IL 71-72; IM, Hines VA Hosp, Chicago, IL 72-74; **FEL:** EDM, Northwestern Mem Hosp, Chicago, IL 74-76; **FAP:** Prof Loyola U-Stritch Sch Med, Maywood; **HOSP:** VA Med Ctr; ***SI:*** *Diabetes Mellitus; Thyroid Disease*; **HMO:** +
2-4 Weeks

Epstein, Paul A. (MD) EDM
Northwest Comm Hlthcare
Suburban Endocronology, 2010 S Arlington Heights Rd Ste 209; Arlington Hts, IL 60005; (847) 228-3200; **BDCERT:** IM 83; EDM 86; **MS:** Yale U Sch Med 80; **RES:** EDM, Hosp of U Penn, Philadelphia, PA 84-87; IM, Northwestern Mem Hosp, Chicago, IL 81-83; **HOSP:** Alexian Brothers Med Ctr; ***SI:*** *Thyroid-Fine needle aspiration; Osteoporosis*; **HMO:** Aetna Hlth Plan, CIGNA, Prudential, United Healthcare +
LANG: Sp, Itl; 2-4 Weeks VISA

Fogelfeld, Leon (MD) EDM
Michael Reese Hosp & Med Ctr
2929 S Ellis St; Chicago, IL 60616; (312) 791-3156; **BDCERT:** IM 96; **MS:** Italy 75; **RES:** IM, Assaf - Haroferh Hospital, Israel 77-82; **FEL:** EDM, Michael Reese Medical Center, Chicago, IL 87-90; ***SI:*** *Diabetis*; **HMO:** HMO, CIGNA
2-4 Weeks

Garcia-Buder, Sofia A (MD) EDM
St Joseph Hosp-Elgin
467 W Deming Pl Ste 712; Chicago, IL 60614; (773) 388-5685; **BDCERT:** EDM 95; IM 89; **MS:** Philippines 83; **RES:** IM, Mount Sinai Hosp Med Ctr, Chicago, IL 86-88; **FEL:** EDM, U IL Med Ctr, Chicago, IL 88-90; EDM, U Chicago Hosp, Chicago, IL 90-91; **FAP:** Clin Instr Northwestern U; ***SI:*** *Thyroid Disease; Diabetes*; **HMO:** +
1 Week

Jameson, James Larry (MD & PhD) EDM
Northwestern Mem Hosp
Northwestern Univ - Ctr Endo Metb & Mole Med, 303 E Chicago Ave Tarry 15; Chicago, IL 60611; (312) 503-0469; **BDCERT:** EDM 87; IM 85; **MS:** U NC Sch Med 81; **RES:** IM, Mass Gen Hosp, Boston, MA 82-83; **FEL:** EDM, Mass Gen Hosp, Boston, MA 83-85; **FAP:** Prof Med Northwestern U; ***SI:*** *Thyroid problems; Pituitary problems*
1 Week VISA

Klugman, Vanessa (MD) EDM
West Suburban Hosp Med Ctr
1 Erie Ct L500; Oak Park, IL 60302; (708) 763-6750; **BDCERT:** EDM 95; IM 92; **MS:** Univ IL Coll Med 89; **RES:** IM, Rush Presbyterian-St Luke's Med Ctr, Chicago, IL 89-92; **FEL:** EDM, U Chicago Hosp, Chicago, IL 92-94; **HOSP:** Oak Park Hosp; ***SI:*** *Osteoporosis; Diabetes*
A Few Days VISA

Landsberg, Lewis (MD) EDM
Northwestern Mem Hosp
250 E Superior St Ste 296; Chicago, IL 60611; (312) 908-8202; **BDCERT:** IM 71; **MS:** Yale U Sch Med 64; **RES:** IM, Yale-New Haven Hosp, New Haven, CT 65-66; Yale-New Haven Hosp, New Haven, CT 68-69; **FEL:** EDM, Nat Inst Health, Bethesda, MD 66-68; **FAP:** Prof Med Northwestern U; ***SI:*** *Hypertension; Diabetes*

Lindquist, John (MD) EDM
Evanston Hosp
2050 Pfingsten Rd Suite 170; Glenview, IL 60025; (847) 570-1410; **BDCERT:** EDM 87; IM 77; **MS:** Northwestern U 74; **RES:** IM, NW U-Evanston Hosp, Evanston, IL 75-76; IM, Mercy Hosp Med Ctr, San Diego, CA 76-78

Litvin, Julia (MD) EDM
Rush North Shore Med Ctr
9669 Kenton Ave Ste 103; Skokie, IL 60076; (847) 676-1333; **BDCERT:** EDM 87; IM 85; **MS:** Russia 71; **RES:** Morristown Meml Hosp, Morristown, NJ 79-80; Hennepin Co Med Ctr, Minneapolis, MN 80-82; **FEL:** EDM, U IL Med Ctr, Chicago, IL 83-85

Madison, Laird (MD) EDM
Northwestern Mem Hosp
Endocrinology of the Northwestern Med Faculty Foundation, 303 E Ohio St; Chicago, IL 60611; (312) 908-7970; **BDCERT:** IM 91; EDM 95; **MS:** Yale U Sch Med 86; **RES:** Brigham & Women's Hosp, Boston, MA 87-88; **FEL:** Mass Gen Hosp, Boston, MA 88-91; **FAP:** Asst Prof Northwestern U

Mazzone, Theodore (MD) EDM
Rush-Presbyterian-St Luke's Med Ctr
(see page 122)
1725 W Harrison St Ste 316; Chicago, IL 60612; (312) 942-6163; **BDCERT:** IM 80; EDM 83; **MS:** Northwestern U 77; **RES:** IM, UCLA Med Ctr, Los Angeles, CA 78-80; **FEL:** Met, U WA Med Ctr, Seattle, WA 80; **FAP:** Asst Prof IM Rush Med Coll

Metzger, Boyd (MD) EDM
Northwestern Mem Hosp
Northwestern University & Hosp-Endo Division, 303 E Ohio St Ste 460; Chicago, IL 60611; (312) 908-8023; **BDCERT:** IM 72; **MS:** U Iowa Coll Med 59; **RES:** EndoMetab, Michael Reese Hosp Med Ctr, Chicago, IL 60-63; **FEL:** Biochemistry, U WA Med Ctr, Seattle, WA 65-67; **FAP:** Prof Med Northwestern U

Molitch, Mark (MD) EDM
Northwestern Mem Hosp
Northwestern U Medical School, 303 E Chicago Ave; Chicago, IL 60611; (312) 503-4130; **BDCERT:** IM 72; EDM 75; **MS:** Univ Penn 69; **RES:** IM, Hosp of U Penn, Philadelphia, PA 70-72; **FEL:** EDM, UCLA Med Ctr, Los Angeles, CA 72-75; **FAP:** Prof Med Northwestern U

Guide to symbols and abbreviations can be found on pages 110-113.

Motto, George S (MD) EDM
Alexian Brothers Med Ctr
(see page 138)
Suburban Endocrinology, 2010 S Arlington Hts Rd Ste 209; Arlington Hts, IL 60005; (847) 228-3200; **BDCERT:** EDM 73; IM 71; **MS:** Loyola U-Stritch Sch Med, Maywood 66; **RES:** IM, U IL Med Ctr, Chicago, IL 67-69; IM, Mayo Clinic, Rochester, MN 69-70; **FEL:** EDM, U IL Med Ctr, Chicago, IL 72-74
LANG: Sp, Pol; VISA

Ruder, Henry (MD) EDM
Northwestern Mem Hosp
680 N Lake Shore Dr Ste 118; Chicago, IL 60611; (312) 503-6000; **BDCERT:** EDM 77; IM 72; **MS:** Northwestern U 67; **RES:** IM, Boston Med Ctr, Boston, MA 68-69; EDM, Nat Inst Health, Bethesda, MD 69-72; **FEL:** EDM, Northwestern Mem Hosp, Chicago, IL 72-74; **FAP:** Assoc Prof of Clin Med Northwestern U; ***SI:*** *Thyroid Cancer; Adrenal Disease*
LANG: Sp; 1 Week VISA

Schickler, Renee (MD) EDM
Ravenswood Hosp Med Ctr
4646 N Marine Dr; Chicago, IL 60640; (773) 275-9545; **BDCERT:** IM 80; EDM 83; **MS:** Med Coll Wisc 77; **RES:** IM, Milwaukee City Hosp, Milwaukee, WI 78-80; **FEL:** EDM, U IL Med Ctr, Chicago, IL 80-82; **FAP:** Asst Clin Prof Univ IL Coll Med; **HMO:** Aetna Hlth Plan, Blue Cross & Blue Shield, Californiacare, CIGNA, Healthamerica

Shah, Upendra (MD) EDM
Resurrection Med Ctr
7447 W Talcott Ave Ste 444; Chicago, IL 60631; (773) 631-8474; **BDCERT:** IM 82; EDM 85; **MS:** India 77; **RES:** Louis A Weiss Mem Hosp, Chicago, IL 78-81; **FEL:** EDM, U Ill Hosp, Chicago, IL 81-83; **FAP:** Asst Clin Prof Med U Chicago-Pritzker Sch Med; ***SI:*** *Diabetes; Thyroid Diseases*; **HMO:** Blue Cross & Blue Shield, HealthStar, HealthNet, CIGNA PPO, Preferred Plan +
2-4 Weeks

Sinsheimer, Erica (MD) EDM
St Francis Hosp
Endocrinology & Metabolism, 9933 N Lawler Ave Ste 228; Skokie, IL 60077; (847) 677-1330; **BDCERT:** IM 83; EDM 89; **MS:** Northwestern U 80; **RES:** IM, McGaw Med Ctr-Evanston Hosp, Evanston, IL 81-83; **FEL:** EDM, U IL Med Ctr, Chicago, IL 84-86; **FAP:** Asst Clin Prof Med Univ IL Coll Med; **HMO:** Aetna Hlth Plan, Blue Cross & Blue Shield, Choicecare, CIGNA, Prudential

Sizemore, Glen (MD) EDM
Loyola U Med Ctr (see page 120)
Loyola University Medical Center, 2160 S 1st Ave Bldg 117 11; Maywood, IL 60153; (708) 216-3238; **BDCERT:** IM 72; EDM 73; **MS:** U Rochester 63; **RES:** IM, U KY Hosp, Lexington, KY 63-67; **FEL:** EDM, Mayo Clinic, Rochester, MN 69-72; **FAP:** Prof Med Loyola U-Stritch Sch Med, Maywood; ***SI:*** *Thyroid Disease and Cancer; Osteoporosis*; **HMO:** +
2-4 Weeks VISA

Werner, Phillip Ladd (MD) EDM
Lutheran Gen Hosp (see page 143)
Advocate Medical Group, 1255 Millwaukee Ave; Park Ridge, IL 60025; (847) 795-2400; **BDCERT:** EDM 77; IM 75; **MS:** Univ IL Coll Med 72; **RES:** IM, U IL Med Ctr, Chicago, IL 73-74; **FEL:** EDM, U WA Med Ctr, Seattle, WA 75-77; **FAP:** Assoc Clin Prof Med Chicago Coll Osteo Med

FAMILY PRACTICE

Arguello, Maria (MD) FP
PCP
St Mary's of Nazareth Hosp Ctr
3556 N Pulaski Rd; Chicago, IL 60641; (773) 545-1866; **BDCERT:** FP 94; **MS:** Nicaragua 88; **RES:** FP, St Mary's of Nazareth Hosp Ctr, Chicago, IL 94-97; ***SI:*** *Diabetes; Hypertension*; **HMO:** HMO Illinois, HMO Blue
LANG: Sp, Pol; Immediately

Arya, Jai (MD) FP
PCP
Roseland Comm Hosp
Roseland Hospital, 67 W 111th St Ste 301; Chicago, IL 60628; (773) 995-3463; **BDCERT:** FP 96; EM 90; **MS:** India 69; **RES:** , Chandigar, India 71-74; Cook Cty Hosp, Chicago, IL 75-77

Bardwell, Jacqueline (MD) FP
PCP
Christ Hosp & Med Ctr (see page 140)
Christ Family Practice Center, 4400 W 95th St; Oak Lawn, IL 60453; (708) 346-5305; **BDCERT:** FP 87; **MS:** Univ IL Coll Med 84; **RES:** Rush Presbyterian-St Luke's Med Ctr, Chicago, IL 84-87; **FAP:** Asst Prof Univ IL Coll Med; **HMO:** Blue Cross & Blue Shield, Humana Health Plan, United Healthcare, Rush Pru

Becker, Bruce (MD) FP
PCP
St Mary's of Nazareth Hosp Ctr
Doctors Office, 5308 W Belmont Ave; Chicago, IL 60641; (773) 205-8200; **BDCERT:** FP 94; **MS:** U Hlth Sci/Chicago Med Sch 78; **RES:** S, U NC Hosp, Chapel Hill, NC 78-79; **FEL:** FP, St Mary's of Nazareth Hosp Ctr, Chicago, IL 79-81; **FAP:** Asst Prof U Chicago-Pritzker Sch Med; ***SI:*** *Preventive Medicine; Herbal Medicine;* **HMO:** Aetna Hlth Plan, Champus, Bay State Health Plan, Humana Health Plan, CIGNA PPO
Immediately

Beusse, Walter (DO) FP
PCP
St Alexius Med Ctr
North Suburban Clinic, 1124 W Stearns Rd; Bartlett, IL 60103; (630) 213-7788; **BDCERT:** FP 92; **MS:** Chicago Coll Osteo Med 80; **HOSP:** Alexian Brothers Med Ctr
VISA

Blair, Kenneth (MD) FP
PCP
West Suburban Hosp Med Ctr
Family Practice Ctr, 7411 Lake St Ste 1120; River Forest, IL 60305; (708) 216-1116; **BDCERT:** FP 93; **MS:** Wayne State U Sch Med 75

Blankemeier, Julie (MD) FP
PCP
Lutheran Gen Hosp **(see page 143)**
Advocate Medical Group, 1 N Broadway St; Des Plaines, IL 60016; (847) 298-3150; **BDCERT:** FP 93; **MS:** Northwestern U 90
LANG: Sp;
1 Week VISA

Blumen, Edward (MD) FP
PCP
Evanston Hosp
ENH, 500 Davis St; Evanston, IL 60201; (847) 866-3700; **BDCERT:** FP 94; **MS:** U Hlth Sci/Chicago Med Sch 73; **RES:** IM, Cook Cty Hosp, Chicago, IL 74; **HMO:** Humana Health Plan
Immediately
VISA

Brander, William (MD) FP
PCP
Lutheran Gen Hosp **(see page 143)**
Advocate Medical Group, 1600 Dempster St Ste 120; Park Ridge, IL 60068; (847) 296-5500; **BDCERT:** FP 95; **MS:** Rush Med Coll 86; **RES:** FP, Lutheran Gen Hosp, Park Ridge, IL 86-89; **HMO:** Blue Cross & Blue Shield, Chicago HMO
VISA

Burns, Elizabeth (MD) FP
PCP
Univ of Illinois at Chicago Med Ctr
Family Medicine Dept, 1919 W Taylor St Ste 145AHP; Chicago, IL 60612; (312) 996-1103; **BDCERT:** FP 97; **MS:** U Mich Med Sch 76; **RES:** FP, Harrisburg Hosp, Harrisburg, PA 77-79; **FEL:** FP, U IA Hosp, Iowa City, IA 79-81

Casey, Gerald M (MD) FP
PCP
Palos Comm Hosp
11824 Southwest Hwy; Palos Heights, IL 60463; (708) 361-2160; **BDCERT:** FP 94; **MS:** Northwestern U 75; **RES:** ObG, Loyola U Med Ctr, Maywood, IL 77-78; FP, Resurrection Med Ctr, Chicago, IL 78-80

Cherny, Yuri (MD) FP
PCP
Swedish Covenant Hosp
Cherny's Medical Ctr, 3217 W Devon Ave; Chicago, IL 60659; (773) 743-6600; **BDCERT:** FP 93; **MS:** Italy 80; **RES:** FP, St Mary's of Nazareth Hosp Ctr, Chicago, IL 81-84; **FAP:** Asst Prof Chicago Coll Osteo Med

Collins, Mark (MD) FP
PCP
Alexian Brothers Med Ctr
(see page 138)
Bonaventure Medical-Elk Grove, 901 Biesterfield Rd Ste 306; Elk Grove Village, IL 60007; (847) 593-6420; **BDCERT:** FP 94; Ger 90; **MS:** Northwestern U 79
VISA

Cullinane, Kevin (MD) FP
PCP
West Suburban Hosp Med Ctr
West Suburban Family Practice, 7411 Lake St Ste 1120; River Forest, IL 60305; (708) 488-1490; **BDCERT:** FP 93; **MS:** Rush Med Coll 84; **HMO:** Blue Cross & Blue Shield, Chicago HMO, Humana Health Plan, Metlife, Prudential

Cupic, Dragana (MD) FP
PCP
Christ Hosp & Med Ctr **(see page 140)**
Advanced Medical, 4201 W 95th St; Oak Lawn, IL 60453; (708) 636-1466; **BDCERT:** FP 94; **MS:** Yugoslavia 64

Daum, Thomas (MD) FP
PCP
Little Company of Mary Hosp & Hlth Care Ctrs **(see page 142)**
Evergreen Medical, 2850 W 95th St Ste 403; Evergreen Park, IL 60805; (708) 423-2662; **BDCERT:** FP 93; **MS:** Univ Ky Coll Med 78; **RES:** FP, St Joseph Med Ctr, South Bend, IN 78-81

Di'Pasquo, Raymond (DO) FP
PCP
St Francis Hosp
14300 Ravenia Ave; Orland Park, IL 60462; (708) 403-5655; **BDCERT:** FP 84; **MS:** Chicago Coll Osteo Med 83; **HOSP:** Palos Comm Hosp
Immediately VISA

Dodda, Lakshmi (MD) FP
PCP
Jackson Park Hosp & Med Ctr
Jackson Park Hospital, 7501 S Stony Island Ave; Chicago, IL 60649; (773) 947-7310; **BDCERT:** FP 90; **MS:** India 78; **RES:** Ger, New York University Med Ctr, New York, NY 85-87; FP, Jackson Park Hosp & Med Ctr, Chicago, IL 87-90; ***SI:*** *Diabetes Mellitus; Hypertension*; **HMO:** Blue Cross & Blue Shield, Chicago HMO, Harmony, American Health Plan +
LANG: Sp, Hin, Tel; Immediately

Doot, Martin (MD) FP
PCP
Lutheran Gen Hosp (see page 143)
Advocate Medical Group, 701 Lee St Ste 220; Des Plaines, IL 60016; (847) 795-2875; **BDCERT:** FP 97; **MS:** Loyola U-Stritch Sch Med, Maywood 73; **RES:** FP, Macneal Mem Hosp, Berwyn, IL 73-76; **FAP:** Asst Prof FP Univ IL Coll Med; ***SI:*** *Addiction Medicine; Physician Health Programs*; **HMO:** Blue Cross & Blue Shield, United Healthcare, Medicare, Blue Choice PPO
1 Week VISA

Early, Michael (MD) FP
PCP
St Mary's of Nazareth Hosp Ctr
Chiao Monticello Medical Center, 3623 W Chicago Ave; Chicago, IL 60651; (773) 722-6171; **BDCERT:** FP 86; **MS:** Wright State U 82; **RES:** Cook Cty Hosp, Chicago, IL 83-85; **HOSP:** Bethany Hosp; **HMO:** Aetna Hlth Plan, United Healthcare, CIGNA, Humana Health Plan, Chicago HMO +
LANG: Sp; 2-4 Weeks

Eisenstein, Steven (MD) FP
PCP
Highland Park Hosp
Family Doctors of Northbrook, 1885 Shermer Rd; Northbrook, IL 60062; (847) 272-4600; **BDCERT:** FP 95; **MS:** Northwestern U 86; **RES:** FP, Riverside Regl Med Ctr, Newport News, VA 86-89; **FAP:** Asst Clin Prof Univ IL Coll Med; **HMO:** Aetna Hlth Plan, Blue Cross & Blue Shield, Californiacare, CIGNA, HealthNet
VISA

Evans-Beckman, Linda (MD) FP
PCP
Christ Hosp & Med Ctr (see page 140)
Family Practice Healthcare, 3913 W 95th St; Evergreen Park, IL 60805; (708) 422-4090; **BDCERT:** FP 94; **MS:** Rush Med Coll 85; **RES:** FP, Christ Hosp & Med Ctr, Oak Lawn, IL 85-88; **HOSP:** Little Company of Mary Hosp & Hlth Care Ctrs

Fischer, Calvin (DO) FP
PCP
St Alexius Med Ctr
Poplar Creek Family Practice Ltd, 1575 Barrington Rd Ste 115; Hoffman Estates, IL 60194; (847) 882-2400; **BDCERT:** FP 76; **MS:** Chicago Coll Osteo Med 69; **RES:** Detroit Osteo Hosp, Detroit, MI 69-70; **FAP:** Instr FP Chicago Coll Osteo Med; ***SI:*** *Back Pain*; **HMO:** Prudential, Blue Shield, Californiacare, Principal Health Care
2-4 Weeks VISA

Freedman, Mark (MD) FP
PCP
Ravenswood Hosp Med Ctr
Field Medical Group, 4025 N Western Ave; Chicago, IL 60618; (773) 588-2292; **BDCERT:** FP 81; **MS:** Univ IL Coll Med 78; **RES:** FP, West Suburban Hosp Med Ctr, Oak Park, IL 78-81; **FAP:** Clin Instr FP Univ IL Coll Med; ***SI:*** *Family Oriented Obstetrics; Preventive Medicine*; **HMO:** Blue Cross & Blue Shield, Humana Health Plan, CIGNA, United Healthcare
LANG: Sp, Heb, Fil, Rus, Bul; A Few Days VISA

Gomez, Carlos Alberto (MD) FP
PCP
St Mary's of Nazareth Hosp Ctr
5308 W Belmont; Chicago, IL 60641; (773) 205-8200; **BDCERT:** FP 94; **MS:** Costa Rica 86; **RES:** St Mary's of Nazareth Hosp Ctr, Chicago, IL 90-93

Goyal, Arvind (MD) FP
PCP
Northwest Comm Hlthcare
Family Doctor Ltd, 3407 Kirchoff Rd Ste 1; Rolling Meadows, IL 60008; (847) 255-0095; **BDCERT:** FP 94; **MS:** India 71; **RES:** FP, Cook Cty Hosp, Chicago, IL 72-75; **FEL:** PHGPM, U IL Med Ctr, Chicago, IL 75; **FAP:** Asst Clin Prof FP U Hlth Sci/Chicago Med Sch

Gros, William (MD) FP
PCP
La Grange Mem Hosp (see page 141)
10215 W Roosevelt Rd; Westchester, IL 60154; (708) 865-0018; **BDCERT:** FP 96; **MS:** Loyola U-Stritch Sch Med, Maywood 80; **HOSP:** Hinsdale Hosp
VISA

Grosdidier, Maureen (MD) FP
PCP
Lutheran Gen Hosp (see page 143)
Affiliated Family Physicians, 3633 W Lake Ave Ste 304; Glenview, IL 60025; (847) 998-0700; **BDCERT:** FP 94; **MS:** Univ IL Coll Med 85; **RES:** FP, Lutheran Gen Hosp, Park Ridge, IL 85-88; **HMO:** Blue Cross & Blue Shield, Chicago HMO, Bay State Health Plan, Humana Health Plan, Prudential

Hannon, Margaret (MD) FP
PCP
La Grange Mem Hosp (see page 141)
Family Medical Ctr, 606 W Burlington Ave; La Grange, IL 60525; (708) 354-6332; **BDCERT:** FP 90; **MS:** U Hlth Sci/Chicago Med Sch 87; **RES:** FP, La Grange Mem Hosp, La Grange, IL 87-90; **HMO:** +

Hernandez, Jose (MD) FP
PCP
Norwegian-American Hosp
2404 W Augusta Blvd; Chicago, IL 60622; (773) 276-1333; **BDCERT:** FP 95; **MS:** Cuba 59; **HMO:** Aetna Hlth Plan, Blue Cross & Blue Shield, Californiacare, Healthplus, Heritage National Healthplan

Homan, Diane (MD) FP
PCP
Christ Hosp & Med Ctr (see page 140)
University Family Physicians, 7000 W 111th St Ste 210; Worth, IL 60482; (708) 923-9810; **BDCERT:** FP 93; **MS:** Ind U Sch Med 84; **RES:** FP, Rush Presbyterian-St Luke's Med Ctr, Chicago, IL 84-87; **FEL:** FP, Rush Presbyterian-St Luke's Med Ctr, Chicago, IL 87-88; **FAP:** Asst Prof Rush Med Coll; **HOSP:** Rush-Presbyterian-St Luke's Med Ctr; **HMO:** Blue Cross & Blue Shield, CIGNA, Bay State Health Plan, Metlife, Prudential

Iagmin, Peter (MD) FP
PCP
St James Hosp & Hlth Ctrs
Horizon Health Care, 2605 W Lincoln Hwy Suite 130; Olympia Fields, IL 60461; (708) 747-9780; **BDCERT:** FP 89; **MS:** U Colo Sch Med 63; **HMO:** Blue Cross & Blue Shield, Choicecare, Healthamerica, MD Individual Practice Assoc, Metlife

Kelly, Derek (MD) FP
PCP
Swedish Covenant Hosp
Sauganash-Health Assoc, 6341 N Pulaski Rd; Chicago, IL 60646; (773) 588-8484; **BDCERT:** FP 96; **MS:** Ireland 78; **RES:** FP, Swedish Covenant Hosp, Chicago, IL 80-82; **HMO:** Aetna Hlth Plan, Blue Cross & Blue Shield, Chicago HMO, CIGNA, Humana Health Plan

Levy, Howard (MD) FP
PCP
Louis A Weiss Mem Hosp
Pediatric Ctr of Chicago, 4646 N Marine Dr; Chicago, IL 60640; (773) 564-7338; **BDCERT:** FP 93; Ped 77; **MS:** Univ IL Coll Med 68; **RES:** Rush Presby-St Luke's Med Ctr, Chicago, IL 70-72; Children's Mem Hosp, Chicago, IL 73-75; **FEL:** PNep, Children's Mem Med Ctr, Chicago, IL 73-75; **FAP:** Assoc Prof Rush Med Coll

Lipsky, Martin (MD) FP
PCP
Evanston Hosp
Glenbrook Hospital - Dept of Family Medicine, 2100 Pfingstein Rd; Glenview, IL 60025; (842) 657-1827; **BDCERT:** FP 94; Ger 90; **MS:** Med Coll PA 79; **RES:** FP, UC Irvine Med Ctr, Orange, CA 79-82; **FEL:** Primary Care, Mich State U, Lansing, MI 86; **FAP:** Prof/Chair FP Northwestern U; **HOSP:** Northwestern Mem Hosp; ***SI:*** *Geriatrics; Type 2 Diabetes*; **HMO:** Blue Cross & Blue Shield, Humana Health Plan, United Healthcare, HMO, Aetna-US Healthcare +
A Few Days

Locke, Susan (MD) FP
PCP
West Suburban Hosp Med Ctr
7411 Lake St Ste 2210; River Forest, IL 60305; (708) 366-8200; **BDCERT:** FP 94; **MS:** Washington U, St Louis 85; **RES:** FP, West Suburban Hosp Med Ctr, Oak Park, IL 85-88

Lubben, Georgia (MD) FP
PCP
Jackson Park Hosp & Med Ctr
Friedell Clinic, 7531 S Stony Island Ave Ste 254; Chicago, IL 60649; (773) 947-7752; **BDCERT:** FP 96; **MS:** U Hlth Sci/Chicago Med Sch 89; **RES:** FP, Jackson Park Hosp & Med Ctr, Chicago, IL 81-84; **HMO:** Chicago HMO

March, Anthony (DO) FP
PCP
Lutheran Gen Hosp (see page 143)
Advocate Medical Grp, 1700 Luther Ln; Park Ridge, IL 60068; (847) 640-9180; **BDCERT:** FP 92; **MS:** Chicago Coll Osteo Med 81

Marchi, Michael (MD) FP
PCP
Resurrection Med Ctr
7447 W Talcott Ste 312; Chicago, IL 60631; (773) 763-7440; **BDCERT:** FP 91; **MS:** Univ IL Coll Med 63; **RES:** Cook Cty Hosp, Chicago, IL 63-64; **HOSP:** Ravenswood Hosp Med Ctr

Mc Donough, Richard (MD) FP
PCP
Good Shepherd Hosp
Barrington Family Physicians, 500 W Il Route 22; Barrington, IL 60010; (847) 381-3000; **BDCERT:** FP 92; **MS:** Univ IL Coll Med 75
Mcr VISA

Mercado, Ramiro (MD) FP
PCP
St Mary's of Nazareth Hosp Ctr
4206 W 26th St; Chicago, IL 60623; (773) 521-4305; **BDCERT:** FP 94; **MS:** Bolivia 75; **RES:** S, St Mary's of Nazareth Hosp Ctr, Chicago, IL 90-93

Guide to symbols and abbreviations can be found on pages 110-113.

O'Neill, Hugh (MD) FP
PCP
Christ Hosp & Med Ctr (see page 140)
Family Practice Healthcare, 3913 W 95th St; Evergreen Park, IL 60805; (708) 422-4090; **BDCERT:** FP 91; **MS:** U Hlth Sci/Chicago Med Sch 81; **RES:** S, Lenox Hill Hosp, New York, NY 73-77

Patel, Kokila (MD) FP
PCP
Resurrection Med Ctr
7447 W Talcott Ave Ste 216; Chicago, IL 60631; (773) 631-0566; **BDCERT:** FP 84; **MS:** Other Foreign Country 73; **RES:** Anes, George Elliot Hosp, Nuneaton, England 75-77; FP, Resurrection Med Ctr, Chicago, IL 79-82

Pector, Steven (DO) FP
PCP
Alexian Brothers Med Ctr (see page 138)
North Suburban Clinic, 701 Biesterfield Rd; Elk Grove Vlg, IL 60007; (847) 228-0712; **BDCERT:** FP 97; **MS:** Chicago Coll Osteo Med 88; **RES:** FP, MacNeal Mem Hosp, Berwyn, IL 88-91

Perish, Cressa (MD) FP
PCP
Ingalls Mem Hosp
Ingalls Family Care Ctr, 4647 Lincoln Hwy; Matteson, IL 60443; (708) 747-7720; **BDCERT:** FP 92; **MS:** Ohio State U 82; **RES:** FP, St Joseph's Hosp, Chicago, IL 83-85

Rothschild, Steven (MD) FP
PCP
Rush-Presbyterian-St Luke's Med Ctr (see page 122)
Neighborhood Family Practice, 1702 S Halsted St; Chicago, IL 60608; (312) 421-4126; **BDCERT:** FP 97; Ger 88; **MS:** U Mich Med Sch 80; **RES:** FP, Cleveland Metro Gen Hosp, Cleveland, OH 80-83; **FAP:** Asst Prof Rush Med Coll

Sadowski, Joseph (MD) FP
PCP
Resurrection Med Ctr
3466 N Pulaski Rd Fl 1; Chicago, IL 60641; (773) 736-7766; **BDCERT:** FP 86; **MS:** Poland 83; **RES:** FP, St Mary's of Nazareth Hosp Ctr, Chicago, IL 83-86; **HOSP:** St Mary's of Nazareth Hosp Ctr; **HMO:** Blue Cross & Blue Shield, Travelers

Sage, John (MD) FP
PCP
Lutheran Gen Hosp (see page 143)
Metro Family Practice, 1247 N Milwaukee Ave; Glenview, IL 60025; (847) 296-3040; **BDCERT:** IM 77; FP 77; **MS:** Loyola U-Stritch Sch Med, Maywood 73; **RES:** IM, St Elizabeth's Med Ctr, Boston, MA 74-75; FP, Lutheran Genl Hosp, Des Plaines, IL 74-75

Schwer, William (MD) FP
PCP
Rush-Presbyterian-St Luke's Med Ctr (see page 122)
7000 W 111th St; Worth, IL 60482; (708) 923-9810; **BDCERT:** FP 81; **MS:** Univ IL Coll Med 78; **RES:** FP, Christ Hosp & Med Ctr, Oak Lawn, IL 78-81; **FEL:** FP, Christ Hosp & Med Ctr, Oak Lawn, IL 81-82; **FAP:** Asst Prof Rush Med Coll

Slusinski, Bernard (DO) FP
PCP
Holy Cross Hosp
Holy Cross Outptnt & Phys Ctr, 6084 S Archer Ave Ste 203; Chicago, IL 60638; (773) 884-4150; **BDCERT:** FP 82; **MS:** Chicago Coll Osteo Med 79; ***SI:*** *Osteopathy; Diabetes*; **HMO:** +
Mcr Mcd Immediately VISA

Spishakoff, Leonard (MD) FP
PCP
St Elizabeth's Hosp
St. Elizabeth Hosp, Professional Bldg, 1431 N Claremont Ave Ste 406; Chicago, IL 60622; (773) 486-2712; **BDCERT:** FP 96; **MS:** Mexico 86; **RES:** FP, St Elizabeth's Hosp, Chicago, IL 93-96; **FAP:** Asst Clin Prof FP Univ IL Coll Med; **HOSP:** St Mary's of Nazareth Hosp Ctr; ***SI:*** *Asthma, Hypertension; Diabetes, HIV/Aids*

Sproul, Stephen (MD) FP
PCP
Lutheran Gen Hosp (see page 143)
Advocate Medical Group, 825 E Golf Rd; Arlington Hts, IL 60005; (847) 640-9180; **BDCERT:** FP 96; Ger 92; **MS:** Penn State U-Hershey Med Ctr 80; **RES:** FP, JFK Med Ctr, Edison, NJ 81-83; **FEL:** FP, Lutheran Gen Hosp, Park Ridge, IL 83-84; **FAP:** Univ IL Coll Med

Veldman, Marie Ann (DO) FP
PCP
Christ Hosp & Med Ctr (see page 140)
16750 S 80th Ave; Tinley Park, IL 60477; (708) 532-5900; **BDCERT:** FP 96; **MS:** Chicago Coll Osteo Med 87; **RES:** FP, Rush Presbyterian-St Luke's Med Ctr, Chicago, IL 87-90

Walsh, Katherine (MD) FP
PCP
West Suburban Hosp Med Ctr
7411 Lake St; River Forest, IL; (708) 488-1490; **BDCERT:** FP 94; **MS:** Loyola U-Stritch Sch Med, Maywood 80; **RES:** FP, West Suburban Hosp Med Ctr, Oak Park, IL 80-83; **FAP:** Clin Prof Loyola U-Stritch Sch Med, Maywood; ***SI:*** *Women's Health Issues; Geriatrics*; **HMO:** HMO Illinois, Rush Prudential, Humana Health Plan, Blue Choice
SA SU Mcr Mcd NFI Immediately VISA

Wollner, Timothy (DO) FP
PCP
Little Company of Mary Hosp & Hlth Care Ctrs (see page 142)
3754 W 95th St; Evergreen Park, IL 60805; (708) 425-9550; **BDCERT:** FP 88; **MS:** Chicago Coll Osteo Med 85

Zalski, Andrew (MD) FP
PCP
Illinois Masonic Med Ctr
(see page 118)
Rush-Illinois Masonic Fmly Ctr, 3048 N Wilton Ave 3rd Fl; Chicago, IL 60657; (773) 296-7400; **BDCERT:** FP 86; **MS:** Poland 82; **RES:** FP, Illinois Masonic Med Ctr, Chicago, IL 82-85; **HOSP:** Columbus Hosp

GASTROENTEROLOGY

Berkelhammer, Charles (MD) Ge
Christ Hosp & Med Ctr (see page 140)
Southwest Gastroenterology, 4400 W 95th St Ste 311; Oak Lawn, IL 60453; (708) 499-5678; **BDCERT:** IM 84; Ge 85; **MS:** Canada 80; **RES:** U Toronto Hosp, Toronto, Canada 80-84; **FEL:** GO, U Chicago Hosp, Chicago, IL 84-86; GO, U Toronto Hosp, Toronto, Canada 86-87; **FAP:** Assoc Prof Univ IL Coll Med; **HOSP:** Little Company of Mary Hosp & Hlth Care Ctrs; ***SI:*** *Digestive Diseases*; **HMO:** Blue Cross, HMO Illinois, CIGNA +
1 Week

Bresnahan, Joseph (MD) Ge
Macneal Mem Hosp
3722 S Harlem Ave Ste 102; Riverside, IL 60546; (708) 783-7000; **BDCERT:** IM 90; Ge 93; **MS:** Creighton U 87; ***SI:*** *Hepatology*; **HMO:** Aetna Hlth Plan, CIGNA, Blue Choice, CCN, Medicare +
2-4 Weeks VISA

Breuer, Richard (MD) Ge
Evanston Hosp
Evanston Northwestern Med Gr, 1000 Central St Ste 615; Evanston, IL 60201; (847) 869-5636; **BDCERT:** Ge 65; **MS:** Yale U Sch Med 57; **RES:** IM, Duke U Med Ctr, Durham, NC 62-65; **FEL:** EDM, Duke U Med Ctr, Durham, NC 64-65; Ge, U Chicago Hosp, Chicago, IL 65-67; ***SI:*** *Inflammatory Bowel Diseases; Liver Disease*; **HMO:** Preferred Plan, Blue Cross & Blue Shield, Californiacare, CIGNA, Humana Health Plan
2-4 Weeks

Castillo, Samuel (MD) Ge
St Elizabeth's Hosp
1431 N Western Ave Ste 133; Chicago, IL 60622; (312) 633-5909; **BDCERT:** IM 79; Ge 89; **MS:** Spain 66; **FAP:** Asst Clin Prof Med Chicago Coll Osteo Med; **HOSP:** St Mary's of Nazareth Hosp Ctr

Craig, Robert (MD) Ge
Northwestern Mem Hosp
Northwestern Medical Faculty, 680 N Lake Shore Dr Ste 822; Chicago, IL 60611; (312) 290-5620; **BDCERT:** Ge 75; IM 72; **MS:** Northwestern U 67; **RES:** IM, VA Rsch Hosp, Chicago, IL 68-69; IM, VA Rsch Hosp, Chicago, IL 71-72; **FEL:** Ge, Northwestern Mem Hosp, Chicago, IL 72-74; **FAP:** Prof Northwestern U; ***SI:*** *Malabsorption; Crohns Disease*; **HMO:** +
A Few Days VISA

Deutsch, Stephen (MD) Ge
West Suburban Hosp Med Ctr
1 Erie Ct; Oak Park, IL 60302; (708) 763-6585; **BDCERT:** Ge 83; IM 81; **MS:** Tufts U 78; **RES:** IM, U Chicago Hosp, Chicago, IL 78-81; **FEL:** Ge, U Chicago Hosp, Chicago, IL 81-83; **FAP:** Asst Clin Prof Loyola U-Stritch Sch Med, Maywood; **HMO:** Humana Health Plan, Rush Health Plans +
Immediately

Franklin, James L (MD) Ge
Rush-Presbyterian-St Luke's Med Ctr
(see page 122)
1725 W Harrison St Ste 358; Chicago, IL 60612; (312) 243-6316; **BDCERT:** IM 70; Ge 72; **MS:** Northwestern U 64; **RES:** IM, Northwestern Mem Hosp, Chicago, IL 65-66; Northwestern Mem Hosp, Chicago, IL 68-70; **FEL:** Ge, U Chicago Hosp, Chicago, IL 70-72; **FAP:** Assoc Prof Rush Med Coll; ***SI:*** *Inflammatory Bowel Disease; Colonoscopy*; **HMO:** Aetna Hlth Plan, Prudential
1 Week VISA

Ghazanfari, K (MD) Ge
Illinois Masonic Med Ctr
(see page 118)
Gastroenterology Assoc SC, 836 W Wellington Ave Ste 1410; Chicago, IL 60657; (773) 296-7071; **BDCERT:** IM 75; Ge 77; **MS:** Iran 70; **RES:** IM, Long Beach VA Hosp, Long Beach, CA 72-74; **FEL:** Ge, Hines VA Hosp, Chicago, IL 74-76; **FAP:** Asst Clin Prof Loyola U-Stritch Sch Med, Maywood; **HOSP:** St Joseph Hosp-Chicago; **HMO:** Share, Rush Prudential
A Few Days

Gluskin, Lawrence (MD) Ge
St Joseph Hosp-Elgin
2800 N Sheridan Rd Ste 506; Chicago, IL 60657; (773) 248-1616; **BDCERT:** IM 81; Ge 83; **MS:** Univ IL Coll Med 78; **RES:** U IL Med Ctr, Chicago, IL 79-81; **FEL:** Ge, Rush Presbyterian-St Luke's Med Ctr, Chicago, IL 81-83; **FAP:** Asst Prof Northwestern U

Hanan, Ira (MD) Ge
U Chicago Hosp (see page 124)
Univ of Chicago Hospitals, 5758 S Maryland Ave MC9028; Chicago, IL 60637; (773) 702-1459; **BDCERT:** IM 83; **MS:** SUNY Downstate 80; **RES:** IM, U Chicago Hosp, Chicago, IL 81-83; **FEL:** Ge, U Chicago Hosp, Chicago, IL 83-85

Guide to symbols and abbreviations can be found on pages 110-113.

Hanauer, Stephen (MD) Ge
U Chicago Hosp (see page 124)
Univ-Chicago-Gastroenterology, 5758 S Maryland Ave MC4076; Chicago, IL 60637; (773) 702-1466; **BDCERT:** IM 80; Ge 83; **MS:** Univ IL Coll Med 77; **RES:** IM, U Chicago Hosp, Chicago, IL 77-80; **FEL:** Ge, U Chicago Hosp, Chicago, IL 80-82; **FAP:** Prof Med U Chicago-Pritzker Sch Med; **SI:** *Inflammatory Bowel Disease*
4+ Weeks VISA

Jacobs, Jeffrey (MD) Ge
Rush North Shore Med Ctr
9555 Gross Point Rd; Skokie, IL 60076; (847) 679-3411; **BDCERT:** Ge 93; IM 88; **MS:** Jefferson Med Coll 85; **RES:** IM, St Francis Hosp, Hartford, CT 85-88; **FEL:** Ge, Lankenau Hosp, Philadelphia, PA 90-92; **HOSP:** Evanston Hosp; **SI:** *Hepatitis*; **HMO:** +
LANG: Rus; Immediately VISA

Jensen, Donald (MD) Ge
Rush-Presbyterian-St Luke's Med Ctr
(see page 122)
University Hepatologists, 1725 W Harrison Street Ste 204; Chicago, IL 60612; (312) 942-8910; **BDCERT:** IM 75; Ge 81; **MS:** Univ IL Coll Med 72; **RES:** IM, Rush Presbyterian-St Luke's Med Ctr, Chicago, IL 72-75; Ge, Rush Presbyterian-St Luke's Med Ctr, Chicago, IL 75-76; **FEL:** Ge, King's College Hosp, London, England 76-78; **FAP:** Associate Prof Ge Rush Med Coll; **SI:** *Liver Disease; Hepatitis*; **HMO:** Aetna-US Healthcare, Rush Health Plans, United Healthcare, CIGNA
A Few Days VISA

Kahrilas, Peter (MD) Ge
Northwestern Mem Hosp
Searle 10541, 320 E Superior St; Chicago, IL 60611; (312) 908-5620; **BDCERT:** IM 82; Ge 87; **MS:** U Rochester 79; **RES:** IM, U Hosp of Cleveland, Cleveland, OH 80-82; **FEL:** Ge, Northwestern Mem Hosp, Chicago, IL 82-84; Ge, Med Coll WI, Milwaukee, WI 84-86; **FAP:** Prof Med Northwestern U; **SI:** *Esophageal Physiology; Pathophysiology*; **HMO:** Northwestern POS, Rush Prudential, HMO Illinois +
LANG: Sp, Lth; 2-4 Weeks VISA

Klamut, Michael (MD) Ge
Loyola U Med Ctr (see page 120)
Loyola University, 2160 S 1st Ave Bldg 117 Rm 20A; Maywood, IL 60153; (708) 216-9229; **BDCERT:** IM 76; **MS:** Loyola U-Stritch Sch Med, Maywood 73; **RES:** IM, Loyola U Med Ctr, Maywood, IL 74-76; **FEL:** Ge, Loyola U Med Ctr, Maywood, IL 76-78; **FAP:** Assoc Prof Med Loyola U-Stritch Sch Med, Maywood; **HMO:** Blue Cross & Blue Shield +
1 Week VISA

Klygis, Linas (MD) Ge
Macneal Mem Hosp
6827 Stanley Ave; Berwyn, IL 60402; (708) 749-4617; **BDCERT:** Ge 93; IM 90; **MS:** Northwestern U 86; **RES:** IM, Northwestern Mem Hosp, Chicago, IL 87-89; **FEL:** Ge, Northwestern Mem Hosp, Chicago, IL 89-92

Konicek, Frank (MD) Ge
Illinois Masonic Med Ctr
(see page 118)
Ill Masonic Med Ctr, 836 W Wellington Ste 1410; Chicago, IL 60657; (773) 296-7071; **BDCERT:** Ge 75; IM 77; **MS:** Loyola U-Stritch Sch Med, Maywood 63; **RES:** IM, St Francis Hosp of Evanston, Evanston, IL 64-65; Hines VA Hosp, Chicago, IL 67-69; **FEL:** Ge, Hines VA Hosp, Chicago, IL 69-71; **FAP:** Assoc Clin Prof Med Loyola U-Stritch Sch Med, Maywood; **SI:** *Liver Diseases; Intestinal Diseases*; **HMO:** Humana Health Plan, Share, Prudential +
LANG: Sp; 1 Week

Lalyre, Yolanda (MD) Ge
Thorek Hosp & Med Ctr
3538 W Fullerton Ave; Chicago, IL 60647; (773) 772-1212; **BDCERT:** IM 97; Ge 81; **MS:** Univ IL Coll Med 74; **RES:** IM, U IL Med Ctr, Chicago, IL 75-77; **FEL:** Ge, Chicago VA Hlth Care System-Westside, Chicago, IL 77-79; **FAP:** Asst Clin Prof Univ IL Coll Med; **SI:** *Ulcers; Gastroesophageal Reflux*
1 Week

Layden, Thomas (MD) Ge
Univ of Illinois at Chicago Med Ctr
840 S Woods MC787; Chicago, IL 60612; (312) 996-5178; **BDCERT:** Ge 77; IM 72; **MS:** Loyola U-Stritch Sch Med, Maywood 69; **RES:** IM, Barnes Hosp, St Louis, MO 70-72; **FEL:** Ge, U Chicago Hosp, Chicago, IL 72-74; **FAP:** Prof Med Univ IL Coll Med

Levitan, Ruven (MD) Ge
Lutheran Gen Hosp (see page 143)
North Shore Gastroenterology, 4709 Golf Rd Ste 1000; Skokie, IL 60076; (847) 677-1170; **BDCERT:** Ge 68; IM 80; **MS:** Israel 53; **RES:** Mt Sinai Med Ctr, New York, NY 56-57; Beth Israel Hosp, Boston, MA 58-59; **FEL:** IM, Mem Sloan Kettering Cancer Ctr, New York, NY 57-58; **FAP:** Clin Prof U Chicago-Pritzker Sch Med; **HOSP:** Rush North Shore Med Ctr; **HMO:** Blue Cross & Blue Shield, Century Medical Health Plan, Choicecare, CIGNA, Compare Health Service

Muscarello, Vincent (MD) Ge
Palos Comm Hosp
9921 Southwest Hwy; Oak Lawn, IL 60453; (708) 425-9456; **BDCERT:** Ge 89; IM 85; **MS:** Loyola U-Stritch Sch Med, Maywood 82; **RES:** IM, Loyola U Med Ctr, Maywood, IL 82-85; **FEL:** Ge, Loyola U Med Ctr, Maywood, IL 86-88; **HOSP:** Little Company of Mary Hosp & Hlth Care Ctrs
4+ Weeks

Olinger, Edward (MD) Ge
Northwestern Mem Hosp
Northwestern Memorial Hosp, 707 N Fairbanks Ct Ste 920; Chicago, IL 60611; (312) 787-3369; **BDCERT:** IM 77; Ge 79; **MS:** Yale U Sch Med 72; **RES:** IM, U Chicago Hosp, Chicago, IL 73-74; Ge, Nat Inst Health, Bethesda, MD 74-76; **FEL:** Ge, Hosp of U Penn, Philadelphia, PA 76-78; **HMO:** +

Plotnick, Bennett (MD) Ge
Rush-Presbyterian-St Luke's Med Ctr
(see page 122)
University Gastroenterologists, 9700 N Kenton St Ste 3; Skokie, IL 60076; (847) 674-2087; **BDCERT:** IM 83; Ge 85; **MS:** Univ IL Coll Med 80; **RES:** IM, Lutheran Gen Hosp, Park Ridge, IL 80-83; **FEL:** Ge, Northwestern Mem Hosp, Chicago, IL 83-85; **FAP:** Asst Prof Med Rush Med Coll; **HMO:** Aetna Hlth Plan, Blue Choice, Blue Cross & Blue Shield, Chicago HMO, HealthNet

Rogers, B H Gerald (MD) Ge
Ravenswood Hosp Med Ctr
505 N Lake Shore Dr Ste 406; Chicago, IL 60611; (312) 828-9747; **BDCERT:** IM 69; Ge 77; **MS:** U Chicago-Pritzker Sch Med 62; **RES:** Ped A&I, U Chicago Hosp, Chicago, IL 65-66; IM, Northwestern Mem Hosp, Chicago, IL 66-68; **FEL:** Ge, U Chicago Hosp, Chicago, IL 69-71; **FAP:** Clin Prof U Chicago-Pritzker Sch Med; **HOSP:** Grant Hosp

Rosenberg, James (MD) Ge
Evanston Hosp
Northshore Gastroenterology, 510 Green Bay Rd; Kenilworth, IL 60043; (847) 256-3400; **BDCERT:** Ge 73; IM 80; **MS:** Northwestern U 67; **RES:** Michael Reese Hosp Med Ctr, Chicago, IL 68-70; **FEL:** Ge, U Chicago Hosp, Chicago, IL 70-73; **FAP:** Asst Clin Prof Med Northwestern U; **HMO:** Blue Cross & Blue Shield, Chicago HMO

Rosenthal, Gayle (MD) Ge
West Suburban Hosp Med Ctr
West Suburban Hosp Med Ctr, Dept of Gastroenterology, One Erie at Austin; Oak Park, IL 60302; (708) 383-6200; **BDCERT:** Ge 89; IM 87; **MS:** Univ IL Coll Med 84; **HMO:** +
LANG: Sp, Itl, Grk; 2-4 Weeks VISA

Ruchim, Michael (MD) Ge
Louis A Weiss Mem Hosp
Mid North Gastroenterlogists, 4646 N Marine Dr Ste 5100; Chicago, IL 60640; (773) 333-7581; **BDCERT:** IM 82; Ge 85; **MS:** Univ IL Coll Med 79; **RES:** IM, U IL Med Ctr, Chicago, IL 79-82; **FEL:** Ge, U IL Med Ctr, Chicago, IL 82-84; **HOSP:** U Chicago Hosp; ***SI:** Colon Cancer; Stomach Pains*; **HMO:** HealthStar, Blue Cross & Blue Shield, Californiacare, United Healthcare, Prudential +
A Few Days VISA

Sabesin, Seymour M (MD) Ge
Rush-Presbyterian-St Luke's Med Ctr
(see page 122)
University Gastroenterologists, 1725 W Harrison St Ste 339; Chicago, IL 60612; (312) 942-5861; **BDCERT:** Path 67; **MS:** NYU Sch Med; **FAP:** Prof Med Rush Med Coll

Sales, David (MD & PhD) Ge
Alexian Brothers Med Ctr
(see page 138)
Northwest Gastroenterologists, 850 Biesterfield Rd Ste 2002; Elk Grove Vlg, IL 60007; (847) 439-1005; **BDCERT:** IM 80; Ge 83; **MS:** U Chicago-Pritzker Sch Med 77; **RES:** IM, U Chicago Hosp, Chicago, IL 77-80; **FEL:** Ge, U Chicago Hosp, Chicago, IL 80-82; **HOSP:** Northwest Comm Hlthcare; ***SI:** Inflammatory Bowel Disease; Cancer Prevention*; **HMO:** +
A Few Days VISA

Schwartz, Jerrold (MD) Ge
Northwest Comm Hlthcare
Northwest Gastroenterologists Sc, 1215 S Arlington Heights Road; Arlington Heights, IL 60005; (847) 439-1005; **BDCERT:** Ge 77; IM 75; **MS:** Univ IL Coll Med 72; **RES:** IM, U IL Med Ctr, Chicago, IL 72-75; **FEL:** Ge, U IL Med Ctr, Chicago, IL 75-77; **HOSP:** Alexian Brothers Med Ctr; ***SI:** Colitis And Crohn's Disease; Ulcer Disease*
LANG: Rus, Heb, Sp; A Few Days VISA

Shah, Nikunj (MD) Ge
Ravenswood Hosp Med Ctr
1945 W Wilson Ave Ste 6117; Chicago, IL 60640; (773) 989-6960; **BDCERT:** IM 80; Ge 83; **MS:** India 73; **RES:** IM, Ravenswood Hosp Med Ctr, Chicago, IL 77-80; **FEL:** Ge, U Chicago Hosp, Chicago, IL 80-82; **FAP:** Clinc.Asst.Prof Ge U Chicago-Pritzker Sch Med; **HOSP:** U Chicago Hosp; ***SI:** Liver Disease; Hepatitis*; **HMO:** Blue Cross, United Healthcare, Californiacare, Humana Health Plan, Most
LANG: Guj; A Few Days VISA

Guide to symbols and abbreviations can be found on pages 110-113.

Sittler, Stephen (MD) Ge
Christ Hosp & Med Ctr (see page 140)
Southwest Gastroenterology, 9921 Southwest Highway; Oak Lawn, IL 60453; (708) 499-5678; **BDCERT:** IM 76; Ge 77; **MS:** Case West Res U 72; **RES:** IM, Cleveland Metro Gen Hosp, Cleveland, OH 73-75; **FEL:** Ge, U Texas SW Med Ctr, Dallas, TX 75-78; **HMO:** Aetna Hlth Plan, Blue Cross & Blue Shield, Chicago HMO, Choicecare, CIGNA

Smith, Matthew (MD) Ge
Westlake Comm Hosp
Associates in Digestive Diseases, 1111 Superior St Ste 307; Melrose Park, IL 60160; (708) 531-5240; **BDCERT:** Ge 93; **MS:** U Chicago-Pritzker Sch Med 87; **RES:** IM, U Chicago Hosp, Chicago, IL 88-90; **FEL:** Ge, U Chicago Hosp, Chicago, IL 90-92; **HMO:** Aetna Hlth Plan, Blue Cross & Blue Shield, Chicago HMO, CIGNA, Health Alliance Plan

Sparberg, Marshall (MD) Ge
Northwestern Mem Hosp
676 N Saint Clair St Ste 1525; Chicago, IL 60611; (312) 944-7080; **BDCERT:** IM 68; Ge 72; **MS:** Northwestern U 60; **RES:** IM, Barnes Hosp, St Louis, MO 61-63; **FEL:** Ge, U Chicago Hosp, Chicago, IL 63-65; **FAP:** Prof Med Northwestern U; ***SI:** Crohn's Disease; Ulcerative Colitis*; **HMO:** Blue Cross, PHCS, Rush Pru, Affordable Hlth Plan
LANG: Hun; 4+ Weeks

Sunbulli, Talal (MD) Ge
Christ Hosp & Med Ctr (see page 140)
G I Assoc, 10500 S Cicero Ave; Oak Lawn, IL 60453; (708) 424-1202; **BDCERT:** IM 76; Ge 81; **MS:** Syria 72; **RES:** IM, Cook Cty Hosp, Chicago, IL 73-76; Ge, Cook Cty Hosp, Chicago, IL 74-77; **HOSP:** Little Company of Mary Hosp & Hlth Care Ctrs

Tsang, Tat-Kin (MD) Ge
Evanston Hosp
North Shore Gastroenterology, 1824 Wilmette Ave; Wilmette, IL 60091; (847) 256-3355; **BDCERT:** IM 81; Ge 83; **MS:** Northwestern U 77; **HMO:** Aetna Hlth Plan, Blue Cross & Blue Shield, Humana Health Plan

Vanagunas, Arvydas (MD) Ge
Northwestern Mem Hosp
Gastroenterology & Hepatology, 675 N St Clair Ste 17-250; Chicago, IL 60611; (312) 908-5620; **BDCERT:** IM 77; Ge 81; **MS:** Univ IL Coll Med 73; **RES:** Ge, Northwestern Mem Hosp, Chicago, IL 78-80; ***SI:** Peptic Ulcer; Colon Cancer Screening*; **HMO:** HMO Illinois, CIGNA, Chicago HMO, Prucare
LANG: Lth, Sp; 2-4 Weeks VISA

Venetos, John (MD) Ge
Swedish Covenant Hosp
John Venetos Ltd, 7126 N Lincoln Ave; Lincolnwood, IL 60646; (847) 679-9900; **BDCERT:** IM 89; Ge 91; **MS:** Univ IL Coll Med 86; **RES:** IM, U IL Med Ctr, Chicago, IL 87-89; **FEL:** Ge, Loyola U Med Ctr, Maywood, IL 89-91; **FAP:** Clin Instr Univ IL Coll Med

Villa, Eduardo (MD) Ge
St Joseph Hosp-Chicago
622 N Milwaukee Ave; Prospect Heights, IL 60070; (847) 520-4887; **BDCERT:** Ge 93; IM 91; **MS:** Chile 83; **RES:** IM, Cook Cty Hosp, Chicago, IL 86-88; **FEL:** Ge, Cook Cty Hosp, Chicago, IL 88-90; **FAP:** Instr U Hlth Sci/Chicago Med Sch; **HOSP:** Holy Family Med Ctr

Wieland, John (MD) Ge
Holy Family Med Ctr
1625 Sheridan Rd; Wilmette, IL 60091; (847) 256-2292; **BDCERT:** Ge 85; IM 83; **MS:** Emory U Sch Med 70; **RES:** IM, Northwestern Mem Hosp, Chicago, IL 70-75; **HOSP:** Evanston Hosp
A Few Days

Winans, Charles (MD) Ge
U Chicago Hosp (see page 124)
University of Chicago, 5758 S Maryland Ave MC 9028; Chicago, IL 60637; (773) 702-6137; **BDCERT:** IM 68; Ge 70; **MS:** Case West Res U 61; **RES:** IM, U Hosp of Cleveland, Cleveland, OH 62-64; **FEL:** Ge, Boston U Med Ctr, Boston, MA 64-66; **FAP:** Prof U Chicago-Pritzker Sch Med

Zahrebelski, George (MD) Ge
St Alexius Med Ctr
Digest Disorders & Liver Ctr, 1575 N Barrington Rd Ste 235; Hoffman Estates, IL 60194; (847) 882-8300; **BDCERT:** Ge 90; IM 90; **MS:** Univ IL Coll Med 87; **RES:** IM, U IL Med Ctr, Chicago, IL 88-90; **FEL:** Hepatology, U NC Sch Med Hosp, Chapel Hill, NC 90-93; **HOSP:** Alexian Brothers Med Ctr; ***SI:** Hepatology*
LANG: Prt, Pol, Sp; 4+ Weeks VISA

Zarling, Edwin (MD) Ge
Loyola U Med Ctr (see page 120)
Loyola University Medical Ctr, 2160 S 1st Ave Bldg 117 25; Maywood, IL 60153; (708) 821-6799; **BDCERT:** IM 81; Ge 82; **MS:** Med Coll Wisc 76; **RES:** IM, Baptist Memorial Hosp, Memphis, TN 76-79; **FEL:** Ge, U KS Med Ctr, Kansas City, KS 79-82; **FAP:** Assoc Prof Loyola U-Stritch Sch Med, Maywood; ***SI:** Heartburn; Irritable Bowel Syndrome*; **HMO:** +
A Few Days

GERIATRIC MEDICINE

Birhanu, Kidanu (MD) Ger
PCP
Little Company of Mary Hosp & Hlth Care Ctrs (see page 142)
4901 W 79th St Ste 5; Burbank, IL 60459; (708) 229-1395; **BDCERT:** IM 88; Ger 90; **MS:** Greece 80; **RES:** IM, Grant Hosp, Chicago, IL 84-88; **FEL:** Ger, U Chicago Hosp, Chicago, IL 88-90; ***SI:*** *Dementia; Wound Care*; **HMO:** Humana Health Plan, Accord, HMO Illinois, Aetna Hlth Plan, American Health Plan
LANG: Grk, Amh; Immediately

Braund, Victoria (MD) Ger
Lutheran Gen Hosp (see page 143)
LGMG Geriatrics, 1775 Ballard St; Park Ridge, IL 60068; (847) 318-2500; **BDCERT:** Ger 89; IM 92; **MS:** U ND Med School 86; **RES:** Ger, U Chicago Hosp, Chicago, IL 89-91; IM, U ND Sch Med Affil Hosp, Fargo, ND 87-89; **FAP:** Asst Clin Prof Med U Chicago-Pritzker Sch Med
4+ Weeks

Fischer, Tessa (MD) Ger
St Francis Hosp
1325 W Howard St; Evanston, IL 60202; (847) 733-1495; **BDCERT:** Ger 90; FP 93; **MS:** Georgetown U 75; **RES:** FP, Cook Cty Hosp, Chicago, IL 75-78; **HOSP:** Evanston Hosp; ***SI:*** *Women's Health; Holistic Health*

Grant, Mark (MD) Ger
PCP
West Suburban Hosp Med Ctr
West Suburban Family Practice, 7411 Lake St Ste 1120; River Forest, IL 60305; (708) 488-1490; **BDCERT:** FP 86; Ger 92; **MS:** Med Coll Wisc 83; **RES:** FP, Cleveland Metro Gen Hosp, Cleveland, OH 84-86; **FEL:** FP, Cook Cty Hosp, Chicago, IL 87-88; **FAP:** Asst Prof Univ IL Coll Med

La Palio, Lawrence (MD) Ger
La Grange Mem Hosp (see page 141)
Geriatric Assessment Ctr, 5101 Willow Springs Rd; La Grange, IL 60525; (708) 579-4073; **BDCERT:** Ger 88; IM 79; **MS:** St Louis U 76; **RES:** IM, U IL Med Ctr, Chicago, IL 76-79; **FEL:** Ctr Ed Development, Chicago, IL 79-80; **FAP:** Assoc Prof Med Loyola U-Stritch Sch Med, Maywood; **HOSP:** Hinsdale Hosp; ***SI:*** *Alzheimer's Disease; Dementia*
A Few Days

Levinson, Monte (MD) Ger
Evanston Hosp
The Presby Homes, 3200 Grant St; Evanston, IL 60201; (847) 492-4842; **BDCERT:** Ger 90; IM 67; **MS:** Univ IL Coll Med 57; **RES:** Michael Reese Hosp Med Ctr, Chicago, IL 58-59; **FAP:** Assoc Prof Med Northwestern U

Pomerantz, Rhoda (MD) Ger
St Joseph Hosp-Elgin
2900 N Lake Shore Dr Fl 12; Chicago, IL 60657; (773) 665-3085; **BDCERT:** IM 71; Ger 88; **MS:** Med Coll PA 63; **RES:** IM, Rush Presbyterian-St Luke's Med Ctr, Chicago, IL 64-69

Repasy, Andrew Bela (MD) Ger
Northwestern Mem Hosp
680 N Lake Shore Drive; Chicago, IL 60611; (312) 503-6000; **BDCERT:** Ger 90; IM 84; **MS:** Loyola U-Stritch Sch Med, Maywood 81; **RES:** Northwestern Meml Hosp, Chicago, IL 81-84; **HMO:** +
LANG: Sp, Hun;
4+ Weeks VISA

Schwartz, Janice (MD) Ger
Northwestern Mem Hosp
Geriatric Evaluation Services, 250 Superior St Ste 148; Chicago, IL 60611; (312) 908-4525; **BDCERT:** Ger 92; Cv 81; **MS:** Tulane U 74; **RES:** IM, Cedars-Sinai Med Ctr, Los Angeles, CA 75-76; **FEL:** Cv, Cedars-Sinai Med Ctr, Los Angeles, CA 77-78; Cv, Stanford Med Ctr, Stanford, CA 78-81; **FAP:** Northwestern U

Sier, Herbert (MD) Ger
PCP
Lutheran Gen Hosp (see page 143)
1775 Ballard Rd; Park Ridge, IL 60068; (847) 318-2500; **BDCERT:** IM 83; Ger 97; **MS:** Med Coll Va 80; **RES:** IM, Lutheran Gen Hosp, Park Ridge, IL 81-83; **FEL:** Ger, UCLA Med Ctr, Los Angeles, CA 83-85; **FAP:** Clinical Profes Ger U Hlth Sci/Chicago Med Sch; ***SI:*** *Dementia*; **HMO:** Blue Cross & Blue Shield, United Healthcare, Health Direct, Humana Health Plan
2-4 Weeks VISA

Weise, Roger A (MD) Ger
Alexian Brothers Med Ctr (see page 138)
810 Biesterfield Rd G09; Elk Grove Village, IL 60007; (847) 364-6724; **BDCERT:** Ger 88; IM 81; **MS:** Univ IL Coll Med 78; **RES:** Rush Presbyterian-St Luke's Med Ctr, Chicago, IL 79-81; **FEL:** Ger, Rush Presbyterian-St Luke's Med Ctr, Chicago, IL 81-82

Guide to symbols and abbreviations can be found on pages 110-113.

GERIATRIC PSYCHIATRY

Buch, Piyush (MD) GerPsy
Christ Hosp & Med Ctr **(see page 140)**
7480 W College Drive Ste 203; Palos Heights, IL 60463; (708) 361-0540; **BDCERT:** GerPsy 91; Psyc 84; **MS:** India 73; **RES:** Psyc, Univ of Illinois at Chicago Psyciatric Institute, Chicago, IL 78-81; **FAP:** Asst Prof Rush Med Coll; **HMO:** +
A Few Days

Lee-Chuy, Ismael (MD & PhD) GerPsy
Alexian Brothers Med Ctr
(see page 138)
955 Beisner Rd; Elk Grove, IL 60007; (630) 695-8401; **BDCERT:** Psyc 90; **MS:** Philippines 79; **RES:** Psyc, U Chicago Hosps, Chicago, IL 82-86; N, Psyc- U Chicaco Hosps, Chicago, IL 86-88; **FEL:** GerPsy, Rush U, Chicago, IL 88-89

Luchins, Daniel (MD) GerPsy
U Chicago Hosp **(see page 124)**
5841 S Maryland Ave MC3007; Chicago, IL 60637; (773) 702-9716; **BDCERT:** GerPsy 92; Psyc 78; **MS:** Canada 73; **RES:** Douglas Hosp, Canada 75; St Mary's Hosp, Canada 76; **FEL:** Allan Mem Inst, Canada 76-77; **FAP:** Chf Psyc U Chicago-Pritzker Sch Med

Mershon, Stephen (MD) GerPsy
Evanston Hosp
1500 Waukegan Rd Ste 213; Glenview, IL 60025; (847) 998-5556; **BDCERT:** Psyc 86; GerPsy 91; **MS:** MC Ohio, Toledo 80; **RES:** Psyc, Northwestern Mem Med Ctr, Chicago, IL 81-84; **FEL:** GerPsy, Rush Presbyterian-St Luke's Med Ctr, Chicago, IL 84-85; **FAP:** Asst Prof Rush Med Coll; ***SI:*** *Depression; Dementia*

GYNECOLOGIC ONCOLOGY

Azizi, Freidoon (MD) GO
Resurrection Med Ctr
Columbus Hosp-ObGyn, 2520 N Lakeview Ave; Chicago, IL 60614; (773) 665-6458; **BDCERT:** ObG 77; GO 82; **MS:** Iran 67; **RES:** ObG, Pahlavi U, India 70-72; ObG, Mount Sinai Hosp Med Ctr, Chicago, IL 72-75; **FEL:** GO, U Chicago Hosp, Chicago, IL 75-78; Cytopathology, U Chicago Hosp, Chicago, IL 75-76; **FAP:** Asst Prof ObG Northwestern U; **HOSP:** St Joseph Hosp-Chicago; ***SI:*** *Radical Gynecologic Cancer Surgery*; **HMO:** Blue Cross & Blue Shield, Aetna Hlth Plan, United Healthcare, One Health Care +
LANG: Sp;
A Few Days

De Geest, Koen (MD) GO
Rush-Presbyterian-St Luke's Med Ctr
(see page 122)
1725 W Harrison St Ste 863; Chicago, IL 60612; (312) 942-6723; **BDCERT:** GO 97; ObG 97; **MS:** Belgium 77; **RES:** ObG, U Ghent, Ghent, Belgium 77-82; **FEL:** GO, Penn State Univ Coll Med, Hershey, PA 87-90; **FAP:** Asst Prof Rush Med Coll; **HMO:** +

Dini, Morteza (MD) GO
Illinois Masonic Med Ctr
(see page 118)
Ob-Gyn Dept, 901 W Wellington Ave; Chicago, IL 60657; (773) 296-7089; **BDCERT:** ObG 89; GO 82; **MS:** Iran 72; **RES:** ObG, Cook Cty Hosp, Chicago, IL 75-78; **FEL:** GO, Cook Cty Hosp, Chicago, IL 78-80; **FAP:** Assoc Prof Univ IL Coll Med; **HOSP:** St Mary's of Nazareth Hosp Ctr; **HMO:** Aetna Hlth Plan, Blue Cross & Blue Shield, Californiacare, CIGNA, Healthamerica

Dolan, James R (MD) GO
Lutheran Gen Hosp **(see page 143)**
Lutheran General Cancer Care, 1700 Luther Lane; Park Ridge, IL 60068; (847) 723-7758; **BDCERT:** GO 98; ObG 98; **MS:** Univ IL Coll Med 83; **RES:** ObG, St Francis Hosp of Evanston, Evanston, IL 83-87; **FEL:** GO, Loyola U Med Ctr, Maywood, IL 87-89; **HOSP:** St Francis Hosp of Evanston; ***SI:*** *Ovarian-Endometrial Cancer; Breast Diseases*; **HMO:** Blue Choice, CIGNA, Humana Health Plan, HMO Illinois, United Healthcare +
LANG: Sp;
A Few Days VISA

Fishman, David A (MD) GO
Northwestern Mem Hosp
333 E Superior St Ste 420; Chicago, IL 60611; (312) 908-7540; **BDCERT:** GO 98; ObG 95; **MS:** Tex Tech U Sch Med 88; **RES:** Yale-New Haven Hosp, New Haven, CT 89-92; **FEL:** ObG, Yale-New Haven Hosp, New Haven, CT 92-94; **FAP:** Asst Prof ObG Northwestern U; ***SI:*** *Ovarian Cancer*

Javaheri, Ghodrat (MD) GO
Mercy Hosp & Med Ctr
2525 S Michigan Ave; Chicago, IL 60616; (312) 791-5722; **BDCERT:** ObG 74; GO 77; **MS:** Iran 63; **RES:** ObG, U of Pittsburgh Med Ctr, Pittsburgh, PA 68-69; ObG, Michael Reese Hosp Med Ctr, Chicago, IL 69-72; **FEL:** GO, Metropolitan Hosp Ctr, New York, NY 72-74; **FAP:** Assoc Prof Univ IL Coll Med; **HMO:** Humana Health Plan, Chicago HMO +
LANG: Sp;

Lurain, John (MD) GO
Northwestern Mem Hosp
Northwestern Memorial Hospital, 333 E Superior St; Chicago, IL 60611; (312) 908-7365; **BDCERT:** ObG 77; GO 81; **MS:** U NC Sch Med 72; **RES:** ObG, U of Pittsburgh Med Ctr, Pittsburgh, PA 72-75; **FEL:** GO, Roswell Park Cancer Inst, Buffalo, NY 77-79; **FAP:** Prof ObG Northwestern U

Waggoner, Steven (MD) GO
U Chicago Hosp **(see page 124)**
University Of Chicago Dept Ob/Gyn, 5841 S Maryland Ave MC2050; Chicago, IL 60637; (773) 702-6123; **BDCERT:** ObG 92; GO 94; **MS:** U Wash, Seattle 84; **RES:** ObG, U Chicago Hosp, Chicago, IL 84-88; **FEL:** GO, Georgetown U Hosp, Washington, DC 88-91; **FAP:** Associate Prof. GO U Chicago-Pritzker Sch Med; **HOSP:** Little Company of Mary Hosp & Hlth Care Ctrs; ***SI:*** *Ovarian Cancer; Cervical Dysplasia*
LANG: Sp; 1 Week

Weiss, Regis (MD) GO
Northwest Comm Hlthcare
Chicago Gynecologic Oncology, 120 W Golf Rd Ste 214; Schaumburg, IL 60195; (847) 843-5100; **BDCERT:** ObG 81; GO 85; **MS:** McGill U 74; **RES:** ObG, Naval Med Ctr, San Diego, CA 76-78; **FEL:** GO, UC San Diego Med Ctr, San Diego, CA 79-81; **HOSP:** Alexian Brothers Med Ctr; ***SI:*** *Cervical Cancer; Ovarian Cancer*; **HMO:** +
A Few Days VISA

Yordan, Edgardo (MD) GO
Lutheran Gen Hosp **(see page 143)**
Luth Gen Hosp-Canc Care Ctr, Advocate Med Gp, 1700 Luther Ln; Park Ridge, IL 60068; (847) 723-8110; **BDCERT:** ObG 80; GO 83; **MS:** U Md Sch Med 72; **RES:** ObG, Columbia-Presbyterian Med Ctr, New York, NY 73-77; GO, Mem Sloan Kettering Cancer Ctr, New York, NY 76; **FEL:** GO, USC Med Ctr, Los Angeles, CA 77-79; **FAP:** Prof ObG Rush Med Coll; **HOSP:** Central DuPage Hosp; ***SI:*** *Ovarian Cancer; Endometrial Cancer*

HAND SURGERY

Bednar, Michael S (MD) HS
Loyola U Med Ctr **(see page 120)**
Loyola Univ Med Ctr - Dept Ortho, 2160 S First Ave Bldg 54; Maywood, IL 60153; (708) 216-3475; **BDCERT:** HS 95; OrS 94; **MS:** Harvard Med Sch 86; **RES:** OrS, Hosp For Special Surgery, New York, NY 87-91; **FEL:** HS, The Indiana Hand Ctr, Indianapolis, IN 91-92; **FAP:** Asst Prof OrS Loyola U-Stritch Sch Med, Maywood; ***SI:*** *Hand and Wrist Problems*
NFI A Few Days
VISA

Benson, Leon (MD) HS
Glenbrook Hosp
Suburban Orthopaedic Assoc Ltd, 3636 Westlake Ave Suite 300; Glenbrook, IL 60025; (847) 724-4197; **BDCERT:** HS 94; OrS 93; **MS:** Northwestern U 85; **RES:** OrS, Northwestern Mem Hosp, Chicago, IL 86-90; **FEL:** HS, Harvard Med Sch, Cambridge, MA 90-91; **HOSP:** Evanston Hosp

Derman, Gordon (MD) HS
Rush-Presbyterian-St Luke's Med Ctr
(see page 122)
800 S Wells St Ste 105; Chicago, IL 60607; (312) 408-0800; **BDCERT:** PlS 84; HS 89; **MS:** Rush Med Coll 75; **RES:** S, Loyola U Med Ctr, Maywood, IL 77-81; PlS, U Mich Hosp, Ann Arbor, IL 81-83; **FEL:** MicSRsch, Rush Med Coll, Chicago, IL 76; **FAP:** Asst Prof Rush Med Coll; **HOSP:** Evanston Hosp; ***SI:*** *Carpal Tunnel Syndrome; Nerve & Tendon Injuries*

Gonzalez, Mark Henry (MD) HS
Cook Cty Hosp
Univ of IL, 1835 W Harrison St; Chicago, IL 60612; (312) 633-6601; **BDCERT:** HS 92; OrS 90; **MS:** U Chicago-Pritzker Sch Med 80; **RES:** OrS, Univ of IL, Chicago, IL 82-85; Ohio State U Hosp, Columbus, OH 86; **FEL:** HS, U Louisville Hosp, Louisville, KY 86-87; **FAP:** Asst Prof Univ IL Coll Med; **HOSP:** Univ of Illinois at Chicago Med Ctr

Harris, Gerald D (MD) HS
Northwestern Mem Hosp
Bell Stromberg Harris & Nagle, 448 E Ontario St Ste 500; Chicago, IL 60611; (312) 337-6960; **BDCERT:** PlS 80; HS 90; **MS:** Univ IL Coll Med 73; **RES:** S, Northwestern Mem Hosp, Chicago, IL 74-77; PlS, Northwestern Mem Hosp, Chicago, IL 77-79; **FEL:** HS, UC San Francisco Med Ctr, San Francisco, CA 79; **FAP:** Asst Prof S Northwestern U

Jablon, Michael (MD) HS
Michael Reese Hosp & Med Ctr
Park Ridge Orthopedic, 401 W Talcott Rd; Park Ridge, IL 60068; (847) 825-2163; **BDCERT:** HS 89; OrS 81; **MS:** U Hlth Sci/Chicago Med Sch 74; **RES:** Michael Reese Hosp Med Ctr, Chicago, IL 75-78; **FEL:** HS, U Louisville Hosp, Louisville, KY 78-79; **FAP:** Asst Prof OrS Univ IL Coll Med; **HOSP:** Resurrection Med Ctr

Kagan, Robert (MD) HS
Alexian Brothers Med Ctr
(see page 138)
Kagan Plastic Surgery, 810 Biesterfield Rd Ste 308; Elk Grove Vlg, IL 60007; (847) 952-9333; **BDCERT:** HS 94; PlS 92; **MS:** Univ IL Coll Med 82; **RES:** PlS, Rush Presbyterian-St Luke's Med Ctr, Chicago, IL 83-87; **FEL:** PlS, Rush Presbyterian-St Luke's Med Ctr, Chicago, IL 87-89; **HOSP:** Condell Med Ctr; **HMO:** Aetna Hlth Plan, Blue Cross & Blue Shield, Californiacare, Chicago HMO, CIGNA

Light, Terry (MD) HS
Loyola U Med Ctr **(see page 120)**
Loyola University Medical Ctr, 2160 S 1st Ave; Maywood, IL 60153; (708) 216-4570; **BDCERT:** OrS 79; HS 99; **MS:** U Hlth Sci/Chicago Med Sch 73; **RES:** OrS, Yale-New Haven Hosp, New Haven, CT 74-77; **FEL:** HS, Hartford Hosp, Hartford, CT 77; **FAP:** Chf Loyola U-Stritch Sch Med, Maywood

Guide to symbols and abbreviations can be found on pages 110-113.

Nagle, Daniel J. (MD) HS
Northwestern Mem Hosp
Bell Stromberg Harris & Nagle, 448 E Ontario St Ste 500; Chicago, IL 60611; (312) 908-3366; **BDCERT:** Oto 86; HS 89; **MS:** Belgium 78; **RES:** OrS, Northwestern Mem Hosp, Chicago, IL 79-83; **FEL:** HS, Christine Kleinert Inst Hand & Microsurgery, Louisville, KY 83-84; **FAP:** Asst Prof S Northwestern U

Schenck, Robert (MD) HS
Rush-Presbyterian-St Luke's Med Ctr
(see page 122)
Hand Surgery Ltd, 1725 W Harrison St Ste 263; Chicago, IL 60612; (312) 243-6250; **BDCERT:** HS 98; PlS 73; **MS:** Univ IL Coll Med 55; **RES:** S, Western Penn Hosp, Pittsburgh, PA 67-69; PlS, Columbia-Presbyterian Med Ctr, New York, NY 69-71; **FEL:** HS, Hosp For Joint Diseases, New York, NY 62; HS, Roosevelt Hosp, Edison, NJ 71-72; **FAP:** Assoc Prof & Dir PlS; ***SI:*** *Carpal Tunnel Syndrome; Work Related Accidents*; **HMO:** Aetna Hlth Plan, Blue Cross & Blue Shield, CIGNA, Humana Health Plan, John Hancock +
LANG: Sp; 2-4 Weeks VISA

Vender, Michael (MD) HS
Alexian Brothers Med Ctr
(see page 138)
Hand Surgery Assoc, 515 Algonquin Rd Ste 120; Arlington Hts, IL 60005; (847) 956-0099; **BDCERT:** OrS 88; HS 89; **MS:** Univ IL Coll Med 79; **RES:** S, Northwestern Mem Hosp, Chicago, IL 80-81; OrS, Northwestern Mem Hosp, Chicago, IL 81-85; **FEL:** HS, Conn Combined Hand Svc, Hartford, CT 85-86

Wiedrich, Thomas (MD) HS
Northwestern Mem Hosp
Bell Stromberg Harris Nagle, 448 E Ontario St Ste 500; Chicago, IL 60611; (312) 337-6960; **BDCERT:** PlS 94; HS 95; **MS:** U Mich Med Sch 85; **RES:** S, Northwestern Mem Hosp, Chicago, IL 85-88; PlS, Northwestern Mem Hosp, Chicago, IL 88-91; **FEL:** HS, Indiana Hand Center, Indianapolis, IN 91-92; **FAP:** Asst Prof Northwestern U; **HOSP:** Highland Park Hosp; ***SI:*** *Hand Surgery; Microvascular Surgery*; **HMO:** Blue Cross & Blue Shield, Aetna Hlth Plan, Bay State Health Plan, Humana Health Plan, Rush Health Plans +
LANG: Sp; A Few Days VISA

HEMATOLOGY

Adler, Solomon (MD) Hem
Rush-Presbyterian-St Luke's Med Ctr
(see page 122)
1753 W Congress Pkwy; Chicago, IL 60612; (312) 942-5978; **BDCERT:** Hem 73; Onc 75; **MS:** Albert Einstein Coll Med 70; **RES:** Hem, Brookdale Univ Hosp Med Ctr, Brooklyn, NY 72-73; IM, Brookdale Univ Hosp Med Ctr, Brooklyn, NY 71-72; **FEL:** Hem, Rush Presbyterian-St Luke's Med Ctr, Chicago, IL 73-75; **FAP:** Prof Med Rush Med Coll; **HMO:** Anchor, Travelers, CIGNA, Blue Cross & Blue Shield +
LANG: Heb, Yd, Ger; A Few Days VISA

Banerji, Manatosh (MD) Hem
Macneal Mem Hosp
Hemotology & Oncology Assoc, 3245 Grove Ave; Berwyn, IL 60402; (708) 484-8400; **BDCERT:** Hem 74; Onc 75; **MS:** India 65; **RES:** IM, Hines VA Hosp, Chicago, IL 68-69; **FEL:** Hem, Hines VA Hosp, Chicago, IL 70-71; **FAP:** Asst Prof Rush Med Coll; **HOSP:** Westlake Comm Hosp

Baron, Joseph M. (MD) Hem
U Chicago Hosp (see page 124)
Univ of Chicago Hospital, 5841 S Maryland MC 2115; Chicago, IL 60637; (773) 702-6114; **BDCERT:** Hem 72; Onc 75; **MS:** U Chicago-Pritzker Sch Med 62; **RES:** IM, U Chicago Hosp, Chicago, IL 63-68; **FEL:** U Chicago Hosp, Chicago, IL 67-68; **FAP:** Assoc Prof Med U Chicago-Pritzker Sch Med; ***SI:*** *Bleeding and Clotting; Anemias and Platelet Problems*; **HMO:** +
VISA

Bitran, Jacob (MD) Hem
Lutheran Gen Hosp (see page 143)
Advocate Medical Group, 1700 Luther Ln; Park Ridge, IL 60068; (847) 723-2500; **BDCERT:** Hem 85; Onc 77; **MS:** Univ IL Coll Med 71; **RES:** Michael Reese Hosp Med Ctr, Chicago, IL 71-75; Rush Presbyterian-St Luke's Med Ctr, Chicago, IL 72-73; **FEL:** U Chicago Hosp, Chicago, IL 75-77; ***SI:*** *Breast Cancer; Malignant Lymphomas*; **HMO:** CIGNA, Humana Health Plan, Aetna Hlth Plan
LANG: Sp, Rus; Immediately VISA

Brown, Susan (MD) Hem
St Joseph Hosp-Chicago
2900 N Lake Shore Drive; Chicago, IL 60657; (773) 665-3290; **BDCERT:** Hem 92; Onc 91; **MS:** St Louis U 84
LANG: Sp; 1 Week VISA

Chediak, Juan (MD) Hem
Illinois Masonic Med Ctr
(see page 118)
Illinois Masonic Med Ctr-Creticos Cancer Ctr, 901 W Wellington Ave Fl 2; Chicago, IL 60657; (773) 296-7068; **MS:** Ecuador 66; **RES:** IM, Hosp Eugenio Espejo, Quito, Ecuador 66-68; Hem, Gen Hosp, Mexico City, Mexico 69-71; **FEL:** Hem, Michael Reese Hosp Med Ctr, Chicago, IL 71-73; **FAP:** Assoc Prof Med Rush Med Coll; ***SI:*** *Bleeding Disorders; Leukemia*

Drazkiewicz, Maciej K. (MD) **Hem**
St Mary's of Nazareth Hosp Ctr
2222 W Division St Ste 215; Chicago, IL 60622; (773) 282-5808; **BDCERT:** IM 94; OM 97; **MS:** Poland 83; **RES:** Hem, Univ Hosp SUNY Bklyn, Brooklyn, NY 92-95; IM, Ravenswood Hosp Med Ctr, Chicago, IL 89-92; **HMO:** CapCare, Blue Cross, Humana Health Plan, United Healthcare, Unicare Primary Plus +
LANG: Rus, Pol, Sp, Czc; Mcr Mcd Immediately

Galvez, Angel Galvez (MD & PhD) **Hem**
Illinois Masonic Med Ctr
(see page 118)
1219 Jackson Galvez; River Forest, IL 60305; (773) 296-7068; **BDCERT:** Hem 96; Onc 95; **MS:** Spain 82; **RES:** IM, Long Island Coll Hosp, Brooklyn, NY 86-89; **FEL:** HO, Columbia-Presbyterian Med Ctr, New York, NY 89-92; **FAP:** Asst Prof Onc Rush Med Coll
LANG: Sp, Cat; Mcr Mcd NFI A Few Days

Gilman, Alan (MD) **Hem**
St Joseph Hosp-Elgin
Hematology Onocology Assoc, 2900 N Lake Shore Dr Ste 9W; Chicago, IL 60657; (773) 665-3259; **BDCERT:** Onc 85; Hem 88; **MS:** Univ IL Coll Med 78; **RES:** IM, Hines VA Hosp, Chicago, IL 78-81; IM, Macneal Mem Hosp, Berwyn, IL 81-82; **FEL:** HO, Rush Presbyterian-St Luke's Med Ctr, Chicago, IL 82-86; **FAP:** Asst Prof Med Rush Med Coll

Gordon, Leo I (MD) **Hem**
Northwestern Mem Hosp
Northwestern Univ Med Sch, 303 E Chicago Ave; Chicago, IL 60611; (312) 908-5284; **BDCERT:** Med 79; Hem 78; **MS:** U Cincinnati 73; **RES:** Hem, U MN Med Ctr, Minneapolis, MN 76-78; Hem, U Chicago Hosp, Chicago, IL 78-79; **FEL:** IM, U Chicago Hosp, Chicago, IL 74-76; **FAP:** Prof Med Northwestern U

Green, David (MD) **Hem**
Northwestern Mem Hosp
Rehabilitation Institute, 345 E Superior St Rm1407; Chicago, IL 60611; (312) 908-4701; **BDCERT:** Hem 72; IM 87; **MS:** Jefferson Med Coll 60; **RES:** IM, Thomas Jefferson U Hosp, Philadelphia, PA 61-63; **FEL:** Hem, Thomas Jefferson U Hosp, Philadelphia, PA 63-64; **FAP:** Prof Northwestern U; ***SI:*** *Hemophilia*; **HMO:** Blue Cross & Blue Shield, Humana Health Plan, Prudential, United Healthcare +
SA SU Mcr Mcd NFI 2-4 Weeks

Gregory, Stephanie (MD & PhD) **Hem**
Rush-Presbyterian-St Luke's Med Ctr
(see page 122)
Consultants in Hematology, 1725 W Harrison St Ste 862; Chicago, IL 60612; (312) 942-5982; **BDCERT:** Hem 72; IM 72; **MS:** Med Coll PA 65; **RES:** IM, Rush Presbyterian-St Luke's Med Ctr, Chicago, IL 65-68; IM, Rush Presbyterian-St Luke's Med Ctr, Chicago, IL 68-69; **FEL:** Hem, Rush Presbyterian-St Luke's Med Ctr, Chicago, IL 69-72; **FAP:** Prof Med Southern IL U; ***SI:*** *Lymphomas; Leukemias*; **HMO:** Blue Cross & Blue Choice, Travelers, Humana Health Plan, United Healthcare, Prudential +
Mcr Mcd 1 Week **VISA**

Kaminer, Lynne (MD) **Hem**
Evanston Hosp
1209 Gregory Ave; Wilmette, IL 60091; (847) 570-2110; **BDCERT:** Hem 92; Onc 87; **MS:** Washington U, St Louis 82; **RES:** IM, Hosp of U Penn, Philadelphia, PA 82-85; **FEL:** HO, U Chicago Hosp, Chicago, IL 85-88; **FAP:** Asst Prof Northwestern U; ***SI:*** *Lymphoma; Bone Marrow Transplantation*; **HMO:** +
Mcr Mcd 2-4 Weeks

Kosova, Leonard (MD) **Hem**
Lutheran Gen Hosp **(see page 143)**
North Suburban Medical Cnsltnt, 8915 W Golf Rd FL 3; Niles, IL 60714; (847) 827-9060; **BDCERT:** Hem 72; Onc 75; **MS:** Univ IL Coll Med 61; **RES:** IM, Hines VA Hosp, Hines, IL 62-64; **FEL:** Hem, Cook Cty Hosp, Chicago, IL 64-65; **HOSP:** Holy Family Med Ctr; ***SI:*** *Breast Carcinoma; Lymphoma*

Lind, Stuart E (MD) **Hem**
Evanston Hosp
2650 Ridge Ave; Evanston, IL 60201; (847) 570-2515; **BDCERT:** Hem 82; IM 79; **MS:** NYU Sch Med 76; **RES:** IM, Northwestern Mem Hosp, Chicago, IL 77-79; **FEL:** Hem, Mass Gen Hosp, Boston, MA 79-81; **FAP:** Prof Northwestern U; ***SI:*** *Lymphoma; Coagulation*; **HMO:** +

Stein, Robert N (MD) **Hem**
Christ Hosp & Med Ctr **(see page 140)**
4400 W 95th St Ste 311; Oak Lawn, IL 60453; (708) 346-5671; **BDCERT:** Hem 78; IM 75; **MS:** U Hlth Sci/Chicago Med Sch 71; **RES:** Univ of Wisc, Milwaukee, WI 72-75; Hem, Mayo Clinic, Rochester, MN 75-77; **FAP:** Asst Prof Med Rush Med Coll; ***SI:*** *Leukemia; Malignant Lymphoma*; **HMO:** United Healthcare, CIGNA, BC/BS PPO, Humana Health Plan, Principal Health Care +
Mcr Mcd A Few Days **VISA**

Telfer, Margaret (MD) **Hem**
Michael Reese Hosp & Med Ctr
Michael Reese Hospital, 2929 S Ellis St Ste 1200RC; Chicago, IL 60616; (312) 791-3132; **BDCERT:** Hem 94; Onc 81; **MS:** Washington U, St Louis 65; **RES:** IM, Michael Reese Hosp Med Ctr, Chicago, IL 66-69; **FEL:** HO, Michael Reese Hosp Med Ctr, Chicago, IL 69-70; **FAP:** Assoc Prof Med Univ IL Coll Med; ***SI:*** *Blood Clotting; Cancer*; **HMO:** Humana Health Plan, United Healthcare, Aetna Hlth Plan, Blue Cross, Prudential +
Mcr Mcd A Few Days

Thomas, Korathu (MD) Hem
St Mary's of Nazareth Hosp Ctr
Cancer Care Ctr, 2222 W Division St Ste 210; Chicago, IL 60622; (312) 770-3205; **BDCERT:** Hem 80; **MS:** India 74; **RES:** St Joseph's Hosp, Chicago, IL 74-77; **FEL:** Hem, U Louisville Hosp, Louisville, KY 77-79; Onc, U Chicago Hosp, Chicago, IL 79-80; **FAP:** Asst Prof U Chicago-Pritzker Sch Med; **HOSP:** St Elizabeth's Hosp; ***SI:*** *Breast Carcinoma; Lung Carcinoma*; **HMO:** United Healthcare, Share
Immediately

Traynor, Ann Elizabeth (MD) Hem
Northwestern Mem Hosp
710 N Fairbanks Ct; Chicago, IL 60611; (312) 908-5284; **BDCERT:** Hem 90; IM 86; **MS:** Geo Wash U Sch Med 83; **RES:** Univ of Vermont, Burlington, VT 86; **FEL:** Hem, Rsch-Univ of Vermont, Burlington, VT 83-86

Wong, Alton (MD) Hem
Mercy Hosp & Med Ctr
5525 S Pulaski Rd; Chicago, IL 60629; (773) 585-1955; **BDCERT:** Hem 86; IM 81; **MS:** Med Coll Wisc 78; **HMO:** +
LANG: Sp; 2-4 Weeks
VISA

INFECTIOUS DISEASE

Andreoni, John (MD) Inf
Little Company of Mary Hosp & Hlth Care Ctrs (see page 142)
Southwest Infectious Disease & Internal Medicine, 11800 Southwest Hwy; Palos Heights, IL 60463; (708) 361-5778; **BDCERT:** Inf 94; IM 88; **MS:** Loyola U-Stritch Sch Med, Maywood 85; **RES:** IM, U Mich Med Ctr, Ann Arbor, MI 85-88; **FEL:** Inf, U IA Hosp, Iowa City, IA 90-94

Balling, David (MD) Inf
Louis A Weiss Mem Hosp
4646 N Marine Dr; Chicago, IL 60640; (773) 878-8700; **BDCERT:** IM 73; Inf 78; **MS:** Jefferson Med Coll 67; **RES:** IM, U IL Med Ctr, Chicago, IL 70-72; **FEL:** Inf, U IL Med Ctr, Chicago, IL 74-76

Citronberg, Robert (MD) Inf
Lutheran Gen Hosp (see page 143)
Advocate Medical Group, 1875 Dempster St Ste 210; Park Ridge, IL 60068; (847) 318-8977; **BDCERT:** IM 92; Inf 94; **MS:** U Conn Sch Med 89; **RES:** IM, Rush Presbyterian-St Luke's Med Ctr, Chicago, IL 90-92; **FEL:** Inf, Rush Presbyterian-St Luke's Med Ctr, Chicago, IL 92

Cook, Francis (MD) Inf
Evanston Hosp
ENH Medical Group, 2100 Pfingsten Rd; Glenview, IL 60025; (847) 657-5959; **BDCERT:** Inf 78; IM 74; **MS:** Med Coll Wisc 70; **HOSP:** Glenbrook Hosp
A Few Days VISA

Costas, Chris (MD) Inf
St Francis Hosp of Evanston
355 Ridge Ave; Evanston, IL 60202; (847) 316-2775; **BDCERT:** Inf 90; Ped 87; **MS:** Loyola U-Stritch Sch Med, Maywood 82; **RES:** Ped, Georgetown U Med Ctr, Washington, DC 83-87; **FEL:** Inf, U Chicago Hosps, Chicago, IL 87-89; **HMO:** Bc/BS, Aetna Hlth Plan +
LANG: Grk;
A Few Days VISA

Creticos, Catherine (MD) Inf
Illinois Masonic Med Ctr
(see page 118)
3019 Old Glenview Rd; Wilmette, IL 60091; (773) 296-7039; **BDCERT:** Inf 86; IM 84; **MS:** U Chicago-Pritzker Sch Med 81; **RES:** IM, Loyola U Med Ctr, Maywood, IL 82-84; **FEL:** Inf, Loyola U Med Ctr, Maywood, IL 84-86; **FAP:** Assoc Prof Med Univ IL Coll Med

Currie, James (MD) Inf
Elmhurst Mem Hosp
4440 W 95th St; Oaklawn, IL 60453; (630) 941-5265; **BDCERT:** IM 87; Inf 96; **MS:** U Iowa Coll Med 84

Deam, Malcolm (MD) Inf
West Suburban Hosp Med Ctr
West Suburban Hospital, 1 Erie Ct L500; Oak Park, IL 60302; (708) 383-6200; **BDCERT:** IM 73; Inf 76; **MS:** Northwestern U 69; **RES:** Rush Presbyterian-St Luke's Med Ctr, Chicago, IL 72-73; IM, Rush Presbyterian-St Luke's Med Ctr, Chicago, IL 74; **FEL:** Inf, Rush Presbyterian-St Luke's Med Ctr, Chicago, IL 74-75; **FAP:** Asst Prof Med Rush Med Coll; **HOSP:** Gottlieb Mem Hosp; ***SI:*** *General Infectious Disease; HIV*; **HMO:** Aetna Hlth Plan, United Healthcare, Humana Health Plan, Most
LANG: Sp, Pol;
A Few Days VISA

Gerding, Dale Nicholas (MD) Inf
Northwestern Mem Hosp
VA Chicago HSC Lakeside Div, 333 E Huron St; Chicago, IL 60611; (312) 640-2193; **BDCERT:** Inf 76; IM 73; **MS:** U Minn 68; **RES:** IM, U MN Med Ctr, Minneapolis, MN 71-73; **FEL:** Inf, VA Med Ctr, Minneapolis, MN 73-74; **FAP:** Prof Med Northwestern U; **HOSP:** VA Hlthcare Systems-Lakeside; ***SI:*** *Clostridium Difficile; Pseudomembranous Colitis*

Goodman, Larry J (MD) Inf
Rush-Presbyterian-St Luke's Med Ctr
(see page 122)
1653 W Congress Pkwy; Chicago, IL 60612; (312) 942-3665; **BDCERT:** Inf 82; IM 79; **MS:** U Mich Med Sch 76; **RES:** Rush Presbyterian-St Luke's Med Ctr, Chicago, IL 76-79; **FEL:** Rush Presbyterian-St Luke's Med Ctr, Chicago, IL 79-81; **FAP:** Prof Rush Med Coll; ***SI:** Central Nervous System Infections; Bowel Infections*; **HMO:** Blue Cross & Blue Shield, Rush Prudential, CIGNA, Humana Health Plan, United Healthcare
LANG: Sp; 1 Week

Jones, Lynwood A (MD) Inf
Alexian Brothers Med Ctr
(see page 138)
850 Biesterfield Rd Ste 30003; Elk Grove Vlg, IL 60007; (847) 981-3694; **BDCERT:** Inf 94; IM 87; **MS:** Creighton U 78; **RES:** IM, Mount Sinai Hosp Med Ctr, Chicago, IL 78-81; **FEL:** Inf, Long Island Jewish Med Ctr, New Hyde Park, NY 86-88

Kessler, Harold (MD) Inf
Rush-Presbyterian-St Luke's Med Ctr
(see page 122)
Rush-Presby-St Lukes Hosp, 600 S Paulina St Ste 143; Chicago, IL 60612; (312) 942-4807; **BDCERT:** IM 77; Inf 82; **MS:** Rush Med Coll 74; **RES:** IM, Rush Presbyterian-St Luke's Med Ctr, Chicago, IL 75-77; **FEL:** Inf, Rush Presbyterian-St Luke's Med Ctr, Chicago, IL 77-79; Inf, London Sch Hygiene & Trop Med, London, England 78-79; **FAP:** Prof Rush Med Coll; **HMO:** +

Levin, Stuart (MD) Inf
Rush-Presbyterian-St Luke's Med Ctr
(see page 122)
1653 W Congress Pkwy; Chicago, IL 60612; (312) 942-6600; **BDCERT:** Inf 76; IM 67; **MS:** Univ IL Coll Med 60; **RES:** IM, Chicago VA Hlth Care System-Westside, Chicago, IL 61-64; Inf, U IL Med Ctr, Chicago, IL 66-67; **FAP:** Chrmn IM Rush Med Coll

Luskin-Hawk, Roberta (MD) Inf
St Joseph Hosp-Elgin
Lake Shore Infectious Disease Associates, 2900 N Lake Shore Dr; Chicago, IL 60657; (773) 665-3261; **BDCERT:** Inf 86; IM 82; **MS:** Univ IL Coll Med 79; **RES:** IM, Michael Reese Hosp Med Ctr, Chicago, IL 80-83; **FEL:** Inf, U Chicago Hosp, Chicago, IL 83-85; **FAP:** Northwestern U; **HOSP:** Illinois Masonic Med Ctr; ***SI:** HIV Infection; AIDS*; **HMO:** Blue Cross & Blue Shield, Chicago HMO, Bay State Health Plan, Compare Health Service, Humana Health Plan
2-4 Weeks VISA

McLeod, Rima (MD) Inf
Michael Reese Hosp & Med Ctr
939 E 57th St; Chicago, IL 60637; (773) 834-4152; **BDCERT:** IM 74; **MS:** UC San Francisco 71; **HOSP:** U Chicago Hosp; ***SI:** Toxoplasmosis*

Noskin, Gary (MD) Inf
Northwestern Mem Hosp
303 E Superior St Ste 8E; Chicago, IL 60611; (312) 908-8358; **BDCERT:** IM 89; Inf 92; **MS:** U Hlth Sci/Chicago Med Sch 86; **RES:** IM, Northwestern Mem Hosp, Chicago, IL 86-89; **FEL:** Inf, Northwestern Mem Hosp, Chicago, IL 89-91; **FAP:** Assoc Prof Med Northwestern U

O'Keefe, James Paul (MD) Inf
Loyola U Med Ctr **(see page 120)**
2160 S 1st Ave; Maywood, IL 60153; (708) 216-3232; **BDCERT:** Inf 78; IM 74; **MS:** Loyola U-Stritch Sch Med, Maywood 71; **RES:** Loyola U Med Ctr, Maywood, IL 72-74; **FEL:** Inf, VA Hosp, Sepulveda, CA 74-75; Inf, Tufts New England Med Ctr, Boston, MA 75-77

Ramakrishna, Bhagavatula (MD) Inf
Little Company of Mary Hosp & Hlth Care Ctrs **(see page 142)**
11800 Southwest Hwy; Palos Heights, IL 60463; (708) 361-5778; **BDCERT:** IM 77; Inf 80; **MS:** India 70; **HOSP:** Christ Hosp & Med Ctr

Santos, Rene (MD) Inf
Ingalls Mem Hosp
Infectious Disease, 71 W 156th St Ste 304; Harvey, IL 60426; (708) 333-3113; **BDCERT:** IM 84; Inf 88; **MS:** Harvard Med Sch 81; **RES:** IM, UCLA Med Ctr, Los Angeles, CA 82-84; **FEL:** Inf, U Chicago Hosp, Chicago, IL 85-87

Semel, Jeffrey (MD) Inf
Highland Park Hosp
9701 Knox Ave Ste 103; Skokie, IL 60076; (847) 675-6466; **BDCERT:** IM 76; Inf 78; **MS:** U Chicago-Pritzker Sch Med 88

Weinstein, Robert Alan (MD) Inf
Cook Cty Hosp
Div Inf Dis, Cook County Hosp, 1835 W Harrison St; Chicago, IL 60612; (312) 633-3237; **BDCERT:** IM 77; Inf 78; **MS:** Cornell U 72; **RES:** IM, Barnes Hosp, St Louis, MO 72-74; Centers for Disease Control, Atlanta, GA 74-76; **FEL:** Inf, U Chicago Hosp, Chicago, IL 76-78; **FAP:** Prof Med Rush Med Coll
NFI 2-4 Weeks

Guide to symbols and abbreviations can be found on pages 110-113.

White, G Wesley (MD) **Inf**
Lutheran Gen Hosp (see page 143)
1775 Dempster St; Park Ridge, IL 60068; (847) 795-2400; **BDCERT:** Inf 80; IM 77; **MS:** Univ IL Coll Med 74; **RES:** IM, U IL Med Ctr, Chicago, IL 74-77; **FEL:** Inf, U IL Med Ctr, Chicago, IL 77-79; **HOSP:** Resurrection Med Ctr; ***SI:*** *Infectious Diseases; Travel Medicine*; **HMO:** +
A Few Days *VISA*

Wurtz, Rebecca (MD) **Inf**
Evanston Hosp
Evanston Hospital, 2650 Ridge Ave; Evanston, IL 60201; (847) 657-5959; **BDCERT:** IM 88; Inf 90; **MS:** Harvard Med Sch 85; **RES:** IM, Rush Presbyterian-St Luke's Med Ctr, Chicago, IL 86-88; **FEL:** UC San Francisco Med Ctr, San Francisco, CA 88-89; **FAP:** Asst Prof Northwestern U; **HOSP:** Glenbrook Hosp; ***SI:*** *Mycobacterial Infections; Pneumonia*; **HMO:** Aetna Hlth Plan, Prudential
Immediately

INTERNAL MEDICINE

Adelson, Bernard (MD) **IM**
PCP
Evanston Hosp
700 Oak St; Winnetka, IL 60093; (847) 446-8082; **BDCERT:** IM 57; **MS:** Northwestern U 51; **RES:** IM, Evanston Hosp, Evanston, IL 51-53; IM, Cook Cty Hosp, Chicago, IL 52-54; **FAP:** Prof of Clin Med Northwestern U; ***SI:*** *Medical Ethics*; **HMO:** Blue Cross, Aetna-US Healthcare, CIGNA +
1 Week *VISA*

Altkorn, Diane (MD) **IM**
PCP
U Chicago Hosp (see page 124)
University Health Svc, 5841 S Maryland Ave Ste 3051; Chicago, IL 60637; (773) 702-2458; **BDCERT:** IM 85; Ger 90; **MS:** U Chicago-Pritzker Sch Med 82; **RES:** IM, U Chicago Hosp, Chicago, IL 83-84; IM, UC San Diego Med Ctr, San Diego, CA 84-85; **FEL:** IM, UC San Diego Med Ctr, San Diego, CA 85-86; **FAP:** Assoc Clin Prof Med U Chicago-Pritzker Sch Med

Argaez, Juvenal (MD) **IM**
Norwegian-American Hosp
1505 W Devon St; Chicago, IL 60660; (773) 235-7455; **BDCERT:** IM 78; **MS:** Colombia 70; **RES:** Charity Hosp, New Orleans, LA 68-70

Aronson, Alan (MD) **IM**
PCP
Rush North Shore Med Ctr
North Suburban Clinic, 9977 Woods Drive; Skokie, IL 60077; (847) 663-0540; **BDCERT:** IM 93; Ger 88; **MS:** Univ IL Coll Med 56; **RES:** U IL Med Ctr, Chicago, IL 57-59; U IL Med Ctr, Chicago, IL 61-62; **FEL:** Ge, U IL Med Ctr, Chicago, IL 58-59

Arteaga, Waldo (MD) **IM**
PCP
Holy Cross Hosp
Holy Cross Family Medical Ctr, 1841 W 47th St; Chicago, IL 60609; (773) 927-5524; **BDCERT:** IM 96; **MS:** Bolivia 74; **RES:** IM, Mercy Hosp & Med Ctr, Chicago, IL 81-82; IM, Hines VA Hosp, Chicago, IL 83-85; ***SI:*** *Asthma; Hypertension*; **HMO:** HMO Illinois, Humana Health Plan, United Healthcare, NYLCare +
LANG: Sp;
Immediately *VISA*

Balandrin, Jorge (MD) **IM**
Christ Hosp & Med Ctr (see page 140)
4340 W 95th St Ste 106; Oak Lawn, IL 60453; (708) 424-1222; **BDCERT:** IM 87; **MS:** Mexico 82; **RES:** IM, Christ Hosp & Med Ctr, Oak Lawn, IL 83-86

Barrocas, Salvador (MD) **IM**
PCP
Alexian Brothers Med Ctr
(see page 138)
850 Biesterfield Rd Ste 2007; Elk Grove Vlg, IL 60007; (847) 437-8833; **BDCERT:** IM 68; **MS:** Cuba 57; **RES:** IM, Mount Sinai Hosp Med Ctr, Chicago, IL 68; IM, Chicago VA Hlth Care System-Westside, Chicago, IL 69; **FEL:** Cv, Michael Reese Hosp Med Ctr, Chicago, IL 62; **FAP:** Assoc Clin Prof Med Loyola U-Stritch Sch Med, Maywood; ***SI:*** *High Cholesterol*; **HMO:** Blue Shield
LANG: Sp; 4+ Weeks

Berkowitz, Gerald (MD) **IM**
Louis A Weiss Mem Hosp
4640 N Marine Dr C6700; Chicago, IL 60640; (773) 728-7877; **BDCERT:** IM 66; **MS:** Northwestern U 59; **HMO:** Blue Cross & Blue Shield, Chicago HMO, Bay State Health Plan, Compare Health Service, FHP Inc

Berlin, Gabriel (MD) **IM**
PCP
Evanston Hosp
3633 W Lake Ave Ste 302; Glenview, IL 60025; (847) 998-5700; **BDCERT:** IM 78; **MS:** Northwestern U 75; **RES:** IM, Evanston Hosp, Evanston, IL 76-78; **FAP:** Instr Northwestern U; **HMO:** Blue Cross & Blue Shield, Californiacare, Rush Health Plans, Sanus

Bhorade, Maruti (MD) **IM**
St Mary's of Nazareth Hosp Ctr
St. Mary's of Nazareth Hosp Ctr, 2233 W Division St; Chicago, IL 60622; (312) 770-2172; **BDCERT:** IM 73; Ger 90; **MS:** India 60; **RES:** IM, KEM Hosp, Bombay, India 61-69; **FEL:** U Chicago Hosp, Chicago, IL 67-70; **FAP:** Assoc Clin Prof Med Loyola U-Stritch Sch Med, Maywood; ***SI:*** *Hypertension, Kidney Failure; Diabetes, Dialysis, Edema*; **HMO:** United Healthcare, Blue Cross & Blue Shield, Americaid, Harmony
1 Week

Bogacz, Kathleen (MD) IM
PCP
Evanston Hosp
8707 Skokie Blvd Ste 216; Skokie, IL 60077; (847) 677-8880; **BDCERT:** IM 86; **MS:** Univ IL Coll Med 83; **RES:** IM, Evanston Hosp, Evanston, IL 83-87; **FAP:** Clin Instr Northwestern U; ***SI:*** *Preventive Medicine; Women's Health Issues*; **HMO:** Aetna Hlth Plan, Blue Cross & Blue Shield, Californiacare, Rush Prudential, PHCS
Mcr Mcd A Few Days

Brill, John (MD) IM
PCP
Rush-Presbyterian-St Luke's Med Ctr
(see page 122)
500 W Madison Ave Suite 400; Chicago, IL 60661; (312) 930-0999; **BDCERT:** IM 98; **MS:** Ohio State U 85; **RES:** IM, Rush Presbyterian-St Luke's Med Ctr, Chicago, IL 86-88; **HMO:** +
Mcr

Brongiel, Alan (MD) IM
PCP
St Alexius Med Ctr
Streamwood Family Medical Ctr, 403 W Irving Park Rd; Streamwood, IL 60107; (630) 830-1900; **BDCERT:** IM 79; **MS:** U Hlth Sci/Chicago Med Sch 76

Bulmash, Jack (MD) IM
PCP
Illinois Masonic Med Ctr
(see page 118)
1725 W Harrison St Ste 352; Chicago, IL 60612; (312) 666-2578; **BDCERT:** IM 75; Ger 88; **MS:** Univ IL Coll Med 70; **RES:** IM, U IL Med Ctr, Chicago, IL 73-75; **FAP:** Asst Prof Med Rush Med Coll; **HOSP:** Vencor Hosp; ***SI:*** *Geriatrics*; **HMO:** Rush Prudential, Aetna Hlth Plan, Humana Health Plan, Humana Health Plan, Blue Cross +
LANG: Sp; Mcr Mcd NFI 1 Week

Burton, Wayne N (MD) IM
PCP
Northwestern Mem Hosp
Northwestern Internists Ltd, 676 N Saint Clair St Ste 415; Chicago, IL 60611; (312) 335-1133; **BDCERT:** IM 77; **MS:** U Oreg/Hlth Sci U, Portland 74; **RES:** IM, Northwestern Mem Hosp, Chicago, IL 74-78; **FAP:** Assoc Clin Prof Med Northwestern U; **HMO:** Aetna Hlth Plan, Blue Cross & Blue Shield, Californiacare, CIGNA, HealthNet
Mcr 4+ Weeks

Candocia, Santiago (MD) IM
PCP
Evanston Hosp
North Grove Internal Medicine, 1215 Mchenry Rd; Buffalo Grove, IL 60089; (847) 913-9092; **BDCERT:** IM 89; **MS:** Univ IL Coll Med 86; **RES:** IM, Evanston Hosp, Evanston, IL 87-89; IM, Evanston Hosp, Evanston, IL 89-90; **FAP:** Instr Med Northwestern U; **HMO:** Blue Choice, Blue Cross & Blue Shield, Chicago HMO, CIGNA, Humana Health Plan

Carlson, Bruce (MD) IM
PCP
Good Shepherd Hosp
Barrington Specialists, 450 W IL Route 22 Ste 16; Barrington, IL 60010; (847) 382-6633; **BDCERT:** IM 78; **MS:** Univ IL Coll Med 75; **HMO:** Blue Cross & Blue Shield, Humana Health Plan, Metlife, Prudential, Rush Health Plans

Clarke, John (MD) IM
PCP
Northwestern Mem Hosp
Geriatric Evaluation Svc, 250 E Superior St Ste 148; Chicago, IL 60611; (312) 908-4525; **BDCERT:** IM 75; Ger 92; **MS:** Northwestern U 68; **RES:** IM, Barnes Hosp, St Louis, MO 69-70; IM, Northwestern Mem Hosp, Chicago, IL 74-75; **FEL:** Inf, U WA Med Ctr, Seattle, WA 72-74

Cobleigh, Melody (MD) IM
Rush-Presbyterian-St Luke's Med Ctr
(see page 122)
1725 W Harrison St; Chicago, IL 60612; (312) 942-3240; **BDCERT:** IM 79; Onc 81; **MS:** Rush Med Coll 76; **RES:** IM, Rush Presbyterian-St Luke's Med Ctr, Chicago, IL 77-79; **FEL:** Onc, Indiana U Med Ctr, Indianapolis, IN 79-81; **FAP:** Assoc Prof Med Rush Med Coll; ***SI:*** *Breast Cancer*

Coe, Fredric (MD) IM
U Chicago Hosp (see page 124)
Univ of Chicago Hospital, 5841 S Maryland Ave; Chicago, IL 60637; (773) 702-1473; **BDCERT:** IM 68; **MS:** U Chicago-Pritzker Sch Med 61; **RES:** IM, Michael Reese Hosp Med Ctr, Chicago, IL 62-65; **FEL:** Renal Disease, U Texas SW Med Ctr, Dallas, TX 67-69; **FAP:** Prof Med U Chicago-Pritzker Sch Med; ***SI:*** *Kidney Stones*
2-4 Weeks

Cole, James (MD) IM
PCP
Northwest Comm Hlthcare
Arlington Medical Assoc, 1009 S Evergreen Ave; Arlington Hts, IL 60005; (847) 255-0800; **BDCERT:** IM 77; **MS:** Loyola U-Stritch Sch Med, Maywood 61; **RES:** Mount Sinai Hosp Med Ctr, Chicago, IL 62-65
Mcr Mcd VISA

Cruz, Sidney (MD) IM
Swedish Covenant Hosp
Cruz, 5300 W Devon Ave; Chicago, IL 60646; (773) 631-2223; **BDCERT:** IM 77; EDM 81; **MS:** Philippines 65; **RES:** IM, Northwestern Mem Hosp, Chicago, IL 67-69; **FEL:** EDM, Northwestern Mem Hosp, Chicago, IL 70-71; **HMO:** Aetna Hlth Plan, Blue Cross & Blue Shield, Californiacare, Humana Health Plan, Metlife

Curry, Raymond (MD) IM
PCP
Northwestern Mem Hosp
303 E Ohio St Ste 300; Chicago, IL 60611; (312) 503-9443; **BDCERT:** IM 85; Ger 92; **MS:** Washington U, St Louis 82; **RES:** IM, Northwestern Mem Hosp, Chicago, IL 83-85; **FAP:** Assoc Prof Med Northwestern U; **HMO:** Blue Choice, Chicago HMO, Bay State Health Plan, Metlife, Prudential

Danon, Joseph (MD) IM
PCP
St Mary's of Nazareth Hosp Ctr
2222 W Division St Ste 205; Chicago, IL 60622; (773) 395-4505; **BDCERT:** Ger 88; Pul 74; **MS:** Israel 58; **RES:** IM, Beilinson Hosp, Tel Aviv, Israel 59-61; IM, Hadassah Hosp, Jerusalem, Israel 62-63; **FEL:** Pul, Hines VA Hosp, Chicago, IL 68-70; ***SI:*** *Asthma; Cholesterol Disorders*; **HMO:** Blue Cross, United Healthcare, Medicare
LANG: Sp, Heb, Itl, Pol; Immediately

De Backer, Noel (MD) IM
Northwestern Mem Hosp
680 N Lakeshore Drive Ste 118; Chicago, IL 60611; (312) 503-6000; **BDCERT:** IM 82; Ger 88; **MS:** Baylor 79; **RES:** IM, Northwestern Meml Hosp, Chicago, IL 80-83; **FAP:** Asst Clin Prof Med Northwestern U; **HMO:** +

Deano, Danilo (MD) IM
PCP
St Mary's of Nazareth Hosp Ctr
Deano Medical Assoc, 4643 N Clark St; Chicago, IL 60640; (773) 989-1099; **BDCERT:** IM 74; Cv 77; **MS:** Philippines 67; **RES:** FP, Grant Hosp, Chicago, IL 70-71; IM, U IL Med Ctr, Chicago, IL 71-73; **FEL:** Cv, U IL Med Ctr, Chicago, IL 73-76

Diamond, Merle (MD) IM
Columbus Hosp
Diamond Headache Clinic, 467 W Deming Pl Ste 500; Chicago, IL 60614; (773) 388-6375; **BDCERT:** IM 84; EM 96; **MS:** Northwestern U 80; **RES:** IM, Northwestern Mem Hosp, Chicago, IL 81-84; ***SI:*** *Headache; Women's Health Issues*

Dillon, Charles (MD) IM
PCP
Rush-Presbyterian-St Luke's Med Ctr **(see page 122)**
1725 W Harrison St Ste 352; Chicago, IL 60612; (312) 829-3533; **BDCERT:** IM 83; **MS:** Georgetown U 80; **RES:** IM, Penn State Univ, Philadelphia, PA 80-83; **FAP:** Asst Prof Rush Med Coll; ***SI:*** *Hypertension; Hypercholesterolemia*; **HMO:** Blue Cross & Blue Shield, Humana Health Plan, Preferred Plan, Private Healthcare
LANG: Sp; 2-4 Weeks
VISA

Fainman, Zachary (MD) IM
PCP
Lutheran Gen Hosp **(see page 143)**
Advocate Medical Group, 960 Rand Rd Ste 205; Des Plaines, IL 60016; (847) 480-1616; **BDCERT:** IM 79; **MS:** Univ IL Coll Med 76; **RES:** IM, Lutheran Gen Hosp, Park Ridge, IL 77-79
VISA

Farrell, Richard (MD) IM
PCP
Little Company of Mary Hosp & Hlth Care Ctrs **(see page 142)**
5660 W 95th St; Oak Lawn, IL 60453; (708) 499-4190; **BDCERT:** IM 86; **MS:** Loyola U-Stritch Sch Med, Maywood 82; **RES:** Mercy Hosp Med Ctr, Chicago, IL 83-85

Foody, James (MD) IM
PCP
U Chicago Hosp **(see page 124)**
University of Chicago Phys, 222 N La Salle St Ste 250; Chicago, IL 60601; (773) 702-0416; **BDCERT:** IM 83; **MS:** U Chicago-Pritzker Sch Med 80; **RES:** IM, U Chicago Hosp, Chicago, IL 81-83; **FAP:** Assoc Prof of Clin Med U Chicago-Pritzker Sch Med

Furey, Warren (MD) IM
PCP
Mercy Hosp & Med Ctr
Medical Associates, 251 E Chicago Ave Ste 1127; Chicago, IL 60611; (312) 642-6868; **BDCERT:** IM 87; Inf 72; **MS:** Northwestern U 60; **RES:** IM, Chicago Wesley Mem Hosp, Chicago, IL 61-66; VA Rsch Hosp, Chicago, IL 66-67; **FAP:** Assoc Prof of Clin Med Northwestern U; **HOSP:** Northwest Comm Hlthcare; **HMO:** Aetna Hlth Plan, Blue Cross & Blue Shield, Californiacare

Gardner, Allen (MD) IM
PCP
Evanston Hosp
Glenview Medical Assoc, 1306 Waukegan Rd; Glenview, IL 60025; (847) 724-5353; **BDCERT:** IM 97; **MS:** SUNY Downstate 78; **RES:** IM, NC Mem Hosp, Chapel Hill, NC 57; IM, Yale-New Haven Hosp, New Haven, CT 60; **FEL:** Cv, Yale-New Haven Hosp, New Haven, CT 61-63; **FAP:** Sr Instr Ped Rush Med Coll; **HMO:** Blue Cross & Blue Shield, Humana Health Plan
VISA

Ginsburg, David Lee (MD) IM
PCP
St Alexius Med Ctr
1786 Moonlake Blvd; Hoffman Estates, IL 60194; (847) 885-7400; **BDCERT:** IM 78; Ger 88; **MS:** Univ IL Coll Med 75; **RES:** IM, U IL Hosp, Chicago, IL 76-78

Grendon, Michael Todd (MD) IM
PCP
St Joseph Hosp-Elgin
Commonwealth Medical Assoc, 2800 N Sheridan Rd Ste 400; Chicago, IL 60657; (773) 472-5803; **BDCERT:** IM 83; Ger 94; **MS:** U Cincinnati 79; **RES:** IM, Northwestern Mem Hosp, Chicago, IL 80-82; **FAP:** Asst Prof of Clin Med U Chicago-Pritzker Sch Med
1 Week VISA

Gupta, Ashutosh (MD) IM
PCP
Jackson Park Hosp & Med Ctr
7531 S Stony Island Ave Ste 158; Chicago, IL 60649; (773) 493-4268; **BDCERT:** IM 81; Nep 88; **MS:** India 69; **RES:** Delhi Univ, India 70-73; Cook Cty Hosp, Chicago, IL 74-76; **FEL:** U Chicago Hosp, Chicago, IL 76-78

Havey, Robert (MD) IM
PCP
St Joseph Hosp-Chicago
Chicago Lakeshore Med Assoc, 2515 N Clark St Ste 900; Chicago, IL 60614; (773) 327-9190; **BDCERT:** IM 83; **MS:** Northwestern U 80; **RES:** Northwestern Mem Hosp, Chicago, IL 81-83; **FEL:** Northwestern Mem Hosp, Chicago, IL 83-84; **HOSP:** Northwest Comm Hlthcare; **HMO:** +
2-4 Weeks VISA

Hedberg, Carl Anderson (MD) IM
Rush-Presbyterian-St Luke's Med Ctr (see page 122)
Hedberg & Assoc, 1725 W Harrison St Ste 762; Chicago, IL 60612; (312) 226-1162; **BDCERT:** IM 74; Ge 72; **MS:** Cornell U 61; **RES:** IM, NY Hosp-Cornell Med Ctr, New York, NY 62-64; **FEL:** Ge, U Chicago Hosp, Chicago, IL 64-68; **FAP:** Assoc Prof Med Rush Med Coll

Hering, Paul (MD) IM
PCP
Loyola U Med Ctr (see page 120)
Loyola University, 2160 S 1st Ave; Maywood, IL 60153; (708) 216-1350; **BDCERT:** IM 77; **MS:** Loyola U-Stritch Sch Med, Maywood 77
VISA

Horowitz, Kenneth (MD) IM
PCP
Northwest Comm Hlthcare
Arlington Heights Medical Associates, 1700 W Central Rd Ste 260; Arlington Heights, IL 60005; (847) 255-7107; **BDCERT:** IM 86; **MS:** Loyola U-Stritch Sch Med, Maywood 83; **RES:** IM, Faulkner Hosp, Boston, MA 83-86; ***SI:*** *Cardiology; Diabetes*; **HMO:** Aetna Hlth Plan, HMO Blue, Aetna-US Healthcare, Humana Health Plan
LANG: Sp; A Few Days VISA

Hoyer, Danuta (MD) IM
PCP
Rush-Presbyterian-St Luke's Med Ctr (see page 122)
Rush Center For Women's Health, 500 W Madison Street Ste 400; Chicago, IL 60660; (312) 551-1301; **BDCERT:** IM 85; **MS:** Rush Med Coll 82; **RES:** IM, Rush Presbyterian-St Luke's Med Ctr, Chicago, IL 82-85; **FEL:** IM, Rush Presbyterian-St Luke's Med Ctr, Chicago, IL 85-86; **FAP:** Asst. Prof. IM Rush Med Coll; **HOSP:** Rush North Shore Med Ctr; ***SI:*** *Women's Health*
LANG: Pol; 1 Week VISA

Jaffe, Harry (MD) IM
PCP
Evanston Hosp
Central Street Partnership, 1713 Central St; Evanston, IL 60201; (847) 475-8888; **BDCERT:** IM 76; **MS:** Georgetown U 71; **RES:** IM, Georgetown U Hosp, Washington, DC 72-73; IM, Georgetown U Hosp, Washington, DC 75-76; **HMO:** Blue Cross & Blue Shield, Chicago HMO, FHP Inc

Kashian, Stephen M (MD) IM
Evanston Hosp
Orchard Medical Group, 64 Old Orchard Shop Ctr Ste LL; Skokie, IL 60077; (847) 679-6707; **BDCERT:** IM 84; **MS:** Univ IL Coll Med 81; **RES:** IM, U IL Med Ctr, Chicago, IL 82-84; **FAP:** Asst Prof Northwestern U

Katz, Richard (MD) IM
PCP
Highland Park Hosp
1275 Shermer Rd; Northbrook, IL 60062; (847) 272-0005; **BDCERT:** IM 83; **MS:** Univ IL Coll Med 80; **RES:** Evanston Hosp, Evanston, IL 81-83; **HMO:** Aetna Hlth Plan, Blue Cross & Blue Shield, Californiacare, CIGNA, Metlife

Kehoe, William (MD) IM
PCP
Rush-Presbyterian-St Luke's Med Ctr (see page 122)
Ramsey Kehoe Palmer, 9669 Kenton Ave Ste 102; Skokie, IL 60076; (847) 675-2040; **BDCERT:** IM 79; **MS:** Loyola U-Stritch Sch Med, Maywood 75; **RES:** IM, Rush Presbyterian-St Luke's Med Ctr, Chicago, IL 76-79; **FAP:** Assoc Prof Med Rush Med Coll

Kerchberger, Vern (MD) IM
PCP
Northwest Comm Hlthcare
1300 E Central Rd C; Arlington Hts, IL 60005; (847) 255-5029; **BDCERT:** IM 82; Inf 84; **MS:** Emory U Sch Med 79; **RES:** IM, Parkland Mem Hosp, Dallas, TX 80-82; **FEL:** Inf, Barnes Hosp, St Louis, MO 82-84

Kerr, William (MD) IM
Evanston Hosp
Medical Group of Evanston, 1000 Central St; Evanston, IL 60201; (847) 570-1410; **BDCERT:** IM 74; Ger 94; **MS:** Johns Hopkins U 60; **RES:** IM, Johns-Hopkins-Oster Med Ctr, Baltimore, MD 61-62; IM, NC Meml Hosp, Chapel Hill, NC 63-65; **FEL:** EDM, U Miami Hosp, Miami, FL 65-67; EDM, Univ of Strasbourg, Strasbourg, France 62-63; **FAP:** Asst Prof Med Northwestern U

Kim, Jinsup (MD) IM
St James Hosp & Hlth Ctrs
333 Dixie Hwy; Chicago Heights, IL 60411; (708) 709-6230; **BDCERT:** IM 84; **MS:** South Korea 72; **RES:** IM, St Francis Hosp of Evanston, Evanston, IL 79-81; **HOSP:** South Suburban Hosp

Kirby, Joanne (MD) IM
PCP
Columbus Hosp
Chicago Lakeshore Medical, 2515 N Clark St Ste 900; Chicago, IL 60614; (773) 327-9190; **BDCERT:** IM 88; Pul 90; **MS:** UMDNJ-RW Johnson Med Sch 85; **RES:** IM, Northwestern Mem Hosp, Chicago, IL 85-88; **FEL:** Pul & CCM, U Ill Med Ctr, Chicago, IL 88-91; **HOSP:** Northwestern Mem Hosp; ***SI:** Asthma; Sleep Disorders*; **HMO:** HMO Illinois, Rush Health Plans +
Mcr A Few Days VISA

Kogan, Edward (MD) IM
PCP
St Alexius Med Ctr
West Brook Intl Med, 1575 Barrington Rd Ste 505; Hoffman Estates, IL 60194; (847) 884-7111; **BDCERT:** IM 81; Ger 88; **MS:** Univ IL Coll Med 78

Kopin, Jeffrey (MD) IM
PCP
Northwestern Mem Hosp
Memorial Physicians Group, 111 W Washington St Ste 1801; Chicago, IL 60602; (312) 357-2280; **BDCERT:** IM 87; **MS:** Northwestern U 84; **RES:** IM, Northwestern Mem Hosp, Chicago, IL; ***SI:** Diabetes-Thyroid Disease; Hypertension-Cholesterol*; **HMO:** HMO Illinois, United Healthcare, Rush Prudential +
$ Mcr Mcd Immediately VISA

Koshy, Mabel (MD) IM
Univ of Illinois at Chicago Med Ctr
University of Illinois, 840 S Wood St Ste 8133; Chicago, IL 60612; (312) 996-5680; **BDCERT:** IM 84; **MS:** Malaysia 64; **RES:** IM, Detroit Meml Hosp, Detroit, MI 68-69; IM, Sinai Hosp, Detroit, MI 69-71; **FEL:** HemOnc, Michael Reese Hosp Med Ctr, Chicago, IL 71-73; **FAP:** Prof Med Univ IL Coll Med; ***SI:** Sickle Cell Disease*

Kreamer, Jeffry (MD) IM
PCP
Good Shepherd Hosp
Regency Medical Ctr, 782 W Euclid Ave; Palatine, IL 60067; (847) 358-1045; **BDCERT:** IM 94; **MS:** Univ Osteo Med & Hlth Sci 87; **RES:** U Chicago Hosp, Chicago, IL 87-90; **HMO:** +

Krishnan, Meera (MD) IM
PCP
Christ Hosp & Med Ctr (see page 140)
Primary Care/Urgent Care, 5019 W 95th St; Oak Lawn, IL 60453; (708) 423-5159; **BDCERT:** IM 96; **MS:** India 75; **RES:** U IL Med Ctr, Chicago, IL 88-92; ***SI:** Allergies & Asthma; Anxiety Disorder*; **HMO:** +
SA SU $ Mcr Mcd

Kroger, Elliott (MD) IM
PCP
West Suburban Hosp Med Ctr
West Suburban Intrnl Medicine, 7411 Lake St L120; River Forest, IL 60305; (708) 488-1919; **BDCERT:** IM 81; **MS:** Rush Med Coll 78; **RES:** IM, Rush Presbyterian-St Luke's Med Ctr, Chicago, IL 78-81; **FAP:** Asst Clin Prof Loyola U-Stritch Sch Med, Maywood; ***SI:** High Blood Pressure; Congestive Heart Failure*; **HMO:** HMO Illinois, Rush Prudential, Humana Health Plan, NYLCare
LANG: Sp, Pol, SCr; SA SU $ Mcr Mcd NFI 1 Week VISA

Lewis, Gerald (MD) IM
PCP
Lutheran Gen Hosp (see page 143)
Primary Care Medical Specs, 960 Rand Rd Ste 205; Des Plaines, IL 60016; (847) 298-0310; **BDCERT:** IM 79; Ger 90; **MS:** Univ IL Coll Med 76; **HOSP:** St Joseph Med Ctr-Joliet; **HMO:** Blue Cross & Blue Shield, Humana Health Plan

Logan, Patrick (MD) IM
PCP
Evanston Hosp
530 Winnetka Ave; Winnetka, IL 60093; (847) 441-6869; **BDCERT:** IM 80; **MS:** Wayne State U Sch Med 76

Madhav, Gopal (MD) IM
PCP
Christ Hosp & Med Ctr (see page 140)
3900 W 95th St Ste 7; Evergreen Park, IL 60805; (708) 423-7733; **BDCERT:** IM 81; **MS:** India 77; **RES:** IM, Christ Hosp & Med Ctr, Oak Lawn, IL 78-79; IM, Christ Hosp & Med Ctr, Oak Lawn, IL 79-81; ***SI:** Diabetes-Mellitus; Cardiovascular Disease*; **HMO:** Blue Choice, Advocate, United Healthcare, Humana Health Plan, CIGNA
LANG: Hin; $ Mcr Mcd 1 Week

Majumdar, Sanjoy (MD) IM
Our Lady Of the Resurrection Med Ctr
Waterford Medical Ltd, 5958 W Lawrence Ave; Chicago, IL 60630; (773) 282-4572; **BDCERT:** IM 80; Ger 90; **MS:** India 72

Markey, W S (MD) IM
Grant Hosp
Professional Medical Svc, 550 W Webster Ave Ste 305; Chicago, IL 60614; (312) 944-1247; **BDCERT:** IM 74; Ge 79; **MS:** Case West Res U 71; **RES:** IM, Rush Presbyterian-St Luke's Med Ctr, Chicago, IL 71-74; **FEL:** Ge, Rush Presbyterian-St Luke's Med Ctr, Chicago, IL 76-78; **FAP:** Asst Prof Rush Med Coll; **HOSP:** Rush-Presbyterian-St Luke's Med Ctr; ***SI:*** *Irritable Bowel Syndrome; Gastrointestinal Malignancy*
LANG: Sp; Mcr Mcd A Few Days

Marwah, Birinder (MD) IM
Grant Hosp
2266 N Lincoln Ave; Chicago, IL 60614; (773) 281-3670; **BDCERT:** IM 84; Ger 88; **MS:** India 78; **RES:** IM, Grant Hosp, Chicago, IL 82-84; **FAP:** Instr Med Rush Med Coll; **HOSP:** Illinois Masonic Med Ctr

Meiselman, Mick (MD) IM
Evanston Hosp
510 Green Bay Rd; Kenilworth, IL 60043; (847) 256-3495; **BDCERT:** IM 82; Ge 85; **MS:** Northwestern U 79; **RES:** IM, Cedars-Sinai Med Ctr, Los Angeles, CA 79-82; **FEL:** Ge, UC San Francisco Med Ctr, San Francisco, CA 82-84; **FAP:** Asst Clin Prof Northwestern U; **HOSP:** Glenbrook Hosp

Meyers, Kim (MD) IM
PCP
Evanston Hosp
Central Street Partnership, 1713 Central St; Evanston, IL 60201; (847) 869-5050; **BDCERT:** IM 80; **MS:** Loyola U-Stritch Sch Med, Maywood 79

Michael, Magdy (MD) IM
PCP
St Mary's of Nazareth Hosp Ctr
Brodech Medical Assoc, 809 N Western Ave; Chicago, IL 60622; (773) 772-9121; **BDCERT:** IM 86; **MS:** Egypt 76; **RES:** IM, Mount Sinai Hosp Med Ctr, Chicago, IL 84-86

Miller, James (MD) IM
PCP
Mount Sinai Hosp Med Ctr
West Chicago Physicians Assoc, 1145 Westgate St; Oak Park, IL 60301; (708) 848-7673; **BDCERT:** IM 84; **MS:** U Chicago-Pritzker Sch Med 80; **RES:** IM, U Chicago Hosp, Chicago, IL 81-83; **HOSP:** Little Company of Mary Hosp & Hlth Care Ctrs

Milner, Larry (MD) IM
PCP
Highland Park Hosp
1500 Shermer Rd Ste 325E; Northbrook, IL 60062; (847) 498-1515; **BDCERT:** IM 80; Onc 77; **MS:** Univ IL Coll Med 66; **RES:** IM, U IL Med Ctr, Chicago, IL 67-68; **FEL:** Hem, Mass Gen Hosp, Boston, MA 70-71; **HMO:** Aetna Hlth Plan, Blue Cross & Blue Shield, Chicago HMO, CIGNA, Humana Health Plan

Morgan, Herman (MD) IM
PCP
Trinity Hosp
Damen Wellness Ctr, 1947 W 95th St; Chicago, IL 60643; (773) 779-1610; **BDCERT:** IM 93; **MS:** Northwestern U 69; **RES:** IM, Cook Cty Hosp, Chicago, IL 70-72; **FEL:** EDM, Northwestern Mem Hosp, Chicago, IL 72-73

Mozwecz, Jeffrey (MD) IM
PCP
Christ Hosp & Med Ctr **(see page 140)**
10522 S Cicero Ave Ste 3A; Oak Lawn, IL 60453; (708) 636-4441; **BDCERT:** IM 84; **MS:** Loyola U-Stritch Sch Med, Maywood 81; **RES:** IM, U IL Med Ctr, Chicago, IL 82-84; **FAP:** Clin Prof IM Rush Med Coll; **HOSP:** Palos Comm Hosp; **HMO:** Blue Cross PPO, Humana PPO

Murphy, Joseph Leroy (MD) IM
PCP
St Joseph Hosp-Elgin
4952 W Irving Park Rd Ste 200; Chicago, IL 60641; (773) 736-8896; **BDCERT:** IM 87; Ge 88; **MS:** Loyola U-Stritch Sch Med, Maywood 65; **RES:** IM, St Joseph Hosp-Chicago, Chicago, IL 66-69; **FAP:** Asst Clin Prof Med Northwestern U

Mutterperl, Robert (DO) IM
PCP
Resurrection Med Ctr
7447 W Talcott Ste 405; Chicago, IL 60631; (773) 763-3033; **BDCERT:** IM 77; Nep 82; **MS:** Univ Osteo Med & Hlth Sci 72; **RES:** IM, Michael Reese Hosp Med Ctr, Chicago, IL 73-74; **FEL:** Nep, Michael Reese Hosp Med Ctr, Chicago, IL 74-76

Newberger, Todd (MD) IM
PCP
Evanston Hosp
Central Street Partnership, 1713 Central St; Evanston, IL 60201; (847) 475-1333; **BDCERT:** IM 88; **MS:** Northwestern U 85

Nora, Maryannette (MD) IM
PCP
Columbus Hosp
Nora Medical Group, 6969 N Lincoln Ave Ste 324; Lincolnwood, IL 60646; (847) 674-1200; **BDCERT:** IM 93; **MS:** Loyola U-Stritch Sch Med, Maywood 83

Guide to symbols and abbreviations can be found on pages 110-113.

Ohri, Arun (MD) IM
PCP
Resurrection Med Ctr
7447 W Talcott Ave Ste 209; Chicago, IL 60631; (773) 631-2728; **BDCERT:** IM 84; Ge 89; **MS:** India 77; **RES:** IM, Lady Hasdinge Hospital, New Delhi, India 77-80; IM, Cook Cty Hosp, Chicago, IL 80-84; **FEL:** Ge, Cook Cty Hosp, Chicago, IL 84-86

Palmer, Scott Bradley (MD) IM
PCP
Rush North Shore Med Ctr
1725 Harrison Ste 318; Chicago, IL 60612; (312) 738-2966; **BDCERT:** IM 88; **MS:** Rush Med Coll 85; **RES:** IM, Rush Presbyterian-St Luke's Med Ctr, Chicago, IL 86-89; **HOSP:** Rush-Presbyterian-St Luke's Med Ctr

Patel, Jayant (MD) IM
PCP
Holy Cross Hosp
4255 W 63rd St; Chicago, IL 60629; (773) 581-7441; **BDCERT:** IM 82; **MS:** India 70; **RES:** St Francis Hosp, Elmhurst, NY 73-76; **FEL:** Cv, Mt Sinai Hosp, Chicago, IL 76-78; *SI: Diabetes; Geriatrics*; **HMO:** +
LANG: Eln;
A Few Days

Patel, Natubhai (MD) IM
PCP
St Mary's of Nazareth Hosp Ctr
North St Lewis Med Ctr, 3441 W North Ave; Chicago, IL 60647; (773) 772-6418; **BDCERT:** Inf 80; Ge 92; **MS:** India 70; **RES:** IM, Catholic Med Ctr Bklyn & Qns, Jamaica, NY 72-74; **FEL:** Inf, Queens Hosp Ctr, Jamaica, NY 74-76; **HMO:** Aetna Hlth Plan, Blue Cross & Blue Shield, Californiacare, Chicago HMO, Healthamerica +

Paul, Tarak (Dharam) (MD) IM
PCP
Grant Hosp
Grant Hosp- Internal Med, 550 W Webster Ave; Chicago, IL 60614; (773) 883-2000; **BDCERT:** IM 72; **MS:** India 55; **RES:** IM, Case West Res Univ Hosp, Cleveland, OH 65-66; IM, Cook Cty Hosp, Chicago, IL 70-72; **HMO:** Blue Cross & Blue Shield, Chicago HMO, Travelers

Pearson, Marilyn (MD) IM
PCP
Illinois Masonic Med Ctr
(see page 118)
Illinois Masonic Hosp, 3000 N Halsted St Ste 607; Chicago, IL 60657; (773) 296-5090; **BDCERT:** IM 80; Onc 83; **MS:** Boston U 77; **RES:** IM, U Chicago Hosp, Chicago, IL 77-81; **FEL:** HO, U IL Med Ctr, Chicago, IL 81-84; **FAP:** Asst Clin Prof Med U Chicago-Pritzker Sch Med; **HMO:** Blue Cross & Blue Shield, Chicago HMO, CIGNA, HIP Network, MD Individual Practice Assoc

Perez, Andrew (MD) IM
PCP
Little Company of Mary Hosp & Hlth Care Ctrs **(see page 142)**
2800 W 95th St; Evergreen Park, IL 60805; (708) 425-9399; **BDCERT:** IM 85; **MS:** Univ IL Coll Med 81; **RES:** IM, Illinois Masonic, Chicago, IL 81-84

Pierce, Warren (MD) IM
PCP
St Alexius Med Ctr
Northwest Health Care Assoc, 1575 Barrington Rd Ste 415; Hoffman Estates, IL 60194; (847) 843-7030; **BDCERT:** IM 81; Ger 94; **MS:** Univ IL Coll Med 78; **HOSP:** Alexian Brothers Med Ctr; **HMO:** Aetna Hlth Plan, Blue Cross & Blue Shield, CIGNA, Rush Health Plans

Pieri, Italo D. (MD) IM
PCP
Resurrection Med Ctr
7447 W Talcott Ave Ste 512; Chicago, IL 60631; (773) 774-3110; **BDCERT:** IM 81; Ge 88; **MS:** Italy 77; **RES:** IM, Illinois Masonic Med Ctr, Chicago, IL 78-81

Polychronopoulos, Soterios G (MD) IM
PCP
Little Company of Mary Hosp & Hlth Care Ctrs **(see page 142)**
Asklepious Medical Group, 11638 S Western Ave; Chicago, IL 60643; (773) 445-2422; **BDCERT:** IM 80; **MS:** Greece 71; **RES:** IM, Cook Cty Hosp, Chicago, IL 75-78; **FEL:** Pul, Hines VA Hosp, Hines, IL 78-80; **HMO:** Aetna Hlth Plan, Blue Choice, Blue Cross & Blue Shield, Chicago HMO, CIGNA

Principe, John R (MD) IM
PCP
Christ Hosp & Med Ctr **(see page 140)**
6234 S Narragansett Ave; Chicago, IL 60638; (773) 586-0843; **BDCERT:** IM 87; **MS:** Rush Med Coll 84; **RES:** IM, Rush Presbyterian-St Luke's Med Ctr, Chicago, IL 84-87; **FAP:** Assoc Prof Rush Med Coll

Raines, Robert (MD) IM
PCP
Christ Hosp & Med Ctr **(see page 140)**
Dale S Raines & Assoc Ltd, 4340 W 95th St Ste 205; Oak Lawn, IL 60453; (708) 636-1601; **BDCERT:** IM 78; **MS:** UC San Diego 75; **RES:** IM, Strong Mem Hosp, Rochester, NY 76-78

Ramsey, Michael (MD) IM
PCP
Rush-Presbyterian-St Luke's Med Ctr
(see page 122)
Ramsey Kehoe & Palmer, 1725 W Harrison St Ste 318; Chicago, IL 60612; (312) 738-2966; **BDCERT:** IM 71; **MS:** Northwestern U 68; **RES:** IM, Rush Presbyterian-St Luke's Med Ctr, Chicago, IL 69-72; **FAP:** Assoc Prof Rush Med Coll
LANG: Sp, Rus, Lth; A Few Days VISA

Reddy, Rajagopal (MD) IM
PCP
St Elizabeth's Hosp
1431 N Western Ave Ste 503; Chicago, IL 60622; (773) 489-7979; **BDCERT:** IM 80; Cv 83; **MS:** Other Foreign Country 73; **RES:** IM, Ill Masonic Med Ctr, Chicago, IL 77-80; **FEL:** Cv, Ill Masonic Med Ctr, Chicago, IL 81-83

Rehusch, Steven (MD) IM
PCP
St Alexius Med Ctr
Streamwood Family Medical Ctr, 403 W Irving Park Rd; Streamwood, IL 60107; (630) 830-1900; **BDCERT:** IM 85; **MS:** Univ IL Coll Med 82; **RES:** IM, Evanston Hosp, Evanston, IL 83-85; **HMO:** Blue Cross & Blue Shield, Rush Health Plans

Ringel, Paul (MD) IM
PCP
Illinois Masonic Med Ctr
(see page 118)
Drs Ringel, Fox & Pearson, 3000 N Halsted St; Chicago, IL 60657; (773) 296-5090; **BDCERT:** IM 81; **MS:** Rush Med Coll 78; **RES:** IM, Cook Cty Hosp, Chicago, IL 79-82; **FAP:** Clin Instr IM Rush Med Coll; **HMO:** Aetna Hlth Plan, Blue Cross & Blue Shield, Chicago HMO, Humana Health Plan, Prudential

Rotenberg, Morry (MD) IM
PCP
Holy Family Med Ctr
Adult Care Specialists, 1538 N Arlington Heights Rd; Arlington Hts, IL 60004; (847) 253-6464; **BDCERT:** IM 75; **MS:** Ohio State U 72; **RES:** IM, Rush Presbyterian-St Luke's Med Ctr, Chicago, IL 72-75; **FAP:** Asst Prof Rush Med Coll; **HOSP:** Northwest Comm Hlthcare; ***SI:** Preventive Care*; **HMO:** Humana Health Plan, United Healthcare, Rush Health Plans, Blue Cross & Blue Shield +
Immediately VISA

Rowley, Guy (MD) IM
PCP
St Joseph Hosp-Elgin
Sage Medical Group, 4811 N Milwaukee Ave Fl 2; Chicago, IL 60630; (773) 725-7557; **BDCERT:** IM 76; EM 83; **MS:** Northwestern U 72; **RES:** IM, Northwestern Meml Hosp, Chicago, IL 73-74; IM, Cook Cty Hosp, Chicago, IL 75-76; **FEL:** CCM, Hosp Foch, Paris, France 74-75; **HMO:** Aetna Hlth Plan, Blue Choice, Blue Cross & Blue Shield, Choicecare, CIGNA

Sabbagh, Haissam (MD) IM
PCP
Macneal Mem Hosp
6738 Cermak Rd; Berwyn, IL 60402; (708) 788-6363; **BDCERT:** IM 75; Pul 76; **MS:** Syria 68

Saheb, Farid (MD) IM
PCP
Our Lady Of the Resurrection Med Ctr
4900 N Cumberland; Norridge, IL 60656; (708) 453-0530; **BDCERT:** IM 76; Nep 76; **MS:** Other Foreign Country 70; **RES:** IM, Mount Sinai Hosp Med Ctr, Chicago, IL 71-73; **FEL:** Nep, Hines VA Hosp, Chicago, IL 73-75

Sattar, Abdul (MD) IM
PCP
Ravenswood Hosp Med Ctr
1945 W Wilson Ave Ste 1115; Chicago, IL 60640; (773) 728-4655; **BDCERT:** IM 73; EDM 75; **MS:** Pakistan 67; **RES:** IM, Wayne Cnty Gen Hosp, Detroit, MI 69-70; IM, Cook Cty Hosp, Chicago, IL 70-72; **FEL:** EDM, Michael Reese Hosp Med Ctr, Chicago, IL 72-73; EDM, Cook Cty Hosp, Chicago, IL 73-74; ***SI:** Diabetes; Thyroid*; **HMO:** Aetna Hlth Plan, Blue Cross & Blue Shield, CIGNA, United Healthcare, Prudential
LANG: Ur, Sp; A Few Days

Serushan, Majid (MD) IM
South Suburban Hosp
2605 Lincoln Hwy Ste 130; Olympia Fields, IL 60461; (708) 747-9780; **BDCERT:** Rhu 80; Ger 92; **MS:** Iran 73; **RES:** IM, Christ Hosp & Med Ctr, Oak Lawn, IL 75-78; **FEL:** Rhu, U IL Med Ctr, Chicago, IL 78-80; **FAP:** Asst Prof Univ IL Coll Med

Shah, Ashok (MD) IM
PCP
Ravenswood Hosp Med Ctr
Montrose Ashland Medical Ctr, 1624 W Montrose Ave; Chicago, IL 60613; (773) 769-3338; **BDCERT:** IM 84; **MS:** India 74; **RES:** IM, Christ Hosp & Med Ctr, Oak Lawn, IL 81-82; IM, Mercy Hosp & Med Ctr, Chicago, IL 82-84; **HOSP:** Swedish Covenant Hosp; ***SI:** Peptic Ulcer; Preventive Medicine*; **HMO:** Aetna Hlth Plan, Blue Cross & Blue Shield, United Healthcare, CIGNA, One Health Care +
LANG: Sp, Guj, Hin; Immediately VISA

Shah, Ranchhodlal (MD) IM
St Mary's of Nazareth Hosp Ctr
903 N Western Ave; Chicago, IL 60622; (773) 252-3113; **BDCERT:** IM 79; CCM 91; **MS:** India 70

Siegler, Mark (MD) IM
PCP
U Chicago Hosp (see page 124)
5841 S Maryland Ave MC 6098; Chicago, IL 60637; (773) 702-1453; **BDCERT:** IM 73; **MS:** U Chicago-Pritzker Sch Med 67; **RES:** IM, U Chicago Hosp, Chicago, IL 68-70; IM, U Chicago Hosp, Chicago, IL 70-71; **FEL:** IM, Royal Postgrad Med Sch, London, England 71-72; **FAP:** Prof Med U Chicago-Pritzker Sch Med

Siglin, Martin (MD) IM
PCP
Louis A Weiss Mem Hosp
Siglin Medical Assoc, 5327 N Sheridan Rd Ste A; Chicago, IL 60640; (773) 989-1111; **BDCERT:** IM 79; Ge 88; **MS:** Rush Med Coll 76; **RES:** IM, Rush Presbyterian-St Luke's Med Ctr, Chicago, IL 77-79; **FAP:** Assoc Clin Instr Med U Chicago-Pritzker Sch Med; **HMO:** Blue Cross & Blue Shield, Chicago HMO, Travelers

Simovic, Predrag (MD) IM
PCP
St Joseph Hosp-Chicago
2800 N Sheridan Ste 500; Chicago, IL 60657; (773) 348-0700; **BDCERT:** IM 96; **MS:** Yugoslavia 79; **RES:** IM, St Joseph's Hosp, Chicago, IL 84-87; ***SI:*** *Hypertension; Cholesterol*; **HMO:** +
LANG: Sp, Srb, Itl; Immediately

Skul, Vesna (MD) IM
PCP
Rush-Presbyterian-St Luke's Med Ctr (see page 122)
The Rush Center for Women's Medicine, 500 W Madison Ave Ste 400; Chicago, IL 60661; (312) 551-1301; **BDCERT:** IM 84; **MS:** Rush Med Coll 81; **RES:** IM, Rush Presbyterian-St Luke's Med Ctr, Chicago, IL 81-84; **FAP:** Asst Prof Rush Med Coll; ***SI:*** *Menopause; Alternative Medicine*; **HMO:** Rush Prudential, Blue Cross & Blue Shield, Aetna Hlth Plan, CIGNA +
LANG: Crt, Pol, Sp; 2-4 Weeks VISA

Sokol, Norton (MD) IM
PCP
Mount Sinai Hosp Med Ctr
Touhy Health Ctr, 2901 W Touhy Ave; Chicago, IL 60608; (773) 973-7350; **BDCERT:** IM 69; **MS:** U Hlth Sci/Chicago Med Sch 61; **RES:** IM, Mount Sinai Hosp Med Ctr, Chicago, IL 62-63; IM, Chicago VA Hlth Care System-Westside, Chicago, IL 64-66; **HMO:** Blue Cross & Blue Shield, Chicago HMO, Maxicare Health Plan

Starr, Byron (MD) IM
PCP
Northwestern Mem Hosp
676 N Saint Clair St Ste 300; Chicago, IL 60611; (312) 787-2772; **BDCERT:** IM 75; **MS:** Ind U Sch Med 72; **RES:** IM, Northwestern Mem Hosp, Chicago, IL 73-75; **FAP:** Assoc Prof Northwestern U
1 Week

Sweeney, Howard (MD) IM
Mercy Hosp & Med Ctr
Mercy Medical In Chicago Ridge, 9830 Ridgeland Ave; Chicago Ridge, IL 60415; (708) 636-8200; **BDCERT:** IM 70; EDM 79; **MS:** Loyola U-Stritch Sch Med, Maywood 62; **RES:** IM, Mercy Hosp & Med Ctr, Chicago, IL 63-64; IM, West Side VA, Chicago, IL 64-67; **FEL:** EndoNum - U IL-West Side VA, Chicago, IL 67-68; **FAP:** Clin Prof Univ IL Coll Med; **HMO:** Blue Cross & Blue Shield, Chicago HMO

Tatar, Arnold M (MD) IM
PCP
Northwestern Mem Hosp
Tatar, Tatar & Buchanan, 111 N Wabash Ave Ste 1919; Chicago, IL 60602; (312) 726-8800; **BDCERT:** IM 74; **MS:** Univ IL Coll Med 57; **RES:** IM/Cv, Michael Reese Hosp Med Ctr, Chicago, IL 57-61; **FAP:** Asst Prof Northwestern U; ***SI:*** *Hypertension*; **HMO:** Blue Choice, Blue Shield, Californiacare, Rush Health Plans, CIGNA
LANG: Sp; 4+ Weeks VISA

Tatar, Audrey (MD) IM
PCP
Northwestern Mem Hosp
111 N Wabash Ave Ste 1919; Chicago, IL 60602; (312) 726-8800; **BDCERT:** IM 91; **MS:** U Chicago-Pritzker Sch Med 88; **RES:** IM, Michael Reese Hosp Med Ctr, Chicago, IL 88-92; **FAP:** Clin Instr Northwestern U; ***SI:*** *Primary Care*; **HMO:** Blue Cross & Blue Shield, United Healthcare, Aetna Hlth Plan, PHCS +
2-4 Weeks VISA

Thomas, Michael (DO) IM
PCP
Little Company of Mary Hosp & Hlth Care Ctrs (see page 142)
2850 W 95th St Ste 106; Evergreen Park, IL 60805; (708) 842-9399; **BDCERT:** IM 86; **MS:** Univ Hlth Sci Coll -Osteo Med 80; **RES:** IM, Chicago Coll Osteopathic Medicine, Chicago, IL 80-84; **HOSP:** St Francis Hosp; ***SI:*** *Geriatrics*; **HMO:** Humana Health Plan, Blue Cross & Blue Shield +
1 Week

Tosetti, Patrick (MD) IM
PCP
Loyola U Med Ctr (see page 120)
Loyola U Med Ctr, 9608 S Roberts Rd; Hickory Hills, IL 60457; (708) 233-5333; **BDCERT:** IM 85; **MS:** U Chicago-Pritzker Sch Med 82; **RES:** IM, U Chicago Hosp, Chicago, IL 83-85; **FAP:** Asst Prof Med Loyola U-Stritch Sch Med, Maywood

Tulley, John E. (MD) IM
PCP
Michael Reese Hosp & Med Ctr
IM Clinic, 2800 S Vernon St; Chicago, IL 60616; (312) 791-5000; **BDCERT:** IM 79; **MS:** Univ IL Coll Med 74; **RES:** IM, Cook Cty Hosp, Chicago, IL 76-79; **FAP:** Asst Clin Prof Univ IL Coll Med

Twaddle, Martha (MD) IM
PCP
Evanston Hosp
Orchard Medical Group - Lower Level, 64 Old Orchard Ctr; Skokie, IL 60077; (847) 679-6707; **BDCERT:** IM 88; **MS:** Ind U Sch Med 85; **RES:** IM, Evanston Hosp, Evanston, IL 85-89

Valaitis, Daiva (MD) IM
Resurrection Med Ctr
Chicago Nephrology Assoc, 7447 W Talcott Ave Ste 245; Chicago, IL 60631; (773) 763-3033; **BDCERT:** IM 90; Nep 96; **MS:** Univ IL Coll Med 84; **RES:** IM, U IL Med Ctr, Chicago, IL 85-88; **FEL:** Nep, U IL Med Ctr, Chicago, IL 87-89; **FAP:** Clin Instr Med Univ IL Coll Med; **HOSP:** Grant Hosp

Wechter, David T (MD) IM
PCP
Michael Reese Hosp & Med Ctr
Hyde Park Assoc In Medicine, 1515 E 52nd Pl Fl 3; Chicago, IL 60615; (773) 493-8212; **BDCERT:** IM 82; **MS:** Univ IL Coll Med 79; **RES:** IM, Michael Reese Hosp Med Ctr, Chicago, IL 79-82; **FAP:** Asst Clin Prof U Chicago-Pritzker Sch Med; **HMO:** Aetna Hlth Plan, Blue Cross & Blue Shield, Chicago HMO, CIGNA, Humana Health Plan

Wistenberg, Lexy (MD) IM
PCP
Rush North Shore Med Ctr
North Shore Medical Specialist, 6131 W Dempster St; Morton Grove, IL 60053; (847) 967-5010; **BDCERT:** IM 91; **MS:** U Wisc Med Sch 88; **HMO:** Aetna Hlth Plan, Blue Cross & Blue Shield, Chicago HMO, Metlife, Prudential

Wyse, Joseph (MD) IM
PCP
Evanston Hosp
Orchard Medical Group, 64 Old Orchard Ctr Ste 210; Skokie, IL 60025; (847) 679-6707; **BDCERT:** IM 94; **MS:** U Chicago-Pritzker Sch Med 90; **RES:** IM, Evanston Hosp-Northwestern, Evanston, IL 91-93; IM, Evanston Hosp-Northwestern, Evanston, IL 93-94; **FAP:** Clin Instr Northwestern U

Yegelwel, Eric (MD) IM
PCP
Lutheran Gen Hosp (see page 143)
Riverside Medical, 3405 N Arlington Heights Rd; Arlington Hts, IL 60004; (847) 577-9300; **BDCERT:** IM 86; Ge 89; **MS:** UMDNJ-NJ Med Sch, Newark 83; **RES:** IM, U Chicago Hosp, Chicago, IL 84-86; **FEL:** Ge, Loyola U Med Ctr, Maywood, IL 87-89; **HOSP:** Northwest Comm Hlthcare
VISA

Zimmanck Jr, Robert D (MD) IM
PCP
Lutheran Gen Hosp (see page 143)
Internal Medicine Dept, 1775 Ballard Rd; Park Ridge, IL 60068; (847) 318-9340; **BDCERT:** IM 84; **MS:** Univ IL Coll Med 81; **RES:** IM, Lutheran Gen Hosp, Park Ridge, IL 82-85; **FAP:** Assoc Prof Med Univ IL Coll Med

MATERNAL & FETAL MEDICINE

Ambrose, Steven (MD) MF
Christ Hosp & Med Ctr (see page 140)
Christ Hospital, 4440 W 95th St; Oak Lawn, IL 60453; (630) 505-9700; **BDCERT:** ObG 91; MF 96; **MS:** Northwestern U 84; **HMO:** +
Mcr Mcd 1 Week

Ismail, Mahmoud (MD) MF
U Chicago Hosp (see page 124)
University-Chicago-Dept of Ob/Gyn, 5841 S Maryland Ave MC 2050; Chicago, IL 60637; (773) 702-6118; **BDCERT:** ObG 97; MF 87; **MS:** Egypt 70; ***SI:*** *Infectious Diseases*

Mangurten, Henry (MD) MF
Lutheran Gen Hosp (see page 143)
Depatrment of Pediatrics, 1775 Dempster St; Park Ridge, IL 60068; (847) 723-6993; **BDCERT:** Ped 70; **MS:** Univ IL Coll Med 65; **RES:** Ped, U IL Med Ctr, Chicago, IL 66-67; Ped, USC Med Ctr, Los Angeles, CA 67-68; **FEL:** NP, U IL Med Ctr, Chicago, IL 70-72; **FAP:** Clin Prof U Chicago-Pritzker Sch Med; ***SI:*** *Maternal Drug Use and the Newborn; Newborns with Birth Injuries*
Mcr Mcd

Strassner, Howard T (MD) MF
Rush-Presbyterian-St Luke's Med Ctr (see page 122)
1725 W Harrison Suite 408; Chicago, IL 60612; (847) 942-6611; **BDCERT:** ObG 81; MF 82; **MS:** U Chicago-Pritzker Sch Med 74; **RES:** ObG, Columbia-Presbyterian Med Ctr, New York, NY 74-78; **FEL:** MF, USC Med Ctr, Los Angeles, CA 78-80; **FAP:** Assoc Prof Rush Med Coll; ***SI:*** *High Risk Pregnancy*; **HMO:** Aetna Hlth Plan, Blue Cross & Blue Shield, Californiacare, Rush Health Plans, Travelers +
LANG: Sp, Pol; Mcr Mcd NFI
A Few Days

Guide to symbols and abbreviations can be found on pages 110-113.

MEDICAL GENETICS

Booth, Carol (MD) MG
Lutheran Gen Hosp (see page 143)
Advocate Medical Group Genetics, 1875 Dempster St Ste 340; Park Ridge, IL 60068; (847) 723-7705; **BDCERT:** CG 82; Ped 73; **MS:** Northwestern U 68; **RES:** Ped, Children's Mem Med Ctr, Chicago, IL 68-71; **FEL:** CG, Children's Mem Med Ctr, Chicago, IL 71-73; **HOSP:** Northwest Comm Hlthcare; ***SI:*** *Prenatal Diagnosis; Cancer Genetics*; **HMO:** Blue Cross & Blue Shield, CIGNA, Prucare, PHCS
A Few Days VISA

Burton, Barbara (MD) MG
Children's Mem Med Ctr (see page 139)
Children's Memorial Hospital, 2300 Children's Plz; Chicago, IL 60612; (773) 880-4000; **BDCERT:** Ped 78; CG 82; **MS:** Northwestern U 73; **RES:** MG, Children's Mem Med Ctr, Chicago, IL 75-77; Ped A&I, Children's Mem Med Ctr, Chicago, IL 74-75; **FAP:** Prof Northwestern U; ***SI:*** *Marfan's Syndrome; Urea Cycle Defects*; **HMO:** +
2-4 Weeks

Hoganson, George E (MD) MG
Univ of Illinois at Chicago Med Ctr
840 S Wood St MC856; Chicago, IL 60612; (312) 996-0963; **BDCERT:** MG 93; Ped 82; **MS:** Univ IL Coll Med 78; **RES:** U Wisc Hosp, Madison, WI 79-81; **FEL:** U Wisc Hosp, Madison, WI 81-84; **FAP:** Assoc Prof Univ IL Coll Med; ***SI:*** *Inborn Errors of Metabolism; Birth Defects*; **HMO:** +
LANG: Sp; 1 Week

Israel, Jeannette (MD) MG
Christ Hosp & Med Ctr (see page 140)
Hope Children's Hospital, 4440 W 95th St Rm 3141 H; Oak Lawn, IL 60453; (708) 346-2529; **BDCERT:** MG 82; Ped 76; **MS:** U Hlth Sci/Chicago Med Sch 71

Wong, Paul (MD) MG
Rush-Presbyterian-St Luke's Med Ctr
(see page 122)
Presbyterian-St Lukes Medical Center, 1750 W Harrison St; Chicago, IL 60612; (312) 942-6298; **BDCERT:** MG 82; Ped 64; **MS:** Hong Kong 58; **RES:** St Boniface Hosp, Winnipeg, Canada 59-60; Childrens Hosp, Winnipeg, Canada 60-61; **FEL:** Children's Mem Med Ctr, Chicago, IL 62-64; Children's Mem Med Ctr, Chicago, IL 65-67; ***SI:*** *Huntington's Disease; Fragility Syndrome*
LANG: Chi; NFI
Immediately VISA

MEDICAL ONCOLOGY

Ahmed, Vasia (MD) Onc
Ingalls Mem Hosp
Horizon Health Care Assoc, 16325 S Harlem Ave Ste 1W; Tinley Park, IL 60477; (708) 429-1960; **BDCERT:** IM 88; Onc 95; **MS:** Pakistan 79; **RES:** IM, Cook Cty Hosp, Chicago, IL 84-86; **FEL:** Onc, U Chicago Hosp, Chicago, IL 86-88; Hem, Rush Presbyterian-St Luke's Med Ctr, Chicago, IL 88-89; **FAP:** Asst Prof Rush Med Coll; **HOSP:** St James Hosp & Hlth Ctrs; ***SI:*** *Oncology; Hematology*; **HMO:** +
A Few Days VISA

Albain, Kathy (MD) Onc
Loyola U Med Ctr (see page 120)
Loyola Univ Medical Ctr, 2160 S 1st Ave Ste 109; Maywood, IL 60153; (708) 327-3102; **BDCERT:** IM 81; Onc 83; **MS:** U Mich Med Sch 78; **RES:** IM, U IL Med Ctr, Chicago, IL 79-81; **FEL:** HO, U Chicago Hosp, Chicago, IL 81-84; **FAP:** Prof Med Loyola U-Stritch Sch Med, Maywood; ***SI:*** *Breast Cancer; Lung Cancer*; **HMO:** +
VISA

Bonomi, Philip (MD) Onc
Rush-Presbyterian-St Luke's Med Ctr
(see page 122)
Rush Cancer Institute, 1725 W Harrison St Ste 821; Chicago, IL 60612; (312) 942-5904; **BDCERT:** Onc 77; IM 75; **MS:** Univ IL Coll Med 70; **RES:** IM, Geisinger Med Ctr, Danville, PA 71-72; Geisinger Med Ctr, Danville, PA 74-75; **FEL:** Onc, Rush Presbyterian-St Luke's Med Ctr, Chicago, IL 75-77; **FAP:** Assoc Prof Rush Med Coll; ***SI:*** *Lung Cancer; Mesothelioma*; **HMO:** Blue Cross & Blue Shield, Rush Prudential, Aetna-US Healthcare
LANG: Sp; NFI

Burt, Richard K. (MD) Onc
Northwestern Mem Hosp
Northwestern Meml Hosp-Olson Pavilion, 710 N Fairbanks Ct FL 8; Chicago, IL 60611; (312) 908-5400; **BDCERT:** IM 89; Onc 93; **MS:** St Louis U 84; ***SI:*** *Bone Marrow Transplant-Allogenic; Auto Immune Disease*; **HMO:** +
LANG: Sp; VISA

Chawla, Manjeet S (MD) Onc
Thorek Hosp & Med Ctr
850 W Irving Park Rd; Chicago, IL 60613; (773) 525-6780; **BDCERT:** Hem 80; Onc 79; **MS:** India 72; **RES:** IM, , India 73-76; **FEL:** Hem&Onc, U IL Med Ctr, Chicago, IL 76-79; **FAP:** Asst Clin Prof Univ IL Coll Med; **HOSP:** Norwegian-American Hosp

Fisher, Richard (MD) Onc
Loyola U Med Ctr (see page 120)
Cardinal Bernardin Cancer Ctr-Rm. 255; Loyola University Medical Center, 2160 S First Ave Rm255; Maywood, IL 60153; (708) 327-3300; **BDCERT:** Onc 77; IM 73; **MS:** Harvard Med Sch 70; **RES:** IM, Mass Gen Hosp, Boston, MA 71-72; Nat Cancer Inst, Bethesda, MD 72-74; **FEL:** Onc, Nat Cancer Inst, Bethesda, MD 74-75; **FAP:** Chrmn Onc Loyola U-Stritch Sch Med, Maywood; ***SI:*** *Hodgkin's Disease; Non-Hodgkin's Lymphoma*; **HMO:** Aetna-US Healthcare, Blue Cross & Blue Shield, First Health
1 Week

Golomb, Harvey (MD) Onc
U Chicago Hosp (see page 124)
5841 S Maryland Ave; Chicago, IL 60637; (773) 702-6115; **BDCERT:** IM 75; Onc 79; **MS:** Univ Pittsburgh 68; **RES:** Johns Hopkins Hosp, Baltimore, MD 71-72; Johns Hopkins Hosp, Baltimore, MD 72-73; **FEL:** HO, U Chicago Hosp, Chicago, IL 73-75; **FAP:** Prof Med U Hlth Sci/Chicago Med Sch; ***SI:*** *Leukemia/Lymphoma; Lung Cancer*
1 Week

Grad, Gary I. (MD) Onc
Alexian Brothers Med Ctr
(see page 138)
Oncology & Hematology, 820 Biesterfield Rd Ste 120; Elk Grove Village, IL 60007; (847) 956-5107; **BDCERT:** Onc 95; IM 92; **MS:** U Chicago-Pritzker Sch Med 89; **RES:** IM, U Chicago Hosp, Chicago, IL 90-92; **FEL:** HO, U Chicago Hosp, Chicago, IL 92-94; **HOSP:** Northwest Comm Hlthcare; ***SI:*** *Autologous Stem Cell Transplant; Breast Cancer*
1 Week VISA

Hannigan, James (MD) Onc
La Grange Mem Hosp (see page 141)
La Grange Oncology Assoc, 1325 Memorial Dr; La Grange, IL 60525; (708) 579-3418; **BDCERT:** Onc 87; IM 84; **MS:** U Chicago-Pritzker Sch Med 81; **RES:** IM, U Chicago Hosp, Chicago, IL 82-84; **FEL:** Onc, Johns Hopkins Hosp, Baltimore, MD 84; **HOSP:** Christ Hosp & Med Ctr

Hoeltgen, Thomas (MD) Onc
Christ Hosp & Med Ctr (see page 140)
Associates In Medical Oncology, 4400 W 95th St Ste 311; Oak Lawn, IL 60453; (708) 424-9710; **MS:** Northwestern U 66; **RES:** IM, Rush Presby-St Lukes, Chicago, IL 68-72; **FEL:** Onc, Rush Presby-St Lukes, Chicago, IL 73; **FAP:** Asst Prof Med Rush Med Coll; ***SI:*** *Breast Cancer; Colorectal Cancer*

Khandekar, Janardan (MD) Onc
Evanston Hosp
Evanston Hospital, 2650 Ridge Ave G355; Evanston, IL 60201; (847) 570-2515; **BDCERT:** IM 74; Onc 75; **MS:** India 69; **RES:** IM, Allegheny Gen Hosp, Pittsburgh, PA 72-73; **FEL:** Onc, Tufts U, Boston, MA 73-75; **HOSP:** Glenbrook Hosp; ***SI:*** *Prevention & Treatment of Breast Cancer; Prostate Cancer*; **HMO:** Aetna Hlth Plan, Blue Cross, Humana Health Plan, CIGNA, United Healthcare
LANG: Hin, Mar;
1 Week VISA

Kies, Merrill (MD) Onc
Northwestern Mem Hosp
Northwestern Medical Faculty Foundation, 233 E Erie St Ste 700; Chicago, IL 60611; (312) 908-8697; **BDCERT:** Onc 76; **MS:** Loyola U-Stritch Sch Med, Maywood 73; **RES:** Walter Reed Army Med Ctr, Washington, DC 74-76; **FEL:** HO, Brooke Army Med Ctr, San Antonio, TX 76-78; **FAP:** Prof Med Northwestern U; ***SI:*** *Head & Neck Cancer; Lung Cancer*; **HMO:** +
1 Week VISA

Klingerman, Hans (MD) Onc
Rush-Presbyterian-St Luke's Med Ctr
(see page 122)
1653 W Congress Pkwy; Chicago, IL 60612; (312) 942-3047; **BDCERT:** Onc 86; IM 84; **MS:** Germany 76; **RES:** IM, Univ Med Sch, Marburg, Germany 78-84; **FEL:** Onc, Fred Hutchinson Cancer Research Ctr, Seattle, WA 84-86; **FAP:** Prof Med Rush Med Coll; ***SI:*** *Bone Marrow Transplant; Immunotherapy*; **HMO:** Aetna Hlth Plan, Rush Prudential +
LANG: Sp, Ger;
A Few Days VISA

Krauss, Stuart (MD) Onc
Louis A Weiss Mem Hosp
4646 N Marine Dr; Chicago, IL 60640; (773) 878-8700; **BDCERT:** IM 75; Onc 77; **MS:** Univ IL Coll Med 72; **RES:** IM, U IL Med Ctr, Chicago, IL 73-75; **FEL:** HO, U IL Med Ctr, Chicago, IL 75-77; **FAP:** Assoc Prof Med U Chicago-Pritzker Sch Med

Leibach, Steven J (MD) Onc
Alexian Brothers Med Ctr
(see page 138)
Northwest Oncology & Hmtlgy, 820 Biesterfield Rd Ste 120; Elk Grove Vlg, IL 60007; (847) 437-3312; **BDCERT:** Onc 85; IM 81; **MS:** Univ IL Coll Med 78; **RES:** Onc, Rush Presbyterian-St Luke's Med Ctr, Chicago, IL 81-83; Ohio State U Hosp, Columbus, OH; **FEL:** Onc, Rush Presbyterian-St Luke's Med Ctr, Chicago, IL; **HOSP:** Northwest Comm Hlthcare

Locker, Gershon (MD) Onc
Evanston Hosp
Evanston Hospital, 2650 Ridge Ave G355; Evanston, IL 60201; (847) 570-2515; **BDCERT:** Onc 77; IM 76; **MS:** Harvard Med Sch 73; **RES:** IM, U Chicago Hosp, Chicago, IL 74-75; **FEL:** Onc, Nat Cancer Inst, Bethesda, MD 75-78; **FAP:** Assoc Prof Med Northwestern U

Guide to symbols and abbreviations can be found on pages 110-113.

Locker, Gershon (MD) **Onc**
Evanston Hosp
Kellogg Cancer Center, 2650 Ridge Ave; Evanston, IL 60201; (847) 570-2515; **BDCERT:** Onc 77; IM 76; **MS:** Harvard Med Sch 73; **RES:** IM, U Chicago Hosp, Chicago, IL 74-75; **FEL:** Onc, Nat Cancer Inst, Bethesda, MD 75-78; **FAP:** Assoc Prof Med Northwestern U; ***SI:*** *Gastrointestinal Cancers; Ovarian and Breast Cancers*
2-4 Weeks

Merkel, Douglas (MD) **Onc**
Evanston Hosp
Evanston Northwestern Healthcare, 2650 Ridge Avenue; Evanston, IL 60201; (847) 570-2515; **BDCERT:** IM 84; Onc 87; **MS:** Northwestern U 81; **RES:** IM, Northwestern Mem Hosp, Chicago, IL 81-84; **FEL:** Path, Northwestern Mem Hosp, Chicago, IL 84-85; Onc, Univ of Texas Health Science Center, San Antonio, TX 85; **FAP:** Asst. Professor Onc Northwestern U; **HOSP:** Glenbrook Hosp; ***SI:*** *Breast Cancer*
1 Week VISA

Mullane, Michael (MD) **Onc**
Univ of Illinois at Chicago Med Ctr
Hem/Onc Dept, 840 Southwood St; Chicago, IL 60619; (312) 996-5585; **BDCERT:** Onc 87; IM 85; **MS:** Wayne State U Sch Med 82; ***SI:*** *Pancreatic Cancer*; **HMO:** +
1 Week

Newman, Steven (MD) **Onc**
Northwestern Mem Hosp
Hematology Oncology Assoc, 676 N Saint Clair St Ste 2140; Chicago, IL 60611; (312) 664-5400; **BDCERT:** Onc 83; Hem 84; **MS:** Tufts U 77; **RES:** IM, U Chicago Hosp, Chicago, IL 77-80; **FEL:** Hem, U Chicago Hosp, Chicago, IL 80-81; Onc, UCLA Med Ctr, Los Angeles, CA 81-82; **FAP:** Asst Prof Northwestern U; ***SI:*** *Leukemia, Lymphoma, Myeloma; Lung, Breast, Colon, Cancers*; **HMO:** Aetna Hlth Plan, Blue Cross & Blue Shield, Californiacare, CIGNA, Metlife +
A Few Days

O'Reilly, William (MD) **Onc**
Palos Comm Hosp
Palos Internal Medicine, 12150 S Harlem Ave; Palos Heights, IL 60463; (708) 361-4778; **BDCERT:** Onc 81; IM 78; **MS:** Loyola U-Stritch Sch Med, Maywood 75; **RES:** IM, Rush Presbyterian-St Luke's Med Ctr, Chicago, IL 76-78; **HOSP:** Little Company of Mary Hosp & Hlth Care Ctrs

Piel, Ira (MD) **Onc**
Illinois Masonic Med Ctr
(see page 118)
Medical Oncology & Hematology, 901 W Wellington Ave; Chicago, IL 60657; (773) 296-7089; **BDCERT:** Onc 75; IM 73; **MS:** Univ IL Coll Med 67; **RES:** IM, St Lukes Hosp, Chicago, IL 70-72; **FEL:** Onc, St Lukes Hosp, Chicago, IL 72-74; **FAP:** Asst Prof Rush Med Coll; **HMO:** Chicago HMO, United Healthcare

Preisler, Harvey (MD) **Onc**
Rush-Presbyterian-St Luke's Med Ctr
(see page 122)
Rush Cancer Institute, 1725 W Harrison St; Chicago, IL 60612; (312) 563-2190; **BDCERT:** IM 72; Onc 75; **MS:** U Rochester 65; **RES:** IM, Buffalo Gen Hosp, Buffalo, NY 66-67; IM, Roswell Park Mem Hosp, Buffalo, NY 66-67; **FEL:** Hem, Columbia-Presbyterian Med Ctr, New York, NY 69-71

Rosen, Steven (MD) **Onc**
Northwestern Mem Hosp
Northwestern Medical Faculty Foundation, 233 E Erie St Ste 700; Chicago, IL 60611; (312) 908-8697; **BDCERT:** Onc 81; Hem 84; **MS:** Northwestern U 76; **RES:** IM, Northwestern Mem Hosp, Chicago, IL 76-79; **FEL:** Onc, Nat Cancer Inst, Bethesda, MD 79-81; **FAP:** Prof Northwestern U; ***SI:*** *Hematologic Malignancies; Breast Cancer*; **HMO:** Aetna Hlth Plan, Rush Prudential, Blue Cross, Humana Health Plan, Private Healthcare +
LANG: Sp;
A Few Days VISA

Rosi, David (MD) **Onc**
Northwestern Mem Hosp
Hematology Oncology Assoc, 676 N Saint Clair St Ste 2140; Chicago, IL 60611; (312) 664-5400; **BDCERT:** Onc 81; IM 78; **MS:** Northwestern U 75; **RES:** IM, Cook Cty Hosp, Chicago, IL 76-78; **FEL:** Onc, MD Anderson Cancer Ctr, Houston, TX 78-79; **HMO:** Aetna Hlth Plan, Chicago HMO, CIGNA

Samuels, Brian (MD) **Onc**
Lutheran Gen Hosp **(see page 143)**
Lutheran General Cancer Center, 1700 Luther Lane; Park Ridge, IL 60068; (847) 723-2500; **BDCERT:** Onc 87; IM 84; **MS:** Zimbabwe 76; **RES:** IM, Albert Einstein Med Ctr, Philadelphia, PA 79-81; IM, Albert Einstein Med Ctr, Philadelphia, PA 83-84; **FEL:** Hem, U Chicago Hosp, Chicago, IL 84-88; **HOSP:** Univ of Illinois at Chicago Med Ctr; ***SI:*** *Sarcomas; Breast Cancer*

Shah, Prabodh (MD) **Onc**
Little Company of Mary Hosp & Hlth Care Ctrs **(see page 142)**
2850 W 95th St; Evergreen Park, IL 60805; (312) 633-7215; **BDCERT:** Hem 74; Onc 77; **MS:** India 62; **RES:** Chicago VA Hlth Care System-Westside, Chicago, IL 65-68; **FEL:** Hem, Chicago VA Hlth Care System-Westside, Chicago, IL 68-70; **HOSP:** Cook Cty Hosp

Shaw, John M (MD) **Onc**
Northwestern Mem Hosp
676 N Saint Clair St Ste 2140; Chicago, IL 60611; (312) 664-5400; **BDCERT:** IM 76; Onc 81; **MS:** U Md Sch Med 68; **RES:** IM, Northwestern Mem Hosp, Chicago, IL 69-72; **FEL:** Hem, Temple U Hosp, Philadelphia, PA 74-76; Onc, Temple U Hosp, Philadelphia, PA 74-76; **FAP:** Asst Prof Northwestern U; ***SI:*** *Cancer Chemotherapy*
A Few Days

Sowray, Paul (MD) **Onc**
Alexian Brothers Med Ctr
(see page 138)
NW Oncology & Hematology, 820 Biesterfield Rd Ste 120; Elk Grove Vlg, IL 60007; (847) 437-3312; **BDCERT:** Hem 96; Onc 87; **MS:** U Tenn Ctr Hlth Sci, Memphis 79; **RES:** IM, Madigan AMC, Tacoma, WA 80-82; **FEL:** HO, Letterman Gen Hosp, San Francisco, CA 84-87

Taylor, Samuel (MD) **Onc**
Illinois Masonic Med Ctr
(see page 118)
Illinois Masonic Cancer Ctr, 901 W Wellington Ave; Chicago, IL 60657; (773) 296-7405; **BDCERT:** IM 73; Onc 75; **MS:** Canada 69; **RES:** Albany Med Ctr, Albany, NY 70-72; **FEL:** Onc, Albany Med Ctr, Albany, NY 72-74; **FAP:** Prof Med Rush Med Coll

Tsarwhas, Dean (MD) **Onc**
Condell Med Ctr
North Shore Oncology, 450 W Il Route 22 G80; Barrington, IL 60010; (847) 842-0850; **BDCERT:** Onc 93; IM 90; **MS:** NE Ohio U 87; **RES:** IM, U Mich Med Ctr, Ann Arbor, MI 87-91; **FEL:** Onc, Dana-Farber Cancer Inst, Boston, MA 91-93; **HMO:** Aetna Hlth Plan, Chicago HMO, Travelers

Vokes, Everett E (MD) **Onc**
U Chicago Hosp **(see page 124)**
5841 S Maryland Ave MC2115; Chicago, IL 60637; (773) 834-3093; **BDCERT:** Onc 85; IM 83; **MS:** Germany 80; **RES:** IM, Ravenswood Hosp Med Ctr, Chicago, IL 81-82; IM, Los Angeles Cty Hosp, Los Angeles, CA 82-83; **FEL:** Hem, U Chicago Hosp, Chicago, IL 83-86; **FAP:** Prof U Chicago-Pritzker Sch Med; ***SI:*** *Head & Neck Cancer; Lung Cancer*

Wade, Elaine (MD) **Onc**
West Suburban Hosp Med Ctr
7420 W Central; River Forrest, IL 60305; (708) 383-6200; **BDCERT:** Onc 95; Hem 96; **MS:** Rush Med Coll 89; **RES:** IM, Rush Presbyterian-St Luke's Med Ctr, Chicago, IL 90-92; **FEL:** Hem/Onc, Northwestern Mem Hosp, Chicago, IL 92-95; **FAP:** Asst Prof Loyola U-Stritch Sch Med, Maywood

Wolter, Janet (MD) **Onc**
Rush-Presbyterian-St Luke's Med Ctr
(see page 122)
Center for Medical Oncology, 1725 W Harrison St Ste 821; Chicago, IL 60612; (312) 563-2512; **BDCERT:** IM 72; **MS:** Univ IL Coll Med 50; **RES:** IM, Duke U Med Ctr, Durham, NC 53-54; IM, U IL Rsch-Ed Hosps, Chicago, IL 54-55; **FEL:** IM, U IL Presby Hosp, Chicago, IL 51-52; **FAP:** Prof Med Rush Med Coll; ***SI:*** *Breast Cancer;* **HMO:** Aetna Hlth Plan, Blue Cross & Blue Shield, Care America Health Plan, Chicago HMO, Humana Health Plan
A Few Days VISA

NEONATAL-PERINATAL MEDICINE

Benawara, Raghbir (MD) **NP**
Lutheran Gen Hosp **(see page 143)**
1775 Dempster St; Park Ridge, IL 60068; (847) 723-5313; **BDCERT:** NP 79; Ped 79; **MS:** Univ IL Coll Med 72; **RES:** Ped, Lutheran Gen Hosp, Park Ridge, IL 75-77; **FEL:** NP, Lutheran Gen Hosp, Park Ridge, IL 77-79; **FAP:** Asst Prof Ped Univ IL Coll Med

Caplan, Michael (MD) **NP**
Evanston Hosp
ENH Evanston Hosp-Dept of Pediatrics, 2650 Ridge Ave; Evanston, IL 60201; (847) 570-2033; **BDCERT:** Ped 88; NP 89; **MS:** U Chicago-Pritzker Sch Med 84; **RES:** Ped, Children's Mem Med Ctr, Chicago, IL 84-87; NP, Children's Mem Med Ctr, Chicago, IL 87-89; **FAP:** Assoc Prof Ped Northwestern U; ***SI:*** *Necrotizing Enterocolitis;* **HMO:** +
VISA

Chaudhry, Urmila (MD) **NP**
Gottlieb Mem Hosp
701 W North Ave; Melrose Park, IL 60010; (773) 883-3555; **BDCERT:** Ped 85; NP 89; **MS:** India 77

Deddish, Ruth B (MD) **NP**
Northwestern Mem Hosp
333 E Superior St Rm326; Chicago, IL 60611; (312) 926-7514; **BDCERT:** Ped 77; NP 77; **MS:** SUNY Syracuse 69; **RES:** NP, Northwestern Mem Hosp, Chicago, IL 73-75; Ped A&I, Children's Mem Med Ctr, Chicago, IL 69-72; **FAP:** Asst Prof ObG Northwestern U; ***SI:*** *Critical Care Pediatrics*
LANG: Sp;

Gardner, Thomas (MD) **NP**
Evanston Hosp
Evanston Hosp, 2650 Ridge Ave; Evanston, IL 60201; (847) 570-2033; **BDCERT:** NP 77; PCd 65; **MS:** Case West Res U 56; **RES:** NC Meml Hosp, Chapel Hill, NC 56; Yale-New Haven Hosp, New Haven, CT 60; **FEL:** Cv, Yale-New Haven Hosp, New Haven, CT 61-63; **FAP:** Prof Ped Northwestern U

George, Jeffrey (DO) **NP**
Lutheran Gen Hosp **(see page 143)**
Lutheran General Hospital, 1775 Dempster St; Park Ridge, IL 60068; (847) 723-5313; **BDCERT:** Ped 90; NP 95; **MS:** U of Hlth Sci, Coll Osteo Med 86

Ghai, Vivek (MD) NP
Illinois Masonic Med Ctr
(see page 118)
Illinois Masonic Med Ctr, 836 W Wellington Rm3613; Chicago, IL 60657; (312) 296-7042; **BDCERT:** NP 89; Ped 87; **MS:** India 81; **RES:** Ped, U IL Med Ctr, Chicago, IL 84-86; **FEL:** NP, U IL Med Ctr, Chicago, IL 86-88; **FAP:** Asst Prof Rush Med Coll; ***SI:*** *PPHN; RDS*
LANG: Sp, Hin, Pun, Tel, Tag; Immediately VISA

Kim, Moon (MD) NP
St James Hosp & Hlth Ctrs
Neonatology & Pediatrics, 2555 Lincoln Hwy Ste 204; Olympia Fields, IL 60461; (708) 748-3360; **BDCERT:** Ped 84; **MS:** South Korea 70; **RES:** Ped, Hanyung U, Korea 74-76; Ped, St Louis City Hosp, St Louis, MO 76-78; **FEL:** NP, U Chicago Hosp, Chicago, IL 78-80; **HOSP:** South Suburban Hosp; ***SI:*** *Respiratory Disease in Newborns; Prematurity*; **HMO:** Blue Cross & Blue Shield, Aetna Hlth Plan, Rush Pru, CIGNA +
LANG: Kor; Immediately

Lee, Kwang-Sun (MD) NP
U Chicago Hosp **(see page 124)**
University of Chicago Children's Hospital - MC6060, 5841 S Maryland Ave; Chicago, IL 60637; (773) 702-6210; **BDCERT:** Ped 71; NP 76; **MS:** South Korea 66; **RES:** Ped, Albert Einstein Med Ctr, Bronx, NY 66-68; **FEL:** PCd, Brookdale Univ Hosp Med Ctr, Brooklyn, NY 69-71; NP, Albert Einstein Med Ctr, Bronx, NY 71-73; **FAP:** Prof ObG U Chicago-Pritzker Sch Med; ***SI:*** *Pediatric Epidemiology*; **HMO:** +
LANG: Kor;

Muraskas, Jonathon (MD) NP
Loyola U Med Ctr **(see page 120)**
Russo Surgical Pav, Loyola U Med Ctr, 2160 S First Ave Rm5806; Maywood, IL 60153; (708) 327-9082; **BDCERT:** NP 87; Ped 86; **MS:** Loyola U-Stritch Sch Med, Maywood 82; **RES:** Ped A&I, Loyola U Med Ctr, Maywood, IL 83-85; **FEL:** NP, Loyola U Med Ctr, Maywood, IL 85-87; **FAP:** Assoc Prof Ped Loyola U-Stritch Sch Med, Maywood

Ogata, Edward (MD) NP
Children's Mem Med Ctr **(see page 139)**
2300 N Childrens Plz Ste 45; Chicago, IL 60614; (773) 880-4012; **BDCERT:** Ped 76; NP 77; **MS:** Northwestern U 71

Paton, John (MD) NP
Michael Reese Hosp & Med Ctr
Michael Reese Hospital & Med Ctr, 2929 S Ellis St Ste 12KC; Chicago, IL 60616; (312) 791-2000; **BDCERT:** Ped 70; NP 75; **MS:** England 64; **RES:** U Edinburgh, Edinburgh, Scotland 66-67; Brigham & Women's Hosp, Boston, MA 67-68; **FEL:** NP, U IL Med Ctr, Chicago, IL 69-71; **FAP:** Assoc Clin Prof Ped Univ IL Coll Med

Polk, Dan (MD) NP
Children's Mem Med Ctr **(see page 139)**
Children's Meml Hosp, 2300 Children's Plz 9FL; Chicago, IL 60614; (773) 880-4142; **BDCERT:** NP 87; Ped 86; **MS:** U Hlth Sci/Chicago Med Sch 80; **RES:** Ped, Harbor-UCLA Med Ctr, Torrance, CA 81-83; **FEL:** NP, Harbor-UCLA Med Ctr, Torrance, CA 83-85; **FAP:** Prof Ped Northwestern U

Rathi, Manohar (MD) NP
Christ Hosp & Med Ctr **(see page 140)**
Midwest Neoped Assoc Ltd, 4440 W 95th St N232; Oak Lawn, IL 60453; (708) 346-5718; **BDCERT:** NP 75; Ped 70; **MS:** India 61; **RES:** IM, Memorial Hosp, Darlington, KY 63-64; Ped, Methodist Hosp, Brooklyn, NY 69-70; **FEL:** NP, NY Methodist Hosp, Brooklyn, NY 70-71; **FAP:** Assoc Prof Ped Rush Med Coll

Wassef, Samir Y (MD) NP
St Mary's of Nazareth Hosp Ctr
Metropolitan Neopediatrix SC, 11786 Lighthouse Lane; Palos Heights, IL 60463; (773) 227-0111; **BDCERT:** NP 97; Ped 94; **MS:** Egypt 86; **RES:** Ped, Childrens Hosp Of WI, Milwaukee, WI 88-90; Ped, Henry Ford Hosp, Detroit, MI 90-92; **FEL:** NP, LSU Med Ctr, Shreveport, LA 92-93; NP, U Chicago Hosp, Chicago, IL 93; **FAP:** Clinical Instr. NP Univ IL Coll Med; **HOSP:** Christ Hosp & Med Ctr; ***SI:*** *Newborn Care; Asthma*; **HMO:** Blue Cross & Blue Shield, Aetna-US Healthcare, Travelers, Rush Health Plans
LANG: Sp, Ar, Pol, SCr, Rus; Immediately

NEPHROLOGY

Agrawal, Rekha (MD) Nep
Hinsdale Hosp **(see page 275)**
Dept of Pediatrics, 2160 S First Ave; Maywood, IL 60153; (708) 327-9149; **BDCERT:** Ped 86; PNep 88; **MS:** India 75; **RES:** Ped, All India Inst Med Science, New Delhi, India 75-77; Ped, Cook Cty Hosp, Chicago, IL 82-84; **FEL:** PNep, U IL Med Ctr, Chicago, IL 84-86; **FAP:** Instr Univ IL Coll Med; **HMO:** +
1 Week

Ahuja, Satya (MD) **Nep**
South Shore Hosp
2534 W 69th St; Chicago, IL 60629; (312) 951-4950; **BDCERT:** Nep 86; IM 75; **MS:** India 68; **RES:** IM, Cook Cty Hosp, Chicago, IL 72-74; Nep, Cook Cty Hosp, Chicago, IL 74-75; **FEL:** Nep, U Chicago Hosp, Chicago, IL 75-76; ***SI:*** *Dialysis*; **HMO:** +

Ball, John T (MD) **Nep**
Illinois Masonic Med Ctr
(see page 118)
3000 N Halstead Ste 405; Chicago, IL 60657; (773) 975-5550; **BDCERT:** Nep 80; IM 77; **MS:** Geo Wash U Sch Med 74; **RES:** Presbyterian U Hosp, Pittsburgh, PA; **FEL:** Tufts U, Boston, MA 78-80; **FAP:** Assoc Clin Prof Univ IL Coll Med

Bansal, Vinod (MD) **Nep**
Loyola U Med Ctr **(see page 120)**
Loyola U MC, Dept Renal/Hypertension, 2160 S First Ave Rm3668; Maywood, IL 60153; (708) 216-3808; **BDCERT:** Nep 76; IM 75; **MS:** India 64; **RES:** IM, Illinois Masonic Med Ctr, Chicago, IL 70-73; **FEL:** Renal Disease, Colorado Med Ctr, Denver, CO 66-67; **FAP:** Prof Loyola U-Stritch Sch Med, Maywood; ***SI:*** *High Blood Pressure; Kidney Transplant Care*; **HMO:** +
2-4 Weeks VISA

Berns, Arnold (MD) **Nep**
St Francis Hosp of Evanston
Lakeside Nephrology, 2277 W Howard St; Chicago, IL 60645; (773) 508-0110; **BDCERT:** IM 74; Nep 78; **MS:** Northwestern U 71; **RES:** IM, Boston Med Ctr, Boston, MA 71-72; IM, Northwestern Mem Hosp, Chicago, IL 72-74; **FEL:** Nep, Colorado Med Ctr, Denver, CO 75-77; **FAP:** Professor Nep Univ IL Coll Med; **HOSP:** Rush North Shore Med Ctr; ***SI:*** *Kidney Failure; Kidney Stones*
2-4 Weeks

Black, Henry (MD) **Nep**
Rush-Presbyterian-St Luke's Med Ctr
(see page 122)
Rush Hypertension Svc, 1725 W Harrison St Ste 119; Chicago, IL 60612; (312) 942-2798; **BDCERT:** IM 72; Nep 74; **MS:** NYU Sch Med 67; **RES:** IM, Johns Hopkins Hosp, Baltimore, MD 67-68; IM, Yale-New Haven Hosp, New Haven, CT 71-72; **FEL:** Nep, Yale-New Haven Hosp, New Haven, CT 72-74; ***SI:*** *High Blood Pressure; Prevention of Heart Disease*
1 Week VISA

Cohen, Edward (MD) **Nep**
Univ of Illinois at Chicago Med Ctr
835 S Wolcott Ave; Chicago, IL 60612; (312) 996-9479; **BDCERT:** IM 74; Nep 74; **MS:** SUNY Downstate 65; **RES:** IM, Montefiore Med Ctr, Bronx, NY 68-71; Nep, Montefiore Med Ctr, Bronx, NY 71-72; **FEL:** Nep, Northwestern Mem Hosp, Chicago, IL 72-73; **HOSP:** St Mary's of Nazareth Hosp Ctr

Crawford, Paul (MD) **Nep**
Trinity Hosp
Associates In Nephrology, 450 E Ohio St; Chicago, IL 60611; (312) 951-4950; **BDCERT:** IM 83; Nep 84; **MS:** Loyola U-Stritch Sch Med, Maywood 74; **RES:** St Joseph Hospital, Chicago, IL 75-77; **FEL:** Nep, Univ Ill Hosp, Chicago, IL 77-79; **HOSP:** Little Company of Mary Hosp & Hlth Care Ctrs

Hamburger, Ronald (MD) **Nep**
Christ Hosp & Med Ctr **(see page 140)**
Southwest Nephrology Assoc, 3650 W 95th St; Evergreen Park, IL 60805; (708) 422-7715; **BDCERT:** Nep 78; IM 78; **MS:** Univ IL Coll Med 75; **RES:** IM, 76-78; **FEL:** Nep, U IL Med Ctr, Chicago, IL 78-80; **FAP:** Asst Clin Prof Med Univ IL Coll Med; **HOSP:** Little Company of Mary Hosp & Hlth Care Ctrs; **HMO:** +
1 Week VISA

Hedger, Robert (MD) **Nep**
Columbus Hosp
Associates In Nephrology, 450 E Ohio St; Chicago, IL 60611; (312) 951-4950; **BDCERT:** Nep 74; IM 77; **MS:** Bowman Gray 64; **RES:** Presbyterian-St Lukes Med Ctr, Chicago, IL 65; Presby-St Lukes Hosp, Chicago, IL 67-69; **FEL:** Nep, Presbyterian-St Lukes Hosp, Chicago, IL 69-71; **FAP:** Asst Clin Prof Med Northwestern U

Hirsch, Sheldon (MD) **Nep**
Michael Reese Hosp & Med Ctr
Lakeside Nephrology Ltd, 1712 S Prairie Ave 2nd Flr; Chicago, IL 60616; (312) 913-0110; **BDCERT:** IM 84; Nep 86; **MS:** Tufts U 81; **RES:** IM, Michael Reese Hosp Med Ctr, Chicago, IL 82-84; **FEL:** Nep, UCLA-Univ Med Ctr, Chicago, IL 84-85; Nep, Jewish Hosp of St Louis, St Louis, MO 86-87

Ivanovich, Peter (MD) **Nep**
VA Hlthcare Systems-Lakeside
North American Headquaters, 333 E Huron St Ste 853; Chicago, IL 60611; (312) 335-8244; **MS:** St Louis U 55; **RES:** IM, St Mary's Hosp, San Francisco, CA 56-58; **FEL:** EDM, U WA Med Ctr, Seattle, WA 61-63; Nep, U WA Med Ctr, Seattle, WA 64-66; **FAP:** Prof Northwestern U; **HOSP:** Northwestern Mem Hosp; **HMO:** +
2-4 Weeks

Josephson, Michelle (MD) **Nep**
U Chicago Hosp **(see page 124)**
University of Chicago Hospitals, 5841 S Maryland; Chicago, IL 60637; (773) 702-1473; **BDCERT:** IM 86; Nep 90; **MS:** Univ Penn 83; **RES:** IM, U Chicago Hosp, Chicago, IL 83-86; **FEL:** Nep, U Chicago Hosp, Chicago, IL 87-91; **FAP:** Asst. Professor Nep U Chicago-Pritzker Sch Med; **HOSP:** Northwestern Mem Hosp; ***SI:*** *Transplantation*
4+ Weeks

Guide to symbols and abbreviations can be found on pages 110-113.

Kuznetsky, Kenneth (MD) **Nep**
Our Lady Of the Resurrection Med Ctr
550 W Webster Ave; Chicago, IL 60614; (773) 348-4640; **BDCERT:** Nep 84; IM 82; **MS:** Rush Med Coll 79; **RES:** IM, Rush Presbyterian-St Luke's Med Ctr, Chicago, IL 79-82; **FEL:** Nep, Rush Presbyterian-St Luke's Med Ctr, Chicago, IL 82-84; **FAP:** Instructor IM Rush Med Coll; **HOSP:** Resurrection Med Ctr; ***SI:** Dialysis; Hypertension*
A Few Days

Levin, Murray (MD) **Nep**
Northwestern Mem Hosp
Northwestern Meml Hosp - Jennings Pav, 707 N Fairbanks Ct Ste 800; Chicago, IL 60611; (312) 908-4609; **BDCERT:** Nep 74; IM 70; **MS:** Tufts U 61; **RES:** IM, Beth Israel Med Ctr, Boston, MA 62-64; **FEL:** Nep, U TX Med Branch Hosp, Galveston, TX 64-66; **FAP:** Sr Prof Med Northwestern U; **HOSP:** VA Hlthcare Systems-Lakeside

Lewis, Edmund (MD) **Nep**
Rush-Presbyterian-St Luke's Med Ctr
(see page 122)
1653 W Congress Pkwy Ste 501; Chicago, IL 60612; (312) 942-6688; **BDCERT:** Nep 69; **MS:** U British Columbia Fac Med 62; **RES:** IM, Johns Hopkins Hosp, Baltimore, MD 62-65; **FEL:** Nep, Peter Bent Brigham Hosp, Boston, MA 65-66; Nep, Peter Bent Brigham Hosp, Boston, MA 68-69; **FAP:** Prof Rush Med Coll; ***SI:** Lupus Nephritis; Diabetic Kidney Disease*; **HMO:** Rush Prudential, Blue Cross & Blue Choice, Aetna Hlth Plan, CIGNA
LANG: Sp; 4+ Weeks VISA

Obasi, Ejikeme (MD) **Nep**
Little Company of Mary Hosp & Hlth Care Ctrs **(see page 142)**
Nephrology, 3650 W 95th St; Evergreen, IL 60805; (708) 422-7715; **BDCERT:** Nep 94; IM 91; **MS:** Nigeria 80; **RES:** IM, U Nigeria Teach Hosps, Enugu, Nigeria 81-88; IM, Cook Cty Hosp, Chicago, IL 88-91; **FEL:** Nep, Rush Presbyterian-St Luke's Med Ctr, Chicago, IL 91-93

Orlowski, Janis (MD) **Nep**
Rush-Presbyterian-St Luke's Med Ctr
(see page 122)
Rush Presbyterian St Lukes, 1653 W Congress Pkwy Ste 501; Chicago, IL 60612; (312) 942-6685; **BDCERT:** IM 85; Nep 90; **MS:** Med Coll Wisc 82; **RES:** IM, Rush Presbyterian-St Luke's Med Ctr, Chicago, IL 83-86; **FEL:** Nep, Rush Presbyterian-St Luke's Med Ctr, Chicago, IL 86; **FAP:** Asst Prof Med Rush Med Coll

Oyama, Joseph (MD) **Nep**
Christ Hosp & Med Ctr **(see page 140)**
Southwest Nephrology Assoc, 3650 W 95th St; Evergreen Park, IL 60805; (708) 422-7715; **BDCERT:** Nep 72; IM 80; **MS:** Univ IL Coll Med 65; **RES:** IM, U IL Med Ctr, Chicago, IL 67-68; **FEL:** Rush Presbyterian-St Luke's Med Ctr, Chicago, IL 68-71; **FAP:** Asst Prof Univ IL Coll Med; **HOSP:** Little Company of Mary Hosp & Hlth Care Ctrs; **HMO:** Rush Prudential, Blue Cross & Blue Shield, Californiacare, CIGNA, Humana Health Plan +
1 Week VISA

Pillsbury, Lisa (MD) **Nep**
Alexian Brothers Med Ctr
(see page 138)
Nephrology Assoc-Northern Il, 901 Biesterfield Rd; Elk Grove Vlg, IL 60007; (847) 952-9332; **BDCERT:** Nep 96; IM 93; **MS:** Univ IL Coll Med 90; **RES:** IM, St Francis Hosp-U IL Coll Med, Peoria, IL 90-93; **FEL:** Nep, U Iowa Coll Med, Iowa City, IA 93-95

Roseman, Melvin K. (MD) **Nep**
St Joseph Hosp-Chicago
2800 N Sheridan Rd Ste 510; Chicago, IL 60657; (773) 248-6700; **BDCERT:** IM 74; **MS:** U Chicago-Pritzker Sch Med 73; **RES:** IM, St Joseph's Hosp, Chicago, IL 73-74; IM, Carney Hosp, Boston, MA 74-76; **FEL:** Nep, U IL Med Ctr, Chicago, IL 76-78; **HOSP:** Resurrection Med Ctr; ***SI:** Dialysis Care; Hypertension*; **HMO:** United Healthcare, Aetna Hlth Plan, CIGNA +
A Few Days

Rydel, James (MD) **Nep**
Little Company of Mary Hosp & Hlth Care Ctrs **(see page 142)**
Southwest Nephrology, 3650 W 95th St; Evergreen Park, IL 60805; (708) 422-7715; **BDCERT:** Nep 94; IM 92; **MS:** Rush Med Coll 88

Salem, Mohamed (MD) **Nep**
St Joseph Hosp-Chicago
Associates In Nephrology, 450 E Ohio St; Chicago, IL 60611; (312) 951-4950; **BDCERT:** IM 88; Nep 90; **MS:** Egypt 78; **RES:** IM, Cook Cty Hosp, Chicago, IL 86-88; **FEL:** Nep, Northwestern Mem Hosp, Chicago, IL 88-91; **FAP:** Asst Prof of Clin Med Northwestern U

Simon, Norman (MD) **Nep**
Evanston Hosp
Evanston Northwestern Healthcare, 2650 Ridge Ave; Evanston, IL 60201; (847) 570-2512; **BDCERT:** Nep 63; **MS:** Northwestern U 55; **RES:** IM, Michael Reese Hosp Med Ctr, Chicago, IL 59-61; **FEL:** Nep, Northwestern Mem Hosp, Chicago, IL 61-63; **FAP:** Prof Med Northwestern U; **HOSP:** Northwestern Mem Hosp; ***SI:** Hypertension*
2-4 Weeks VISA

Soifer, Neil (MD) Nep
Mercy Hosp & Med Ctr
Lakeside Nephrology, 55 E Washington St Ste 1100; Chicago, IL 60602; (312) 345-0110; **BDCERT:** IM 88; **MS:** U Mich Med Sch 85; **RES:** IM, Michael Reese Hosp Med Ctr, Chicago, IL 85-89; **FEL:** Nep, Yale-New Haven Hosp, New Haven, CT 90-94; **HOSP:** Michael Reese Hosp & Med Ctr; **HMO:** Blue Cross & Blue Shield, Chicago HMO +

Sprague, Stuart (MD) Nep
Evanston Hosp
Evanston Hospital - Division of Nephrology, 2650 Ridge Ave; Evanston, IL 60201; (847) 570-2512; **BDCERT:** Nep 88; IM 86; **MS:** Mich St U 82; **RES:** IM, Rush Presbyterian-St Luke's Med Ctr, Chicago, IL 83-86; **FEL:** Nep, U Chicago Hosp, Chicago, IL 86-89; **FAP:** Asst Prof U Chicago-Pritzker Sch Med; **HOSP:** U Chicago Hosp

Vilbar, Remegio (MD) Nep
St Elizabeth's Hosp
1431 N Western Ave Ste 202; Chicago, IL 60622; (773) 489-6605; **BDCERT:** IM 77; Nep 78; **MS:** Philippines 69; **RES:** IM, Hines VA Hosp, Chicago, IL 73-75; **FEL:** N, Hines VA Hosp, Chicago, IL 75-77; **HOSP:** St Mary's of Nazareth Hosp Ctr

Yohay, Daniel (MD) Nep
St James Hosp & Hlth Ctrs
Horizon Health Care, 2601 W Lincoln Hwy Ste 108; Olympia Fields, IL 60461; (708) 747-6815; **BDCERT:** Nep 92; IM 91; **MS:** Duke U 87; **HOSP:** South Suburban Hosp
Mcr Mcd 2-4 Weeks VISA

Zikos, Demetrios (MD) Nep
Christ Hosp & Med Ctr (see page 140)
3650 W 95th St; Evergreen Park, IL 60805; (708) 422-7715; **BDCERT:** IM 82; Nep 86; **MS:** Greece 77; **RES:** IM, Christ Hosp & Med Ctr, Oak Lawn, IL 79-82; **FEL:** Nep, U Chicago Hosp, Chicago, IL 82-84; **FAP:** Assoc Clin Prof Med U Hlth Sci/Chicago Med Sch; **HOSP:** Little Company of Mary Hosp & Hlth Care Ctrs; ***SI:*** *Kidney Stones; Hypertension*; **HMO:** CIGNA, Aetna Hlth Plan, UHC, Humana Health Plan, Blue Cross PPO +
LANG: Grk, Pol; Mcr Mcd
1 Week VISA

NEUROLOGICAL SURGERY

Anderson, Douglas E (MD) NS
Loyola U Med Ctr (see page 120)
Loyola Med Center - Neurosurgery-Bldg 54, 2160 S 1st Ave Rm 261; Maywood, IL 60153; (708) 216-8235; **BDCERT:** NS 87; **MS:** U Hlth Sci/Chicago Med Sch 77; **RES:** NS, Loyola U Med Ctr, Maywood, IL 78-83; **FAP:** Assoc Prof Loyola U-Stritch Sch Med, Maywood; **HMO:** +
Mcr Mcd

Ausman, James (MD) NS
Univ of Illinois at Chicago Med Ctr
Neurosurgery Dept MC-799, 912 S Wood St; Chicago, IL 60612; (312) 996-4842; **BDCERT:** NS 72; **MS:** Johns Hopkins U 63; **RES:** NS, Minnesota Hosp, Minneapolis, MN 64-66; NS, Minnesota Hosp, Minneapolis, MN 68-72; **FAP:** Prof NS Univ IL Coll Med

Batjer, Hunt (MD) NS
Northwestern Mem Hosp
Northwestern U Med Sch, 233 E Erie Ste 614; Chicago, IL 60611; (312) 908-8170; **BDCERT:** NS 86; **MS:** U Tex SW, Dallas 77; **RES:** NS, Parkland Mem Hosp, Dallas, TX 78-81; **FEL:** NS, U West Ontario, London, Canada 81-82; **FAP:** Prof NS Northwestern U; ***SI:*** *Aneurysm Vascular Malformation; AVM Stroke*; **HMO:** +
LANG: Sp, Man; Mcr Mcd

Bauer, Jerry (MD) NS
Lutheran Gen Hosp (see page 143)
Center-Brain & Spine Surgery, 1875 Dempster St Ste 605; Park Ridge, IL 60068; (847) 698-1088; **BDCERT:** NS 81; **MS:** Univ IL Coll Med 74; **RES:** NS, Northwestern Mem Hosp, Chicago, IL 74-75; NS, U IL Med Ctr, Chicago, IL 75-79; ***SI:*** *Brain Tumor Surgery; Back Pain*
Mcr Mcd A Few Days VISA

Brown, Frederick (MD) NS
U Chicago Hosp (see page 124)
University of Chicago Phys, 5841 S Maryland Ave J341; Chicago, IL 60637; (773) 702-2123; **BDCERT:** NS 82; **MS:** Ohio State U 72; **RES:** NS, U Chicago Hosp, Chicago, IL 74-78; **FAP:** Assoc Prof NS U Chicago-Pritzker Sch Med; ***SI:*** *Spinal Surgery; Pain Management*; **HMO:** Blue Cross & Blue Shield

Cerullo, Leonard (MD) NS
Columbus Hosp
Chicago Institute of Neurosurgery, 2515 N Clark St Ste 801; Chicago, IL 60614; (773) 883-8500; **BDCERT:** NS 79; **MS:** Jefferson Med Coll 70; **RES:** Lankenau Hosp, Philadelphia, PA 71-72; Northwestern Mem Hosp, Chicago, IL 72-77; **FEL:** NS, Hosp Foch, Paris, France 73; **FAP:** Assoc Prof NS Northwestern U; **HOSP:** Northwestern Mem Hosp

Ciric, Ivan (MD) NS
Evanston Hosp
North Shore Neurosurgeons, 1000 Central St Ste 800; Evanston, IL 60201; (847) 570-1444; **BDCERT:** NS 69; **MS:** Yugoslavia 58; **RES:** NS, U Cologne, Cologne, Germany 62-63; NS, Wesley Mem Hosp, Chicago, IL 63-66; **FEL:** Montefiore Med Ctr, Bronx, NY 67; Notre Dame Hosp, Montreal, Quebec 67; **FAP:** Prof S Northwestern U; **HOSP:** Highland Park Hosp

Cozzens, Jeffrey (MD) NS
Evanston Hosp
Evanston Hospital, 2650 Ridge Ave; Evanston, IL 60201; (847) 757-1440; **BDCERT:** NS 88; **MS:** Univ IL Coll Med 78; **RES:** NS, Northwestern Mem Hosp, Chicago, IL 79-84; NS, Cook Cty Hosp, Chicago, IL 84; **FEL:** NS, U Minn, Minneapolis, MN 85; **FAP:** Asst Clin Prof Northwestern U; ***SI:*** *Brain Tumors; Epilepsy Surgery*
1 Week

Cybulski Jr., George R. (MD) NS
Northwestern Mem Hosp
251 E Chicago Ave; Chicago, IL 60611; (312) 908-2731; **BDCERT:** NS 88; **MS:** Univ IL Coll Med 79

Eller, Theodore (MD) NS
Evanston Hosp
2650 Ridge Ave Ste 4220; D.N Evantston Hosp, IL 60201; (847) 570-1440; **BDCERT:** NS 81; **MS:** U Iowa Coll Med 70; **RES:** Northwestern Mem Hosp, Chicago, IL 74-75; Northwestern Mem Hosp, Chicago, IL 73-78; **FEL:** Harvard Med Sch, Cambridge, MA 74-75; Mayo Clinic, Rochester, MN; **FAP:** Assoc Prof S Northwestern U; **HOSP:** Glenbrook Hosp; ***SI:*** *Aneurysms/Thalamic & Sub Stimulator Implants for Dystonia; Pallidotomy for Parkinson's*; **HMO:** Aetna Hlth Plan, Select, HMO Illinois, CIGNA
VISA

Ferguson, R Lawrence (MD) NS
Michael Reese Hosp & Med Ctr
Chicago Inst of Neurosurgery & Neuroresearch, 71 W 156th St Ste 208; Harvey, IL 60426; (708) 331-6669; **BDCERT:** NS 76; **MS:** Queens U 67; **HOSP:** Ingalls Mem Hosp; ***SI:*** *Brain Aneurysm; Arteriovenous Malformation*

Geisler, Fred (MD) NS
Columbus Hosp
Chicago Institute of Neurosurgery, 2515 N Clark St Ste 801; Chicago, IL 60614; (773) 388-7600; **BDCERT:** NS 87; **MS:** SUNY Buffalo 78; **RES:** NS, Univ Hosp SUNY Buffalo, Buffalo, NY 79-83; **FEL:** Ntrauma, MD Inst EM Med Svcs Sys, Baltimore, MD 83-84; **HMO:** Aetna Hlth Plan, AV-MED Health Plan, Bay State Health Plan, Blue Choice, Blue Cross & Blue Shield

Hahn, Yoon (MD) NS
Christ Hosp & Med Ctr (see page 140)
4440 W 95th St; Oak Lawn, IL 60453; (708) 346-1013; **BDCERT:** NS 86; **MS:** South Korea 67; **RES:** NS, Yonsei U Med Ctr, Seoul, South Korea 67; NS, Northwestern Mem Hosp, Chicago, IL 79; **FEL:** NS, Hosp Foch, Paris, France 76; **FAP:** Prof NS Loyola U-Stritch Sch Med, Maywood; **HMO:** Blue Cross & Blue Shield, CIGNA, Bay State Health Plan, Metlife, Prudential

Hekmatpanah, Javad (MD) NS
U Chicago Hosp (see page 124)
University of Chicago Phys, 5841 S Maryland Ave; Chicago, IL 60637; (773) 702-6157; **BDCERT:** NS 66; N 67; **MS:** Iran 56; **RES:** N, U WI Sch Med, Milwaukee, WI 58-61; NS, U Chicago Hosp, Chicago, IL 61-64; **FAP:** Prof NS U Chicago-Pritzker Sch Med; ***SI:*** *Spine Diseases; Brain Tumors*; **HMO:** CCN, CIGNA, HMO Blue, Blue Choice, One Health Care
LANG: Fr, Sp;
A Few Days VISA

Karasick, Jeffrey (MD) NS
St Francis Hosp
Service Corp, 9700 Kenton St Ste K401; Skokie, IL 60076; (847) 674-9394; **BDCERT:** NS 76; **MS:** U Hlth Sci/Chicago Med Sch 66; **RES:** NS, Chicago Hosp-Clins, Chicago, IL 66-67; NS, Chicago Hosp-Clins, Chicago, IL 68-73; **HOSP:** Rush North Shore Med Ctr; ***SI:*** *Spinal Disorders; Brain Tumors*; **HMO:** Aetna Hlth Plan, Blue Cross & Blue Shield, Chicago HMO, CIGNA, HealthNet +
A Few Days

Kranzler, Leonard (MD) NS
Illinois Masonic Med Ctr
(see page 118)
Neurosurgical Specialists Ltd, 3000 N Halstead Ste 701; Chicago, IL 60657; (773) 296-6666; **BDCERT:** NS 74; **MS:** Northwestern U 63; **RES:** Northwestern Mem Hosp, Chicago, IL 64-69; **FEL:** NS, , Zurich, Switzerland 71; **HOSP:** St Joseph Hosp-Chicago
VISA

Le Compte, Benjamin (MD) NS
St Alexius Med Ctr
1575 N Barrington Rd Ste 325; Hoffman Estates, IL 60194; (847) 843-7743; **BDCERT:** NS 83; **MS:** U Va Sch Med 74; **RES:** Rush Presbyterian-St Luke's Med Ctr, Chicago, IL 75-80; **FAP:** Asst Prof Rush Med Coll

Luken, Martin (MD) NS
Rush-Presbyterian-St Luke's Med Ctr
(see page 122)
Chicago Institute of Neurosurgery, 71 W 156th St Ste 208; Harvey, IL 60426; (708) 331-6669; **BDCERT:** NS 83; **MS:** Columbia P&S 73; **RES:** U IL Med Ctr, Chicago, NY 75-76; NS, Neuro Inst-Columbia Presby, Chicago, IL 76-80

Maltezos, Stavros (MD) NS
Christ Hosp & Med Ctr (see page 140)
CNS Neurological Surgery, 11824 SW Highway St Ste 230; Palos Heights, IL 60463; (708) 361-9890; **BDCERT:** NS 93; **MS:** Rush Med Coll 81; **RES:** NS, Rush Presbyterian-St Luke's Med Ctr, Chicago, IL 82-87; **FAP:** Instr NS Rush Med Coll

McLone, David (MD) NS
Children's Mem Med Ctr (see page 139)
Pediatric Neurosurgery - Childrens Hosp, 2300 N Childrens Plz Ste 28; Chicago, IL 60614; (773) 880-4373; **BDCERT:** NS 78; **MS:** U Mich Med Sch 65; **RES:** NS, Northwestern Mem Hosp, Chicago, IL; **FAP:** Prof NS Northwestern U; ***SI:*** *Spinal Dysraphism; Brain Tumors*

McLone, David (MD) NS
Children's Mem Med Ctr (see page 139)
Children's Memorial Hospital, 2300 Children's Plaza; Chicago, IL 60614; (773) 880-4373; **BDCERT:** NS 78; **MS:** U Mich Med Sch 65

Moser, Richard P (MD) NS
Northwest Comm Hlthcare
Wimmer Medical Plaza - Surg Neuro Assoc Ltd, 810 Biesterfield Rd Ste 404; Elk Grove Vlg, IL 60007; (847) 593-6363; **BDCERT:** NS 85; **MS:** Loyola U-Stritch Sch Med, Maywood 74; **RES:** S, U MN Med Ctr, Minneapolis, MN 76-77; NS, U MN Med Ctr, Minneapolis, MN 77-82; **FEL:** N Onc, Karolinska Institute, Stockholm, Sweden 81-82; **HOSP:** Alexian Brothers Med Ctr; ***SI:*** *Brain Surgery; Spinal Surgery*

Panchal, Kanu (MD) NS
St Alexius Med Ctr
1575 Barrington Rd Ste 325; Hoffman Estates, IL 60194; (847) 784-7066; **BDCERT:** NS 85; **MS:** India 73; **RES:** NS, Boston Med Ctr, Boston, MA 75-76; NS, U Ill Med Ctr, Chicago, IL 78-82; **FAP:** Asst Clin Prof NS Univ IL Coll Med; **HOSP:** Northern Illinois Med Ctr; ***SI:*** *Back Pain; Neck Pain*; **HMO:** Blue Cross & Blue Shield, Chicago HMO, Healthamerica, Healthcare America, PHS
Mcr A Few Days

Pupillo, Louis (MD) NS
Resurrection Med Ctr
Neurological & Neurosurgical, 1400 E Golf Rd Ste 121; Des Plaines, IL 60016; (847) 635-7650; **BDCERT:** NS 81; **MS:** Loyola U-Stritch Sch Med, Maywood 71; **RES:** NS, Loyola U Med Ctr, Maywood, IL 72-77; **HOSP:** Holy Family Med Ctr; **HMO:** Blue Cross & Blue Shield, Chicago HMO, Bay State Health Plan, Compare Health Service, Health Options

Ruge, John (MD) NS
Lutheran Gen Hosp (see page 143)
Center-Brain & Spine Surgery, 1875 Dempster St Ste 605; Park Ridge, IL 60068; (847) 698-1088; **BDCERT:** NS 93; **MS:** Northwestern U 83; **RES:** Northwestern Mem Hosp, Chicago, IL 84-89; **FEL:** Ped NS, Children's Mem Med Ctr, Chicago, IL 89-90; **FAP:** Asst Prof S U Chicago-Pritzker Sch Med

Salazar, Jose (MD) NS
Illinois Masonic Med Ctr
(see page 118)
3000 N Halsted St; Chicago, IL 60657; (773) 525-7678; **BDCERT:** NS 73; **MS:** Mexico 67; **RES:** NS, Neuropsych Inst-U IL Med Ctr, Chicago, IL 68-71

Shea, John (MD) NS
Loyola U Med Ctr (see page 120)
2160 S First Ave; Maywood, IL 60153; (708) 216-3480; **BDCERT:** NS 82; **MS:** St Louis U 72; **RES:** St Louis U Hosp, St Louis, MO 74-78; **FAP:** Assoc Prof NS Loyola U-Stritch Sch Med, Maywood; ***SI:*** *Spine*; **HMO:** +
4+ Weeks

Thapedi, Isaac (MD) NS
St Francis Hosp
9730 S Western Ave Ste 230; Evergreen Park, IL 60805; (708) 422-4944; **BDCERT:** NS 76; **MS:** Howard U 66; **RES:** NS, U Hospital, Saskatoon, Canada 68-72; NS, Hosp For Sick Children, Toronto, Canada 72

Tomita, Tadanori (MD) NS
Children's Mem Med Ctr (see page 139)
Children's Memorial Hospital, 2300 Children's Plaza; Chicago, IL 60614; (773) 880-4373; **BDCERT:** NS 84; **MS:** Japan 70; **RES:** NS, Kobe Univ Hosp, Kobe, Japan 72-74; NS, Northwestern Mem Hosp, Chicago, IL 74-80; **FEL:** S, Mem Sloan Kettering Cancer Ctr, New York, NY 80-81; **HOSP:** Northwestern Mem Hosp; ***SI:*** *Pediatric Brain Tumor; Hydrocephalus*; **HMO:** Blue Cross & Blue Shield, CIGNA, Humana Health Plan, United Healthcare
LANG: Jpn; Mcr Mcd
Immediately VISA

Weir, Bryce (MD) NS
U Chicago Hosp (see page 124)
Univ-Chicago Section-Neurosurg, 5841 S Maryland Ave J341; Chicago, IL 60637; (773) 702-9385; **BDCERT:** NS 69; **MS:** Canada 60; **RES:** NS, Montreal Neurological Inst, Montreal, Canada 62-66; N, Neurological Inst, New York, NY 64-65; ***SI:*** *Brain Aneurysms; Brain Tumors*; **HMO:** Rush Prudential, United Healthcare, Blue Choice, One Health Care +
Mcr Mcd

Guide to symbols and abbreviations can be found on pages 110-113.

Whisler, Walter (MD) NS
Rush-Presbyterian-St Luke's Med Ctr
(see page 122)
Neurological Surgery, 1653 W Congress Pkwy; Chicago, IL 60612; (847) 942-6644; **BDCERT:** NS 67; **MS:** Univ IL Coll Med 59; **RES:** S, Rush Presby-St Lukes Hosp, Chicago, IL 60-61; NS, IL Rsch-Ed Hosps, Chicago, IL 61-64; **FAP:** Chrmn & Prof Rush Med Coll

Yapor, Wesley (MD) NS
Northwestern Mem Hosp
Northwestern Neurosurgical, 707 N Fairbanks Ct Ste 911; Chicago, IL 60611; (312) 951-9092; **BDCERT:** NS 92; **MS:** Univ IL Coll Med 82; **RES:** NS, U IL Med Ctr, Chicago, IL; **HOSP:** St Mary's of Nazareth Hosp Ctr; **HMO:** Blue Cross & Blue Shield, Humana Health Plan +
1 Week VISA

NEUROLOGY

Ahmad, Shahida (MD) N
Trinity Hosp
2315 E 93rd St Ste 320; Chicago, IL 60617; (773) 768-6400; **BDCERT:** N 81; **MS:** Pakistan 72; **RES:** N, NJ Coll Med, Newark, NJ 76-79; **FEL:** EEG, Coll Hosp, Newark, NJ 79-81; ***SI:*** *Seizures; Headaches*; **HMO:** Humana Health Plan, Blue Cross & Blue Shield, Californiacare, Champus, United Healthcare
A Few Days

Allen, Neil (MD) N
Highland Park Hosp
Consultants In Neurology Ltd, 3545 Lake Ave Ste 100; Wilmette, IL 60091; (847) 251-1800; **BDCERT:** N 75; IM 71; **MS:** Univ IL Coll Med 65; **RES:** IM, Cook Cty Hosp, Chicago, IL 68-71; N, U Chicago Hosp, Chicago, IL 71-73; **FAP:** Clin Prof N U Chicago-Pritzker Sch Med; **HOSP:** Edgewater Med Ctr
1 Week VISA

Bennett, David A (MD) N
Rush-Presbyterian-St Luke's Med Ctr
(see page 122)
1653 W Congress Pkwy; Chicago, IL 60612; (312) 942-3350; **BDCERT:** N 90; **MS:** Rush Med Coll 84

Bernstein, Lawrence (MD) N
Evanston Hosp
Division of Neurology /EEG, 2650 Ridge Ave; Evanston, IL 60201; (847) 570-2570; **BDCERT:** N 80; **MS:** U Chicago-Pritzker Sch Med 70; **RES:** N, U Chicago Hosp, Chicago, IL 72-75; **FEL:** Neurophysiology, U Chicago Hosp, Chicago, IL 75-77; **FAP:** Asst Prof Northwestern U

Bikshorn, Barry (MD) N
St Alexius Med Ctr
2260 W Higgins Rd Ste 201; Hoffman Estates, IL 60195; (847) 882-6604; **BDCERT:** N 89; **MS:** Rush Med Coll 83; **RES:** N, Rush Presbyterian-St Luke's Med Ctr, Chicago, IL 84-87; **HMO:** Blue Cross & Blue Shield, Humana Health Plan, Prudential, Rush Health Plans, United Healthcare
2-4 Weeks VISA

Burke, Allan (MD) N
Ingalls Mem Hosp
Neurology Associates Ltd, 71 W 156th St Ste 308; Harvey, IL 60426; (708) 331-6617; **BDCERT:** N 82; **MS:** Columbia P&S 76; **RES:** IM, NY Hosp-Cornell Med Ctr, New York, NY 77-78; N, Columbia-Presbyterian Med Ctr, New York, NY 78-81; **FEL:** Hosp of U Penn, Philadelphia, PA 81-83; **FAP:** Assoc Clin Prof N Northwestern U; **HOSP:** Northwestern Mem Hosp; ***SI:*** *Stroke; MS*; **HMO:** +
Immediately VISA

Burnstine, Thomas (MD) N
Lake Forest Hosp **(see page 309)**
Consultants In Neurology Ltd, 3545 Lake Ave Ste 100; Wilmette, IL 60091; (847) 251-1800; **BDCERT:** N 89; **MS:** Rush Med Coll 84; **RES:** N, Case Western Reserve U Hosp, Cleveland, OH 85-88; **FEL:** Epilepsy, Johns Hopkins Hosp, Baltimore, MD 88-90; **HOSP:** Ravenswood Hosp Med Ctr
VISA

Cohen, Bruce (MD) N
Northwestern Mem Hosp
233 E Erie St Ste 500; Chicago, IL 60611; (312) 908-7950; **BDCERT:** N 86; **MS:** Univ IL Coll Med 78; **RES:** IM, Lutheran Gen Hosp, Park Ridge, IL 79-81; N, Northwestern Mem Hosp, Chicago, IL 81-84; **FAP:** Assoc Prof Northwestern U; ***SI:*** *Multiple Sclerosis; Neurologic Infectious Disease*; **HMO:** +
2-4 Weeks VISA

Davis, Floyd (MD) N
Rush-Presbyterian-St Luke's Med Ctr
(see page 122)
Msc Neurologic Consultants, 1725 W Harrison St Ste 309; Chicago, IL 60612; (312) 942-8011; **BDCERT:** N 70; **MS:** Univ Penn 60; **RES:** Mount Sinai Med Ctr, New York, NY 63-66; **FEL:** N, Columbia-Presbyterian Med Ctr, New York, NY 61-63; **FAP:** Prof N Rush Med Coll

Davis, Lloyd S (MD) N
Lutheran Gen Hosp **(see page 143)**
Advocate Medical Group, 9301 Golf Rd Ste 201; Des Plaines, IL 60016; (847) 298-3540; **BDCERT:** N 86; IM 80; **MS:** Univ IL Coll Med 77; **RES:** N, Harbor Gen Hosp, Los Angeles, CA 81-84; IM, Lutheran Gen Hosp, Park Ridge, IL 78-80; **FAP:** Asst Clin Prof U Chicago-Pritzker Sch Med; ***SI:*** *Parkinson's Disease; Multiple Sclerosis*

Fox, Jacob H (MD) N
Rush-Presbyterian-St Luke's Med Ctr
(see page 122)
710 S Paulina St Ste 8N; Chicago, IL 60612; (312) 942-4463; **BDCERT:** N 74; **MS:** Univ IL Coll Med 67; **RES:** N, Barnes Hosp, St Louis, MO 68-71; ***SI:*** *Alzheimer's Disease*; **HMO:** +
LANG: Sp; VISA

Goodwin, James (MD) N
Univ of Illinois at Chicago Med Ctr
University of IL Eye & Ear, 1855 W Taylor St Ste 144; Chicago, IL 60612; (312) 996-9120; **BDCERT:** N 75; **MS:** Univ IL Coll Med 69; **RES:** U MN Med Ctr, Minneapolis, MN 70-73; **FEL:** Neurophthalmology, Bascom Palmer Eye Inst, Miami, FL 75-76; **FAP:** Prof Oph Univ IL Coll Med

Gorelick, Philip (MD & PhD) N
Rush-Presbyterian-St Luke's Med Ctr
(see page 122)
Neuro Science Institute, 1725 W Harrison St Ste 755; Chicago, IL 60612; (312) 563-2030; **BDCERT:** N 82; **MS:** Loyola U-Stritch Sch Med, Maywood 77; **RES:** Loyola Univ Med Ctr, Maywood, IL 78-81; **FEL:** Cerebral Diseases, Michael Reese Hosp Med Ctr, Chicago, IL 81-82; **FAP:** Prof & Dir Rush Med Coll; **HMO:** Aetna Hlth Plan, Chicago HMO, Choicecare, CIGNA, Compare Health Service

Helgason, Cathy (MD) N
Univ of Illinois at Chicago Med Ctr
Univ IL - Dept of Neurology, 912 S Wood St Rm 855N; Chicago, IL 60612; (312) 996-6497; **BDCERT:** N 88; **MS:** Iceland 78; **RES:** N, U Chicago Hosp, Chicago, IL 80-83; **FEL:** Cerebrovascular Disease, Michael Reese Hosp Med Ctr, Chicago, IL 83-84; EEG/EP, Rush Presbyterian-St Luke's Med Ctr, Chicago, IL 84-85; **FAP:** Prof N Univ IL Coll Med; ***SI:*** *Stroke; Migraine*

Hier, Daniel (MD) N
Univ of Illinois at Chicago Med Ctr
Univ Illinois-Dept of Neurolgy, 912 S Wood St Ste 655N; Chicago, IL 60612; (312) 996-1757; **BDCERT:** N 78; **MS:** Harvard Med Sch 73; **RES:** N, Mass Gen Hosp, Boston, MA 74-77; **FEL:** N, Mass Gen Hosp, Boston, MA 77-79; **FAP:** Professor N Univ IL Coll Med; ***SI:*** *Dementia; Stroke*
Mcr Mcd NFI A Few Days

Ho, Sam (MD) N
Northwestern Mem Hosp
251 E Chicago Ave Ste 1228; Chicago, IL 60611; (312) 787-9499; **BDCERT:** N 78; NP 92; **MS:** Northwestern U 73; **RES:** N, Northwestern Mem Hosp, Chicago, IL 74-77; **FAP:** Assoc Clin Prof N Northwestern U

Homer, Daniel (MD) N
Evanston Hosp
ENH, 2650 Ridge Ave; Evanston, IL 60201; (847) 570-2570; **BDCERT:** N 90; **MS:** Northwestern U 79

Joshi, Nalinaksha (MD) N
St Mary's of Nazareth Hosp Ctr
2222 W Division St Ste 310; Chicago, IL 60622; (773) 395-8200; **BDCERT:** N 81; **MS:** India 71; **RES:** N, Mount Sinai Hosp Med Ctr, Chicago, IL 74-77; **FEL:** NS, Cook Cty Hosp, Chicago, IL 73-74

Kelly, James (MD) N
Rehab Institute of Chicago
Rehabilitation Institute, 345 E Superior St; Chicago, IL 60611; (312) 908-8512; **BDCERT:** N 91; **MS:** Northwestern U 83; **RES:** N, U of Colorado Hosp, Denver, CO 85-88; **FEL:** N, U of Colorado Hosp, Denver, CO 88-89; **FAP:** Assoc Prof Northwestern U; **HOSP:** Northwestern Mem Hosp; ***SI:*** *Brain Injury*; **HMO:** Aetna Hlth Plan, Blue Cross & Blue Shield, Californiacare, CIGNA, Rush Pru
Mcr Mcd A Few Days VISA

Markovitz, David (MD) N
Palos Comm Hosp
Berger Neurological Assoc, 7350 W College Dr; Palos Heights, IL 60463; (708) 361-3880; **BDCERT:** N 81; **MS:** U Ariz Coll Med 75; **RES:** N, Univ of Arizona, Tucson, AZ 77-80; **FEL:** U of VA Health Sci Ctr, Charlottesville, VA 80-81; **HOSP:** Little Company of Mary Hosp & Hlth Care Ctrs

Mohan, Jagan (MD) N
Holy Cross Hosp
Consultants In Neurology Ltd, 3545 Lake Ave Ste 100; Wilmette, IL 60091; (847) 251-1800; **BDCERT:** N 80; **MS:** India 64; **RES:** N, U KS Med Ctr, Kansas City, KS 75-77; Psyc, Menninger Clinic, Topeka, KS 69-72; **FEL:** U MN Med Ctr, Minneapolis, MN 77-78

Rezak, Michael (MD) N
Evanston Hosp
Glenbrook Hosp - Neurology, 2100 Pfingsten Rd B110; Glenview, IL 60025; (847) 657-5875; **BDCERT:** N 90; **MS:** Loyola U-Stritch Sch Med, Maywood 85; **RES:** N, Rush Presby-St Lukes Hosp, Chicago, IL 86-87; N, Yale-New Haven Hosp, New Haven, CT 87-89; **FAP:** Asst Clin Prof Northwestern U; **HMO:** Blue Cross & Blue Shield

Rozental, Jack M. (MD & PhD) N
Northwestern Mem Hosp
Dept of Neurology, 233 E Erie St Ste 500; Chicago, IL 60611; (312) 908-7950; **BDCERT:** N 91; **MS:** Dominican Republic 79; **RES:** N, U WI Sch Med, Milwaukee, WI 82-85; **FAP:** Northwestern U
Mcr

Rubin, Susan (MD) N
Highland Park Hosp
Lake Cook Neurolgical Consultants, 8780 W Golf Rd Ste 202; Niles, IL 60062; (847) 298-4590; **BDCERT:** N 96; **MS:** Univ IL Coll Med 88; **RES:** N, Northwestern Mem Hosp, Chicago, IL 90-93; **FEL:** N, Northwestern Mem Hosp, Chicago, IL 93-94; **HOSP:** Lutheran Gen Hosp; ***SI:*** *Epilepsy/Seizures in Women; Migraines*; **HMO:** HMO Illinois, Humana Health Plan, Blue Cross & Blue Shield, Aetna Hlth Plan, CIGNA +
2-4 Weeks VISA

Rubinstein, Wayne (MD) N
Lutheran Gen Hosp (see page 143)
Advocate Medical Group, 9301 Golf Rd Ste 201; Des Plaines, IL 60016; (847) 298-3540; **BDCERT:** N 93; NP 94; **MS:** U Chicago-Pritzker Sch Med 86; ***SI:*** *Myasthenia Gravis*
VISA

Schwartz, Michael (MD) N
Christ Hosp & Med Ctr (see page 140)
Neurologic Associates, 11824 Southwest Hwy; Palos Heights, IL 60463; (708) 361-0222; **BDCERT:** N 79; **MS:** NY Med Coll 71; **RES:** N, U Oregon Health Sci U Hosp, Portland, OR 72-75; **FAP:** Asst Prof Rush Med Coll; **HOSP:** Little Company of Mary Hosp & Hlth Care Ctrs

Siddique, Teepu (MD) N
Northwestern Mem Hosp
Dept of Neurology, 233 E Erie St Ste 500; Chicago, IL 60611; (312) 908-7950; **BDCERT:** N 80; **MS:** Pakistan 73; **RES:** N, UMDNJ-RW Johnson, Plainfield, NJ 76-79; **FEL:** Neuromuscular, Hosp For Special Surgery, New York, NY 79-80; Neuromuscular, Nat Inst Health, Bethesda, MD 80-81; **FAP:** Prof N Northwestern U

Stobnicki, Aleksandra (MD) N
Resurrection Med Ctr
7447 W Talcott Ave Ste 427; Chicago, IL 60631; (773) 775-2323; **BDCERT:** N 89; **MS:** Poland 77; **RES:** N, Cook Cty Hosp, Chicago, IL 81-82; **HMO:** Aetna Hlth Plan, Blue Cross & Blue Shield, Californiacare, HealthNet, Humana Health Plan

Swisher, Charles (MD) N
Children's Mem Med Ctr (see page 139)
2300 Children's Plz; Chicago Heights, IL 60614; (708) 756-0100; **BDCERT:** Ped 75; ChiN 78; **MS:** McGill U 65; **RES:** Ped, Montreal Children's Hosp, Montreal, Canada 65-67; N, Barnes Hosp, St Louis, MO 69-70; **FEL:** ChiN, St Louis Children's Hosp, St Louis, MO 70-72; **FAP:** Assoc Prof Northwestern U; ***SI:*** *Behavioral Neurology; Developmental Neurology*; **HMO:** +
2-4 Weeks

Vick, Nicholas A (MD) N
Evanston Hosp
Div of Neur-Evanston Hosp-Burch Rm 309, 2650 Ridge Ave; Evanston, IL 60201; (847) 570-2570; **BDCERT:** N 71; **MS:** U Chicago-Pritzker Sch Med 65; **RES:** N, U Chicago Hosp, Chicago, IL 66-68; **FEL:** N, Nat Inst Health, Bethesda, MD 68-70; **FAP:** Prof N Northwestern U; ***SI:*** *Brain Tumors*; **HMO:** CIGNA, Blue Cross, Humana Health Plan +
2-4 Weeks

Wasserman, Michael (MD) N
Highland Park Hosp
Lake Cook Neurological Assoc, 8780 W Golf Rd Ste 102; Niles, IL 60714; (847) 298-4590; **BDCERT:** N 73; **MS:** Northwestern U 64; **RES:** Ped, Children's Mem Med Ctr, Chicago, IL 65; N, Northwestern Mem Hosp, Chicago, IL 66-68; **FAP:** Asst Clin Prof N Northwestern U; **HOSP:** Lutheran Gen Hosp; **HMO:** Aetna Hlth Plan, Chicago HMO, CIGNA, Health Alliance Plan, Humana Health Plan

Wichter, Melvin (MD) N
Christ Hosp & Med Ctr (see page 140)
11800 Southwest Hwy; Palos Heights, IL 60463; (708) 361-0222; **BDCERT:** N 79; **MS:** NY Med Coll 71; **RES:** N, Bellevue Hosp Ctr, New York, NY 73-75; **FAP:** Assoc Prof NS Rush Med Coll

Wright, Robert (MD) N
Rush-Presbyterian-St Luke's Med Ctr (see page 122)
1653 W Congress Pkwy; Chicago, IL 60612; (312) 942-4500; **BDCERT:** N 88; **MS:** Univ IL Coll Med 82; **RES:** N, Rush Presbyterian-St Luke's Med Ctr, Chicago, IL 83-86; **FEL:** N, Rush Presbyterian-St Luke's Med Ctr, Chicago, IL 86-87; ***SI:*** *Headache; Myasthenia*

Young, I James (MD) N
Northwest Comm Hlthcare
Northwest Neurological Associates Ltd, 2010 S Arlington Hghts Rd Ste 200; Arlington Hts, IL 60005; (847) 437-9176; **BDCERT:** N 65; **MS:** Univ IL Coll Med 54; **RES:** N, VA Rsch Hosp, Chicago, IL 59-62; **FEL:** Psyc, VA Research Hosp, Chicago, IL 59-62
2-4 Weeks

NEURORADIOLOGY

Duda, Eugene (MD) NRad
Christ Hosp & Med Ctr (see page 140)
Christ Hosp - Dept of Radiology - Chairman, 4440 W 95th St; Oak Lawn, IL 60453; (708) 425-8000; **BDCERT:** NR 96; DR 73; **MS:** Loyola U-Stritch Sch Med, Maywood 66; **RES:** DR, U Chicago Hosp, Chicago, IL 69-72; **FEL:** NRad, U Chicago Hosp, Chicago, IL 72-73; **FAP:** Assoc Prof Rush Med Coll

NUCLEAR MEDICINE

Bekerman, Carlos (MD) **NuM**
Michael Reese Hosp & Med Ctr
2929 S Ellis Ave Fl 2; Chicago, IL 60616; (312) 791-2520; **BDCERT:** NuM 73; **MS:** Uruguay 68; **RES:** IM, U Montevideo, Montevideo, Chile 68-72; **FEL:** NuM, U Chicago Hosp, Chicago, IL 68-69; **FAP:** Prof Univ IL Coll Med; ***SI:*** *Thyroid Gland; Nuclear Oncology*
Immediately

Conway, James (MD) **NuM**
Children's Mem Med Ctr **(see page 139)**
2300 Childrens Plz Ste 42; Chicago, IL 60614; (773) 880-4000; **BDCERT:** Rad 68; NuM 72; **MS:** Northwestern U 63; **RES:** Hosp Med College of PA, Philadelphia, PA 64-68; **FAP:** Prof Rad Northwestern U; **HMO:** Aetna Hlth Plan, Blue Cross & Blue Shield, Chicago HMO, CIGNA, Prudential

Dillehay, Gary (MD) **NuM**
Loyola U Med Ctr **(see page 120)**
2160 S 1st Ave; Maywood, IL 60153; (708) 216-3559; **BDCERT:** NuM 85; DR 87; **MS:** Mayo Med Sch 79; **RES:** DR, Northwestern Mem Hosp, Chicago, IL 79-83; NuM, Northwestern Mem Hosp, Chicago, IL 83-84; **FAP:** Assoc Prof Loyola U-Stritch Sch Med, Maywood

Frank, Stasia (MD) **NuM**
Resurrection Med Ctr
Resurrection Radiology, 7435 W Talcott Ave; Chicago, IL 60631; (773) 792-5188; **BDCERT:** Rad 67; NuM 72; **MS:** Univ IL Coll Med 60; **RES:** Rad, Cook Cty Hosp, Chicago, IL 63-67; **FEL:** NuM, Cook Cty Hosp, Chicago, IL 67-68; **FAP:** Asst Clin Prof Rad Loyola U-Stritch Sch Med, Maywood

Martinez, Charles J. (MD) **NuM**
Lutheran Gen Hosp **(see page 143)**
Lutheran General Hospital, 1775 Dempster St; Park Ridge, IL 60068; (847) 723-6080; **BDCERT:** NuM 72; IM 73; **MS:** St Louis U 61; **RES:** NuM, Hines VA Hosp, Hines, IL 68; IM, Hines VA Hosp, Hines, IL 65-68; **FAP:** Assoc Prof Med U Chicago-Pritzker Sch Med; ***SI:*** *PET Scanning; Thyroid Cancer*

Pavel, Dan (MD) **NuM**
Univ of Illinois at Chicago Med Ctr
University-Illinois Hospital, 1740 W Taylor St Ste 2500; Chicago, IL 60612; (312) 996-3966; **BDCERT:** NuM 74; **MS:** Romania 57; **RES:** Northwestern Mem Hosp, Chicago, IL 72-74; **FAP:** Prof Univ IL Coll Med

Peller, Patrick (MD) **NuM**
Lutheran Gen Hosp **(see page 143)**
Luthern General Hospital, 1775 Dempster St; Park Ridge, IL 60068; (847) 723-6080; **BDCERT:** NuM 91; IM 86; **MS:** U Minn 83; **RES:** IM, Fitzsimons AMC, Aurora, IL 84-86; **FEL:** NuM, Walter Reed Army Med Ctr, Washington, DC 89-91; **FAP:** Asst Clin Prof U Chicago-Pritzker Sch Med

Perlman, Reid (MD) **NuM**
Evanston Hosp
2849 Birchwood Ave; Wilmette, IL 60091; (847) 570-2591; **BDCERT:** DR 80; **MS:** U Hlth Sci/Chicago Med Sch 76; **RES:** DR, Michael Reese Hosp Med Ctr, Chicago, IL 77-80; NuM, Michael Reese Hosp Med Ctr, Chicago, IL 80-81; **HOSP:** Glenbrook Hosp; **HMO:** Aetna Hlth Plan, Blue Cross & Blue Shield, CIGNA, Humana Health Plan, Principal Health Care

Rosenblum, Leigh (MD) **NuM**
Rush North Shore Med Ctr
9669 Kenton Ave Ste 203; Skokie, IL 60076; (847) 677-0212; **BDCERT:** NuM 72; IM 63; **MS:** Univ IL Coll Med 52; **RES:** Mount Sinai Hosp Med Ctr, Chicago, IL 53; **FAP:** Assoc Clin Prof Med Univ IL Coll Med; **HMO:** Chicago HMO, Rush Health Plans

Spies, Stewart (MD) **NuM**
Northwestern Mem Hosp
Dept of Nuclear Medicine, 251 E Huron St 8th Flr; Chicago, IL 60611; (312) 926-2514; **BDCERT:** NuM 74; IM 73; **MS:** Northwestern U 70; **RES:** IM, UCLA Med Ctr, Los Angeles, CA 71-73; NuM, UCLA Med Ctr, Los Angeles, CA 73-74

OBSTETRICS & GYNECOLOGY

Acharya, Vasant (MD) **ObG**
PCP
West Suburban Hosp Med Ctr
Archie & Acharya, 1 Erie Ct Ste 7040; Oak Park, IL 60302; (708) 488-2611; **BDCERT:** ObG 79; **MS:** India 71; **RES:** ObG, Rush Presbyterian-St Luke's Med Ctr, Chicago, IL 72-75; **FEL:** MF, Rush Presbyterian-St Luke's Med Ctr, Chicago, IL 75-77; **HOSP:** Rush-Presbyterian-St Luke's Med Ctr; ***SI:*** *Surgery*; **HMO:** Blue Cross & Blue Shield, Rush Prudential, Humana Health Plan, United Healthcare +
1 Week ***VISA***

Albion, Timothy (MD) **ObG**
Alexian Brothers Med Ctr **(see page 138)**
810 Biesterfield Rd Ste 102; Elk Grove Vlg, IL 60007; (847) 364-0040; **BDCERT:** ObG 92; **MS:** U Hlth Sci/Chicago Med Sch 86; **HMO:** Aetna Hlth Plan, Blue Cross & Blue Shield, Californiacare, CIGNA, Health Alliance Plan
4+ Weeks ***VISA***

Archie, Julian (MD) ObG
PCP
Rush-Presbyterian-St Luke's Med Ctr
(see page 122)
Archie & Acharya, 1 Erie Ct Ste 7040; Oak Park, IL 60302; (708) 386-8008; **BDCERT:** ObG 72; **MS:** SUNY Buffalo 60; **RES:** Millard Fillmore Health Sys, Buffalo, NY 63-64; Univ Hosp SUNY Buffalo, Buffalo, NY 64-68; **FAP:** Asst Prof Rush Med Coll

Axelrod, Edward (MD) ObG
Christ Hosp & Med Ctr (see page 140)
Southwest Obstetrics Gyn Ltd, 4225 W 95th St; Oak Lawn, IL 60453; (708) 423-2300; **BDCERT:** ObG 72; **MS:** Univ IL Coll Med 63; **RES:** Cook Cty Hosp, Chicago, IL 66-69; **FAP:** Assoc Clin Prof ObG Univ IL Coll Med; **HMO:** Humana Health Plan, Blue Cross & Blue Shield +
4+ Weeks

Barriuso, Eduardo (MD) ObG
Norwegian-American Hosp
B & B Partnership, 6035 W Cermak Rd; Cicero, IL 60650; (708) 222-6800; **BDCERT:** ObG 76; **MS:** Bolivia 63; **RES:** West Suburban Hosp Med Ctr, Oak Park, IL 66-70; **HMO:** Aetna Hlth Plan, Blue Cross & Blue Shield, Californiacare, Choicecare, CIGNA

Barton, John (MD) ObG
Illinois Masonic Med Ctr
(see page 118)
836 W Wellington Ave Ste 5723; Chicago, IL 60657; (773) 296-7045; **BDCERT:** ObG 83; **MS:** Univ IL Coll Med 61; **RES:** ObG, Cook Cty Hosp, Chicago, IL 62-65; **FAP:** Prof ObG Rush Med Coll; **HMO:** +
LANG: Sp; A Few Days
VISA

Bayly Jr, Melvyn (MD) ObG
Northwestern Mem Hosp
Northwestern Gynecology & Ob, 1535 Lake Cook Rd Ste 600; Northbrook, IL 60062; (847) 559-1881; **BDCERT:** ObG 77; **MS:** Northwestern U 71; **RES:** ObG, Parkland Mem Hosp, Dallas, TX 72-75; **FAP:** Asst Clin Prof ObG Northwestern U
4+ Weeks VISA

Beck, Herbert (MD) ObG
PCP
Evanston Hosp
1000 Central St Ste 730; Evanston, IL 60201; (847) 570-0005; **BDCERT:** ObG 85; **MS:** Northwestern U 76; **RES:** Northwestern Mem Hosp, Chicago, IL 77-80; **FEL:** GO, Loyola U Med Ctr, Maywood, IL 80-83; **FAP:** Instr ObG Northwestern U; **HMO:** Aetna Hlth Plan, Blue Cross & Blue Shield, Chicago HMO, CIGNA, HealthNet

Blanks, Mary (MD) ObG
Little Company of Mary Hosp & Hlth Care Ctrs (see page 142)
Wellness Connections, 10725 S Western Ave; Chicago, IL 60643; (773) 233-6500; **BDCERT:** ObG 85; **MS:** Howard U 79; **RES:** ObG, U Chicago Hosp, Chicago, IL 80-83; **HOSP:** Christ Hosp & Med Ctr; ***SI:*** *Holistic Medicine*; **HMO:** Blue Cross PPO, Blue Choice, Aetna Hlth Plan, United Healthcare, Preferred Plan
Immediately VISA

Blankstein, Josef (MD) ObG
Mount Sinai Hosp Med Ctr
Mt Sinai Hosp Med Ctr - ObGyn, California Ave at 15th St; Chicago, IL 60608; (773) 354-2000; **BDCERT:** ObG 81; **MS:** Israel 70; **RES:** ObG, Chaim Sheba Med Ctr, Tel Aviv, Israel 70-76; ObG, U Manitoba Hlth Sci Ctr, Winnipeg, Canada 77-79; **FEL:** RE, Cleveland Clinic Hosp, Cleveland, OH 88-89; ***SI:*** *Infertility; Menopause*
A Few Days

Boatwright, Patricia (MD) ObG
PCP
Rush-Presbyterian-St Luke's Med Ctr
(see page 122)
1725 W Harrison St Ste 351; Chicago, IL 60612; (312) 738-0055; **BDCERT:** ObG 87; **MS:** U Mich Med Sch 85
VISA

Bray, James (MD) ObG
Christ Hosp & Med Ctr (see page 140)
Glenwood Medical Corp, 9651 W 153rd St; Orland Park, IL 60462; (708) 873-7775; **BDCERT:** ObG 83; **MS:** Loyola U-Stritch Sch Med, Maywood 77; **RES:** ObG, Columbus Hosp, Chicago, IL 78-81; **FAP:** Clin Instr Rush Med Coll; **HOSP:** Palos Comm Hosp

Brubaker, Linda (MD) ObG
Rush-Presbyterian-St Luke's Med Ctr
(see page 122)
University Urogynecologists, 1725 W Harrison St Ste 818; Chicago, IL 60612; (312) 733-5551; **BDCERT:** ObG 91; **MS:** Rush Med Coll 84; **RES:** ObG, Rush Presbyterian-St Luke's Med Ctr, Chicago, IL 84-88; **FEL:** U, Rush Presbyterian-St Luke's Med Ctr, Chicago, IL 88-90; **FAP:** Assoc Prof Rush Med Coll; ***SI:*** *Bladder Problems and Conditions*
LANG: Sp; VISA

Bubala, Paul (MD) ObG
Lutheran Gen Hosp (see page 143)
Ellinwood Medical Assoc, 701 Lee St Ste 670; Des Plaines, IL 60016; (847) 297-5500; **BDCERT:** ObG 79; **MS:** Northwestern U 59; **HMO:** Blue Cross & Blue Shield

Carson, Maureen (MD) ObG
Lutheran Gen Hosp (see page 143)
Associates In Ob-Gyn, 1875 Dempster St Ste 360; Park Ridge, IL 60068; (847) 825-7030; **BDCERT:** ObG 91; **MS:** Univ IL Coll Med 85; **RES:** ObG, U Chicago Hosp, Chicago, IL 85-87; ObG, Lutheran Gen Hosp, Park Ridge, IL 87-89

Charles, Allan (MD) ObG
PCP
Michael Reese Hosp & Med Ctr
Women's Health Consultants, 55 E Washington Ste 3700; Chicago, IL 60602; (312) 263-5517; **BDCERT:** ObG 63; **MS:** NYU Sch Med 52; **RES:** ObG, Mount Sinai Med Ctr, New York, NY 55-57; ObG, Michael Reese Hosp Med Ctr, Chicago, IL 57-59; **FAP:** Clin Prof ObG Univ IL Coll Med; ***SI:*** *Management of Menopause; Second Opinions*

Chiranand, Pinit (MD) ObG
PCP
St Bernard Hosp
Century Medical Ctr, 758 W 69th St; Chicago, IL 60621; (773) 783-4700; **BDCERT:** ObG 75; **MS:** Thailand 62; **RES:** ObG, , Thailand 63-64; **FEL:** GO, Albany Med Ctr, Albany, NY 73-74; ***SI:*** *Surgery (Tubal Ligation); Fibroid Removal*; **HMO:** Harmony, United Healthcare, Family Med Net, NYLCare, American Health Plan
LANG: Thai; Immediately

Cislak, Carol (MD) ObG
PCP
Evanston Hosp
Obstetrics & Gynecology, 2500 Ridge Ave Ste 311; Evanston, IL 60201; (847) 869-5800; **BDCERT:** ObG 89; **MS:** Northwestern U 83; **HMO:** Aetna Hlth Plan, Blue Cross & Blue Shield, Chicago HMO, CIGNA, Metlife

Collins, Karen L. (MD) ObG
St Alexius Med Ctr
Northwest Associates-Womens, 1585 Barrington Rd Ste 302; Hoffman Estates, IL 60194; (847) 884-1800; **BDCERT:** ObG 85; **MS:** Univ IL Coll Med 79; **RES:** ObG, Rush Presbyterian-St Luke's Med Ctr, Chicago, IL 80-83; ***SI:*** *Premenstrual Syndrome; Menopause Health*

Coupet, Edouard (MD) ObG
St Francis Hosp
14229 Chicago Rd; Dolton, IL 60419; (708) 849-4004; **BDCERT:** ObG 85; **MS:** Univ IL Coll Med 79

Crandall, David (MD) ObG
Good Shepherd Hosp
27401 W Il Route 22 Ste 107; Barrington, IL 60010; (847) 382-7330; **BDCERT:** ObG 91; **MS:** U Iowa Coll Med 84; **RES:** ObG, U IA Hosp, Iowa City, IA 85-89; **HMO:** Blue Cross & Blue Shield, Californiacare, Metlife, Principal Health Care
LANG: Sp; VISA

Cromer, David (MD) ObG
PCP
Evanston Hosp
Assocs Gynec Surg & ObGyn, 1000 Central St Ste 700; Evanston, IL 60201; (847) 869-3300; **BDCERT:** ObG 89; **MS:** Northwestern U 61; **RES:** ObG, Evanston Hosp, Evanston, IL 62-65; **FAP:** Assoc Prof ObG Northwestern U; **HOSP:** Glenbrook Hosp; ***SI:*** *Menopause; Pelvic Surgery*; **HMO:** Aetna Hlth Plan, Humana Health Plan, Prudential, Bc/BS +
2-4 Weeks VISA

Darrell, Brenda A (MD) ObG
Illinois Masonic Med Ctr
(see page 118)
Women's Health Resources, 836 W Wellington Ave; Chicago, IL 60611; (773) 296-3500; **BDCERT:** ObG 98; **MS:** UMDNJ-RW Johnson Med Sch 82

Dooley, Sharon L (MD) ObG
PCP
Northwestern Mem Hosp
Prentice Womens Hosp-ObG Northwestern U Med Sch, 333 E Superior St Room 410; Chicago, IL 60611; (312) 908-7519; **BDCERT:** ObG 89; MF 81; **MS:** U Va Sch Med 73; **FAP:** Prof ObG Northwestern U; ***SI:*** *Maternal Fetal Medicine*

Drachler, A Michael (MD) ObG
Rush North Shore Med Ctr
9669 Kenton Ave Ste 606; Skokie, IL 60076; (847) 933-3950; **BDCERT:** ObG 94; **MS:** Univ Hlth Sci Coll -Osteo Med 78; **RES:** ObG, Cook County Hospital, Chicago, IL 79-82; **FAP:** Asst Prof Rush Med Coll

Duboe, Fred (MD) ObG
PCP
St Alexius Med Ctr
NW Associates for Womens Healthcare, 1585 Barrington Rd Ste 302; Hoffman Estates, IL 60194; (847) 884-1800; **BDCERT:** ObG 97; **MS:** Univ IL Coll Med 80; **RES:** ObG, Northwestern Mem Hosp, Chicago, IL 80-84; **HOSP:** Alexian Brothers Med Ctr; ***SI:*** *High Risk Obstetrics; Laparoscopic Surgery*; **HMO:** Aetna Hlth Plan, Blue Cross & Blue Shield, Californiacare, HMO Illinois, PHCS +
LANG: Pol, Sp; A Few Days VISA

Feingold, Michael (MD) ObG
Palos Comm Hosp
Hygeia Medical Group, 12211 S Harlem Ave; Palos Heights, IL 60463; (708) 361-4211; **BDCERT:** ObG 89; **MS:** Univ IL Coll Med 82; **HOSP:** Christ Hosp & Med Ctr

Fiakpui, E Z (MD) ObG
Trinity Hosp
2315 E 93rd St Ste 337; Chicago, IL 60617; (773) 731-2700; **BDCERT:** ObG 76; **MS:** U Chicago-Pritzker Sch Med 70; **RES:** ObG, Chicago Lying In Hosp, Chicago, IL 71-74; **FAP:** Assoc Clin Instr U Chicago-Pritzker Sch Med

Frederiksen, Marilynn (MD) **ObG**
PCP
Northwestern Mem Hosp
NW Med Faculty Foundation-General Obstetrics, Superior St and Fairbanks CT Ste 1000; Chicago, IL 60611; (312) 908-7382; **BDCERT:** ObG 82; MF 83; **MS:** Boston U 74; **RES:** ObG, Brigham & Women's Hosp, Boston, MA 76-79; Ped, U MD Hosp, Baltimore, MD 75-76; **FEL:** MF, Northwestern Mem Hosp, Chicago, IL 79-81; **FAP:** Assoc Prof ObG Northwestern U

Gerbie, Melvin (MD) **ObG**
Northwestern Mem Hosp
680 N Lakeshore Dr Ste 1000; Chicago, IL 60611; (312) 908-5656; **BDCERT:** ObG 91; **MS:** Northwestern U 60; **RES:** ObG, Passavant Pavillion, Chicago, IL 61-64; **FEL:** GO, NY Med Coll, New York, NY 64-65; **FAP:** Prof of Clin ObG Northwestern U; **HMO:** Blue Cross & Blue Shield, Principal Health Care

Gianopoulos, John (MD) **ObG**
Loyola U Med Ctr **(see page 120)**
Loyola University Medical Ctr, 2160 S 1st Ave Ste 103-1019; Maywood, IL 60153; (708) 216-6233; **BDCERT:** ObG 93; MF 85; **MS:** Loyola U-Stritch Sch Med, Maywood 77; **RES:** ObG, Loyola U Med Ctr, Maywood, IL 77-81; **FEL:** MF, Loyola U Med Ctr, Maywood, IL 81-83; **HMO:** Aetna Hlth Plan, Blue Cross & Blue Shield, Chicago HMO, CIGNA, Prudential

Haag, Mary (MD) **ObG**
Macneal Mem Hosp
Riverside Ob-Gyn Ltd, 3722 Harlem Ave; Riverside, IL 60546; (708) 447-1003; **BDCERT:** ObG 90; **MS:** Rush Med Coll 84; **RES:** ObG, Rush Presbyterian-St Luke's Med Ctr, Chicago, IL 84-88; **HMO:** +
2-4 Weeks

Hass, Marsie (MD) **ObG**
Ingalls Mem Hosp
Reproductive Health Assoc, 16241 Wausau Ave; South Holland, IL 60473; (708) 596-7070; **BDCERT:** ObG 88; **MS:** Northwestern U 82; **RES:** ObG, Michael Reese Hosp Med Ctr, Chicago, IL 82-86; **HMO:** Aetna Hlth Plan, Blue Cross & Blue Shield, Californiacare, HealthNet, Metlife

Hasson, Harith M (MD) **ObG**
Louis A Weiss Mem Hosp
Weiss Health Center, 2551 N Clark St Ste 201; Chicago, IL 60614; (773) 477-8877; **BDCERT:** ObG 78; **MS:** Egypt 55; **RES:** ObG, Rush Presbyterian-St Luke's Med Ctr, Chicago, IL 60-61; West Suburban Hosp Med Ctr, Oak Park, IL 61-66; **FAP:** Clinical Prof ObG U Chicago-Pritzker Sch Med; **HOSP:** Grant Hosp; ***SI:** Laparoscopic Surgery; Endometriosis/Fibroids*; **HMO:** Blue Cross & Blue Shield, United Healthcare, Humana Health Plan, Rush Health Plans
LANG: Ar, Fr, Itl, Sp; Immediately VISA

Hayes, Ernest (MD) **ObG**
PCP
Bethany Hosp
Hayes & Moss Ltd, 3435 W Van Buren St; Chicago, IL 60624; (773) 722-0013; **BDCERT:** ObG 77; **MS:** Meharry Med Coll 69; **RES:** ObG, Cook Cty Hosp, Chicago, IL 70-74; **HOSP:** South Shore Hosp; **HMO:** Blue Cross & Blue Shield, CIGNA, Aetna Hlth Plan, Prudential
1 Week

Herbst, Arthur (MD) **ObG**
U Chicago Hosp **(see page 124)**
U Chicago Sch Med Dept Obg, 5841 S Maryland Ave MC2050; Chicago, IL 60637; (773) 702-6123; **BDCERT:** ObG 83; GO 74; **MS:** Harvard Med Sch 59; **RES:** S, Mass Gen Hosp, Boston, MA 60-62; ObG, Brigham & Women's Hosp, Boston, MA 62-65; **FAP:** Prof U Chicago-Pritzker Sch Med; ***SI:** DES*; **HMO:** +
2-4 Weeks VISA

Herndon, Karyn (MD) **ObG**
Evanston Hosp
Assocs Gyn Surg & Ob, 1000 Central St Ste 700; Evanston, IL 60201; (847) 869-3300; **BDCERT:** ObG 92; **MS:** U Fla Coll Med 86; **RES:** ObG, Northwestern Mem Hosp, Chicago, IL 87-90; **FAP:** Instr Clin ObG Northwestern U; **HOSP:** Glenbrook Hosp; ***SI:** Pap Smear Abnormalities; Breast Cancer Screening*; **HMO:** Blue Cross & Blue Shield, Aetna Hlth Plan +
LANG: Sp; 4+ Weeks VISA

Hobart, John (MD) **ObG**
Evanston Hosp
Evanston Hospital, 2650 Ridge Ave; Evanston, IL 60201; (847) 570-2280; **BDCERT:** ObG 79; MF 83; **MS:** Tulane U 73; **RES:** ObG, Northwestern Mem Hosp, Chicago, IL 73-77; **FEL:** MF, Prentice Women's Hosp, Chicago, IL 77-79; **FAP:** Asst Prof ObG Northwestern U; ***SI:** High Risk Obstetrics*

Hobbs, John (MD) **ObG**
Illinois Masonic Med Ctr
(see page 118)
Female Health Care Assoc, 1725 W Harrison St Ste 740; Chicago, IL 60612; (312) 421-1555; **BDCERT:** ObG 82; **MS:** U Minn-Duluth Sch Med 75; **HOSP:** St Joseph Hosp-Elgin
LANG: Sp;

Holt, Linda (MD) **ObG**
Rush North Shore Med Ctr
Women's Medical Group, 64 Old Orchard Ctr; Skokie, IL 60077; (847) 673-3130; **BDCERT:** ObG 94; **MS:** U Chicago-Pritzker Sch Med 77; **RES:** ObG, U Chicago Hosp, Chicago, IL 78-81; **FAP:** Asst Prof Northwestern U; **HOSP:** Evanston Hosp

Hosseinian, Abdol (MD) ObG
St Joseph Hosp-Elgin
Ob Gyn Consultants, 2800 N Sheridan Ste 304; Chicago, IL 60657; (773) 525-4500; **BDCERT:** ObG 72; RE 74; **MS:** Iran 59; **RES:** ObG, Metro General Hospital, Cleveland, OH 66-70; **FAP:** Prof U Chicago-Pritzker Sch Med

Hussey, Michael J. (MD) ObG
PCP
Rush-Presbyterian-St Luke's Med Ctr
(see page 122)
Womens Hlth Con, 1725 W Harrison Ste 408; Chicago, IL 60612; (312) 942-6611; **BDCERT:** ObG 94; MF 98; **MS:** Univ IL Coll Med 86; **RES:** MF, Rush Presbyterian-St Luke's Med Ctr, Chicago, IL -93; ObG, Loyola U Med Ctr, Maywood, IL 91-93; **FAP:** Asst Prof Rush Med Coll; **HOSP:** Central DuPage Hosp

Hutter, Loren (MD) ObG
Evanston Hosp
Associates for Gynecology, 1000 Central St Ste 700; Evanston, IL 60201; (847) 869-3300; **BDCERT:** ObG 84; **MS:** Northwestern U 78

Jabamoni, Reena (MD) ObG
Good Samaritan Hosp (see page 274)
1585 Barrington Rd Ste 401; Hoffman Estates, IL 60194; (847) 843-7090; **BDCERT:** ObG 80; **MS:** India 64; **RES:** S, Jeanes Hosp, Philadelphia, PA 70-71; ObG, Albert Einstein Med Ctr, Bronx, NY 68-70; **FEL:** Loyola U Med Ctr, Maywood, IL 72-73; **FAP:** Assoc Clin Prof Loyola U-Stritch Sch Med, Maywood

Kennedy, Lofton (MD) ObG
Trinity Hosp
Kennedy Medical Svc Corp, 2301 E 93rd St Ste 115; Chicago, IL 60617; (773) 768-4114; **BDCERT:** ObG 76; **MS:** U Tex Med Br, Galveston 70; **RES:** ObG, Chicago Med Sch-Mt Sinai Hosp, Chicago, IL 71-74; ***SI:*** *Bleeding Disorders; Adolescent Gynecology*; **HMO:** Blue Cross, Prudential, United Healthcare, Aetna Hlth Plan, Travelers +
LANG: Sp; A Few Days *VISA*

Kim, Kee Chong (MD) ObG
PCP
Westlake Comm Hosp
1111 Superior St Ste 304; Melrose Park, IL 60160; (708) 344-7800; **BDCERT:** ObG 85; **MS:** South Korea 66; **RES:** ObG, Hosp of U Penn, Philadelphia, PA 77; **HMO:** Blue Cross & Blue Shield, Chicago HMO, CIGNA, Compare Health Service, Humana Health Plan

Kismartoni, Karoly R (MD) ObG
Resurrection Med Ctr
Ob-Gyn Affiliates, 7447 W Talcott Ave Ste 221; Chicago, IL 60631; (773) 763-6800; **BDCERT:** ObG 82; **MS:** Hungary 63; **RES:** ObG, W. Germany 66-68; ObG, Marion Hosp, Germany 68-70; **FEL:** ObG, St Francis Hosp of Evanston, Evanston, IL 74-75; **HMO:** Blue Cross & Blue Shield, Rush Prudential, United Healthcare, Aetna Hlth Plan +
LANG: Sp, Pol, Hun, Rus;

Koduri, Anur (MD) ObG
PCP
Ravenswood Hosp Med Ctr
Ravenswood Health Care Ctr, 4600 N Ravenswood Ave; Chicago, IL 60640; (773) 275-7700; **BDCERT:** ObG 85; **MS:** India 74; **RES:** ObG, Cook Cty Hosp, Chicago, IL 76-83; **HMO:** Blue Cross & Blue Shield, United Healthcare, Humana Health Plan, American Health Plan
LANG: Sp, Tel, Hin, Ur; A Few Days *VISA*

Krawczyk, Mitchell (MD) ObG
Ingalls Mem Hosp
H F Medical Assoc Inc, 17901 Governors Hwy Ste 102; Homewood, IL 60430; (708) 799-8880; **BDCERT:** ObG 98; **MS:** Univ IL Coll Med 82; **RES:** ObG, Franklin Sq Hosp, Baltimore, MD 85; ObG, Johns Hopkins Hosp, Baltimore, MD 82-86; ***SI:*** *Obstetrics; Norplant*; **HMO:** Aetna Hlth Plan, Blue Cross & Blue Shield, Californiacare, Prudential, United Healthcare +
LANG: Sp, Pol; A Few Days *VISA*

La Pata, Robert (MD) ObG
Evanston Hosp
Associates In Obstetrics, 1000 Central St Ste 700; Evanston, IL 60201; (847) 869-3300; **BDCERT:** ObG 72; **MS:** Marquette U 63; **RES:** ObG, Evanston Hosp, Evanston, IL 66-70; **HMO:** Aetna Hlth Plan, Blue Cross & Blue Shield, Chicago HMO, CIGNA, Metlife

Larson, Paul (MD) ObG
Swedish Covenant Hosp
5140 N California Ave Ste 780; Chicago, IL 60625; (773) 878-7787; **BDCERT:** ObG 79; **MS:** U Mich Med Sch 56

Layman, Lawrence (MD) ObG
U Chicago Hosp (see page 124)
University of Chicago, 5841 S Maryland Ave; Chicago, IL 60637; (773) 702-6642; **BDCERT:** ObG 89; **MS:** U Cincinnati 81; **RES:** IM, Jewish Hosp, Cincinnati, OH 81-82; ObG, U Louisville Hosp, Louisville, KY 82-86; **FEL:** RE, Med Coll of GA Hosp, Augusta, GA 86-88; **FAP:** Assoc Prof U Chicago-Pritzker Sch Med; ***SI:*** *Hypogonadism; Premature Menopause*; **HMO:** Humana Health Plan, United Healthcare, UHC, CIGNA +
1 Week *VISA*

Lee, Seung Soo (MD) ObG
St Mary's of Nazareth Hosp Ctr
1945 W Wilson Ave Ste 5113; Chicago, IL 60640; (773) 728-1443; **BDCERT:** ObG 80; **MS:** Other Foreign Country 64; **RES:** ObG, St Joseph's Hosp, Chicago, IL 69-72

Levine, Elliot (MD) **ObG**
Illinois Masonic Med Ctr
(see page 118)
3000 N Halsted St Ste 209; Chicago, IL 60657; (773) 296-3300; **BDCERT:** ObG 84; **MS:** U Hlth Sci/Chicago Med Sch 78; **RES:** ObG, Illinois Masonic Med Ctr, Chicago, IL 78-82; **FAP:** Asst Clin Prof ObG Rush Med Coll; ***SI:*** *Sexually Transmitted Disease; Painful Intercourse*
2-4 Weeks

Lifchez, Aaron (MD) **ObG**
Illinois Masonic Med Ctr
(see page 118)
Fertility Centers of Illinois, 3703 W Lake; Glenview, IL 60025; (847) 998-8200; **BDCERT:** ObG 76; **MS:** U Hlth Sci/Chicago Med Sch 69; **RES:** Michael Reese Hosp Med Ctr, Chicago, IL 70-74; **FAP:** Asst Clin Prof Univ IL Coll Med; **HMO:** Aetna Hlth Plan, Blue Cross & Blue Shield, Chicago HMO, Humana Health Plan, Maxicare Health Plan

Linn, Edward S (MD) **ObG**
Lutheran Gen Hosp **(see page 143)**
Advocate Medical-Ob/Gyn Dept, 1775 N Dempster St; Park Ridge, IL 60068; (847) 318-2843; **BDCERT:** ObG 94; **MS:** U Chicago-Pritzker Sch Med 74; **RES:** ObG, Michael Reese Hosp Med Ctr, Chicago, IL 74-78; **FAP:** Asst Clin Prof Northwestern U

Locher, Stephen (MD) **ObG**
Illinois Masonic Med Ctr
(see page 118)
3000 N Halsted Ste 209; Chicago, IL 60657; (773) 296-3300; **BDCERT:** ObG 91; **MS:** Univ IL Coll Med 85; **RES:** ObG, U IL Med Ctr, Chicago, IL 85-89

Lopata, Randee (MD) **ObG**
Lutheran Gen Hosp **(see page 143)**
Advocate Medical Group, 1775 Dempster St Ste 145; Park Ridge, IL 60068; (847) 318-9350; **BDCERT:** ObG 91; **MS:** Univ IL Coll Med 85; **RES:** ObG, U Chicago Hosp, Chicago, IL 86-89

Merrick, Frank (MD) **ObG**
Rush-Presbyterian-St Luke's Med Ctr
(see page 122)
1725 W Harrison St Ste 738; Chicago, IL 60612; (312) 829-4405; **BDCERT:** ObG 67; **MS:** U Mich Med Sch 58; **RES:** ObG, Chicago Lying In Hosp, Chicago, IL 59-62

Miller, Ronald W (MD) **ObG**
Evanston Hosp
A G S O, 1000 Central St Ste 700; Evanston, IL 60201; (847) 869-3300; **BDCERT:** ObG 82; **MS:** Univ IL Coll Med 75; **RES:** ObG, Northwestern Mem Hosp, Chicago, IL; **HOSP:** Glenbrook Hosp; ***SI:*** *Childbirth; Menopause*; **HMO:** +
1 Week

Moawad, Atef (MD) **ObG**
U Chicago Hosp **(see page 124)**
University Chicago Hospital, 5841 S Maryland MC 1072; Chicago, IL 60637; (773) 702-6118; **BDCERT:** ObG 89; **MS:** Egypt 57; **RES:** ObG, Thomas Jefferson U Hosp, Philadelphia, PA 61-64; **FEL:** ObG, U Lund Hospitals, Sweden 66-67; Case Western Reserve U Hosp, Cleveland, OH 65-66; **FAP:** Prof ObG U Chicago-Pritzker Sch Med

Mullin, Kimberly Anne (MD) **ObG**
Christ Hosp & Med Ctr **(see page 140)**
7800 W College Dr; Palos Heights, IL 60463; (708) 361-2400; **BDCERT:** ObG 92; **MS:** U Tenn Ctr Hlth Sci, Memphis 86; **RES:** ObG, Rush Presbyterian-St Luke's Med Ctr, Chicago, IL 87-90; **HOSP:** Palos Comm Hosp

Munoz, Maria (MD) **ObG**
St Joseph Hosp-Elgin
Clark Oak Health Specialists, 1001 N Clark St; Chicago, IL 60610; (312) 337-2626; **BDCERT:** ObG 88; **MS:** Univ IL Coll Med 75; **HOSP:** Illinois Masonic Med Ctr

Nye, Elizabeth (MD) **ObG**
Rush-Presbyterian-St Luke's Med Ctr
(see page 122)
500 N Michigan Ave Ste 1046; Chicago, IL 60611; (312) 670-2530; **BDCERT:** ObG 92; **MS:** Rush Med Coll 85; **RES:** ObG, Rush Presbyterian-St Luke's Med Ctr, Chicago, IL 86-89; **FAP:** Assistant Profe ObG Rush Med Coll; **HOSP:** Rush North Shore Med Ctr; ***SI:*** *Hormone Replacement Therapy*; **HMO:** Aetna Hlth Plan, PHCS, United Healthcare, CIGNA PPO
2-4 Weeks **VISA**

O'Connor, Therese Marie (MD) **ObG**
PCP
Lutheran Gen Hosp **(see page 143)**
AMG Ob Gyn, 1875 Dempster Ste 145; Park Ridge, IL 60068; (847) 318-9350; **BDCERT:** ObG 97; **MS:** Univ IL Coll Med 81; **RES:** ObG, Illinois Masonic Med Ctr, Chicago, IL 81-85; **FAP:** Asst Clin Prof ObG Univ IL Coll Med; ***SI:*** *Menopause; Vulvar & Vaginal Diseases*; **HMO:** +
A Few Days **VISA**

Olsen, Norman (MD) **ObG**
PCP
Swedish Covenant Hosp
5140 N California Ave Ste 780; Chicago, IL 60625; (773) 878-7787; **BDCERT:** ObG 68; **MS:** Baylor 61; **RES:** Baylor Med Ctr, Houston, TX 62-65; **HMO:** Aetna Hlth Plan, Blue Cross & Blue Shield, CIGNA, Metlife, Prudential

Pavese, Joseph (MD) ObG
Christ Hosp & Med Ctr (see page 140)
Southwest Obstetrics Gyn Ltd, 4225 W 95th St; Oak Lawn, IL 60453; (708) 423-2300; **BDCERT:** ObG 94; **MS:** Southern IL U 80; **RES:** Rush Presby-St Lukes, Chicago, IL 80-84; **FAP:** Asst Clin Prof Univ IL Coll Med; **HMO:** Aetna Hlth Plan, Blue Cross & Blue Shield, CIGNA, HealthNet, Prudential

Pielet, Bruce (MD) ObG
Lutheran Gen Hosp (see page 143)
Lutheran Genl Hosp-Advocate Medical Group, 1875 Dempster St Ste 325; Park Ridge, IL 60068; (847) 723-8610; **BDCERT:** ObG 90; MF 91; **MS:** Loyola U-Stritch Sch Med, Maywood 81; **RES:** ObG, U Chicago Hosp, Chicago, IL 81-85; **FEL:** MF, Northwestern Mem Hosp, Chicago, IL 85-87; ***SI:*** *High Risk Pregnancies*

Pierce, Scott (MD) ObG
Gottlieb Mem Hosp
Pildes & Pierce, 675 W North Ave Ste 505; Melrose Park, IL 60160; (708) 450-4545; **BDCERT:** ObG 83; **MS:** Northwestern U 77; **FEL:** ObG, Mount Sinai Hosp Med Ctr, Chicago, IL 77-81

Poma, Pedro A (MD) ObG
Ravenswood Hosp Med Ctr
Ravenswood Occupational Health, 1945 W Wilson Ave Ste 5114; Chicago, IL 60640; (773) 907-7411; **BDCERT:** ObG 93; **MS:** Peru 65; **RES:** ObG, Cook Cty Hosp, Chicago, IL 68-71; Path CP, Northwestern Mem Hosp, Chicago, IL 69; **FAP:** Clin Prof ObG Loyola U-Stritch Sch Med, Maywood

Pozzi, Patrick (MD) ObG
PCP
Alexian Brothers Med Ctr
(see page 138)
Catrambone, Pozzi & Forcier Ltd, 810 Biesterfield Rd Ste 106; Elk Grove Vlg, IL 60007; (847) 981-8866; **BDCERT:** ObG 89; **MS:** Univ IL Coll Med 83; **RES:** ObG, Loyola U Med Ctr, Maywood, IL 83-87; **HOSP:** St Alexius Med Ctr; ***SI:*** *Laparoscopic Procedures*; **HMO:** Blue Cross & Blue Choice, CIGNA, HealthStar
LANG: Sp, Ger; Mcr Mcd
Immediately VISA

Regan, Michael (MD) ObG
Christ Hosp & Med Ctr (see page 140)
Christ Hospital, 4440 W 95th St; Oak Lawn, IL 60453; (708) 346-5630; **BDCERT:** ObG 92; **MS:** Univ IL Coll Med 84; **RES:** ObG, Michael Reese Hosp Med Ctr, Chicago, IL 84-88; **FEL:** GO, Loyola U Med Ctr, Maywood, IL 89-91; **FAP:** Assoc Clin Prof Univ IL Coll Med; ***SI:*** *Cervical Dysplasia; Uterine Cancer*
Mcr Mcd A Few Days VISA

Robinson, Barbara (MD) ObG
Lutheran Gen Hosp (see page 143)
Advocate Medical Group, 1875 W Dempster St; Park Ridge, IL 60068; (847) 318-9350; **BDCERT:** ObG 90; **MS:** Univ IL Coll Med 83; **RES:** ObG, Mount Sinai Hosp Med Ctr, Chicago, IL 83-86; ObG, Lutheran Gen Hosp, Park Ridge, IL 86-87

Rotmensch, Jacob (MD) ObG
U Chicago Hosp (see page 124)
Not a primary care practice. S Maryland Ave MC2050; Chicago, IL 60637; (773) 702-6721; **BDCERT:** ObG 94; GO 90; **MS:** Meharry Med Coll 77; **RES:** Johns Hopkins Hosp, Baltimore, MD 78-81; **FEL:** GO, Johns Hopkins Hosp, Baltimore, MD 81-84; **FAP:** Asst Prof U Chicago-Pritzker Sch Med

Rubin, Michael (MD) ObG
Lutheran Gen Hosp (see page 143)
Ellinwood Medical Assoc, 701 Lee St Ste 670; Des Plaines, IL 60016; (847) 297-5500; **BDCERT:** ObG 73; **MS:** Univ IL Coll Med 67; **RES:** U IL Med Ctr, Chicago, IL 68-71; **FAP:** Assoc Northwestern U; **HMO:** Blue Cross & Blue Shield

Schy, Susan (MD) ObG
Lutheran Gen Hosp (see page 143)
1875 Dempster St Ste 550; Park Ridge, IL 60068; (847) 698-7660; **BDCERT:** ObG 94; **MS:** Univ IL Coll Med 80; **RES:** Parkland Mem Hosp, Dallas, TX 81-84

Sciarra, John (MD) ObG
Northwestern Mem Hosp
NW Medical Faculty Foundation, 680 N Lake Shore Dr Ste 1000; Chicago, IL 60611; (312) 908-5656; **BDCERT:** ObG 67; **MS:** Columbia P&S 57; **RES:** ObG, Columbia-Presbyterian Med Ctr, New York, NY 58-64; **FAP:** Prof & Chrmn ObG Northwestern U; ***SI:*** *Gynecological Surgery; Menopause*
Mcr Mcd A Few Days
VISA

Shashoua, Abe (MD) ObG
Louis A Weiss Mem Hosp
4640 N Marine Dr; Chicago, IL 60640; (773) 564-5250; **BDCERT:** ObG 98; **MS:** U Miami Sch Med 92; **RES:** U Chicago Hosp, Chicago, IL 93-97; **FAP:** Clin Instr U Chicago-Pritzker Sch Med; **HOSP:** Evanston Hosp; ***SI:*** *Uterine Fibroids; Urinary Incontinence*; **HMO:** Blue Cross & Blue Shield, United Healthcare, Aetna Hlth Plan, PHCS +
LANG: Sp; Mcr Mcd NFI
A Few Days VISA

Silver, Richard (MD) ObG
Evanston Hosp
Evanston Hospital - ObGyn, 2650 Ridge Ave Ste 1600; Evanston, IL 60201; (847) 570-2280; **BDCERT:** ObG 88; MF 89; **MS:** Northwestern U 81; ***SI:*** *High Risk Obstetrics*

Guide to symbols and abbreviations can be found on pages 110-113.

Socol, Michael (MD) **ObG**
Northwestern Mem Hosp
Northwestern Univ Hospital, 333 E Superior St Ste 410; Chicago, IL 60611; (312) 908-7518; **BDCERT:** ObG 79; MF 81; **MS:** Univ IL Coll Med 74; **RES:** ObG, U IL Med Ctr, Chicago, IL 74-77; **FEL:** MF, USC Med Ctr, Los Angeles, CA 77-79; **FAP:** Dir NP Northwestern U; **HMO:** +
Mcr

Streicher, Lauren F (MD) **ObG**
Northwestern Mem Hosp
680 N Lake Shore Dr Ste 117; Chicago, IL 60611; (312) 654-1166; **BDCERT:** ObG 97; **MS:** Univ IL Coll Med 82; **RES:** ObG, Michael Reese Hosp Med Ctr, Chicago, IL 82-86

Thomas, Joseph (MD) **ObG**
PCP
Little Company of Mary Hosp & Hlth Care Ctrs (see page 142)
9727 S Western Ave; Chicago, IL 60643; (773) 881-3400; **BDCERT:** ObG 86; **MS:** Howard U 79; **RES:** ObG, Howard U Hosp, Washington, DC 80-84; **HOSP:** Trinity Hosp; ***SI:*** *Advanced Laparoscopic Surgery; Myomectomy*; **HMO:** Blue Cross & Blue Shield, Rush Prudential, CIGNA, UHC +
NFI Immediately VISA

Tyler, Lamarr (DO) **ObG**
PCP
Highland Park Hosp
Evanston Northwestern Healthcare, 830 W End Ave Ste 600; Vernon Hills, IL 60022; (847) 680-7900; **BDCERT:** ObG 94; **MS:** Chicago Coll Osteo Med 86; **RES:** ObG, Cook Cty Hosp, Chicago, IL 87-91; **FAP:** Assoc Prof Northwestern U; **HOSP:** Evanston Hosp; ***SI:*** *Advanced Laparoscopic Surgery*; **HMO:** Aetna Hlth Plan, Humana Health Plan, Blue Cross & Blue Shield, HMO Illinois +
SA SU Mcr A Few Days
VISA

Vaziri, Ira (MD) **ObG**
St James Hosp & Hlth Ctrs
2555 Lincoln Hwy Ste 113; Olympia Fields, IL 60461; (708) 748-2835; **BDCERT:** ObG 74; **MS:** Iran 64; **RES:** Wayne Cnty Gen Hosp, Detroit, MI; **FEL:** Wayne Cnty Gen Hosp, Detroit, MI; **HOSP:** South Suburban Hosp; **HMO:** Blue Cross & Blue Shield, CIGNA
SA SU Mcr 1 Week

Wagner, Arnold (MD) **ObG**
Evanston Hosp
Obstetrics & Gynecology, 1215 Old Mchenry Rd; Buffalo Grove, IL 60089; (847) 913-9400; **BDCERT:** ObG 77; **MS:** Northwestern U 69; **RES:** ObG, Evanston Hosp, Evanston, IL 73-75; **HMO:** Aetna Hlth Plan, Blue Cross & Blue Shield, Chicago HMO, CIGNA, Humana Health Plan

Zimmerman, Randy (MD) **ObG**
Good Shepherd Hosp
Good Shepherd Hosp - DOB 11, 450 W Highway #22 Ste 120; Barrington, IL 60010; (847) 277-0500; **BDCERT:** ObG 86; **MS:** Univ IL Coll Med 79; **RES:** ObG, St Francis Hosp of Evanston, Evanston, IL 79-83; ***SI:*** *Patient/Physician Conservative Collaboration*; **HMO:** Aetna Hlth Plan, Blue Cross & Blue Shield, CIGNA, HealthNet, Principal Health Care +
LANG: Sp; SA SU Mcr Mcd
1 Week VISA

OCCUPATIONAL MEDICINE

Woody, Lisa (MD) **OM**
Loyola U Med Ctr (see page 120)
Loyola U Med Ctr-Bldg 105, Occupational Hlth Svcs, 2160 S First Ave Rm 2943; Maywood, IL 60153; (708) 216-4397; **BDCERT:** OM 97; IM 87; **MS:** U Tex SW, Dallas 83; **RES:** IM, U New Mexico Medical Center, Albuquerque, NM 84-87; **FAP:** Asst Prof Loyola U-Stritch Sch Med, Maywood; ***SI:*** *Occupational Disease Prevention; Latex Allergy*
Mcr Mcd NFI Immediately

OPHTHALMOLOGY

Anstadt, Brad (MD) **Oph**
Gottlieb Mem Hosp
Gottlieb Eye Ctr, 675 W North Ave Ste 107; Melrose Park, IL 60160; (708) 450-4510; **BDCERT:** Oph 86; **MS:** Univ IL Coll Med 81; **RES:** Oph, Michael Reese Hosp Med Ctr, Chicago, IL 82-85; **HOSP:** Westlake Comm Hosp; ***SI:*** *Glaucoma; Cataract*

Bello, John (MD) **Oph**
Resurrection Med Ctr
Advanced Vision Specialists, 7447 W Talcott Ave Ste 406; Chicago, IL 60631; (773) 775-9755; **BDCERT:** Oph 89; **MS:** Northwestern U 80; **RES:** Oph, Tulane U Med Ctr, New Orleans, LA 81-84; **FEL:** King Khaled Eye Hosp, Riyadh, Saudi Arabia 84-85; ***SI:*** *Corneal Disease*; **HMO:** United Healthcare, Blue Cross & Blue Shield, Aetna Hlth Plan +
LANG: Sp, Pol, Itl; Mcr VISA

Berman, Andrew (MD) **Oph**
Rush North Shore Med Ctr
Eye Care Ltd, 9630 Kenton Ave; Skokie, IL 60076; (847) 677-1631; **BDCERT:** Oph 86; **MS:** Loyola U-Stritch Sch Med, Maywood 81; **RES:** Oph, Cook Cty Hosp, Chicago, IL 82-85; **FEL:** Neurophthalmology, Northwestern Mem Hosp, Chicago, IL 85-86; **HMO:** Aetna Hlth Plan, Blue Cross & Blue Shield, Californiacare, CIGNA, Humana Health Plan
VISA

Brown, Steven (MD) **Oph**
Evanston Hosp
1800 Sherman Ave Ste 511; Evanston, IL 60201; (847) 492-3250; **BDCERT:** Oph 86; **MS:** Rush Med Coll 79; **RES:** Oph, U NC Hosp, Chapel Hill, NC 80-83; **FEL:** Glaucoma, Mass Eye & Ear Infirmary, Boston, MA 83-85; **FAP:** Assoc Prof Rush Med Coll; **HOSP:** Rush-Presbyterian-St Luke's Med Ctr; ***SI:*** *Cataract & Related Anterior Segment Disorders; Glaucoma*; **HMO:** +
LANG: Rus, Sp; Mcr NFI Immediately VISA

Chapman, Lawrence (MD) **Oph**
St James Hosp & Hlth Ctrs
Arbor Center For Eye Care, 2640 W 183rd St; Homewood, IL 60430; (708) 798-6633; **BDCERT:** Oph 70; **MS:** Univ IL Coll Med 64; **RES:** Oph, Cook Cty Hosp, Chicago, IL 65-68; **FEL:** Ped Oph, IL Eye & Ear Infirmary, Chicago, IL 68-69; **FAP:** Assoc Prof Oph Univ IL Coll Med; **HMO:** Aetna Hlth Plan, Blue Cross & Blue Shield, Californiacare, Humana Health Plan, Prudential
LANG: Sp, Fr; SA SU Mcr Mcd NFI 4+ Weeks VISA

Curnyn, Arnold D (MD) **Oph**
Northwest Comm Hlthcare
Alexian Brothers Medical Ctr, 810 Biesterfield Rd G03; Elk Grove Village, IL 60007; (847) 290-0202; **BDCERT:** Oph 67; **MS:** Univ IL Coll Med 59; **RES:** U IL Med Ctr, Chicago, IL 62-65; **FAP:** Asst Clin Prof Univ IL Coll Med; **HOSP:** Alexian Brothers Med Ctr
SA SU Mcr Mcd VISA

Deutsch, Thomas (MD) **Oph**
Rush-Presbyterian-St Luke's Med Ctr
(see page 122)
University Ophthalmology Assoc, 1725 W Harrison St Ste 918; Chicago, IL 60612; (312) 942-2734; **BDCERT:** Oph 84; **MS:** Rush Med Coll 79; **RES:** Oph, IL Eye & Ear Infirmary, Chicago, IL 80-83; **FAP:** Prof/Chairman Oph Rush Med Coll; **HOSP:** Rush North Shore Med Ctr; ***SI:*** *Cataract; Refractive Surgery*; **HMO:** Rush Health Plans, Aetna-US Healthcare, Californiacare, CIGNA, United Healthcare
LANG: Sp, SCr; SA SU Mcr Mcd A Few Days VISA

Dougal, Mary (MD) **Oph**
Resurrection Med Ctr
Skowron Dougal Mc Clellan, 7447 W Talcott Ave Ste 300; Chicago, IL 60631; (773) 775-0811; **BDCERT:** Oph 83; **MS:** Loyola U-Stritch Sch Med, Maywood 78; **RES:** Loyola U Med Ctr, Maywood, IL 79-82

Epstein, Randy J (MD) **Oph**
Rush-Presbyterian-St Luke's Med Ctr
(see page 122)
Chicago Cornea Consultants ltd, 1585 N Barrington Rd Ste 502; Hoffman Estates, IL 60194; (847) 882-5900; **BDCERT:** Oph 86; **MS:** Rush Med Coll 80; **RES:** Emory U Hosp, Atlanta, GA 85-86; Emory U Hosp, Atlanta, GA 84-85; **FEL:** Emory U Hosp, Atlanta, GA 85-86; **FAP:** Assoc Prof Med Rush Med Coll; **HOSP:** Highland Park Hosp; ***SI:*** *Refractive Corneal Surgery; LASIK*; **HMO:** Prudential, Aetna Hlth Plan, United Healthcare
SA SU Mcr Mcd Immediately

Fishman, Gerald (MD) **Oph**
Univ of Illinois at Chicago Med Ctr
UIC Eye Center, 1855 W Taylor St Ste 385; Chicago, IL 60612; (312) 996-8938; **BDCERT:** Oph 75; **MS:** Ohio State U 69; **RES:** U IL Eye & Ear Infirmary, Chicago, IL 70-73; **FEL:** U IL Eye & Ear Infirmary, Chicago, IL 73-74; **FAP:** Prof Oph Univ IL Coll Med; ***SI:*** *Retinitus Pigmentosa*

Guastella, Frank (MD) **Oph**
Christ Hosp & Med Ctr **(see page 140)**
Southwest Ophthalmology, 5716 W 95th St; Oak Lawn, IL 60453; (708) 425-8485; **BDCERT:** Oph 73; **MS:** Univ IL Coll Med 61; **RES:** Oph, IL Eye & Ear Infirmary, Chicago, IL 68-72; **HOSP:** Mercy Hosp & Med Ctr; ***SI:*** *Cataract & Implant Surgery; Glaucoma*; **HMO:** United Healthcare, Blue Cross & Blue Choice +
Mcr A Few Days

Hanlon, John P (MD) **Oph**
Little Company of Mary Hosp & Hlth Care Ctrs **(see page 142)**
2850 W 95th St Ste 401; Evergreen Park, IL 60805; (708) 499-5500; **BDCERT:** Oph 89; **MS:** Univ IL Coll Med 83; **RES:** Oph, Loyola U Med Ctr, Maywood, IL 84-87; **HMO:** Aetna Hlth Plan, Blue Cross & Blue Shield, Californiacare, Choicecare, Healthamerica +
Mcr 4+ Weeks

Hillman, David (MD) **Oph**
Our Lady Of the Resurrection Med Ctr
Lieberman Eye Assoc, 5600 W Addison St Fl 1; Chicago, IL 60634; (773) 736-1717; **BDCERT:** Oph 91; **MS:** Duke U 86; **RES:** Oph, U IL Med Ctr, Chicago, IL 87-90; **FEL:** Glaucoma, Barnes Hosp, St Louis, MO 90-91; **FAP:** Asst Prof Univ IL Coll Med

Guide to symbols and abbreviations can be found on pages 110-113.

Jampol, Lee (MD) **Oph**
Northwestern Mem Hosp
645 N Michigan Ave Ste 440; Chicago, IL 60611; (312) 908-8152; **BDCERT:** Oph 75; **MS:** Yale U Sch Med 69; **RES:** Oph, Yale-New Haven Hosp, New Haven, CT 70-73; **FEL:** RE, U IL Med Ctr, Chicago, IL 74-75; **FAP:** Prof Chrmn Oph Northwestern U; ***SI:** Macular Degeneration; Retinal Disease*
LANG: Pol, Rus, Sp; 2-4 Weeks **VISA**

Jay, Walter (MD) **Oph**
Loyola U Med Ctr **(see page 120)**
2160 S 1st Ave Ste 102-2603; Maywood, IL 60153; (708) 216-3408; **BDCERT:** Oph 79; **MS:** U Chicago-Pritzker Sch Med 76; **RES:** Oph, U Chicago Hosp, Chicago, IL 76-79; **FEL:** Neurophthalmology, UC San Francisco Med Ctr, San Francisco, CA 79-80; **FAP:** Prof/Chair Loyola U-Stritch Sch Med, Maywood; ***SI:** Cataract Surgery; Laser Surgery of Eye*; **HMO:** Aetna Hlth Plan, Blue Cross & Blue Shield, NYLCare, Humana Health Plan, Principal Health Care +
LANG: Sp, Pol, Rus, Hin; A Few Days **VISA**

Kaplan, Bruce (MD) **Oph**
Lutheran Gen Hosp **(see page 143)**
Ridge Optical Opticians Inc, 444 N Northwest Hwy Ste 360; Park Ridge, IL 60068; (847) 823-2140; **BDCERT:** Oph 94; **MS:** Loyola U-Stritch Sch Med, Maywood 89; **RES:** Mayo Clinic, Rochester, MN 90-93; **FEL:** IL Eye & Ear Infirmary, Chicago, IL 93-94; **FAP:** Asst Prof Univ IL Coll Med

Kearns, William (MD) **Oph**
St Alexius Med Ctr
1575 Barrington Rd Ste 120; Hoffman Estates, IL 60194; (847) 843-3242; **BDCERT:** Oph 73; **MS:** Loyola U-Stritch Sch Med, Maywood 65; **RES:** Cook Cty Hosp, Chicago, IL 68-72; **HMO:** Blue Cross & Blue Shield

Knepper, Paul (MD) **Oph**
Northwestern Mem Hosp
166 E Superior St Ste 402; Chicago, IL 60611; (312) 337-1285; **BDCERT:** Oph 78; **MS:** Northwestern U 68; **RES:** Oph, Northwestern Mem Hosp, Chicago, IL 70-73; **HOSP:** Children's Mem Med Ctr
4+ Weeks **VISA**

Kohn, Arthur (MD) **Oph**
Swedish Covenant Hosp
6801 N California Ave; Chicago, IL 60645; (773) 743-4300; **BDCERT:** Oph 77; **MS:** Univ IL Coll Med 72; **RES:** IM, Illinois Masonic Med Ctr, Chicago, IL 72-73; Oph, Michael Reese Hosp Med Ctr, Chicago, IL 73-76; **HMO:** Aetna Hlth Plan

Kraft, Bertram (MD) **Oph**
Grant Hosp
Total Eye Care, 111 N Wabash Ave Ste 1610; Chicago, IL 60602; (312) 263-6350; **BDCERT:** Oph 75; **MS:** Univ IL Coll Med 69; **RES:** Oph, Michael Reese Hosp Med Ctr, Chicago, IL 70-73; **HOSP:** Highland Park Hosp; ***SI:** Cataract and Glaucoma; Refractive Vision-Laser*; **HMO:** Blue Cross & Blue Choice, CIGNA, United Healthcare +
LANG: Sp; A Few Days **VISA**

Lewicky, Andrew O (MD) **Oph**
Illinois Masonic Med Ctr **(see page 118)**
Chicago Eye Institute, 3982 N Milwaukee; Chicago, IL 60641; (773) 282-2000; **BDCERT:** Oph 76; **MS:** Northwestern U 70; **RES:** Oph, Rush Presbyterian-St Luke's Med Ctr, Chicago, IL 71-74; Oph, IL Eye & Ear Infirmary, Chicago, IL 71-74; **FAP:** Asst Prof Oph Rush Med Coll; ***SI:** Cataract Surgery; Refractive Surgery*

Lieberman, Howard (MD) **Oph**
Our Lady Of the Resurrection Med Ctr
Lieberman Eye Assoc, 5600 W Addison St Fl 1; Chicago, IL 60634; (773) 736-1717; **BDCERT:** Oph 53; **MS:** Univ IL Coll Med 46; **RES:** Oph, Cook Cty Hosp, Chicago, IL 50-52; **FEL:** Northwestern Mem Hosp, Chicago, IL; **FAP:** Prof Northwestern U; **HOSP:** Resurrection Med Ctr; ***SI:** Small Incision Cataract Surgery; Cornea*

Lindberg, C Ronald (MD) **Oph**
La Grange Mem Hosp **(see page 141)**
915 W 55th St Ste 200; Western Springs, IL 60558; (708) 579-3090; **BDCERT:** Oph 81; **MS:** Univ IL Coll Med 76; **RES:** Pacific Presbyterian, San Francisco, CA 76-77; Oph, U IL Med Ctr, Chicago, IL 77-80; **FAP:** Cl Assist Prof. Oph Univ IL Coll Med; **HOSP:** La Grange Mem Hosp; ***SI:** Cataract Surgery; Diabetic Retinopathy*; **HMO:** Aetna-US Healthcare, CIGNA, Blue Cross, Medicare
4+ Weeks **VISA**

Lopez, Osvaldo (MD) **Oph**
Illinois Masonic Med Ctr **(see page 118)**
Chicago Eye Institute, 836 W Wellington Ave Fl 5; Chicago, IL 60657; (773) 296-8000; **BDCERT:** Oph 76; **MS:** Northwestern U 70; **RES:** Michael Reese Hosp Med Ctr, Chicago, IL 71-74; **FEL:** Oph, 74-75; **HOSP:** Norwegian-American Hosp

Lubeck, David (MD) **Oph**
St James Hosp & Hlth Ctrs
Arbor Center For Eye Care, 2640 183rd St; Homewood, IL 60430; (708) 798-6633; **BDCERT:** Oph 90; **MS:** Northwestern U 84; **RES:** Oph, IL Eye & Ear Infirmary, Chicago, IL 85-88; **FEL:** Flinders Medical Center, Bedford Park, Australia 88-89; **FAP:** Asst Clin Prof Oph Univ IL Coll Med; **HOSP:** Univ of Illinois at Chicago Med Ctr; ***SI:** Refractive Surgery; Cornea; Transplantation*; **HMO:** Blue Cross & Blue Shield, Aetna Hlth Plan, PHCS +
LANG: Sp, Fr; 2-4 Weeks **VISA**

Lyon, Alice (MD) Oph
Northwestern Mem Hosp
Northwestern Medical Faculty, 675 N St Clair Fl 15; Chicago, IL 60611; (312) 908-8150; **BDCERT:** Oph 92; **MS:** U Chicago-Pritzker Sch Med 87; **RES:** IM, NY Hosp-Cornell Med Ctr, New York, NY 87-88; Oph, Northwestern Mem Hosp, Chicago, IL 88-91; **FEL:** Retina, Harvard Med Sch, Cambridge, MA 91-93; Schepens Eye Research Inst, Boston, MA 91-93; **FAP:** Instr Oph Northwestern U; ***SI:*** *Diabetic Retinopathy; Macular Degeneration*; **HMO:** + **LANG:** Ger, Pol, Rus;

Mets, Marilyn (MD) Oph
Children's Mem Med Ctr (see page 139)
2300 Children's Plaza; Chicago, IL 60614; (773) 880-4000; **BDCERT:** Oph 81; **MS:** Geo Wash U Sch Med 76; **RES:** Cleveland Clinic Hosp, Cleveland, OH 77-80; **FEL:** Children's Hosp Nat Med Ctr, Washington, DC 80-81; **FAP:** Assoc Prof Northwestern U; ***SI:*** *Pediatric Ophthalmology*
4+ Weeks VISA

Miller, Marilyn T (MD) Oph
Univ of Illinois at Chicago Med Ctr
University-Illinois At Chicago, 1855 W Taylor St Ste 205; Chicago, IL 60612; (312) 996-7445; **BDCERT:** Oph 66; **MS:** Univ IL Coll Med 59; **RES:** U IL Hosps, Chicago, IL 64; IL Eye & Ear Infirmary, Chicago, IL 64; **FEL:** Ped Oph, IL Eye & Ear Infirmary, Chicago, IL 67; **FAP:** Prof Oph Univ IL Coll Med
A Few Days VISA

Millman, Leonard (MD) Oph
Good Shepherd Hosp
Northwest Eye Ctr, 450 W Il Route 22; Barrington, IL 60010; (847) 382-3640; **BDCERT:** Oph 80; **MS:** Univ IL Coll Med 74; **RES:** Oph, Evanston Hosp, Evanston, IL 75-78; **HMO:** Blue Cross & Blue Shield, Metropolitan, Choicecare

Myers, William (MD) Oph
Evanston Hosp
Evanston Opthalmologists, 2500 Ridge Ave Ste 104; Evanston, IL 60201; (847) 328-2020; **BDCERT:** Oph 83; **MS:** Dartmouth Med Sch 78; **RES:** Oph, Northwestern Mem Hosp, Chicago, IL 79-82; **FEL:** Oculoplastics, Med Coll WI, Milwaukee, WI 82-83; **FAP:** Instr Northwestern U; **HOSP:** Northwestern Mem Hosp; ***SI:*** *Cataract and Laser Surgery; Refractive Eye Surgery*; **HMO:** Humana Health Plan, Blue Cross & Blue Shield, Californiacare
A Few Days VISA

Nadimpalli, Chitra (MD) Oph
Mercy Hosp & Med Ctr
Wicker Park Eye Ctr Ltd, 1431 N Western Ave; Chicago, IL 60622; (773) 235-1164; **BDCERT:** Oph 86; **MS:** India 69; **RES:** FP, Sarojini Devi Eye Hospital-Institute, India 72-76; **FEL:** Oph, Mercy Hosp & Med Ctr, Chicago, IL 85-87; **HOSP:** St Mary's of Nazareth Hosp Ctr

Nootens, Raymond (MD) Oph
Macneal Mem Hosp
7120 Cermak Rd; Berwyn, IL 60402; (708) 788-3400; **BDCERT:** Oph 76; **MS:** Univ IL Coll Med 70; **RES:** Rush Presbyterian-St Luke's Med Ctr, Chicago, IL 71-74; **FAP:** Asst Prof Oph Rush Med Coll; **HMO:** CIGNA, Group Health Cooperative, Health Options, MD Individual Practice Assoc, PHS

O'Grady, Richard (MD) Oph
Holy Family Med Ctr
Mullenix & O'Grady, 1775 Glenview Rd Ste 114; Glenview, IL 60025; (847) 724-6617; **BDCERT:** Oph 68; **MS:** Loyola U-Stritch Sch Med, Maywood 58

Orth, David (MD) Oph
Ingalls Mem Hosp
Illinois Retina Assoc, 71 W 156th St Ste 400; Harvey, IL 60426; (708) 596-8710; **BDCERT:** Oph 75; **MS:** U Hlth Sci/Chicago Med Sch 69; **RES:** Michael Reese Hosp Med Ctr, Chicago, IL 71-73; **FEL:** Oph, Wilmer Inst-Johns Hopkins Hosp, Baltimore, MD 74-75; **FAP:** Assoc Prof Rush Med Coll

Palmer, David (MD) Oph
Michael Reese Hosp & Med Ctr
8901 W Golf Rd Ste 201; Des Plaines, IL 60016; (847) 390-8660; **BDCERT:** Oph 85; **MS:** U Chicago-Pritzker Sch Med 80; **RES:** Oph, IL Eye & Ear Infirmary, Chicago, IL 81-84; **FEL:** Mass Eye & Ear Infirmary, Boston, MA 84-85; **FAP:** Asst Prof Northwestern U; **HOSP:** Northwestern Mem Hosp; **HMO:** Aetna Hlth Plan, Blue Cross & Blue Shield, Chicago HMO, Choicecare, CIGNA

Resnick, Kenneth (MD) Oph
Univ of Illinois at Chicago Med Ctr
Retina Associates, 6677 N Lincoln Ave; Lincolnwood, IL 60645; (847) 673-7101; **BDCERT:** Oph 86; **MS:** U Chicago-Pritzker Sch Med 81; **RES:** Oph, Yale-New Haven Hosp, New Haven, CT 82-85; **FEL:** Retinal Surg, Baylor Coll Med, Houston, TX 85-87; **FAP:** Assoc Prof Oph Univ IL Coll Med; **HOSP:** Christ Hosp & Med Ctr

Rosanova, Mark (MD) Oph
Swedish Covenant Hosp
Advanced Eyecare Assoc, 5872 N Milwaukee Ave; Chicago, IL 60646; (773) 594-0000; **BDCERT:** Oph 88; **MS:** Northwestern U 82; **RES:** Northwestern U Hosp, Chicago, IL 84-87

Guide to symbols and abbreviations can be found on pages 110-113.

Rubin, Gary (MD) **Oph**
Holy Cross Hosp
7001 W Archer Ave; Chicago, IL 60638; (773) 229-8818; **BDCERT:** Oph 90; **MS:** U Hlth Sci/Chicago Med Sch 76; **RES:** Cook Cty Hosp, Chicago, IL 76-81; **HOSP:** Mercy Hosp & Med Ctr; ***SI:*** *Cataracts; Glaucoma*; **HMO:** Blue Cross, Aetna Hlth Plan, Share
LANG: Sp, Pol; A Few Days

Scelzo, Frederick (MD) **Oph**
Evanston Hosp
North Suburban Ophthlmlgsts, 1015 Central St; Evanston, IL 60201; (847) 328-6060; **BDCERT:** Oph 75; **MS:** Loyola U-Stritch Sch Med, Maywood 69; **RES:** Oph, Evanston Hosp, Evanston, IL 70-73; **FAP:** Instructor Oph Northwestern U; **HOSP:** Glenbrook Hosp; ***SI:*** *Cataract Surgery; Intraocular Lens Implants*
4+ Weeks

Sloane, Herman (MD) **Oph**
Ingalls Mem Hosp
South Suburban Eye Surgeons, 19950 Governors Hwy; Olympia Fields, IL 60461; (708) 748-0909; **BDCERT:** Oph 86; **MS:** Rush Med Coll 80

Springer, David (MD) **Oph**
West Suburban Hosp Med Ctr
West Suburban Eye Assoc, 1 Erie Ct Ste 6140; Oak Park, IL 60302; (708) 848-2400; **BDCERT:** Oph 88; **MS:** U Cincinnati 83; **RES:** Oph, Michael Reese Hosp Med Ctr, Chicago, IL 84-87; **FEL:** Cornea, U of Pittsburgh Med Ctr, Pittsburgh, PA 87-88; **FAP:** Asst Clin Prof U Chicago-Pritzker Sch Med; **HMO:** Aetna Hlth Plan, Blue Cross & Blue Shield, Chicago HMO, CIGNA, Humana Health Plan

Stock, E Lee (MD) **Oph**
Northwestern Mem Hosp
Cornea Consultant Ltd, 1420 Renaissance Dr Ste 315; Park Ridge, IL 60068; (847) 390-0758; **BDCERT:** Oph 76; **MS:** U Mich Med Sch 68; **RES:** Oph, U KY Hosp, Lexington, KY 71-74; **FEL:** Cornea, Moorfields Eye Hosp, London, England 74-76; **FAP:** Assoc Prof Northwestern U; **HOSP:** Holy Family Med Ctr

Sugar, Joel (MD) **Oph**
Univ of Illinois at Chicago Eye & Ear Infirmary
University Of Illinois Eye Center, 1855 W Taylor St Ste 385; Chicago, IL 60612; (312) 996-8937; **BDCERT:** Oph 75; **MS:** U Mich Med Sch 69; **RES:** Oph, Barnes Hosp, St Louis, MO 70-73; **FEL:** Oph, U FL Shands Hosp, Gainesville, FL 72-73; Oph, Barnes Hosp, St Louis, MO 73; **FAP:** Professor Oph Univ IL Coll Med; **HOSP:** Univ of Illinois at Chicago Med Ctr; ***SI:*** *Corneal Transplants; Eye Infections*; **HMO:** Chicago HMO, United Healthcare
LANG: Sp, Rus; 2-4 Weeks

Taub, Susan J (MD) **Oph**
St Joseph Hosp-Elgin
Taub Eye Center, 104 S Michigan Ave Ste 410; Chicago, IL 60603; (312) 553-1818; **BDCERT:** Oph 88; **MS:** Ind U Sch Med 82; **RES:** Indiana U Med Ctr, Indianapolis, IN 83-86; **FAP:** Instr Rush Med Coll; ***SI:*** *Laser Corrective Surgery; Cataract Surgery*; **HMO:** Blue Cross, Aetna Hlth Plan, FHP Inc +
LANG: Sp, Fr; A Few Days

Thoms, Monica (MD) **Oph**
Northwest Comm Hlthcare
Koziol & Thoms, 1211 S Arlington Heights Rd; Arlington Hts, IL 60005; (847) 259-2777; **BDCERT:** Oph 88; **MS:** Univ IL Coll Med 82; **RES:** Oph, Michael Reese Hosp Med Ctr, Chicago, IL 83-86; ***SI:*** *Small Incision Cataract Surgery*; **HMO:** Aetna Hlth Plan, Blue Cross & Blue Shield, Californiacare, Share, Humana Health Plan
A Few Days

Ticho, Benjamin (MD) **Oph**
Christ Hosp & Med Ctr **(see page 140)**
4400 W 95th St Ste 102; Oak Lawn, IL 60453; (708) 423-4070; **BDCERT:** Oph 92; **MS:** U Mich Med Sch 87; **RES:** Oph, U IL Med Ctr, Chicago, IL 88-91; **FEL:** Ped Oph, Northwestern Mem Hosp, Chicago, IL 91-92; **FAP:** Asst Prof Univ IL Coll Med; **HOSP:** Mercy Hosp & Med Ctr; ***SI:*** *Strabismus & Cataract; Pediatric Ophthalmology*; **HMO:** Aetna Hlth Plan, Blue Cross & Blue Shield, Californiacare, Rush Health Plans, Health Alliance Plan +
2-4 Weeks

Weiss, Robert (MD) **Oph**
Illinois Masonic Med Ctr
(see page 118)
Chicago Eye Institute, 3982 N Milwaukee Ave; Chicago, IL 60641; (773) 328-2000; **BDCERT:** Oph 87; **MS:** U Hlth Sci/Chicago Med Sch 82; **RES:** Oph, NY Hosp-Cornell Med Ctr, New York, NY 83-86; **FEL:** Oph, NY Hosp-Cornell Med Ctr, New York, NY 86-87; Oph, Emory U Hosp, Atlanta, GA 87-88; **FAP:** Assoc Clin Prof Oph Univ IL Coll Med; **HOSP:** Mercy Hosp & Med Ctr; ***SI:*** *Cosmetic EyeLid Surgery; Thyroid Eye Disease*; **HMO:** Rush Health Plans, United Healthcare, PHCS, Blue Cross/Blue Shield, Unicare Primary Plus +
LANG: Sp, Pol, Ukr, Chi, Itl; 2-4 Weeks

Wilensky, Jacob (MD) **Oph**
Univ of Illinois at Chicago Med Ctr
Univ-IL At Chicago-Glaucoma, 1855 W Taylor St Ste 210; Chicago, IL 60612; (312) 996-7030; **BDCERT:** Oph 74; **MS:** Tulane U 68; **RES:** Oph, Tulane U Med Ctr, New Orleans, LA 69-72; **FEL:** Glaucoma, Barnes Hosp, St Louis, MO 72-73; **FAP:** Prof Univ IL Coll Med; ***SI:*** *Glaucoma*; **HMO:** Chicago HMO, Humana Health Plan
2-4 Weeks

Zaret, Cheryl Riva (MD) Oph
Northwestern Mem Hosp
111 N Wabash Ave Ste 911; Chicago, IL 60602; (312) 236-4892; **BDCERT:** Oph 77; **MS:** Jefferson Med Coll 72; **RES:** Oph, Northwest Comm Hlthcare, Chicago, IL 73-76; Children's Mem Med Ctr, Chicago, IL 74-75; **FEL:** Neurophthalmology, Columbia-Presbyterian Med Ctr, New York, NY 76-77; **FAP:** Asst Prof N Northwestern U

ORTHOPAEDIC SURGERY

Abraham, Edward (MD) OrS
Ravenswood Hosp Med Ctr
Uptown Orthopedic Ctr, 4211 N Cicero Ave Ste 201; Chicago, IL 60641; (773) 794-1338; **BDCERT:** OrS 77; **MS:** Lebanon 69; **RES:** OrS, American U Hosp, Beirut, Lebanon 70-71; OrS, U IL Med Ctr, Chicago, IL 71-75; **FEL:** Ped OrS, U Sheffield, Sheffield, England 75-76

Al-Aswad, Basel (MD) OrS
Little Company of Mary Hosp & Hlth Care Ctrs (see page 142)
2850 W 95th St Ste 406; Evergreen Park, IL 60805; (708) 499-4844; **BDCERT:** OrS 78; **MS:** Iraq 68; **RES:** OrS, Michael Reese Hosp Med Ctr, Chicago, IL 73-76; OrS, Shriners Hosp, Chicago, IL 76; **FAP:** Instr Rush Med Coll; ***SI:*** *Hip Replacement; Knee Replacement*; **HMO:** HMO Illinois, Share
LANG: Ar; 1 Week

Andersson, Gunnar (MD) OrS
Rush-Presbyterian-St Luke's Med Ctr
(see page 122)
1725 W Harrison St Ste 1063; Chicago, IL 60612; (312) 243-4244; **BDCERT:** OrS 90; **MS:** Sweden 67; **RES:** OrS, Univ Hosp, Goteborg, Sweden 68-74; **FAP:** Prof & Chrmn Rush Med Coll; ***SI:*** *Lower Back Pain; Spine Surgery*; **HMO:** Blue Cross & Blue Shield, Rush Prudential, Humana Health Plan, Aetna Hlth Plan, CIGNA +
LANG: Ger, Swd, Nwg; 2-4 Weeks VISA

Bach, Bernard (MD) OrS
Rush-Presbyterian-St Luke's Med Ctr
(see page 122)
Midwest Orthopaedics, 1725 W Harrion St Suite 1063; Chicago, IL 60612; (708) 383-0770; **BDCERT:** OrS 89; **MS:** U Cincinnati 79; **RES:** S, New England Deaconess Hosp, Boston, MA 80-81; OrS, Harvard Med Sch, Cambridge, MA 81-85; **FEL:** SM, Hosp For Special Surgery, New York, NY 85-86; **FAP:** Prof OrS Rush Med Coll

Beigler, David (MD) OrS
Illinois Masonic Med Ctr
(see page 118)
Spine & Orthopaedic Surgery, 3000 N Halsted St Ste 611; Chicago, IL 60657; (773) 296-3900; **BDCERT:** OrS 84; **MS:** Loyola U-Stritch Sch Med, Maywood 77; **RES:** OrS, Loyola U Med Ctr, Maywood, IL 78-81; Brigham & Women's Hosp, Boston, MA 81-82; **FEL:** Trauma, U Toronto Hosp, Toronto, Canada 82; **FAP:** Asst Clin Prof OrS Loyola U-Stritch Sch Med, Maywood; **HOSP:** Evanston Hosp; ***SI:*** *Sports/Arthroscopy; Joint Replacement*; **HMO:** Blue Cross & Blue Shield, Principal Health Care, Medicare, Most +
LANG: Sp; A Few Days VISA

Bush-Joseph, Charles (MD) OrS
Rush-Presbyterian-St Luke's Med Ctr
(see page 122)
Midwest Orthopaedics, 1725 W Harrison St Ste 1063; Chicago, IL 60612; (312) 243-4244; **BDCERT:** OrS 92; **MS:** U Mich Med Sch 83; **RES:** OrS, Bush Med Ctr, Chicago, IL 83-88; **FEL:** SM, Cincinnati Sports Med, Cincinnati, OH 88-89; **FAP:** Assoc Prof Rush Med Coll; **HMO:** +
1 Week VISA

Carroll, Charles (MD) OrS
Northwestern Mem Hosp
Northwestern Center for Orthopedics, 676 N Saint Clair St Ste 450; Chicago, IL 60611; (312) 943-7850; **BDCERT:** OrS 90; HS 92; **MS:** U Md Sch Med 82; **RES:** OrS, Johns Hopkins Hosp, Baltimore, MD 83-84; S, Johns Hopkins Hosp, Baltimore, MD 84-87; **FEL:** Indiana U Sch Med, Indianapolis, IN 87-88; **FAP:** Asst Prof of Clin OrS Northwestern U

Chand, Kishan (MD) OrS
Trinity Hosp
Southeastern Medical Ctr, 10559 S Torrence Ave; Chicago, IL 60617; (773) 375-2200; **BDCERT:** OrS 72; **MS:** India 59; **RES:** OrS, Heatherwood Hospital 64-66; ***SI:*** *Total Hip Replacement; Knee Surgery*; **HMO:** Aetna Hlth Plan, Blue Cross & Blue Shield, Chicago HMO, CIGNA, HealthNet
LANG: Hin, Sp; Immediately VISA

Cohen, Mark (MD) OrS
Rush-Presbyterian-St Luke's Med Ctr
(see page 122)
1725 W Harrison St Ste 1063; Chicago, IL 60612; (312) 243-4244; **BDCERT:** OrS 95; HS 96; **MS:** Harvard Med Sch 86; **RES:** S, UC San Diego Med Ctr, San Diego, CA 87-92; **FEL:** HS, Indianapolis Hand Center, Indianapolis, IN 92-93; **FAP:** Asst Prof OrS Rush Med Coll

Guide to symbols and abbreviations can be found on pages 110-113.

Dias, Luciano (MD) OrS
Children's Mem Med Ctr (see page 139)
680 N Lake Shore Dr Ste 924; Chicago, IL 60611; (312) 951-5468; **BDCERT:** OrS 75; **MS:** Brazil 68; **RES:** OrS, Henry Ford Hosp, Detroit, MI 71-74; **FEL:** Ped OrS, Children's Mem Med Ctr, Chicago, IL 74-75; **FAP:** Prof OrS Northwestern U

Egwele, Richard (MD) OrS
Trinity Hosp
Exchange Medical Ctr, 9135 S Exchange Ave; Chicago, IL 60617; (773) 374-2441; **BDCERT:** OrS 79; HS 95; **MS:** Spain 73; **RES:** OrS, Cook Cty Hosp, Chicago, IL 74-78; ***SI:*** *Knee Surgery; Carpal Tunnel Syndrome*

Finn, Henry A (MD) OrS
Louis A Weiss Mem Hosp
Univ of Chicago, Bone and Jnt Rplcmnt Ctr at Weiss, 4646 N Marine Dr; Chicago, IL 60640; (773) 564-5888; **BDCERT:** OrS 88; **MS:** Hahnemann U 80; **RES:** OrS, Hahnemann U Hosp, Philadelphia, PA 81-85; OrS, U Chicago Hosp, Chicago, IL 85-86; **FAP:** Prof of Clin S U Chicago-Pritzker Sch Med; ***SI:*** *Joint Replacement; Limb Salvage*; **HMO:** Blue Cross & Blue Shield, Aetna Hlth Plan, Humana Health Plan, Rush Pru +
LANG: Sp; Immediately VISA

Freedberg, Howard (MD) OrS
St Alexius Med Ctr
1786 Moon Lake Blvd; Hoffman Estates, IL 60194; (847) 674-9800; **BDCERT:** OrS 90; **MS:** Univ IL Coll Med 81; **RES:** OrS, U IL Med Ctr, Chicago, IL 81-86; **FEL:** SM, , Cincinnati, OH 86-87; **HOSP:** Alexian Brothers Med Ctr; ***SI:*** *Arthroscopic Surgery; Sports Medicine*; **HMO:** Blue Cross & Blue Shield, CIGNA
LANG: Sp, Pol, Rus; Immediately VISA

Fuentes, Henry (MD) OrS
Ingalls Mem Hosp
Ortho & Sports Med Hlth Ctr, 16345 Harlem Ave; Tinley Park, IL 60477; (708) 633-8333; **BDCERT:** OrS 94; **MS:** Colombia 82; **RES:** OrS, Cook Cty Hosp, Chicago, IL 86-89; OrS, U IL Med Ctr, Chicago, IL 89-90; **FEL:** SM, St Francis Hosp, Blue Island, IL 90-91; **HOSP:** Palos Comm Hosp; ***SI:*** *Sports Medicine; Hip & Knee Joint Replacement*; **HMO:** Blue Cross & Blue Shield, Aetna-US Healthcare, United Healthcare, CIGNA, Wellmark Health +
LANG: Sp; A Few Days VISA

Galante, Jorge O (MD) OrS
Rush-Presbyterian-St Luke's Med Ctr (see page 122)
Rush Arthritis & Orthopedics, 1725 W Harrison St Ste 1063; Chicago, IL 60612; (312) 243-4244; **BDCERT:** OrS 68; **MS:** Argentina 58; **RES:** Orth, Michael Reese Hosp Med Ctr, Chicago, IL 59-61; **FEL:** Rsrch, U Goteborg, Sweden 64-67

Girzadas, Daniel (MD) OrS
Christ Hosp & Med Ctr (see page 140)
Midwest Orthopaedic Consultant, 4545 W 103rd St; Oak Lawn, IL 60453; (708) 425-3494; **BDCERT:** OrS 71; **MS:** Loyola U-Stritch Sch Med, Maywood 63; **RES:** OrS, U IL Med Ctr, Chicago, IL 64-69; **HMO:** CIGNA, Aetna Hlth Plan, Advocate, Chicago HMO +
LANG: Lth, Sp; VISA

Gitelis, Steven (MD) OrS
Rush-Presbyterian-St Luke's Med Ctr (see page 122)
1725 W Harrison St Ste 440; Chicago, IL 60612; (312) 563-2600; **BDCERT:** OrS 82; **MS:** Rush Med Coll 75; **RES:** OrS, Mayo Clinic, Rochester, MN 81; ***SI:*** *Bone Cancer; Soft Tissue Cancer*

Goldflies, Mitchell (MD) OrS
Columbus Hosp
Sports Medicine Ltd, 6445 N Central Ave; Chicago, IL 60646; (773) 792-3311; **BDCERT:** OrS 82; **MS:** U Hlth Sci/Chicago Med Sch 75; **RES:** OrS, Cook Cty Hosp, Chicago, IL 76-80; **FEL:** Rush Presbyterian-St Luke's Med Ctr, Chicago, IL 80; **FAP:** Asst Clin Prof Chicago Coll Osteo Med; ***SI:*** *Sports Medicine*

Goldstein, Wayne (MD) OrS
Lutheran Gen Hosp (see page 143)
Center For Orthopaedic, 1875 Dempster St Ste 301; Park Ridge, IL 60068; (847) 234-1159; **BDCERT:** OrS 86; **MS:** Univ IL Coll Med 78; **RES:** OrS, U IL Med Ctr, Chicago, IL 79-83; **FEL:** Arthritis, Harvard Med Sch, Cambridge, MA 83-84; **FAP:** Assoc Clin Prof U Chicago-Pritzker Sch Med

Hayek, Richard (MD) OrS
Resurrection Med Ctr
Northwest Orthopaedic Assoc, 7447 W Talcott Ave Ste 411; Chicago, IL 60631; (773) 631-7898; **BDCERT:** OrS 94; **MS:** Georgetown U 86

Hefferon, John (MD) OrS
Northwestern Mem Hosp
Northwestern Center for Orthopedics, 676 N Saint Clair Ste 450; Chicago, IL 60611; (312) 943-7850; **BDCERT:** OrS 80; **MS:** Northwestern U 72; **RES:** OrS, Univ of NY, Buffalo, NY 74-78; **FEL:** OrS, , Los Angelas, CA 78-79; **HOSP:** St Joseph Hosp-Chicago; ***SI:*** *Knee, Ankle Injuries; Shoulder Injuries*

Hill, James (MD) OrS
Northwest Comm Hlthcare
Orthopaedic Associates-Central, 1300 E Central Rd; Arlington Hts, IL 60005; (847) 870-6100; **BDCERT:** OrS 93; **MS:** Northwestern U 74; **RES:** OrS, McGaw Med Ctr-Northwestern, Chicago, IL 75-79; **FEL:** SM, Natl Athletic Inst Hlth, Inglewood, CA 79-80; **FAP:** Prof Northwestern U
1 Week VISA

Hopkinson, William J (MD) **OrS**
Loyola U Med Ctr (see page 120)
Loyola U Med Ctr - Dept Orth Surg, 2160 S First Ave; Maywood, IL 60153; (708) 216-4992; **BDCERT:** OrS 83; **MS:** Loyola U-Stritch Sch Med, Maywood 77; **RES:** OrS, Fitzsimons AMC, Aurora, IL 78-82; SM, Keller Army Hosp, West Point, NY 82-83; **FEL:** Joint Replacement Surg, Nat Hosp for Orth and Rehab, Washington, DC -87; **FAP:** Assoc Prof S Loyola U-Stritch Sch Med, Maywood; **HOSP:** VA Hlthcare Systems-Lakeside; ***SI:*** *Joint Replacement; Hip and Knee Arthritis*; **HMO:** +
4+ Weeks VISA

Kolb, Louis (MD) **OrS**
Illinois Masonic Med Ctr
(see page 118)
Orthopedic Surgery Ltd, 3525 W Peterson Ave Ste 424; Chicago, IL 60659; (773) 588-5550; **BDCERT:** OrS 69; **MS:** U Chicago-Pritzker Sch Med 62; **RES:** S, U Chicago Hosp, Chicago, IL 63-67; **FAP:** Assoc Clin Prof U Chicago-Pritzker Sch Med; **HMO:** Blue Cross & Blue Shield, Chicago HMO, Bay State Health Plan, Humana Health Plan, Metlife

Kuderna, James (MD) **OrS**
Evanston Hosp
Suburban Orthopaedic Assoc Ltd, 1000 Central St Ste 880; Evanston, IL 60201; (847) 475-4040; **BDCERT:** OrS 81; **MS:** Northwestern U 79

Levin, Jay (MD) **OrS**
Condell Med Ctr
Adult & Pediatric Orthopedics, 125 E Lake Cook Rd Ste 120; Buffalo Grove, IL 60089; (847) 541-5050; **BDCERT:** OrS 99; **MS:** Rush Med Coll 80; **RES:** OrS, Rush Presbyterian-St Luke's Med Ctr, Chicago, IL 80-85; **FEL:** S, Rush Presbyterian-St Luke's Med Ctr, Chicago, IL 85-86; **FAP:** Instr Rush Med Coll; **HOSP:** Northwest Comm Hlthcare; **HMO:** Blue Cross & Blue Shield, Metlife

Locher, Frederick G (MD) **OrS**
Good Shepherd Hosp
Lake Cook Orthopedic Assoc, 27401 W Il Route 22 Ste 125; Barrington, IL 60010; (847) 381-0388; **BDCERT:** OrS 81; **MS:** Northwestern U 75; **RES:** OrS, Northwestern Mem Hosp, Chicago, IL 67-80

Lopez, Eugene (MD) **OrS**
Alexian Brothers Med Ctr
(see page 138)
Midwest Sports Medicine, 901 Biesterfield Rd Ste 300; Elk Grove Vlg, IL 60007; (847) 437-9889; **BDCERT:** OrS 92; **MS:** Univ IL Coll Med 85; **RES:** U Chicago Hosp, Chicago, IL 86-90
VISA

Lubicky, John (MD) **OrS**
Shriners Hosp for Children
2211 N Oak Park Ave; Chicago, IL 60635; (773) 385-5500; **BDCERT:** OrS 93; **MS:** Jefferson Med Coll 74; **RES:** S, Med Coll VA Hosp, Richmond, VA 74-75; OrS, Med Coll VA Hosp, Richmond, VA 76-79; **FEL:** PdOrS, Shriners Hosp, Chicago, IL 79; SpCdInj, Rush Presbyterian-St Luke's Med Ctr, Chicago, IL 80; **HOSP:** Rush-Presbyterian-St Luke's Med Ctr; ***SI:*** *Spinal Deformities-Scollosis; Pediatric Bone/Joint Problems*
LANG: Sp, Pol; Immediately

Martell, John (MD) **OrS**
U Chicago Hosp (see page 124)
5758 S Maryland Ave MC3079; Chicago, IL 60637; (773) 702-7297; **BDCERT:** OrS 91; **MS:** U Chicago-Pritzker Sch Med 83; **RES:** U Chicago Hosp, Chicago, IL 87-88; **FEL:** OrS, Rush Presbyterian-St Luke's Med Ctr, Chicago, IL 88-89; **FAP:** Asst Prof OrS U Chicago-Pritzker Sch Med

Meisles, Jeffrey (MD) **OrS**
Gottlieb Mem Hosp
Orthopedic Specialists, 675 W North Ave Ste 402; Melrose Park, IL 60160; (708) 450-5744; **BDCERT:** OrS 93; **MS:** Rush Med Coll 86; **RES:** OrS, Rush Presbyterian-St Luke's Med Ctr, Chicago, IL 87-91; **HOSP:** Elmhurst Mem Hosp; ***SI:*** *Hip and Knee Replacements; Sports Medicine*; **HMO:** Blue Cross, United Healthcare, Aetna Hlth Plan, PHCS +
LANG: Sp; Immediately
VISA

Meltzer, William (MD) **OrS**
Rush North Shore Med Ctr
Schafer, Meltzer & Lewis, 3520 Lake Ave; Wilmette, IL 60091; (847) 256-4000; **BDCERT:** OrS 66; **MS:** Univ IL Coll Med 57; **RES:** Cook Cty Hosp, Chicago, IL 57-58; OrS, U IL Med Ctr, Chicago, IL 58-62; **FEL:** Ortho Rehab, Rancho Los Amigos Med Ctr, Downey, CA 62; **FAP:** Clin Prof OrS Univ IL Coll Med; **HOSP:** Highland Park Hosp; ***SI:*** *Hip Replacement; Knee Replacement*; **HMO:** Aetna Hlth Plan, Blue Cross & Blue Shield, Californiacare, CIGNA, Humana Health Plan +
1 Week

Miz, George (MD) **OrS**
Ingalls Mem Hosp
Orthopedic Specialists, 5540 W 111th St; Oak Lawn, IL 60453; (708) 423-8440; **BDCERT:** OrS 98; **MS:** Loyola U-Stritch Sch Med, Maywood 79; **RES:** OrS, So Ill U Hosp, Springfield, IL 80-84; **FEL:** SpnScolios, NYU Hosp-Cornell Med Ctr, New York, NY 84-85; **HOSP:** Little Company of Mary Hosp & Hlth Care Ctrs; ***SI:*** *Lower Back Disorders; Cervical Spine Disorders*; **HMO:** +
Immediately VISA

Guide to symbols and abbreviations can be found on pages 110-113.

Moran, Michael (MD) **OrS**
Provena Mercy Ctr
Midland Orthopedics Associates, 2850 S Michigan; Chicago, IL 60616; (312) 326-2660; **BDCERT:** OrS 94; **MS:** Rush Med Coll 76; **RES:** OrS, Hosp For Special Surgery, New York, NY 86-90; **FEL:** Harvard Med Sch, Cambridge, MA 90-91; **HOSP:** La Grange Mem Hosp; ***SI:*** *Total Joint Replacement; Reconstructive Surgery-Adult*

Newman, Daniel (MD) **OrS**
St Joseph Hosp-Elgin
Midwest Orthopaedics, 3000 N Halsted St; Chicago, IL 60657; (773) 327-8300; **BDCERT:** OrS 77; **MS:** U Mich Med Sch 70; **RES:** OrS, Rush Presbyterian-St Luke's Med Ctr, Chicago, IL 71-74; **FEL:** Rush Presbyterian-St Luke's Med Ctr, Chicago, IL 75; **HOSP:** Illinois Masonic Med Ctr; **HMO:** Aetna Hlth Plan, Blue Cross & Blue Shield, Chicago HMO, CIGNA, HealthNet

Nuber, Gordon (MD) **OrS**
Northwestern Mem Hosp
680 Lake Shore Dr Ste 1028; Chicago, IL 60611; (312) 664-6812; **BDCERT:** OrS 86; **MS:** Wayne State U Sch Med 78; **RES:** OrS, Northwestern Mem Hosp, Chicago, IL 78-83; **FEL:** SM, Kerlan-Jobe Orthopaedic Clinic, Los Angeles, CA 83-84; **FAP:** Assoc Prof Northwestern U; ***SI:*** *Shoulder Injuries; Knee Injuries*; **HMO:** Blue Cross, Aetna Hlth Plan
LANG: Sp;
A Few Days

Patek, Robert (MD) **OrS**
Lutheran Gen Hosp (see page 143)
IL Bone & Joint Inst, 150 River Rd Ste 100; Des Plains, IL 60016; (847) 375-3000; **BDCERT:** OrS 91; **MS:** U Mich Med Sch 83; **RES:** OrS, Northwestern Mem Hosp, Chicago, IL 83-88; ***SI:*** *Anterior Cruciate Ligament*; **HMO:** Blue Cross & Blue Shield
A Few Days VISA

Pottenger, Lawrence (MD) **OrS**
U Chicago Hosp (see page 124)
5841 S Maryland mc3079 St MC3079; Chicago, IL 60637; (773) 702-6216; **BDCERT:** OrS 93; **MS:** U Chicago-Pritzker Sch Med 74; **RES:** OrS, Johns Hopkins Hosp, Baltimore, MD 75-79; **FAP:** Assoc Prof U Chicago-Pritzker Sch Med; **HMO:** Aetna Hlth Plan, Blue Cross & Blue Shield, CIGNA

Redondo, Luis J (MD) **OrS**
Christ Hosp & Med Ctr (see page 140)
Midwest Orthopaedic Consultant, 4545 W 103rd St; Oak Lawn, IL 60453; (708) 425-3494; **BDCERT:** OrS 71; **MS:** Univ IL Coll Med 85; **RES:** OrS, Rush Presbyterian 85-91; ***SI:*** *Reconstructive Surgery - Adult; Reconstruction - Ligament*

Reider, Bruce (MD) **OrS**
U Chicago Hosp (see page 124)
University of Chicago Sports Medicine, 5841 S Maryland Rd; Chicago, IL 60637; (773) 702-6346; **BDCERT:** OrS 92; **MS:** Harvard Med Sch 75; **RES:** SM, U WI Sch Med, Milwaukee, WI 80-81; SM, Hosp For Special Surgery, New York, NY 76-77; **FAP:** Prof OrS U Chicago-Pritzker Sch Med; ***SI:*** *Sports Medicine*

Rosenberg, Aaron (MD) **OrS**
Rush-Presbyterian-St Luke's Med Ctr (see page 122)
1725 W Harrison St Ste 1063; Chicago, IL 60612; (312) 243-4244; **BDCERT:** OrS 86; **MS:** Albany Med Coll 78; **RES:** OrS, Rush Presbyterian-St Luke's Med Ctr, Chicago, IL 78-83; **FEL:** OrS, Harvard Med Sch, Cambridge, MA 83-84; **FAP:** Prof Rush Med Coll; ***SI:*** *Hip and Knee Replacement; Hip and Knee Reconstruction*; **HMO:** +
2-4 Weeks VISA

Scafuri, Ralph (MD) **OrS**
St Joseph Hosp-Elgin
Orthopedic & Spine Surgery, 450 W Il Route 22 Ste 33; Barrington, IL 60010; (847) 382-6766; **BDCERT:** OrS 84; **MS:** Univ IL Coll Med 76; **RES:** OrS, Rush Presbyterian-St Luke's Med Ctr, Chicago, IL 77-81; **FAP:** Instr Rush Med Coll

Schroeder, Keith E (MD) **OrS**
Alexian Brothers Med Ctr (see page 138)
Barrington Orthopedics Specs, 901 Biesterfield Rd Ste 101; Elk Grove Vlg, IL 60007; (847) 437-1200; **BDCERT:** OrS 77; **MS:** Loyola U-Stritch Sch Med, Maywood 71; **RES:** OrS, Northwestern Mem Hosp, Chicago, IL 72-76; **FEL:** Ped OrS, Northwestern Mem Hosp, Chicago, IL; **FAP:** Assoc OrS Northwestern U; **HMO:** Aetna Hlth Plan, Blue Cross & Blue Shield, Chicago HMO, CIGNA, FHP Inc

Suk, Churl-Soo (MD) **OrS**
St James Hosp & Hlth Ctrs
2555 Lincoln Hwy Ste 108; Olympia Fields, IL 60461; (708) 747-2900; **BDCERT:** OrS 71; **MS:** South Korea 64; **RES:** S, Mary Immaculate Hosp, Jamaica, NY 66-67; OrS, Jersey City Med Ctr, Jersey City, NJ 67-70; **FEL:** Ped OrS, Newark Crippled Chldns Hosp, Newark, NJ 70-71; **HOSP:** South Suburban Hosp

Sweeney, Howard J (MD) **OrS**
Evanston Hosp
Healthsouth Sports Medicine, 1144 Wilmette Ave; Wilmette, IL 60091; (847) 853-9400; **BDCERT:** OrS 60; **MS:** Northwestern U 62; ***SI:*** *Knees and Shoulders*; **HMO:** Blue Cross & Blue Shield, Chicago HMO

Tonino, Pietro (MD) **OrS**
Loyola U Med Ctr **(see page 120)**
Loyola University Medical Ctr, 2160 S 1st Ave Ste 137; Maywood, IL 60153; (708) 216-8730; **BDCERT:** OrS 89; **MS:** Northwestern U 81; **RES:** OrS, Northwestern Mem Hosp, Chicago, IL 81-86; **FAP:** Asst Prof Loyola U-Stritch Sch Med, Maywood; ***SI:*** *Shoulder and Knee Injuries; Sports Medicine*; **HMO:** Blue Cross & Blue Shield
LANG: Sp, Itl;
4+ Weeks VISA

Treister, Michael (MD) **OrS**
St Mary's of Nazareth Hosp Ctr
Treister Orthopedic Svc Ltd, 1431 N Western Ave; Chicago, IL 60622; (773) 327-5866; **BDCERT:** OrS 74; **MS:** Washington U, St Louis 67; **RES:** OrS, St Francis Hosp of Evanston, Evanston, IL 69-70; OrS, Cook Cty Hosp, Chicago, IL 71; **FEL:** HS, Passavant Pavillion, Chicago, IL 71; **FAP:** Asst Prof OrS Chicago Coll Osteo Med; **HOSP:** St Elizabeth's Hosp; ***SI:*** *Spine Surgery; Hand Surgery*; **HMO:** Century Medical Health Plan, SEMS

Visotsky, Jeffrey (MD) **OrS**
Lutheran Gen Hosp **(see page 143)**
Center For Orthopaedic Surgery, 1875 Dempster St Ste 301; Park Ridge, IL 60068; (847) 375-3000; **BDCERT:** OrS 92; **MS:** Northwestern U 84; **RES:** OrS, Northwestern Mem Hosp, Chicago, IL 84-89; **FEL:** HS, Methodist Hosp, Houston, TX 89-90; **HOSP:** Lake Forest Hosp; ***SI:*** *Shoulder Reconstruction; Carpal Tunnel Syndrome*; **HMO:** +
Immediately VISA

Wehner, Julie (MD) **OrS**
Loyola U Med Ctr **(see page 120)**
2160 S 1st Ave; Maywood, IL 60153; (708) 216-3475; **BDCERT:** OrS 93; **MS:** Loyola U-Stritch Sch Med, Maywood 84; **RES:** OrS, Loyola U Med Ctr, Maywood, IL 85-90; S, Loyola U Med Ctr, Maywood, IL 90-91; **FAP:** Asst Clin Prof Loyola U-Stritch Sch Med, Maywood; **HOSP:** Illinois Masonic Med Ctr; ***SI:*** *Herniated Disc*
LANG: Sp; 1 Week
VISA

OTOLARYNGOLOGY

Applebaum, Edward (MD) **Oto**
Univ of Illinois at Chicago Med Ctr
Department of Otolaryngology, 1855 W Taylor St Ste 242; Chicago, IL 60612; (312) 996-6582; **BDCERT:** Oto 70; **MS:** Wayne State U Sch Med 64; **RES:** S, Bon Secours Hosp, Grosse Pointe, MI 65-66; Oto, Mass Eye & Ear Infirmary, Boston, MA 66-69; **FAP:** Prof Oto Univ IL Coll Med
1 Week VISA

Bailey, Larry (MD) **Oto**
Macneal Mem Hosp
Suburban Otolaryngology, 3340 S Oak Park Ave Ste 204; Berwyn, IL 60402; (708) 749-3070; **BDCERT:** Oto 76; **MS:** Univ Kans Sch Med 68; **RES:** S, Hines VA Hosp, Chicago, IL 72-73; Oto, IL Eye & Ear Infirmary, Chicago, IL 73-76; **FAP:** Asst Prof Rush Med Coll; **HOSP:** Gottlieb Mem Hosp; **HMO:** Aetna Hlth Plan, Blue Cross & Blue Shield, Californiacare, Compare Health Service, Health Alliance Plan

Baim, Howard (MD) **Oto**
Illinois Masonic Med Ctr
(see page 118)
2532 W Lincoln Ave; Chicago, IL 60614; (773) 883-1177; **BDCERT:** Oto 78; **MS:** Univ IL Coll Med 73; **RES:** S, IL Med Ctr, Chicago, IL 73-75; Oto, IL Eye & Ear Infirm, Chicago, IL 75-78; **FAP:** Assoc Clin Prof Oto Univ IL Coll Med; **HOSP:** Highland Park Hosp; ***SI:*** *Sinus Disease; Head And Neck Tumors*; **HMO:** Blue Cross & Blue Shield, PHCS, Bay State Health Plan, Beech Street, Prudential
LANG: Sp;
A Few Days VISA

Bastian, Robert (MD) **Oto**
Loyola U Med Ctr **(see page 120)**
Loyola University Medical Ctr, 2160 S 1st Ave Ste 105-1870; Maywood, IL 60153; (708) 216-9183; **BDCERT:** Oto 83; **MS:** Washington U, St Louis 78; **RES:** S, Barnes Hosp, St Louis, MO 78-79; Oto, Barnes Hosp, St Louis, MO 79-83; **FEL:** Oto, , Paris, France -83; **FAP:** Assoc Prof Loyola U-Stritch Sch Med, Maywood; ***SI:*** *Voice Disorders; Larynx Surgery*; **HMO:** +
2-4 Weeks VISA

Caldarelli, David (MD) **Oto**
Rush-Presbyterian-St Luke's Med Ctr
(see page 122)
1725 W Harrison St Ste 308; Chicago, IL 60612; (312) 733-4341; **BDCERT:** Oto 70; **MS:** U Hlth Sci/Chicago Med Sch 65; **RES:** S, Rush Presbyterian-St Luke's Med Ctr, Chicago, IL 66-67; Oto, IL Eye & Ear Infirmary, Chicago, IL 67-70; **FAP:** Prof & Chrmn Oto Rush Med Coll; **HMO:** Aetna Hlth Plan, Blue Cross & Blue Shield, Prudential, Rush Health Plans

Guide to symbols and abbreviations can be found on pages 110-113.

Clemis, Jack (MD) Oto
Mercy Hosp & Med Ctr
Physicians Hearing Aid Svc, 151 N Michigan Ave Ste 914; Chicago, IL 60601; (312) 938-4250; **BDCERT:** Oto 64; **MS:** Canada 58; **RES:** S, Cleveland Clinic Hosp, Cleveland, OH 59; Oto, Cleveland Clinic Hosp, Cleveland, OH 60-62; **FEL:** Oto, Northwestern Mem Hosp, Chicago, IL 62; **FAP:** Lecturer Oto Northwestern U

Cozzi, Laura (MD) Oto
Gottlieb Mem Hosp
Gottlieb Memorial Hospital, 675 W North Ave Ste 301; Melrose Park, IL 60160; (708) 450-4938; **BDCERT:** Oto 90; **MS:** Loyola U-Stritch Sch Med, Maywood 85

DeLeon, Antonio (MD) Oto
St Mary's of Nazareth Hosp Ctr
2552 S Pulaski Rd; Chicago, IL 60623; (773) 277-9600; **BDCERT:** Oto 73; **MS:** Spain 66

Desai, Narendra (MD) Oto
Westlake Comm Hosp
W Suburbn Head & Neck Speclsts, 1111 Superior St Ste 411; Melrose Park, IL 60160; (847) 662-4442; **BDCERT:** Oto 81; IM 79; **MS:** India 69; **RES:** IM, Doctors Hospital, Washington, DC 71-74; S, Albert Einstein Med Ctr, Bronx, NY 76-77; **FAP:** Asst Prof Univ IL Coll Med; **HOSP:** Victory Mem Hosp

Friedman, Michael (MD) Oto
Illinois Masonic Med Ctr
(see page 118)
Advanced Ctr For Specialty Care, 3000 N Halsted St Ste 401; Chicago, IL 60657; (312) 236-3642; **BDCERT:** Oto 77; **MS:** Univ IL Coll Med 72; **RES:** S, Illinois Masonic Med Ctr, Chicago, IL 73-74; Oto, U IL Med Ctr, Chicago, IL 74-77

Girgis, Samuel (MD) Oto
Hinsdale Hosp **(see page 275)**
Doctors Girgis & Assoc, 5201 Willow Springs Rd Ste 240; La Grange, IL 60525; (708) 354-9575; **BDCERT:** Oto 87; **MS:** Mexico 79; **RES:** S, Loyola U Med Ctr, Maywood, IL 81-82; Oto, Loyola U Med Ctr, Maywood, IL 82-86

Goldman, Michael (MD) Oto
St Francis Hosp
111 N Wabash Ave Ste 1100; Chicago, IL 60602; (312) 297-1000; **BDCERT:** Oto 79; **MS:** U Hlth Sci/Chicago Med Sch 74; **RES:** S, Cook Cty Hosp, Chicago, IL 75-76; Oto, Northwestern Mem Hosp, Chicago, IL 76-79; **FEL:** S, Northwestern Mem Hosp, Chicago, IL 79-80; **HOSP:** Northwestern Mem Hosp; ***SI:*** *Head and Neck Surgery; Facial Plastic Surgery*
1 Week

Grossman, Bruce (MD) Oto
St Alexius Med Ctr
990 Grand Canyon Pkwy Ste 120; Hoffman Estates, IL 60194; (847) 882-5888; **BDCERT:** Oto 83; **MS:** Univ IL Coll Med 78; **RES:** S, Northwestern Mem Hosp, Chicago, IL; Oto, Northwestern Mem Hosp, Chicago, IL 80-83; **HOSP:** Alexian Brothers Med Ctr

Hanson, David (MD) Oto
Northwestern Mem Hosp
Northwestern Dept Oto Searle 12-561, 303 E Chicago Ave; Chicago, IL 60611; (312) 908-8182; **BDCERT:** Oto 75; **MS:** U Wash, Seattle 70; **RES:** S, U MN Med Ctr, Minneapolis, MN 70-71; Oto, U MN Med Ctr, Minneapolis, MN 72-75; **FAP:** Chrmn Oto Northwestern U; ***SI:*** *Voice Disorders*; **HMO:** +
2-4 Weeks VISA

Holinger, Lauren (MD) Oto
Children's Mem Med Ctr **(see page 139)**
Childrens Memorial Hosp, 2300 N Childrens Plz Ste 25; Chicago, IL 60614; (773) 880-4457; **BDCERT:** Oto 76; **MS:** U Hlth Sci/Chicago Med Sch 71; **RES:** S, U CO Affil Hosps, Denver, CO 71-72; Oto, U CO Affil Hosps, Denver, CO 72-75; **FEL:** IL Eye & Ear Infirmary, Chicago, IL 75-76; **FAP:** Prof Northwestern U; ***SI:*** *Pediatric Otolaryngology*

Horowitz, Steven (MD) Oto
St James Hosp & Hlth Ctrs
Suburban Heights Medical Ctr, 333 Dixie Hwy; Chicago Heights, IL 60411; (708) 709-6050; **BDCERT:** Oto 81; **MS:** Jefferson Med Coll 75; **RES:** S, Hahnemann U Hosp, Philadelphia, PA 75-76; Oto, U IL Med Ctr, Chicago, IL 76-79; **HOSP:** South Suburban Hosp; ***SI:*** *Facial Plastic Surgery; Snoring: Laser, Surgery*
LANG: Sp;
A Few Days VISA

Hotaling, Andrew J (MD) Oto
Loyola U Med Ctr **(see page 120)**
Loyola University Medical Ctr, 2160 S 1st Ave Bldg105; Maywood, IL 60153; (708) 216-9183; **BDCERT:** Oto 85; **MS:** Case West Res U 79; **RES:** S, Case Western Reserve U Hosp, Cleveland, OH 80-81; Oto, Northwestern Mem Hosp, Chicago, IL 81-84; **FEL:** Ped Oto, U of Pittsburgh Med Ctr, Pittsburgh, PA 84-85; **FAP:** Assoc Prof Oto Loyola U-Stritch Sch Med, Maywood; ***SI:*** *Pediatric Otolaryngology*

Hutchinson Jr, James C (MD) Oto
West Suburban Hosp Med Ctr
Associates Head & Neck Surgery, 3722 Harlem Ave Ste 201; Riverside, IL 60546; (708) 442-1616; **BDCERT:** Oto 74; **MS:** Canada 66; **RES:** S, Mayo Grad Sch Med, Rochester, MN 70-71; Oto, Rush Presby-St Lukes MC, Chicago, IL 71-74; **FAP:** Assoc Prof Oto Rush Med Coll; **HOSP:** Rush-Presbyterian-St Luke's Med Ctr

Jones, Paul John (MD) Oto
St Joseph Hosp-Chicago
Paul J Jones & Assoc, 25 E Washington St Fl 18; Chicago, IL 60602; (312) 553-0152; **BDCERT:** Oto 89; **MS:** Rush Med Coll 83; **RES:** Oto, Rush Presbyterian-St Luke's Med Ctr, Chicago, IL 84-88; **FAP:** Asst Prof Rush Med Coll; **HOSP:** Rush-Presbyterian-St Luke's Med Ctr

Kurtzman, Daniel (MD) Oto
Macneal Mem Hosp
Suburban Otolaryngology, 3340 Oak Park Ave Ste 204; Berwyn, IL 60402; (708) 749-3070; **BDCERT:** Oto 90; **MS:** U Mich Med Sch 85; **RES:** Oto, U IL Med Ctr, Chicago, IL 86-90; **FAP:** Instr Rush Med Coll; **HOSP:** Gottlieb Mem Hosp; ***SI:*** *Sinusitis; Nasal Reconstruction*; **HMO:** Blue Cross & Blue Shield, United Healthcare, Aetna-US Healthcare, CIGNA, Humana Health Plan +
LANG: Sp;
A Few Days VISA

Leonetti, John (MD) Oto
Loyola U Med Ctr (see page 120)
Bldg 105, 2160 S 1st Ave Rm 1870; Maywood, IL 60153; (708) 216-4804; **BDCERT:** Oto 87; **MS:** Loyola U-Stritch Sch Med, Maywood 82; **RES:** Oto, Loyola U Med Ctr, Maywood, IL 82-87; **FEL:** Skull Base Surg, Barnes Hosp, St Louis, MO 87-89; **FAP:** Prof Loyola U-Stritch Sch Med, Maywood; ***SI:*** *Acoustic Neuroma; Hearing Loss*
1 Week VISA

Licameli, Greg (MD) Oto
Univ of Illinois at Chicago Med Ctr
U Ill Chicago, 1855 W Taylor St; Chicago, IL 60612; (312) 413-8821; **BDCERT:** Oto 98; **MS:** Med Coll Ga 91; **RES:** Oto, Boston U Med Ctr, Boston, MA 92-96; **FEL:** PHO, Johns Hopkins Hosp, Baltimore, MD 96-97; **FAP:** Asst Prof Oto Univ IL Coll Med; ***SI:*** *Pediatrics*; **HMO:** +
LANG: Sp; 2-4 Weeks
VISA

Lygizos, Nicholas (MD) Oto
Lutheran Gen Hosp (see page 143)
Audiological Laboratory Ltd, 64 Old Orchard Shopping Ctr; Skokie, IL 60077; (847) 674-5585; **BDCERT:** Oto 86; **MS:** U Mich Med Sch 81; **RES:** Oto, U IL Med Ctr, Chicago, IL 82-86; **FAP:** Asst Clin Prof Univ IL Coll Med; **HOSP:** Highland Park Hosp; **HMO:** Blue Cross & Blue Shield, Chicago HMO, Humana Health Plan, Rush Health Plans, Sanus

Lyon, Susan (MD) Oto
Christ Hosp & Med Ctr (see page 140)
Southwest Head/Neck Surg Assoc, 1000 Ravinia Pl; Orland Park, IL 60462; (708) 460-6663; **BDCERT:** Oto 85; **MS:** Rush Med Coll 80; **RES:** S, Northwestern Mem Hosp, Chicago, IL 80-82; Oto, Northwestern Mem Hosp, Chicago, IL 82-85; **HOSP:** Palos Comm Hosp; ***SI:*** *Pediatric Ent; Sinus & Apnea & ENT Tumors*; **HMO:** Blue Cross & Blue Shield, Humana Health Plan, HealthNet
1 Week VISA

Matz, Gregory (MD) Oto
Loyola U Med Ctr (see page 120)
2160 S First Ave; Maywood, IL 60153; (708) 216-9183; **BDCERT:** Oto 67; **MS:** Loyola U-Stritch Sch Med, Maywood 62; **RES:** Oto, Chicago Hosp, Chicago, IL 63-67; **FAP:** Chrmn Oto Loyola U-Stritch Sch Med, Maywood; ***SI:*** *Head and Neck Cancer*; **HMO:** +
1 Week

Miller, Robert (MD) Oto
Lutheran Gen Hosp (see page 143)
Audiological Laboratory Ltd, 64 Old Orchard Shopping Ctr; Skokie, IL 60077; (847) 674-5585; **BDCERT:** Oto 78; **MS:** Loyola U-Stritch Sch Med, Maywood 74; **RES:** Oto, U IL Med Ctr, Chicago, IL 75-78; **FEL:** Ped Oto, Children's Hosp Med Ctr, Cincinnati, OH 86-87; **FAP:** Asst Clin Prof Univ IL Coll Med; **HOSP:** Children's Mem Med Ctr; ***SI:*** *Pediatric Ear Disease; Airway Problems*; **HMO:** PHCS, Blue Cross & Blue Shield, United Healthcare, CIGNA, Aetna Hlth Plan +
2-4 Weeks

Mokarry, Victor Peter (MD) Oto
Resurrection Med Ctr
Buckingham, 145 S Northwest Hwy; Park Ridge, IL 60068; (847) 825-2115; **BDCERT:** Oto 96; **MS:** Loyola U-Stritch Sch Med, Maywood 90; **RES:** S, Loyola U Med Ctr, Maywood, IL 90-91; Oto, Loyola U Med Ctr, Maywood, IL 91-95; **HMO:** PHCS, CCN, Blue Cross & Blue Shield, Blue Choice +
VISA

Moore, Dennis (MD) Oto
Lutheran Gen Hosp (see page 143)
Ear Nose & Throat Ctr, 444 N Northwest Hwy Ste 150; Park Ridge, IL 60068; (847) 298-4327; **BDCERT:** Oto 88; **MS:** Loyola U-Stritch Sch Med, Maywood 82

Panje, William (MD) Oto
Rush-Presbyterian-St Luke's Med Ctr (see page 122)
University Head & Neck Assoc, 1725 W Harrison St Ste 340; Chicago, IL 60612; (312) 664-6715; **BDCERT:** Oto 77; **MS:** U Iowa Coll Med 71; **RES:** S, U IA Hosp, Iowa City, IA 72-73; Oto, U IA Hosp, Iowa City, IA 73-76; **FEL:** Head, Neck & Pls, U IA Hosp, Iowa City, IA 76-77; **FAP:** Prof Rush Med Coll; **HOSP:** U Chicago Hosp; **HMO:** Blue Choice, Blue Cross & Blue Shield, Californiacare, Metlife, Prudential

Guide to symbols and abbreviations can be found on pages 110-113.

Petchenik, Lon (MD) Oto
Northwest Comm Hlthcare
Suburban Ear Nose & Throat, 1100 W Central Rd Ste 202; Arlington Hts, IL 60005; (847) 259-2530; **BDCERT:** Oto 94; **MS:** Univ IL Coll Med 88; **RES:** UIL Eye & Ear Infirmary, Chicago, IL 89-93

Portugal, Louis (MD) Oto
Univ of Illinois at Chicago Med Ctr
Department of Otolaryngology, 1855 W Taylor St Ste 242; Chicago, IL 60612; (312) 996-6582; **BDCERT:** Oto 93; **MS:** U MO-Kansas City Sch Med 87

Soltes, Steven (MD) Oto
Christ Hosp & Med Ctr (see page 140)
10522 S Cicero Ave Fl 3; Oak Lawn, IL 60453; (708) 422-0500; **BDCERT:** Oto 81; **MS:** Loyola U-Stritch Sch Med, Maywood 77; **RES:** Oto, U IL Med Ctr, Chicago, IL 77-78; **FAP:** Univ IL Coll Med

Tardy, M Eugene (MD) Oto
St Joseph Hosp-Elgin
Head & Neck Surgery Ltd, 2913 N Commonwealth Ave Ste 430; Chicago, IL 60657; (773) 472-7559; **BDCERT:** Oto 68; **MS:** Ind U Sch Med 60; **RES:** Oto, U IL Med Ctr, Chicago, IL 63-67; **FEL:** Head, Neck & PlS, U IL Med Ctr, Chicago, IL 67-68; **FAP:** Clin Prof Oto Univ IL Coll Med; **HOSP:** Univ of Illinois at Chicago Med Ctr

Tojo, David (MD) Oto
Lutheran Gen Hosp (see page 143)
1775 Dempster St; Park Ridge, IL 60068; (847) 674-5585; **BDCERT:** Oto 93; **MS:** U Cincinnati 87; **RES:** Oto, U IL Med Ctr, Chicago, IL 88-92; **FEL:** Skull Base Surg, Univ Zurich, Switzerland 92; **FAP:** Assoc Prof Univ IL Coll Med

Toriumi, Dean (MD) Oto
Univ of Illinois at Chicago Med Ctr
University of Illinois, 1855 W Taylor St Ste 242; Chicago, IL 60612; (312) 996-8897; **BDCERT:** Oto 88; **MS:** Rush Med Coll 81; **RES:** S, U IL Med Ctr, Chicago, IL 83-85; Oto, Northwestern Mem Hosp, Chicago, IL 85-87; **FEL:** Facial PlS, Tulane U Med Ctr, New Orleans, LA 88; Facial PlS, Virginia Mason Hosp, Seattle, WA 89; **FAP:** Assoc Prof Univ IL Coll Med; ***SI:** Facial Plastic Surgery*

Weingarten, Charles (MD) Oto
Evanston Hosp
Otolaryngology Group Ltd, 5140 N California Ave Ste 650; Chicago, IL 60625; (773) 271-7150; **BDCERT:** Oto 69; **MS:** Tulane U 63; **RES:** Oto, Northwestern Mem Hosp, Chicago, IL 64-68; **FAP:** Asst Clin Prof Northwestern U

Yeh, Stephen (MD) Oto
Evanston Hosp
1000 Central St; Evanston, IL 60201; (847) 492-8800; **BDCERT:** Oto 76; **MS:** Northwestern U 71; **RES:** S, Rush Presbyterian-St Luke's Med Ctr, Chicago, IL 71-73; Oto, Northwestern Mem Hosp, Chicago, IL 73-76; **FAP:** Lecturer Northwestern U; **HOSP:** Glenbrook Hosp; ***SI:** Pediatric ENT; Sinus Disease*; **HMO:** Aetna Hlth Plan, Blue Cross & Blue Shield, Californiacare, HealthNet, Humana Health Plan
A Few Days

Young, Nancy (MD) Oto
Children's Mem Med Ctr (see page 139)
Dept Pediatric Oto, 2300 Chldns Plz Ste 25; Chicago, IL 60614; (773) 388-3496; **BDCERT:** Oto 87; **MS:** NYU Sch Med 82; **RES:** S, Montefiore Med Ctr, Bronx, NY 82-84; Oto, Northwestern Mem Hosp, Chicago, IL 84-87; **FEL:** NOto, Hinsdale Hosp, Hinsdale, IL 87-88; **FAP:** Asst Prof Northwestern U; ***SI:** Cochlear Implantation; Cholesteatoma (Congenital)*; **HMO:** +
2-4 Weeks VISA

PAIN MANAGEMENT

Carobene, Holly (MD) PM
Ingalls Mem Hosp
1551 Huntington Drive; Calumet City, IL 60409; (708) 862-3344; **BDCERT:** Anes 91; PM 96; **MS:** Northwestern U 84

Cupic, Milorad (MD) PM
Mercy Hosp & Med Ctr
Pain Management Dept, 2525 S Michigan Ave; Chicago, IL 60616; (312) 567-5657; **BDCERT:** Anes 73; PM 96; **MS:** Yugoslavia 64; **RES:** U Chicago Hosp, Chicago, IL 67; **FAP:** Clin Prof Anes Univ IL Coll Med; **HMO:** Aetna Hlth Plan, Blue Cross & Blue Shield, Californiacare, CIGNA, Humana Health Plan

Harden, R. Norman (MD) PM
Rehab Institute of Chicago
345 E Superior St Ste 1190; Chicago, IL 60611; (312) 908-2845; **BDCERT:** PM 90; **MS:** Med Coll Ga 84; **RES:** N & IM, Med U of SC Med Ctr, Charleston, SC 84-88; **FEL:** PM, Emory U Hosp, Atlanta, GA 88-89; ***SI:** Chronic Pain Management; Headache*; **HMO:** +
A Few Days VISA

Katz, Jeffrey (MD) PM
Rehab Institute of Chicago
Department of Anesthesiology, 303 E Chicago Ave; Chicago, IL 60611; (312) 908-2500; **BDCERT:** PM 94; Anes 87; **MS:** Northwestern U 83; **RES:** Anes, Northwestern Mem Hosp, Chicago, IL 84-86; **FEL:** Northwestern U, Chicago, IL 86-87; PM, Univ Cincinnati, Cincinnati, OH 87-88; **FAP:** Asst Prof

Worwag, Ewelina (MD) PM
Louis A Weiss Mem Hosp
4646 N Marine Dr; Chicago, IL 60640; (773) 564-5678; **BDCERT:** Anes 92; PM 96; **MS:** Poland 80; **RES:** Anes, U Chicago Hosp, Chicago, IL 86-90; **FEL:** PM, U Chicago Hosp, Chicago, IL 89-90; **HOSP:** U Chicago Hosp; ***SI:*** *Low Back Pain; Chronic Pain*; **HMO:** +
LANG: Pol, Rus, Sp, Ger; 2-4 Weeks VISA

PEDIATRIC ALLERGY & IMMUNOLOGY

Dold, Henry (MD) PA&I
Northwest Comm Hlthcare
1100 W Central Rd Ste 409; Arlington Hts, IL 60005; (847) 392-0400; **BDCERT:** Ped 65; A&I 74; **MS:** Loyola U-Stritch Sch Med, Maywood 60; **RES:** Ped, Children's Mem Med Ctr, Chicago, IL 61-63; **FEL:** Rush Presbyterian-St Luke's Med Ctr, Chicago, IL 65-67

Evans, Richard (MD) PA&I
Children's Mem Med Ctr (see page 139)
Children's Memorial Medical Ctr, 2300 N Childrens Plz Ste 60; Chicago, IL 60614; (773) 880-4233; **BDCERT:** A&I 72; Ped 67; **MS:** U Chicago-Pritzker Sch Med 58; **RES:** A&I, Walter Reed Army Med Ctr, Washington, DC 69-70; Children's Hosp of Buffalo, Buffalo, NY 70-71; **FAP:** Prof PA&I Northwestern U; **HMO:** Aetna Hlth Plan, Blue Cross & Blue Shield, Chicago HMO, CIGNA, Humana Health Plan

Gotoff, Samuel (MD) PA&I
Rush-Presbyterian-St Luke's Med Ctr (see page 122)
Rush Presbyterian, 1653 W Congress Pkwy Ste 770; Chicago, IL 60612; (312) 942-8928; **BDCERT:** Ped 63; PA&I 76; **MS:** U Rochester 58; **RES:** Ped, Yale-New Haven Hosp, New Haven, CT 58-61; **FEL:** A&I, Children's Hosp, Boston, MA 63-65; **FAP:** Prof Rush Med Coll; ***SI:*** *Pediatric Rheumatology; Immune Deficiency Diseases*; **HMO:** +
1 Week VISA

Park, C Lucy (MD) PA&I
Univ of Illinois at Chicago Med Ctr
Dept PD, 840 S Wood St Ste 1224; Chicago, IL 60612; (312) 996-6714; **BDCERT:** A&I 88; Ped 83; **MS:** South Korea 75; **RES:** Ped, Baltimore City Hosp, Baltimore, MD 77-80; A&I, Scripps Clin Rsch Fdn, La Jolla, CA 80-82; **FEL:** A&I, Children's Hosp of Philadelphia, Philadelphia, PA 82-84; **FAP:** Asst Prof Univ IL Coll Med

Rich, Kenneth (MD) PA&I
Univ of Illinois at Chicago Med Ctr
University of Illinois Chicago, 840 S Wood St; Chicago, IL 60612; (312) 996-6714; **BDCERT:** A&I 77; **MS:** Tulane U 70; **RES:** Ped, UCLA Med Ctr, Los Angeles, CA 70-73; **FEL:** Ped A&I, UCLA Med Ctr, Los Angeles, CA 73-75; **FAP:** Prof Univ IL Coll Med; ***SI:*** *Immune Deficiency; Pediatric Rheumatology*
1 Week VISA

PEDIATRIC CARDIOLOGY

Agarwala, Brojendra N (MD) PCd
U Chicago Hosp (see page 124)
5841 S Maryland; Chicago, IL 60637; (773) 702-1000; **BDCERT:** Ped 70; PCd 78; **MS:** India 65; **RES:** Ped, St Vincents Hosp & Med Ctr NY, New York, NY 67-69; **FEL:** PCd, New York University Med Ctr, New York, NY 69-72; **HMO:** +
1 Week

Cole, Roger (MD) PCd
Children's Mem Med Ctr (see page 139)
2350 N Lincoln Ave; Chicago, IL 60614; (773) 871-5800; **BDCERT:** Ped 63; PCd 65; **MS:** U Cincinnati 57; **RES:** Ped, Stanford, San Francisco, CA 58-59; Ped, Mt Zion, San Francisco, CA 59-60; **FEL:** PCd, Children's Mem Hosp, Chicago, IL 62-64; **FAP:** Clin Prof Ped Northwestern U; **HOSP:** Evanston Hosp; ***SI:*** *Congenital Heart Disease; Cardiac Arrhythmias*

Dubrow, Ira (MD) PCd
Lutheran Gen Hosp (see page 143)
1675 Dempster St; Park Ridge, IL 60068; (847) 723-6465; **BDCERT:** Ped 89; PCd 89; **MS:** Univ IL Coll Med 66; **RES:** Ped, Illinois Hosp, Chicago, IL 67-69; **FEL:** PCd, U IL Hosp, Chicago, IL 71-73

Fisher, Elizabeth (MD) PCd
Loyola U Med Ctr (see page 120)
Loyola University Medical Ctr, 2160 S 1st Ave Ste 105-3319; Maywood, IL 60153; (708) 327-9102; **BDCERT:** PCd 72; Ped 71; **MS:** Ind U Sch Med 66; **RES:** Ped, Children's Mem Med Ctr, Chicago, IL 67-68; **FEL:** PCd, Childrens Meml Hosp, Chicago, IL 68-71; **FAP:** Clin Prof Ped Univ IL Coll Med

Guide to symbols and abbreviations can be found on pages 110-113.

Gidding, Samuel (MD) PCd
Children's Mem Med Ctr (see page 139)
2300 Childrens Plz; Chicago, IL 60614; (773) 880-4000; **BDCERT:** Ped 83; PCd 85; **MS:** Rutgers U 78; **RES:** Ped, Univ Hosp SUNY Syracuse, Syracuse, NY 79-81; **FEL:** PCd, U Mich Med Ctr, Ann Arbor, MI 81-84; **FAP:** Assoc Prof Ped Northwestern U; **HOSP:** Evanston Hosp
LANG: Sp;

Griffin, Andrew (MD) PCd
Illinois Masonic Med Ctr (see page 118)
Illinois Masonic Medical Ctr, 836 W Wellington Ave Ste 3604; Chicago, IL 60657; (773) 296-7147; **BDCERT:** PCd 77; PCCM 90; **MS:** U Chicago-Pritzker Sch Med 67; **RES:** Ped, Chicago Hosp, Chicago, IL 68-69; **FEL:** PCd, Chicago Hosp, Chicago, IL; **FAP:** Assoc Prof Ped Univ IL Coll Med; **HOSP:** Rush-Presbyterian-St Luke's Med Ctr; ***SI:*** *Heart Disease-Pediatric; Children's Intensive Care*; **HMO:** Blue Cross & Blue Shield, United Healthcare, Rush Pru, CIGNA

Husayni, Tarek Saad (MD) PCd
Christ Hosp & Med Ctr (see page 140)
Hope Children's Hosp, Heart Institute for Children, 4400 W 95th St; Oak Lawn, IL 60453; (708) 346-5580; **BDCERT:** Ped 83; PCd 85; **MS:** Spain 75; **RES:** Ped, U Hosp, Jacksonville, FL 78-81; PCd, U IA Hosp, Iowa City, IA 81-84; **FEL:** NuM, U IA Hosp, Iowa City, IA 83-85; **FAP:** Asst Prof Rush Med Coll

Ow, Earl Phillip (MD) PCd
Good Samaritan Hosp (see page 274)
Heart Inst for Children-Christ Hosp Med Ctr, 4440 W 95th St; Oak Lawn, IL 60453; (708) 346-5580; **BDCERT:** PCd 83; PCCM 90; **MS:** Loyola U-Stritch Sch Med, Maywood 73; **RES:** Ped, Loyola U Foster Med Ctr, Maywood, IL 74-76; **FEL:** Pcd, Wyler Childrens Mem Med Ctr, Chicago, IL 78-81; **FAP:** Assoc Prof Ped Loyola U-Stritch Sch Med, Maywood; **HOSP:** Christ Hosp & Med Ctr

Pahl, Elfriede (MD) PCd
Children's Mem Med Ctr (see page 139)
Childrens Memorial Med Ctr, 2300 N Childrens Plz Fl 5; Chicago, IL 60614; (773) 880-4553; **BDCERT:** Ped 87; PCd 96; **MS:** Northwestern U 83; **RES:** Ped, Northwestern Mem Hosp, Chicago, IL 84-86; **FEL:** PCd, U of Pittsburgh Med Ctr, Pittsburgh, PA 86-88; **FAP:** Asst Prof Northwestern U

Sodt, Peter (MD) PCd
Rush-Presbyterian-St Luke's Med Ctr (see page 122)
Midwest Children's Heart Spec, 1575 Barrington Rd Ste 430; Hoffman Estates, IL 60194; (847) 884-1212; **BDCERT:** PCd 95; Ped 86; **MS:** Northwestern U 80; **RES:** Ped, Oregon Health Sci U Hosp, Portland, OR 81-84; **FEL:** PCd, U Chicago Hosp, Chicago, IL 84-86; **FAP:** Asst Prof Rush Med Coll; **HOSP:** St Anthony Hosp; ***SI:*** *Birth Defects of the Heart; Childhood Heart Rhythm*; **HMO:** Blue Cross & Blue Shield, CIGNA, Bay State Health Plan, United, PHCS +
LANG: Sp;
A Few Days VISA

Thoele, David G (MD) PCd
Univ of Illinois at Chicago Med Ctr
Pediatric Cardiology (M/C 856), 840 S Wood St; Chicago, IL 60612; (312) 996-6605; **BDCERT:** Ped 89; PCd 94; **MS:** U Minn 83

Weigel, Thomas (MD) PCd
Children's Mem Med Ctr (see page 139)
2350 N Lincoln Ave; Chicago, IL 60614; (773) 871-5800; **BDCERT:** Ped 88; **MS:** Loyola U-Stritch Sch Med, Maywood 84; **RES:** PCd, Mayo Clinic, Rochester, MN 84-87; **HOSP:** Evanston Hosp; ***SI:*** *Congenital Heart Disease; Echocardiography*; **HMO:** Aetna Hlth Plan, Blue Cross & Blue Shield, Guardian, United Healthcare, PHCS +
Immediately

PEDIATRIC CRITICAL CARE MEDICINE

Green, Thomas P (MD) PCCM
Children's Mem Med Ctr (see page 139)
Children's Mem Hosp, Dept of Pulmonology/Critical Care Med, 2300 Childrens Plz No 73; Chicago, IL 60614; (773) 880-4549; **BDCERT:** PCCM 96; PPul 94; **MS:** Stanford U 74; **RES:** U MN Med Ctr, Minneapolis, MN 77-79; **FEL:** U MN Med Ctr, Minneapolis, MN 75-77; **FAP:** Prof Ped Northwestern U; **HOSP:** Evanston Hosp; ***SI:*** *Lung Problems-Pediatric; Critical Care*; **HMO:** +
VISA

Naidu, Shrinivas (MD) PCCM
Lutheran Gen Hosp (see page 143)
Pediatrics Dept, 1775 Dempster St; Park Ridge, IL 60068; (847) 723-7682; **BDCERT:** Ped 77; **MS:** India 63; **RES:** Michael Reese Hosp, Chicago, IL 72-73; Lutheran Gen Hosp, Chicago, IL 73-74; **FAP:** Assoc Clin Prof Ped U Chicago-Pritzker Sch Med; ***SI:*** *Intensive Care*

PEDIATRIC ENDOCRINOLOGY

Duck, Stephen C (MD) PEn
Evanston Hosp
Evanston Hospital, 2650 Ridge Ave Rm 1612; Evanston, IL 60201; (847) 757-2034; **BDCERT:** PEn 78; Ped 76; **MS:** Cornell U 71; **RES:** Barnes Hosp, St Louis, MO 73-75; **FEL:** St Louis Children's Hosp, St Louis, MO 72-74; **HOSP:** Glenbrook Hosp; ***SI:*** *Diabetes Control & Complications; Short Stature*; **HMO:** Blue Cross, CIGNA, Aetna Hlth Plan, Humana Health Plan, United Healthcare +
A Few Days VISA

Edidin, Deborah V (MD) PEn
Children's Mem Med Ctr (see page 139)
Childrens Meml Hosp Div Endo, 2300 Childrens Plaza MB54; Chicago, IL 60614; (773) 880-4440; **BDCERT:** EDM 80; Ped 79; **MS:** Univ IL Coll Med 74; **RES:** Kunstadter Children's Center, Chicago, IL 75-79; **FAP:** Asst Prof Ped Northwestern U; **HOSP:** Evanston Hosp; ***SI:*** *Diabetes; Growth and Puberty*; **HMO:** +
LANG: Fr, Ger, Sp; A Few Days

Levy, Richard (MD) PEn
Rush-Presbyterian-St Luke's Med Ctr (see page 122)
1725 W Harrison St Ste 938; Chicago, IL 60612; (312) 942-8989; **BDCERT:** PEn 86; EDM 85; **MS:** LSU Sch Med, New Orleans 71; **RES:** IM, U Mass Med Ctr, Worcester, MA 75-77; Ped, Beth Israel Med Ctr, New York, NY 77-78; **FEL:** EDM, Barnes Hosp, St Louis, MO 79-82; **FAP:** Asst Prof Rush Med Coll; **HOSP:** St Joseph Hosp-Chicago; ***SI:*** *Growth; Thyroid*; **HMO:** Aetna Hlth Plan, United Healthcare, Blue Cross & Blue Shield, Principal Health Care +
LANG: Sp; 1 Week

Rosenfield, Robert (MD) PEn
Children's Mem Med Ctr (see page 139)
University of Chicago Children's Hospital, 5841 S Maryland Ave; Chicago, IL 60637; (312) 947-6349; **BDCERT:** Ped 86; PEn 86; **MS:** Northwestern U 60; **RES:** Children's Hosp of Philadelphia, Philadelphia, PA 61-63; **FEL:** PEn, Children's Hosp of Philadelphia, Philadelphia, PA 65-68; **FAP:** Prof Ped U Chicago-Pritzker Sch Med; ***SI:*** *Puberty Disorders; Growth Disorders*
2-4 Weeks VISA

Silverman, Bernard (MD) PEn
Children's Mem Med Ctr (see page 139)
2300 N Childrens Plz Ste 54; Chicago, IL 60614; (773) 880-4000; **BDCERT:** Ped 85; PEn 86; **MS:** Mt Sinai Sch Med 80; **RES:** Ped, Children's Mem Med Ctr, Chicago, IL 80-84; **FEL:** PEn, UC San Francisco Med Ctr, San Francisco, CA 84-87; **FAP:** Assoc Professor PEn Northwestern U; **HOSP:** Glenbrook Hosp; ***SI:*** *Growth Disorders; Diabetes in Children*
LANG: Sp, Fr, Ger, Itl; 2-4 Weeks

Ziai, Fuad (MD) PEn
St Mary's of Nazareth Hosp Ctr
4440 W 95th St; Oak Lawn, IL 60453; (708) 346-5670; **BDCERT:** Ped 74; PEn 78; **MS:** U Mich Med Sch 67; **HOSP:** Christ Hosp & Med Ctr

PEDIATRIC GASTROENTEROLOGY

Berman, James (MD) PGe
Lutheran Gen Hosp (see page 143)
Yacktman Children's Pavilion, 1675 Dempster St; Park Ridge, IL 60068; (847) 723-7700; **BDCERT:** PGe 90; Ped 86; **MS:** Univ Pittsburgh 81; **RES:** Ped, Children's Hosp of Pittsburgh, Pittsburgh, PA 81-84; **FEL:** PGe, Children's Hosp, Boston, MA 84-87; **FAP:** Asst Professor Ped Loyola U-Stritch Sch Med, Maywood; **HOSP:** Loyola U Med Ctr; ***SI:*** *Crohn's And Colitis; Feeding And Nutrition*; **HMO:** Blue Choice, HMO, Californiacare, Humana Health Plan, Aetna Hlth Plan
LANG: Sp; 1 Week
VISA

Gunasekaran, T S (MD) PGe
Lutheran Gen Hosp (see page 143)
Luth General Hospital-Dept Peds, 1675 Dempster St; Park Ridge, IL 60068; (847) 318-9330; **BDCERT:** Ped 91; PGe 92; **MS:** India 77; **RES:** Ped, Hospitals in United Kingdom, Boston, MA 83-87; Ped, BC Children's Hospital, Boston, MA 90-91; **FEL:** Pge, BC Children's Hospital Canada 91-92; **FAP:** Asst Clin Prof Ped U Chicago-Pritzker Sch Med

Kirschner, Barbara (MD) PGe
U Chicago Hosp (see page 124)
Univ of Chicago Childrns Hosp - MC-4065, 5841 S Maryland Ave; Chicago, IL 60637; (773) 702-6152; **BDCERT:** Ped 72; PGe 91; **MS:** Univ Penn 67; **RES:** Ped, U Chicago Hosp, Chicago, IL 67-70; **FEL:** Ped Ge, U Chicago Hosp, Chicago, IL 75; **FAP:** Prof U Chicago-Pritzker Sch Med; ***SI:*** *Inflammatory Bowel Disease; Chronic Diarrheal Disease*; **HMO:** Blue Cross & Blue Shield, CIGNA, Affordable Hlth Plan, HealthStar, United Healthcare +
LANG: Itl, Fr, Sp;
A Few Days VISA

Guide to symbols and abbreviations can be found on pages 110-113.

Nagpal, Rajeev (MD) PGe
Children's Mem Med Ctr **(see page 139)**
4440 W 95th St; Oak Lawn, IL 60453; (708) 346-5650; **BDCERT:** PGe 95; Ped 98; **MS:** India 78; **FEL:** Childrens, Philadelphia, PA; **HOSP:** Good Samaritan Hosp; ***SI:*** *Crohns Colitis; Liver Disease*; **HMO:** Blue Cross & Blue Shield, Humana Health Plan, United Healthcare, Rush Pru, Aetna Hlth Plan
Immediately

Nelson, Suzanne P (MD) PGe
Children's Mem Med Ctr **(see page 139)**
Children's Meml Hosp, 2300 Chldn's Plz Box 65; Chicago, IL 60614; (773) 880-4354; **BDCERT:** PGe 97; Ped 91; **MS:** Northwestern U 88; **RES:** Ped, Children's Mem Med Ctr, Chicago, IL 88-91; **FEL:** GO, Harvard Med Sch, Cambridge, MA 91-94; **FAP:** Asst Prof Ped Northwestern U; **HOSP:** Evanston Hosp; ***SI:*** *Gastroesophageal- Reflux; Failure to Thrive*; **HMO:** Blue Cross & Blue Shield, Humana Health Plan, CIGNA, United +
LANG: Sp; 1 Week
VISA

Sandler, Richard (MD) PGe
Rush-Presbyterian-St Luke's Med Ctr
(see page 122)
Rush Children's Hospital, 1725 W Harrison St Ste 710; Chicago, IL 60612; (312) 942-2889; **BDCERT:** Ped 89; PGe 95; **MS:** Mich St U 79; **RES:** Ped, Michigan State Univ, Lansing, MI 84-86; **FEL:** Ped GI/Nutrition, Children's Hosp, Boston, MA 87-90; **FAP:** Asst Prof Rush Med Coll; **HOSP:** Lake Forest Hosp; ***SI:*** *Abdominal Pain-Constipation; Failure to Thrive*; **HMO:** Aetna Hlth Plan, Blue Cross & Blue Shield, CIGNA, United Healthcare, Rush Prudential +
LANG: Fr; NFI
A Few Days VISA

PEDIATRIC HEMATOLOGY-ONCOLOGY

Cohn, Susan (MD) PHO
Children's Mem Med Ctr **(see page 139)**
2300 Children's Plz Box 30; Chicago, IL 60614; (773) 880-4586; **BDCERT:** Ped 85; PHO 87; **MS:** Univ IL Coll Med 80; **HOSP:** Evanston Hosp

Morgan, Elaine (MD) PHO
Children's Mem Med Ctr **(see page 139)**
Children's Meml Med Ctr, 2300 Children's Plaza; Chicago, IL 60614; (773) 880-4562; **BDCERT:** Ped 76; PHO 78; **MS:** Univ Penn 71; **RES:** Ped, Children's Hosp of Los Angeles, Los Angeles, CA 72-74; **FEL:** Children's Hosp, Boston, MA 74-75; Children's Mem Med Ctr, Chicago, IL 75-76; **FAP:** Assoc Prof Ped Northwestern U; **HOSP:** Evanston Hosp; ***SI:*** *Leukemia-Aplastic Anemia; Pediatric Cancer*; **HMO:** Aetna Hlth Plan, Blue Cross & Blue Shield, Chicago HMO, Maxicare Health Plan, Principal Health Care +
LANG: Sp; Immediately

Murphy, Sharon (MD) PHO
Children's Mem Med Ctr **(see page 139)**
Pediatric Oncology Group, 645 N Michigan Ave Ste 910; Chicago, IL 60611; (312) 482-9944; **BDCERT:** Ped 74; PHO 74; **MS:** Harvard Med Sch 69; **RES:** Ped, U CO Hosp, Denver, CO 70-71; **FEL:** PHO, Children's Hosp of Philadelphia, Philadelphia, PA 71-73; **FAP:** Prof Ped Northwestern U; **HMO:** Aetna Hlth Plan, Blue Cross & Blue Shield, Chicago HMO

Salvi, Sharad (MD) PHO
Christ Hosp & Med Ctr **(see page 140)**
Pediatric Cancer Institute, 4440 W 95th St; Oak Lawn, IL 60453; (708) 346-4094; **BDCERT:** Ped 82; PHO 82; **MS:** India 74; **RES:** Ped, Lincoln Med & Mental Hlth Ctr, Bronx, NY 77-79; **FEL:** PHO, Children's Hosp of Buffalo, Buffalo, NY 79-81; **HOSP:** Hinsdale Hosp; ***SI:*** *Leukemias & Cancers; Blood Disorders*; **HMO:** +
LANG: Hin, Guj, Ar, Sp;
A Few Days

Seeler, Ruth A (MD) PHO
Michael Reese Hosp & Med Ctr
840 S Wood St Fl 12; Chicago, IL 60612; (312) 567-7294; **BDCERT:** Ped 67; PHO 74; **MS:** Univ Vt Coll Med 62; **RES:** Ped, Bronx Muncipal Hosp Ctr, Bronx, NY 62-65; **FEL:** PHO, U IL Med Ctr, Chicago, IL 65-67; **FAP:** Prof Ped Univ IL Coll Med

Valentino, Leonard (MD) PHO
Rush-Presbyterian-St Luke's Med Ctr
(see page 122)
Rush Presbyterian St Luke's, 1725 W Harrison St Ste 718; Chicago, IL 60612; (312) 942-8114; **BDCERT:** Ped 88; **MS:** Creighton U 84; **RES:** Ped, U IL Med Ctr, Chicago, IL 84-87; **FEL:** PHO, UCLA Med Ctr, Los Angeles, CA 87-90; **HOSP:** Rush-Copley Med Ctr; ***SI:*** *Blood Clotting and Bleeding; Hemophilia*; **HMO:** +
LANG: Sp, Pol, Fr, Ger;
NFI A Few Days VISA

PEDIATRIC INFECTIOUS DISEASE

Daum, Robert S (MD) **Ped Inf**
Children's Mem Med Ctr **(see page 139)**
5426 S East View Park; Chicago, IL 60615; (773) 702-6176; **BDCERT:** Ped 91; **MS:** McGill U 72; **RES:** Ped, Montreal Children's Hosp, Montreal, Canada; **FEL:** Inf, Children's Hosp, Boston, MA; ***SI:*** *Antibiotic Resistance*
Immediately

Johnson, Daniel (MD) **Ped Inf**
Mount Sinai Hosp Med Ctr
Mt Sinai Hospital, California Ave at 15th St; Chicago, IL 60608; (773) 257-6474; **BDCERT:** Ped Inf 94; Ped 87; **MS:** Geo Wash U Sch Med 82; **RES:** Ped, Children's Hosp Med Ctr, Oakland, CA 82-85; **FEL:** Ped Inf, Children's Hosp Med Ctr, Oakland, CA 85-86; **HOSP:** U Chicago Hosp; ***SI:*** *HIV; Infectious Diseases*
LANG: Sp; A Few Days VISA

PEDIATRIC NEPHROLOGY

Clardy, Christopher (MD) **PNep**
Rush-Presbyterian-St Luke's Med Ctr **(see page 122)**
Pediatric Nephrology, 1725 W Harrison St Ste 718; Chicago, IL 60612; (312) 942-5000; **BDCERT:** Ped 87; PNep 88; **MS:** U Va Sch Med 81; **RES:** Ped, Vanderbilt U Med Ctr, Nashville, TN 82-84; **FEL:** Nep, Children's Hosp Med Ctr, Cincinnati, OH 84-87; **FAP:** Asst Prof Rush Med Coll

Kaplan, Richard (MD) **PNep**
Lutheran Gen Hosp **(see page 143)**
Avocate Medical Group, 1675 Dempster St; Park Ridge, IL 60068; (847) 318-9330; **BDCERT:** PNep 95; Ped 98; **MS:** Univ SD Sch Med 87; **HMO:** Blue Choice, Blue Cross & Blue Shield, HIP Network, HealthNet, Humana Health Plan

Langman, Craig (MD) **PNep**
Children's Mem Med Ctr **(see page 139)**
Childrens Memorial Hospital, 2300 N Childrens Plz Ste 69; Chicago, IL 60614; (773) 880-4326; **BDCERT:** Ped 82; PNep 92; **MS:** Hahnemann U 77; **RES:** Ped, Children's Hosp of Philadelphia, Philadelphia, PA 77-79; **FEL:** PNep, Children's Hosp of Philadelphia, Philadelphia, PA 79-81; **FAP:** Prof Ped Northwestern U; **HOSP:** Evanston Hosp; ***SI:*** *Metabolic bone diseases; Kidney Stones*; **HMO:** Aetna Hlth Plan, Blue Choice, Blue Cross & Blue Shield, Care America Health Plan, Century Medical Health Plan +
2-4 Weeks VISA

Lewy, Peter (MD) **PNep**
Evanston Hosp
Pediatric Assoc-The North Shr, 1149 Wilmette Ave; Wilmette, IL 60091; (847) 256-6480; **BDCERT:** PNep 74; Ped 69; **MS:** Case West Res U 64; **RES:** Ped, IL Rsch-Ed Hosps, Chicago, IL 65-67; **FEL:** Ped, Renal Dis-Michael Reese Hosp, Chicago, IL 69-70; Renal Dis - Northwestern U, Chicago, IL 70-71; **FAP:** Assoc Clin Prof Ped Northwestern U; **HMO:** Aetna Hlth Plan, Blue Cross & Blue Shield, Chicago HMO, CIGNA, Humana Health Plan

Miller, Kenneth (MD) **PNep**
Lutheran Gen Hosp **(see page 143)**
Nephrology & Hypertension, 1550 N Northwest Hwy Ste 221; Park Ridge, IL 60068; (847) 297-6374; **BDCERT:** Ped 74; PNep 76; **MS:** U Hlth Sci/Chicago Med Sch 68; **RES:** Ped A&I, Minnesota Hosp, Minneapolis, MN 71-73; **FEL:** Ped A&I, Minnesota Hosp, Minneapolis, MN 73-75; **FAP:** Asst Prof Ped Rush Med Coll; ***SI:*** *Hypertension; Enuresis*; **HMO:** Aetna Hlth Plan, Blue Cross & Blue Shield, Californiacare, Humana Health Plan, CIGNA +
A Few Days VISA

PEDIATRIC OTOLARYNGOLOGY

Dunham, Michael E (MD) **POto**
Children's Mem Med Ctr **(see page 139)**
2300 Children's Plz; Chicago, IL 60614; (773) 880-4533; **BDCERT:** Oto 83; **MS:** Tulane U 78; **RES:** Oto, Tulane U, New Orleans, LA 79-82; **FEL:** Ped Oto, Children's Mem Hosp, Chicago, IL 90-91; **HOSP:** Glenbrook Hosp; **HMO:** +
LANG: Sp; 2-4 Weeks VISA

PEDIATRIC PULMONOLOGY

Thomas, Dolly (MD) **PPul**
Illinois Masonic Med Ctr
(see page 118)
520 E Northwest Hwy; Mt Prospect, IL 60056; (847) 255-3050; **BDCERT:** A&I 87; PPul 98; **MS:** India 77; **RES:** Ped, Illinois Masonic Med Ctr, Chicago, IL 79-82; **FEL:** A&I, U Chicago Hosp, Chicago, IL 82-84; **FAP:** Asst Prof Rush Med Coll; **HOSP:** Northwest Comm Hlthcare; ***SI:*** *Asthma; Lung Diseases of Children*; **HMO:** Blue Cross & Blue Shield, Aetna Hlth Plan, United Healthcare, Prudential +
LANG: Sp, Mly;
A Few Days

PEDIATRIC RADIOLOGY

Fernbach, Sandra (MD) **PR**
Evanston Hosp
Evanston Hospital, 2650 Ridge Ave; Evanston, IL 60201; (847) 570-2475; **BDCERT:** Rad 79; PR 94; **MS:** Johns Hopkins U 75; **RES:** Rad, Montefiore Med Ctr, Bronx, NY 76-79; **FEL:** PR, Children's Hosp, Boston, MA 79-90; **FAP:** Prof Rad Northwestern U

Poznanski, Andrew (MD) **PR**
Children's Mem Med Ctr **(see page 139)**
Childrens Memorial Hospital, 2300 N Childrens Plz Ste 69; Chicago, IL 60614; (773) 880-3520; **BDCERT:** Rad 61; PR 94; **MS:** Canada 56; **RES:** Henry Ford Hosp, Detroit, MI 57-60; **FAP:** Prof Rad Northwestern U; ***SI:*** *Pediatric Radiology*; **HMO:** Blue Choice, Chicago HMO, CIGNA, United Healthcare

Ramilo, Jose (MD) **PR**
Christ Hosp & Med Ctr **(see page 140)**
Oaklawn Radiology, 4440 W 95th St; Oak Lawn, IL 60453; (708) 346-5520; **BDCERT:** PR 95; DR 76; **MS:** Philippines 64; **RES:** Ped, Cook Cty Hosp, Chicago, IL 68-69; DR, Cook Cty Hosp, Chicago, IL 72-75

Shkolnik, Arnold (MD) **PR**
Children's Mem Med Ctr **(see page 139)**
Childrens Memorial Med Ctr, 2300 Childrens Plz; Chicago, IL 60614; (773) 880-3532; **BDCERT:** Ped 64; Rad 71; **MS:** U Hlth Sci/Chicago Med Sch 55; **RES:** Ped, Cook Cty Hosp, Chicago, IL 56-61; Rad, Cook Cty Hosp, Chicago, IL 66-69; **FEL:** PR, Children's Mem Med Ctr, Chicago, IL 69-70; **FAP:** Prof Rad Northwestern U

PEDIATRIC RHEUMATOLOGY

Klein-Gitelman, Marisa (MD) **Ped Rhu**
Children's Mem Med Ctr **(see page 139)**
Children's Memorial Hosp, 2300 Children's Plaza Ste 50; Chicago, IL 60614; (773) 880-4360; **BDCERT:** Ped 89; Ped Rhu 94; **MS:** Washington U, St Louis 85; **RES:** Ped, Columbia-Presbyterian Med Ctr, New York, NY 86-88; Ped, Columbia-Presbyterian Med Ctr, New York, NY 88-89; **FEL:** Ped Rhu, Tufts U, Boston, MA 89-93; **FAP:** Asst Prof Ped Northwestern U; ***SI:*** *Lupus; Childhood Arthritis*; **HMO:** Blue Cross & Blue Shield, Blue Choice, Humana Health Plan, HMO Illinois +
A Few Days VISA

Spencer, Charles (MD) **Ped Rhu**
La Rabida Children's Hosp
La Rabida Hosp, E 65th at Lake Michigan; Chicago, IL 60649; (773) 363-6700; **BDCERT:** Ped Rhu 94; Ped 79; **MS:** LSU Med Ctr, Shreveport 73; **RES:** Ped A&I, USC Med Ctr, Los Angeles, CA 74-77; **FEL:** Ped Rhu, Children's Hosp, Los Angeles, CA 77-79; **HOSP:** Lutheran Gen Hosp

PEDIATRIC SURGERY

Arensman, Robert (MD) **PdS**
Children's Mem Med Ctr **(see page 139)**
Children's Mem Hosp, 2300 Children's Plz Ste 115; Chicago, IL 60614; (773) 880-4999; **BDCERT:** PdS 89; S 79; **MS:** Univ IL Coll Med 69; **RES:** S, U IL Med Ctr, Chicago, IL 70-72; S, U IL Med Ctr, Chicago, IL 74-76; **FEL:** PdS, Children's Hosp Nat Med Ctr, Washington, DC 76-78; **FAP:** Prof PdS U Chicago-Pritzker Sch Med
LANG: Fr, Sp;
Immediately VISA

Backer, Carl (MD) **PdS**
Children's Mem Med Ctr **(see page 139)**
Childrens Surgical Foundation, 2300 N Childrens Plaza Box 22; Chicago, IL 60614; (773) 880-4378; **BDCERT:** S 86; TS 88; **MS:** Mayo Med Sch 80; **RES:** S, Northwestern Mem Hosp, Chicago, IL 80-85; Northwestern Mem Hosp, Chicago, IL 85-87; **FEL:** PCd, Children's Mem Med Ctr, Chicago, IL 87-88; **FAP:** Assoc Prof S Northwestern U; **HOSP:** Northwestern Mem Hosp; ***SI:*** *Cardiac Transplantation; Tracheal Surgery*; **HMO:** Blue Cross, Aetna Hlth Plan, United Healthcare, Private Healthcare +
LANG: Sp, Ger, Fr, Grk;
Immediately

Bassuk, Angel (MD) **PdS**
Christ Hosp & Med Ctr **(see page 140)**
15000 S Califorina Ave; Chicago, IL 60608; (773) 257-6058; **BDCERT:** PdS 97; S 76; **MS:** Argentina 68; **RES:** IM, Albert Einstein Med Ctr, Philadelphia, PA 69-70; Hosp Med College of PA, Philadelphia, PA 70-73; **FEL:** PdS, Temple U Hosp, Philadelphia, PA 73-75; **FAP:** Asst Prof Rush Med Coll; **HOSP:** Mount Sinai Hosp Med Ctr

Chwals, Walter (MD) **PdS**
U Chicago Hosp **(see page 124)**
Children's Hospital, 5841 S Maryland Ave; Chicago, IL 60637; (773) 702-6175; **BDCERT:** S 95; PdS 90; **MS:** Poland 80; **RES:** S, U Mass Med Ctr, Worcester, MA 81-85; PdS, Children's Hosp of Los Angeles, Los Angeles, CA 86-88; **FEL:** S, New England Deaconess Hosp, Boston, MA 85-86; **HMO:** +
LANG: Pol; 2-4 Weeks

Loeff, Deborah (MD) **PdS**
Lutheran Gen Hosp **(see page 143)**
4400 W 95th St Ste 108; Oak Lawn, IL 60453; (708) 424-7541; **BDCERT:** S 96; PdS 90; **MS:** Rush Med Coll 77; **RES:** S, U UT Hosp, Salt Lake City, UT 78-79; S, U UT Hosp, Salt Lake City, UT 79-84; **FEL:** Ped S, Hosp For Sick Children, Toronto, Canada 84-86; **FAP:** Asst Prof S Rush Med Coll; **HOSP:** Rush-Presbyterian-St Luke's Med Ctr; ***SI:*** *Congenital Anomalies; Cancer Surgery in Children*; **HMO:** Blue Cross & Blue Shield, Aetna Hlth Plan, Bay State Health Plan, John Hancock, Rush Health Plans +
Immediately

Radhakrishnan, Jayant (MD) **PdS**
Univ of Illinois at Chicago Med Ctr
2454 E Dempster St Ste 406; Des Plaines, IL 60016; (847) 390-0330; **BDCERT:** S 77; **MS:** India 67; **RES:** S, Cook Cty Hosp, Chicago, IL 72-76; **FEL:** PdS, Cook Cty Hosp, Chicago, IL 76-78; **HOSP:** Lutheran Gen Hosp

Reyes, Hernan M (MD) **PdS**
Rush-Presbyterian-St Luke's Med Ctr **(see page 122)**
1835 W Harrison St Ste M-2200; Chicago, IL 60612; (312) 633-8207; **BDCERT:** S 65; PdS 95; **MS:** Philippines 57; **RES:** S, Cook Cty Hosp, Chicago, IL 59-65; **FEL:** PdS, Cook Cty Hosp, Chicago, IL 64-65; **FAP:** Prof S Rush Med Coll; **HOSP:** Cook Cty Hosp; ***SI:*** *Pediatric Tumors; Pediatric Anomalies/Trauma*; **HMO:** Rush Prudential, Aetna Hlth Plan, CIGNA, Humana Health Plan, Private Healthcare +
Immediately

Sarwark, John (MD) **PdS**
Children's Mem Med Ctr **(see page 139)**
Pediatric Orthopaedic Surgery, 2300 Children's Plaza Ste 69; Chicago, IL 60614; (773) 880-4271; **BDCERT:** OrS 98; **MS:** Northwestern U 79; **RES:** OrS, Northwestern Mem Hosp, Chicago, IL 80-84; **FEL:** Ped, Alfred Du Point Inst, Wilmington, DE 84-85; **FAP:** Assoc Prof Northwestern U; **HOSP:** Evanston Hosp; ***SI:*** *Pediatric Orthopaedics; Scoliosis*; **HMO:** Aetna-US Healthcare, Blue Choice, Humana Health Plan, United Healthcare
LANG: Sp, Pol; 2-4 Weeks
VISA

PEDIATRICS

Barrows, William (MD) **Ped**
PCP
Michael Reese Hosp & Med Ctr
233 E Erie St Ste 304; Chicago, IL 60611; (312) 280-1480; **BDCERT:** Ped 85; **MS:** U Hlth Sci/Chicago Med Sch 80; **RES:** Michael Reese Hosp Med Ctr, Chicago, IL 80-83; **FAP:** Instr Northwestern U; **HOSP:** Rush-Presbyterian-St Luke's Med Ctr; **HMO:** +

Benuck, Irwin (MD) **Ped**
PCP
Children's Mem Med Ctr **(see page 139)**
Traisman Benuck & Traisman, 1325 Howard St Ste 203; Evanston, IL 60202; (847) 869-4300; **BDCERT:** Ped 84; **MS:** Northwestern U 79; **RES:** Children's Mem Med Ctr, Chicago, IL 80-82; **FAP:** Assoc Prof of Clin Ped Northwestern U; **HMO:** Aetna Hlth Plan, Blue Cross & Blue Shield

Blackwell, Mable (MD) **Ped**
Univ of Illinois at Chicago Med Ctr
2121 W Sailer Ave; Chicago, IL 60612; (773) 413-0182; **BDCERT:** Ped 84; **MS:** Univ IL Coll Med 78

Boblick, John (MD) **Ped**
PCP
Elmhurst Mem Hosp
7005 North Ave; Oak Park, IL 60302; (708) 383-8888; **BDCERT:** Ped 96; IM 86; **MS:** Univ IL Coll Med 82; **HOSP:** Loyola U Med Ctr

Boyer, Kenneth (MD) **Ped**
Rush-Presbyterian-St Luke's Med Ctr **(see page 122)**
Rush Presbyterian-St Lukes Hosp, 1653 W Congress Pkwy Ste 718; Chicago, IL 60612; (312) 942-6396; **BDCERT:** Ped 77; Ped Inf 94; **MS:** Univ Penn 70; **RES:** IM, Cleveland Metro Gen Hosp, Cleveland, OH 70-71; Ped, Rainbow Babies & Children's Hosp, Cleveland, OH 71-75; **FEL:** Ped Inf, UCLA Med Ctr, Los Angeles, CA 75-77; **FAP:** Prof Rush Med Coll; **HOSP:** Cook Cty Hosp; ***SI:*** *Pediatric HIV Infection; Travel Immunizations*; **HMO:** Humana Health Plan, United Healthcare, CIGNA, Bc/BS, Aetna Hlth Plan +
LANG: Sp, Fil;
A Few Days

Brown, Donald (MD) Ped
PCP
Children's Mem Med Ctr (see page 139)
233 E Erie Street Ste 304; Chicago, IL 60611; **BDCERT:** Ped 97; **MS:** Univ IL Coll Med 84; **RES:** Ped, U Chicago Hosp, Chicago, IL 84-88; **FAP:** Assoc Clin Prof Ped Northwestern U; **HOSP:** Rush-Presbyterian-St Luke's Med Ctr; ***SI:** Child Development; Respiratory Disorders*
Immediately VISA

Burnet, Deborah (MD) Ped
PCP
U Chicago Hosp (see page 124)
University of Chicago Phys, 5841 S Maryland Ave Ste 3051; Chicago, IL 60637; (773) 702-6840; **BDCERT:** Ped 93; IM 93; **MS:** U Chicago-Pritzker Sch Med 89; **RES:** Ped, U Chicago Hosp, Chicago, IL 90-93; **FAP:** Asst Prof Ped U Chicago-Pritzker Sch Med

Burnstine, Richard (MD) Ped
PCP
Evanston Hosp
North Suburban Pediatrics, 1215 Old McHenry Rd; Buffalo Grove, IL 60089; (847) 913-9120; **BDCERT:** Ped 89; **MS:** Harvard Med Sch 54; **RES:** Ped, NY Hosp-Cornell Med Ctr, New York, NY 55-56; Ped, Children's Hosp, Boston, MA 56-57; **FEL:** Liver Disease, Boston Med Ctr, Boston, MA 60-61; **FAP:** Asst Prof of Clin Ped Northwestern U; **HOSP:** Children's Mem Med Ctr; ***SI:** Digestion Problems; Allergies*; **HMO:** Blue Cross & Blue Shield, CIGNA, Preferred Plan, Rush Prudential +
Immediately VISA

Cabrera, Bertha (MD) Ped
PCP
St Mary's of Nazareth Hosp Ctr
2569 W Fullerton Ave; Chicago, IL 60647; (773) 252-8050; **BDCERT:** Ped 96; **MS:** Dominican Republic 80; **RES:** Cook Cty Hosp, Chicago, IL 82-84; **FEL:** Cook Cty Hosp, Chicago, IL 84-85

Chande, Sumitra (MD) Ped
PCP
Christ Hosp & Med Ctr (see page 140)
Southwest Physicians Group, 4861 W 95th St; Oak Lawn, IL 60453; (708) 425-4488; **BDCERT:** Ped 80; **MS:** India 67; **RES:** Ped, St Jude Children's Hosp, Memphis, TN 76; Ped, Christ Hosp & Med Ctr, Oak Lawn, IL 77; **HMO:** Aetna Hlth Plan, Blue Cross & Blue Shield

Chaudhary, Mohammad Y (MD) Ped
PCP
Bethany Hosp
Bethany Hosp, 3435 W Van Buren St; Chicago, IL 60624; (773) 265-3579; **BDCERT:** Ped 76; **MS:** Pakistan 66; **RES:** Ped, Cook Co Hosp, Chicago, IL 72-74; **FEL:** Cook Co Hosp, Chicago, IL 74-75; ***SI:** Ambulatory Pediatrics*; **HMO:** +
Mcr Mcd A Few Days VISA

Ciskoski, Ronald (MD) Ped
PCP
St Francis Hosp
Northshore Medical Group, 800 Austin St Ste 463; Evanston, IL 60202; (847) 475-8711; **BDCERT:** Ped 68; **MS:** Univ IL Coll Med 62; **RES:** St Francis Hosp of Evanston, Evanston, IL 63-65; **HMO:** Blue Cross & Blue Shield, CIGNA, Metlife

Clark, Aleta (MD) Ped
PCP
Northwestern Mem Hosp
Child & Adolescent Health, 1030 N Clark St Ste 400; Chicago, IL 60610; (312) 943-6964; **BDCERT:** Ped 79; **MS:** Northwestern U 74; **RES:** Ped, Children's Mem Med Ctr, Chicago, IL 74-76; Ped, Children's Mem Med Ctr, Chicago, IL 76-78; **HOSP:** Children's Mem Med Ctr; **HMO:** HealthNet, Principal Health Care +
Immediately VISA

Cohn, Richard (MD) Ped
PCP
Children's Mem Med Ctr (see page 139)
Childrens Memorial Med Ctr, 2300 Childrens Plaza; Chicago, IL 60614; (773) 880-4326; **BDCERT:** Ped 78; PNep 79; **MS:** Albert Einstein Coll Med 72; **RES:** Ped, Johns Hopkins Hosp, Baltimore, MD 73-75; PNep, Minnesota Hosp, Minneapolis, MN 75-78; **FAP:** Assoc Prof Ped Northwestern U

Collins, Mary Ann (MD) Ped
PCP
Christ Hosp & Med Ctr (see page 140)
Pediatric Health Partners, 3900 W 95th St Ste 1; Evergreen Park, IL 60805; (708) 636-0700; **BDCERT:** Ped 85; **MS:** Ind U Sch Med 80; **RES:** U Chicago Hosp, Chicago, IL 81-83; **FEL:** Ped Inf, U Chicago Hosp, Chicago, IL 83-85; **FAP:** Asst Prof of Clin Ped U Chicago-Pritzker Sch Med

Cueva, John Paul (MD) Ped
PCP
Christ Hosp & Med Ctr (see page 140)
Preventive Pediatrics, 3456 W 79th St; Chicago, IL 60652; (773) 737-1990; **BDCERT:** Ped 97; **MS:** Mexico 85; **RES:** Christ Hosp & Med Ctr, Oak Lawn, IL 91-93

Cupeles, Angela B (MD) Ped
PCP
St Mary's of Nazareth Hosp Ctr
2056 W Division; Chicago, IL 60622; (773) 235-4822; **BDCERT:** Ped 83; **MS:** Northwestern U 78; **HMO:** United Healthcare, Aetna Hlth Plan, Prudential +
LANG: Sp; Immediately

De Bofsky, Harvey (MD) Ped
PCP
Trinity Hosp
Harvey De Bofsky Ltd, 2315 E 93rd St Ste 300; Chicago, IL 60617; (773) 978-2000; **BDCERT:** Ped 64; **MS:** Univ IL Coll Med 57; **RES:** Ped, Michael Reese Hosp Med Ctr, Chicago, IL 58-60; **FAP:** Assoc Clin Prof U Chicago-Pritzker Sch Med; **HOSP:** Michael Reese Hosp & Med Ctr; ***SI:** Infectious Diseases*; **HMO:** Aetna Hlth Plan, Blue Cross & Blue Shield, Californiacare, CIGNA, PHCS +
LANG: Sp;
A Few Days

De Paul, Virginia (MD) Ped
PCP
Evanston Hosp
North Suburban Pediatrics, 2530 Ridge Ave Ste 201; Evanston, IL 60201; (847) 869-0892; **BDCERT:** Ped 87; **MS:** Univ IL Coll Med 81; **RES:** Ped, Michael Reese Hosp Med Ctr, Chicago, IL 85; **FAP:** Instr Northwestern U

De Stefani, Thomas (MD) Ped
PCP
Loyola U Med Ctr (see page 120)
Loyola University Medical Center, 2160 S 1st Ave; Maywood, IL 60402; (630) 627-7399; **BDCERT:** Ped 86; **MS:** Loyola U-Stritch Sch Med, Maywood 81; **RES:** Ped, Loyola U Med Ctr, Maywood, IL 81-84; **FAP:** Asst Prof Ped Loyola U-Stritch Sch Med, Maywood

Dechovitz, Arthur (MD) Ped
PCP
Evanston Hosp
North Suburban Pediatrics, 2530 Ridge Ave Ste 201; Evanston, IL 60201; (847) 869-0892; **BDCERT:** Ped 69; **MS:** Emory U Sch Med 64; **RES:** Ped, Children's Mem Med Ctr, Chicago, IL 64-67; **FAP:** Asst Clin Prof Ped Northwestern U; **HOSP:** Children's Mem Med Ctr; ***SI:** Infections Disease; Ear Infections*; **HMO:** Blue Cross & Blue Shield, Chicago HMO, FHP Inc, Aetna Hlth Plan, CIGNA +
LANG: Sp, Itl, Pol;
A Few Days VISA

Delach, Anthony (MD) Ped
PCP
Christ Hosp & Med Ctr (see page 140)
South West Pediatrics Ltd, 8100 W 119th St; Palos Park, IL 60464; (708) 361-3300; **BDCERT:** Ped 85; **MS:** Mexico 78; **RES:** Ped, U Ill Med Ctr, Chicago, IL 79-82; **FAP:** Sr Clin Instr Rush Med Coll; **HOSP:** Palos Comm Hosp

Diamond, Sean (MD) Ped
PCP
Loyola U Med Ctr (see page 120)
Orland Pediatrics, 15300 West Ave Ste 303; Orland Park, IL 60462; (708) 403-0167; **BDCERT:** Ped 96; **MS:** Loyola U-Stritch Sch Med, Maywood 84; **HOSP:** Palos Comm Hosp

Downey, James (MD) Ped
PCP
Evanston Hosp
North Suburban Pediatrics, 2530 Ridge Ave Ste 201; Evanston, IL 60201; (847) 869-0892; **BDCERT:** Ped 65; **MS:** Columbia P&S 60; **RES:** Ped, Columbia-Presbyterian Med Ctr, New York, NY 61-63; **FAP:** Asst Clin Prof Ped Northwestern U

Espinosa, Roberto (MD) Ped
PCP
Swedish Covenant Hosp
5140 N California Ave Ste 705; Chicago, IL 60625; (773) 561-0088; **BDCERT:** Ped 71; **MS:** Colombia 61; **RES:** Ped, Children's Mem Med Ctr, Chicago, IL 66-68; **FEL:** PNep, Children's Mem Med Ctr, Chicago, IL 69; ***SI:** Asthma; Allergy*; **HMO:** Aetna Hlth Plan, CIGNA, Blue Cross & Blue Shield, Health Preferred, Northwestern POS +
LANG: Sp; 1 Week
VISA

Esposito, Patrick (MD) Ped
PCP
St Alexius Med Ctr
Associates In Pediatrics, 1020 E Schaumburg Rd; Streamwood, IL 60107; (630) 830-1930; **BDCERT:** Ped 93; **MS:** U Hlth Sci/Chicago Med Sch 88; **RES:** Lutheran Gen Hosp, Park Ridge, IL 88-91; **HOSP:** Sherman Hosp; **HMO:** Blue Cross & Blue Shield, Aetna Hlth Plan, Rush Prudential, Prudential, CIGNA

Frank, Arthur L (MD) Ped
Univ of Illinois at Chicago Med Ctr
Univ of Illinois-Chicago Med Ctr-Pd Infectious Disease, 840 S Wood St Ste 1224; Chicago, IL 60612; (312) 996-8109; **BDCERT:** Ped 75; Ped Inf 94; **MS:** Stanford U 69; **RES:** Ped, Children's Hosp, Boston, MA 72-74; **FEL:** Inf, Yale-New Haven Hosp, New Haven, CT 74-77; **FAP:** Assoc Prof Ped Univ IL Coll Med; ***SI:** Infectious Disease*

Freed, Marc (DO) Ped
PCP
Macneal Mem Hosp
University of Chicago, 3245 Grove Ave Ste 206; Berwyn, IL 60402; (708) 795-7005; **BDCERT:** Ped 97; **MS:** Philadelphia Coll Osteo Med 80; **RES:** Ped, Rush Presbyterian-St Luke's Med Ctr, Chicago, IL 81-85

Gruszka, Mary (MD) Ped
PCP
Macneal Mem Hosp
Mukhopadhyay & Assoc, 3245 Grove Ave Ste 206; Berwyn, IL 60402; (708) 795-7005; **BDCERT:** Ped 84; **MS:** Rush Med Coll 79; **RES:** Ped, Children's Mem Med Ctr, Chicago, IL 80-82; **FAP:** Asst Prof Loyola U-Stritch Sch Med, Maywood; **HOSP:** La Grange Mem Hosp; **HMO:** Blue Cross & Blue Shield, Prudential, Travelers
2-4 Weeks VISA

Hankin, Bernard (MD) Ped
PCP
Evanston Hosp
Doblin Hankin & Lee, 9669 Kenton Ave Ste 403; Skokie, IL 60076; (847) 674-4730; **BDCERT:** Ped 62; **MS:** Univ IL Coll Med 53; **RES:** Ped, Cook Cty Hosp, Chicago, IL 54-55; Ped, Children's Mem Med Ctr, Chicago, IL 57-58

Hanna, Wafaa (MD) Ped
PCP
South Suburban Hosp
Richton Park Medical Offices, 4511 Sauk Trail; Richton Park, IL 60471; (708) 283-0300; **BDCERT:** Ped 94; **MS:** Egypt 83; **RES:** Ped, Christ Hosp & Med Ctr, Oak Lawn, IL; Ped, South Suburban Hosp, Hazel Crest, IL; **HOSP:** Christ Hosp & Med Ctr; **HMO:** +
LANG: Sp, Hin; 1 Week
VISA

Harris, George (MD) Ped
PCP
Christ Hosp & Med Ctr (see page 140)
South West Pediatrics Ltd, 8100 W 119th St; Palos Park, IL 60464; (708) 361-3300; **BDCERT:** Ped 98; **MS:** Univ IL Coll Med 75; **RES:** Illinois Masonic Med Ctr, Chicago, IL 75-78; **FAP:** Asst Clin Prof Rush Med Coll; **HMO:** Aetna Hlth Plan, Blue Cross & Blue Shield, Californiacare, Humana Health Plan, Metlife

Havalad, Suresh (MD) Ped
Lutheran Gen Hosp (see page 143)
1775 Dempster St; Park Ridge, IL 60068; (847) 696-2210; **BDCERT:** Ped 89; PCCM 92; **MS:** India 74; **RES:** Ped, Lutheran Gen Hosp, Park Ridge, IL 83-85; NP, Lutheran Gen Hosp, Park Ridge, IL 85-87

Hoess, Cynthia (MD) Ped
PCP
Rush-Presbyterian-St Luke's Med Ctr (see page 122)
1645 W Jackson St Ste 200; Chicago, IL 60612; (312) 492-7337; **BDCERT:** Ped 92; **MS:** MC Ohio, Toledo 88; **RES:** Children's Hosp of Pittsburgh, Pittsburgh, PA 89-91

Holland, Julie (MD) Ped
PCP
Evanston Hosp
1000 Central Ste 765; Evanston, IL 60201; (847) 570-1507; **BDCERT:** Ped 92; **MS:** Northwestern U 89; **RES:** Ped, UC San Francisco Med Ctr, San Francisco, CA

Honig, George (MD) Ped
Univ of Illinois at Chicago Med Ctr
University of IL Medical Ctr - Ped Dept, 840 S Wood St; Chicago, IL 60612; (312) 996-8297; **BDCERT:** Ped 86; PHO 86; **MS:** Univ IL Coll Med 61; **RES:** Johns Hopkins Hosp, Baltimore, MD 62-63; PHO, U IL Med Ctr, Chicago, IL 66-68; **FAP:** Prof Univ IL Coll Med; ***SI:*** *Hematology Oncology*

Hrycelak, Maria (MD) Ped
PCP
Lutheran Gen Hosp (see page 143)
Parkridge Pediatrics, 101 S Washington Ave Ste 122; Park Ridge, IL 60068; (847) 692-6628; **BDCERT:** Ped 86; **MS:** Loyola U-Stritch Sch Med, Maywood 80; **RES:** Ped, Lutheran Gen Hosp, Park Ridge, IL 77-80; **HMO:** Blue Cross & Blue Shield, Principal Health Care

Ingall, David (MD) Ped
Evanston Hosp
Department of Pediatrics, 2650 Ridge Ave Ste 1610WH; Evanston, IL 60201; (847) 570-2530; **BDCERT:** Ped 62; NP 77; **MS:** Boston U 57; **RES:** Ped, Boston Med Ctr, Boston, MA 57-60; **FAP:** Prof Northwestern U; ***SI:*** *Neonatology*
2-4 Weeks

Jacob, Molly (MD) Ped
PCP
Illinois Masonic Med Ctr
(see page 118)
4315 N Lincoln Ave; Chicago, IL 60618; (773) 528-3403; **BDCERT:** Ped 80; **MS:** India 68; **RES:** Ped, Illinois Masonic Med Ctr, Chicago, IL 75-79; **FEL:** Ambulatory Care, Illinois Masonic Med Ctr, Chicago, IL 78-79

Jaudes, Paula (MD) Ped
PCP
La Rabida Children's Hosp
La Rabida Children's Hosp & Research Ctr, E 65th St; Chicago, IL 60649; (773) 363-6700; **BDCERT:** Ped 80; **MS:** Rush Med Coll 75; **RES:** Ped A&I, U Chicago Hosp, Chicago, IL 76-78; **FEL:** Ambulatory Ped, U Chicago Hosp, Chicago, IL 78-79; **FAP:** Prof U Chicago-Pritzker Sch Med

Jay, Mary Susan (MD) Ped
Loyola U Med Ctr (see page 120)
Loyola U-Stritch School of Med, 2160 S 1st Ave; Maywood, IL 60153; (708) 327-9119; **BDCERT:** Ped 81; AM 94; **MS:** Univ IL Coll Med 76; **FAP:** AM Loyola U-Stritch Sch Med, Maywood
Immediately

John, Eunice (MD) Ped
PCP
Univ of Illinois at Chicago Med Ctr
840 S Wood St MC856; Chicago, IL 60612; (312) 996-6711; **BDCERT:** Ped 73; PNep 76; **MS:** India 64; **RES:** Ped, McCook Hosp, Hartford, CT 70-71; Ped, Charity Hosp, New Orleans, LA 71-73; **FEL:** PNep, Albert Einstein Med Ctr, Bronx, NY 73-76; **FAP:** Chf PNep Univ IL Coll Med; **HOSP:** Michael Reese Hosp & Med Ctr; **SI:** *Bed Wetting; Kidney Failure Dialysis*; **HMO:** Humana Health Plan, United Healthcare, American Health Plan
LANG: Kan, Sp, Pol, Hin; A Few Days VISA

Johnstone, Helen (MD) Ped
Univ of Illinois at Chicago Med Ctr
University of IL Hospital, 840 S Wood St Ste 1001; Chicago, IL 60612; (312) 299-6143; **BDCERT:** Ped 70; PHO 74; **MS:** Univ IL Coll Med 64; **RES:** Ped, Children's Hosp Med Ctr, Cincinnati, OH 65-67; **FEL:** PHO, U IL Med Ctr, Chicago, IL 67-70; **FAP:** Assoc Prof Univ IL Coll Med; **HOSP:** Michael Reese Hosp & Med Ctr; **SI:** *Acute Leukemia; Sickle Cell Disease*; **HMO:** Humana Health Plan, United Healthcare, American HMO, Advocate, Aetna Hlth Plan +
Mcd A Few Days

Kalichman, Miriam (MD) Ped
Univ of Illinois at Chicago Med Ctr
Center For Handicapped Children, 820 S Wood St Ste 145; Chicago, IL 60612; (312) 996-7202; **BDCERT:** Ped 82; **MS:** U Mich Med Sch 77; **RES:** Ped A&I, Children's Mem Med Ctr, Chicago, IL 77-80; **FEL:** Develpmental Disabilities, Children's Hosp of Philadelphia, Philadelphia, PA 80-82; **FAP:** Assoc Clin Prof Univ IL Coll Med; **SI:** *Cerebral Palsy & Developmental Disabilities; Spina Bifida*; **HMO:** +
LANG: Sp; Mcr Mcd NFI 2-4 Weeks

Kaufman, Jonathan (MD) Ped
PCP
Good Shepherd Hosp
Pediatric Associates, 450 W State Route 22 Ste 2; Barrington, IL 60010; (847) 381-6700; **BDCERT:** Ped 97; **MS:** U Hlth Sci/Chicago Med Sch 85; **RES:** Ped, U IL Med Ctr, Chicago, IL 88-89; Ped, U IL Med Ctr, Chicago, IL 85-88; **HMO:** Aetna Hlth Plan, Blue Cross & Blue Shield, Travelers, United Healthcare

Kaye, Bennett (MD) Ped
PCP
Children's Mem Med Ctr (see page 139)
Childrens Health Care Assoc, 2551 N Clark St Ste 200; Chicago, IL 60614; (773) 348-8300; **BDCERT:** Ped 83; **MS:** Univ IL Coll Med 78; **RES:** Ped, Michael Reese Hosp Med Ctr, Chicago, IL 78-81; **FAP:** Assistant Prof Ped Northwestern U; **HOSP:** Northwestern Mem Hosp; **SI:** *Preventive Medicine; Growth And Development*; **HMO:** Blue Choice, Blue Cross, Bay State Health Plan, Prudential, Guardian
SA SU Mcd 1 Week VISA

Kramer, Jane (MD) Ped
PCP
Rush-Presbyterian-St Luke's Med Ctr (see page 122)
Rush Presby St Lukes, 1653 W Congress Pkwy; Chicago, IL 60612; (312) 942-4978; **BDCERT:** Ped 83; Ped EM 94; **MS:** Northwestern U 76; **RES:** pPed, Michael Reese Hosp Med Ctr, Chicago, IL 76-79; **FAP:** Asst Prof Rush Med Coll

Lantos, John David (MD) Ped
PCP
U Chicago Hosp (see page 124)
5841 S Maryland Ave W732; Chicago, IL 60637; (773) 702-9107; **BDCERT:** Ped 86; **MS:** Univ Pittsburgh 81; **RES:** Ped, Children's Hosp Natl Med Ctr, Washington, DC 82-84; **FEL:** Clinical Ethics, U Chicago Hosp, Chicago, IL 86

Linares, Oscar (MD) Ped
PCP
St Anthony Hosp
5401 W Cermack Rd; Cicero, IL 60804; (708) 652-2442; **BDCERT:** Ped 95; **MS:** Colombia 84; **RES:** Columbus Hosp, Chicago, IL 92-94; **HMO:** +
LANG: Sp; SA SU Mcd 2-4 Weeks

Listernick, Robert (MD) Ped
Children's Mem Med Ctr (see page 139)
2300 Children's Plz; Chicago, IL 60614; (773) 880-3830; **BDCERT:** Ped 84; **MS:** Univ Penn 79

Lotsu, Solace (MD) Ped
PCP
Columbus Hosp
467 W Deming Place; Glencoe, IL 60614; (773) 327-7238; **BDCERT:** Ped 79; **MS:** Ghana 72; **RES:** Ped, Waterbury Hosp, Waterbury, CT 75-76; Ped, U Conn Hlth Ctr, Farmington, CT 76-77

Matray, Mark (MD) Ped
PCP
La Grange Mem Hosp (see page 141)
La Grange Pediatrics Ltd, 51 Garden Market St; Western Springs, IL 60558; (708) 784-1700; **BDCERT:** Ped 85; **MS:** Loyola U-Stritch Sch Med, Maywood 80; **RES:** Children's Mem Med Ctr, Chicago, IL 81-83

Narayan, M S Laxmi (MD) Ped
PCP
Rush-Presbyterian-St Luke's Med Ctr (see page 122)
1725 W Harrison St Ste 940; Chicago, IL 60612; (312) 421-5076; **BDCERT:** Ped 71; PEn 78; **MS:** India 66; **RES:** Cook Cty Hosp, Chicago, IL 68-70; **FEL:** PEn, Cook Cty Hosp, Chicago, IL 70-71; **FAP:** Asst Prof Rush Med Coll
Mcr

Noah, Zehava (MD) Ped
PCP
Children's Mem Med Ctr (see page 139)
Childrens Memorial Hospital, 2300 N Childrens Plz Ste 69; Chicago, IL 60614; (773) 880-4000; **BDCERT:** Ped 81; PCCM 96; **MS:** Israel 69; **RES:** Ped A&I, Shaarei Zedek Genl Hosp, Jersualem, Israel 70-73; NP, John Radcliffe Hosp, Oxford, England 73-74; **FEL:** PdAnes, Chldns Meml Hosp, Chicago, IL; **FAP:** Asst Prof Ped Northwestern U

Paterek, Malgorzata (MD) Ped
PCP
Columbus Hosp
Catholic Health Partners - Pediatrics, 2520 N Lakeview Ave; Chicago, IL 60614; (773) 725-5400; **BDCERT:** Ped 97; **MS:** Poland 80

Pervos, Richard (MD) Ped
PCP
Lutheran Gen Hosp (see page 143)
4113 Dundee Rd; Park Ridge, IL 60062; (847) 272-1005; **BDCERT:** Ped 87; **MS:** U Hlth Sci/Chicago Med Sch 82; **RES:** Ped, Lutheran Gen Hosp, Park Ridge, IL 83-85

Polin, Kenneth (MD) Ped
PCP
Children's Mem Med Ctr (see page 139)
Town & Country Pediatrics, 1775 Walters Ave; Northbrook, IL 60062; (847) 480-6122; **BDCERT:** Ped 87; EM 89; **MS:** St Louis U 81; **RES:** Ped, U IL Med Ctr, Chicago, IL 84-85; Ped, Children's Mem Med Ctr, Chicago, IL 82-84; **FAP:** Asst Clin Prof Ped Northwestern U; **HMO:** Metropolitan, Principal Health Care, Prudential, Rush Health Plans

Qamar, Izhar Ui (MD) Ped
PCP
La Rabida Children's Hosp
La Rabida Children's Hospital & Research Ctr, E 65th St; Chicago, IL 60649; (773) 363-6700; **BDCERT:** Ped 92; **MS:** Pakistan 76; **RES:** Ped, King George Hosp, Essex, England 87-89; Ped A&I, Hosp For Sick Children, Toronto, Canada 91-92; **FEL:** PNep, Hosp For Sick Children, Toronto, Canada 89-91; **FAP:** Asst Prof Ped U Chicago-Pritzker Sch Med
Mcd

Radfar, Baroukh (MD) Ped
PCP
St Francis Hosp
16264 Prince Dr; South Holland, IL 60473; (708) 331-9755; **BDCERT:** Ped 76; **MS:** Iran 66; **RES:** Ped, Michael Reese Hosp Med Ctr, Chicago, IL 71; Ped, Michael Reese Hosp Med Ctr, Chicago, IL 72-74; **FAP:** Asst Prof Rush Med Coll; **HOSP:** Ingalls Mem Hosp; ***SI:** Asthma and Allergies; Skin Problems*; **HMO:** Rush Prudential, Humana Health Plan, United Healthcare +
SA SU Mcd NFI

Rangsithienchai, Pisit (MD) Ped
PCP
Little Company of Mary Hosp & Hlth Care Ctrs (see page 142)
Angspatt-Pisit Md SC, 10401 S Kedzie Ave C; Chicago, IL 60655; (773) 233-7187; **BDCERT:** A&I 77; Ped 76; **MS:** Thailand 70; **RES:** Ped, Michael Reese Hosp, Chicago, IL 72-74; **FEL:** A&I, La Rabida Childrens Hosp, Chicago, IL 74-76

Rauen, Mary (MD) Ped
PCP
Children's Mem Med Ctr (see page 139)
Childrens Health Care Assoc, 2551 N Clark St Ste 200; Chicago, IL 60614; (773) 348-8300; **BDCERT:** Ped 84; **MS:** Loyola U-Stritch Sch Med, Maywood 79; **RES:** Ped, Michael Reese Hosp Med Ctr, Chicago, IL 79-82; **HOSP:** Northwestern Mem Hosp

Reifman, Cathy (MD) Ped
PCP
Macneal Mem Hosp
Mac Neal Health Care, 7020 W 79th St; Bridgeview, IL 60455; (708) 599-8200; **BDCERT:** Ped 97; **MS:** U Miami Sch Med 85; **RES:** Ped, Rush Presby-St Lukes, Chicago, IL 86-89; **FEL:** Inf, Childrens Meml Hosp, Chicago, IL; **HMO:** Aetna Hlth Plan, Blue Cross & Blue Shield, Chicago HMO, Maxicare Health Plan, Principal Health Care

Roth, Susan (MD) Ped
PCP
Children's Mem Med Ctr (see page 139)
Children's Memorial Medical Center, 2300 Children's Plaza; Chicago, IL 60614; (773) 880-4000; **BDCERT:** Ped 97; **MS:** Rush Med Coll 85; **RES:** Ped, Children's Mem Med Ctr, Chicago, IL 85-88; **FAP:** Clin Instr Ped Northwestern U; **HOSP:** Evanston Hosp; **HMO:** +
Mcr

Salafsky, Ira (MD) Ped
PCP
Evanston Hosp
North Suburban Pediatrics, 2530 Ridge Ave Ste 201; Evanston, IL 60201; (847) 869-0892; **BDCERT:** Ped 70; Ge 82; **MS:** Northwestern U 65; **RES:** Ped A&I, Children's Mem Med Ctr, Chicago, IL 66-68; **FEL:** MG, Children's Mem Med Ctr, Chicago, IL 70-72; **FAP:** Asst Prof Ped Northwestern U; **HOSP:** Children's Mem Med Ctr; ***SI:** Birth Defects; Mental Retardation*; **HMO:** Blue Cross & Blue Shield, Chicago HMO, CIGNA, Aetna Hlth Plan, PHCS
VISA

Saleh, Nabil (MD) Ped
PCP
Gottlieb Mem Hosp
927 S Mannheim Rd; Westchester, IL 60154; (708) 450-0112; **BDCERT:** Ped 84; **MS:** Egypt 66; **RES:** Ped A&I, Rush Presbyterian-St Luke's Med Ctr, Chicago, IL 77-79; Ped A&I, Kettering Hosp, England 73-77; **FAP:** Asst Prof Rush Med Coll; **HOSP:** Westlake Comm Hosp

Saul, Richard (MD) Ped
PCP
Highland Park Hosp
Associated Pediatrics Ltd, 1310 Shermer Rd; Northbrook, IL 60062; (847) 498-3434; **BDCERT:** Ped 66; **MS:** U Hlth Sci/Chicago Med Sch 61; **RES:** Ped, Children's Mem Med Ctr, Chicago, IL 62-64; **FEL:** N, -88; **FAP:** Prof U Hlth Sci/Chicago Med Sch; ***SI:** Behavior; Development in Childhood*
A Few Days VISA

Sheftel, David (MD) Ped
Lutheran Gen Hosp (see page 143)
Lutheran General Hospital - Dept Neonatology, 1775 Dempster St; Park Ridge, IL 60068; (847) 723-5313; **BDCERT:** Ped 81; NP 83; **MS:** Univ Kans Sch Med 77; **RES:** Ped A&I, U Chicago Hosp, Chicago, IL 78-80; **FEL:** NP, U Wisc Hosp, Madison, WI 80-82; **FAP:** Asst Clin Prof Univ IL Coll Med

Shulman, Stanford (MD) Ped
Children's Mem Med Ctr (see page 139)
Children's Memorial Hospital, 2300 Children Plaza Ste 20; Chicago, IL 60614; (773) 880-4187; **BDCERT:** Ped 72; Ped Inf 94; **MS:** U Chicago-Pritzker Sch Med 67; **RES:** Ped, U Chicago Hosp, Chicago, IL 68-70; **FEL:** Inf, U FL Shands Hosp, Gainesville, FL 70-73; **FAP:** Prof Inf Northwestern U; ***SI:** Kawasaki Disease; Streptococcal Infections*; **HMO:** +
LANG: Sp; Med A Few Days
VISA

Simpson, Elda (MD) Ped
PCP
Ingalls Mem Hosp
Child Health Assoc, 18430 S Halsted St Ste 202; Glenwood, IL 60425; (708) 754-4950; **BDCERT:** Ped 96; PNep 79; **MS:** Tulane U 72; **RES:** Ped A&I, Columbia-Presbyterian Med Ctr, New York, NY 73-75; **FEL:** PNep, Albert Einstein Med Ctr, Bronx, NY 76-78

Skarpathiotis, Georgios I (MD) Ped
PCP
Christ Hosp & Med Ctr (see page 140)
7110 W 127th St; Palos Heights, IL 60463; (708) 923-6300; **BDCERT:** Ped 94; **MS:** Greece 76

Slavik, Charles (MD) Ped
PCP
Northwest Comm Hlthcare
Buffalo Grove, 125 E Lake Cook Rd Ste 107; Buffalo Grove, IL 60089; (847) 352-9910; **BDCERT:** Ped 70; **MS:** Univ IL Coll Med 63; **RES:** Ped A&I, Children's Mem Med Ctr, Chicago, IL 66-68; **FAP:** Asst Clin Prof Ped Northwestern U

Slivnick, Barbara Yates (MD) Ped
PCP
Children's Mem Med Ctr (see page 139)
Childrens Health Care Assoc, 2551 N Clark St Ste 200; Chicago, IL 60614; (773) 348-8300; **BDCERT:** Ped 88; **MS:** Univ IL Coll Med 83; **RES:** Ped, Michael Reese Hosp Med Ctr, Chicago, IL 83-86; **FAP:** Asst Prof Rush Med Coll

Sud, Madhupa (MD) Ped
PCP
Ingalls Mem Hosp
Dixie Medical & Surgical Assoc, 17901 Governors Hwy Ste 103; Homewood, IL 60430; (708) 335-1400; **BDCERT:** Ped 84; **MS:** India 72; **RES:** Ped A&I, Cook Cty Hosp, Chicago, IL 79-82

Sulayman, Rabi F (MD) Ped
Christ Hosp & Med Ctr (see page 140)
4440 W 95th St; Oak Lawn, IL 60453; (708) 425-8000; **BDCERT:** Ped 75; **MS:** Lebanon 68; **RES:** U Chicago Hosp, Chicago, IL 72-75; Children's Hosp, Boston, MA

Guide to symbols and abbreviations can be found on pages 110-113.

Surati, Natverlal B (MD) Ped
PCP
Ravenswood Hosp Med Ctr
Ravenswood Med Pre-Paid Group, 4211 N Cicero Ste 300; Chicago, IL 60641; (773) 685-1111; **BDCERT:** Ped 87; **MS:** India 82; **RES:** Ped, Mercy Hosp & Med Ctr, Chicago, IL 83-86; ***SI:*** *Asthma; Rashes*; **HMO:** Blue Cross & Blue Shield, United Healthcare, Aetna Hlth Plan, Rush Prudential, American Health Plan
LANG: Hin; A Few Days

Traisman, Edward (MD) Ped
PCP
Children's Mem Med Ctr **(see page 139)**
Traisman Benuck & Traisman, 1325 Howard St Ste 203; Evanston, IL 60202; (847) 869-4300; **BDCERT:** Ped 86; **MS:** Northwestern U 81; **RES:** Ped, Children's Mem Med Ctr, Chicago, IL 82-84; **FAP:** Clin Prof Ped Northwestern U; **HOSP:** Evanston Hosp; **HMO:** Blue Cross & Blue Shield, Aetna Hlth Plan, Rush Prudential, CCN/EPI QUAL +
2-4 Weeks VISA

Typlin, Bonnie (MD) Ped
PCP
Northwestern Mem Hosp
Child & Adol Hlth, 1030 N Clark S Ste 400; Chicago, IL 60610; (312) 943-6964; **BDCERT:** Ped 79; **MS:** Northwestern U 74; **RES:** Ped A&I, Ohio State U Hosp, Columbus, OH 75-76; **FEL:** Ambulatory Ped, Ohio State U Hosp, Columbus, OH 76-78; **FAP:** Clin Instr Northwestern U; **HOSP:** Children's Mem Med Ctr; **HMO:** +

Wheeler, Wendell (MD) Ped
PCP
Trinity Hosp
10814 S Halsted; Chicago, IL 60628; (773) 995-0401; **BDCERT:** Ped 87; **MS:** Northwestern U 82; **RES:** Ped, Michael Reese Hosp Med Ctr, Chicago, IL 82-85; **HMO:** Humana Health Plan, American Health Plan, Blue Cross PPO, HMO of IL +
A Few Days

Whitington, Peter (MD) Ped
PCP
Northwestern Mem Hosp
2300 Children's Plaza Ste 57; Chicago, IL 60614; (773) 880-4643; **BDCERT:** Ped 77; PGe 90; **MS:** U Tenn Ctr Hlth Sci, Memphis 71; **RES:** Ped, U Tenn Hosp, Memphis, TN 73-74; **FEL:** Ge, Johns Hopkins Hosp, Baltimore, MD 75-78; **FAP:** Prof U Chicago-Pritzker Sch Med; **HOSP:** Children's Mem Med Ctr; ***SI:*** *Liver Disease; Liver Transplantation*; **HMO:** CIGNA, Humana Health Plan, United Resource Network, PHCS, Alliance Life Trac
A Few Days

Yanong, Procopio U (MD) Ped
PCP
Ravenswood Hosp Med Ctr
4925 Northwestern Ave Bldg E; Chicago, IL 60618; (773) 275-7700; **BDCERT:** Ped 67; **MS:** Philippines 67; **RES:** Ped, Grant Hosp, Chicago, IL 63-64; Ped, Cook Cty Hosp, Chicago, IL 64-67; **FEL:** PCd, Cook Co Hosp, Chicago, IL 67-69; **HOSP:** Norwegian-American Hosp

Yao, Tito (MD) Ped
PCP
Loretto Hosp
RJ Medical Center, 5351 W North Ave; Chicago, IL 60639; (773) 287-0751; **BDCERT:** Ped 75; Ped 83; **MS:** Philippines 69; **RES:** Ped, NY Methodist Hosp, Brooklyn, NY 71-72; Ped, Baroness Erlanger Hosp, Chattanooga, TN 72-73; **FEL:** PCd, St Christopher's Hosp for Children, Philadelphia, PA 73-74; PCd, Cook Cty Hosp, Chicago, IL 74-75; **HOSP:** St Anthony Hosp; ***SI:*** *Physical Examination & Immunization; Bronchial Asthma*; **HMO:** United Healthcare, HMO Illinois, Bay State Health Plan, Harmony, Blue cross & blue +
LANG: Sp, Tag, Chi; Immediately

Yogev, Ram (MD) Ped
PCP
Children's Mem Med Ctr **(see page 139)**
Childrens Memorial Hospital, 2300 N Childrens Plz Ste 69; Chicago, IL 60614; (773) 880-4757; **BDCERT:** Ped 81; Inf; **MS:** Israel 69; **RES:** Ped, Hadassah Hosp, Jerusalem, Israel 72-75; **FEL:** Ped Inf, Children's Mem Med Ctr, Chicago, IL 75-77; **FAP:** Prof Northwestern U; ***SI:*** *AIDS; Infection-Nervous System*; **HMO:** Blue Cross & Blue Shield, Humana Health Plan, Choicecare, Rush Pru, United Healthcare +
LANG: Sp, Heb; Immediately VISA

Zieserl, Edward (MD) Ped
PCP
Evanston Hosp
1000 Central St Ste 765; Evanston, IL 60201; (847) 570-1507; **BDCERT:** Ped 72; **MS:** Med Coll Wisc 66; **RES:** Ped, Children's Mem Med Ctr, Chicago, IL 67-72; **FAP:** Asst Prof Ped Northwestern U; **HOSP:** Children's Mem Med Ctr; **HMO:** Blue Cross & Blue Shield, Humana Health Plan, Aetna Hlth Plan, CIGNA, Rush Pru +
LANG: Sp, Fr; VISA

Ziring, Philip (MD) Ped
Cook Cty Hosp
Cook County Childrens Hospital, 700 S Wood St; Chicago, IL 60612; (312) 633-5640; **BDCERT:** Ped 67; **MS:** NYU Sch Med 62; **HOSP:** Bethany Hosp

Zollar, Lowell (MD) Ped
PCP
Provena Mercy Ctr
2011 E 75th St Ste 101; Chicago, IL 60649; (773) 288-4824; **BDCERT:** Ped 69; **MS:** Howard U 64; **RES:** Ped A&I, Cook Cty Hosp, Chicago, IL 65-67; **HOSP:** Michael Reese Hosp & Med Ctr; **HMO:** Blue Cross & Blue Shield, CIGNA, Rush Pru, Aetna Hlth Plan, United Healthcare +
Mcd 2-4 Weeks

PHYSICAL MEDICINE & REHABILITATION

Adair, Roy (MD) PMR
Christ Hosp & Med Ctr (see page 140)
4440 W 95th St; Oak Lawn, IL 60453; (708) 346-5431; **BDCERT:** PMR 87; **MS:** Rush Med Coll 82; **RES:** FP, Lutheran Gen Hosp, Park Ridge, IL 82-83; PMR, Rehab Institute of Chicago, Chicago, IL 83-85; **FAP:** Asst Prof Rush Med Coll; ***SI:*** *Spinal Cord Injury; Strokes*; **HMO:** +
Mcr Mcd 2-4 Weeks

Alexander, Bonita (MD) PMR
Alexian Brothers Med Ctr
(see page 138)
Rehab Dept-Alexian Brothers, 800 Biesterfield Rd; Elk Grove Village, IL 60007; (847) 437-5500; **BDCERT:** PMR 89; **MS:** Loyola U-Stritch Sch Med, Maywood 84; **HOSP:** Rehab Institute of Chicago

Cavanaugh, Jean A (MD) PMR
Northwestern Mem Hosp
2650 Ridge Ave; Evanston, IL 60201; (847) 570-2066; **BDCERT:** PMR 77; **MS:** Northwestern U 69; **RES:** PMR, Rehab Inst Chicago, Chicago, IL 70-72; PMR, Georgetown U Hosp, Washington, DC 72-73; **FAP:** Asst Prof of Clin PMR Northwestern U; **HOSP:** Evanston Hosp; ***SI:*** *Stroke; Amputation*; **HMO:** +
Mcr Mcd

Chen, David (MD) PMR
Rehab Institute of Chicago
Rehabilitation Institute, 345 E Superior St; Chicago, IL 60611; (312) 908-0764; **BDCERT:** PMR 92; **MS:** Univ IL Coll Med 87; **RES:** PMR, Rehab Institute of Chicago, Chicago, IL 87-91; **FAP:** Asst Professor PMR Northwestern U; **HOSP:** Northwestern Mem Hosp; ***SI:*** *Spinal Cord Medicine*
Mcr Mcd NFI A Few Days
VISA

Feldman, Joseph (MD) PMR
Evanston Hosp
2650 Ridge Ave; Evanston, IL 60201; (847) 570-2066; **BDCERT:** PMR 71; **MS:** Univ IL Coll Med 65; **RES:** PMR, U IL-Michael Reese Hosp, Chicago, IL 66-69; **FAP:** Asst Prof Northwestern U; **HOSP:** Highland Park Hosp; ***SI:*** *Spine Dysfunction*

Gittler, Michelle (MD) PMR
Schwab Rehab Hosp and Care Network
1401 S California; Chicago, IL 60608; (773) 522-2010; **BDCERT:** PMR 93; **MS:** Univ IL Coll Med 88; **RES:** Northwestern Mem Hosp, Chicago, IL; **FAP:** Asst Clin Prof U Chicago-Pritzker Sch Med; ***SI:*** *Spinal Cord Injury; Amputation*
LANG: Sp; Mcr Mcd 2-4 Weeks

Harvey, Richard (MD) PMR
Rehab Institute of Chicago
The Rehabilitation Institute Of Chicago, 345 E Superior St Ste 1120; Chicago, IL 60611; (312) 908-1975; **BDCERT:** PMR 93; **MS:** U Mich Med Sch 88; **HOSP:** Northwestern Mem Hosp; ***SI:*** *Stroke Rehabilitation; Geriatric Rehabilitation*; **HMO:** Bc/BS, Medicare
Mcr Mcd NFI 1 Week

Jedrychowska, Krystyna (MD) PMR
St Mary's of Nazareth Hosp Ctr
2233 W Division St; Chicago, IL 60622; (312) 770-2202; **BDCERT:** PMR 79; **MS:** Poland 63; **RES:** PMR, New York University Med Ctr, New York, NY 75-78; ***SI:*** *Leg Amputation; Stroke*; **HMO:** St Mary HMO
LANG: Pol; SA SU Mcr Mcd
A Few Days

Kirschner, Kristi (MD) PMR
Rehab Institute of Chicago
Rehabilitation Institute of Chicago, 345 E Superior St Rm1122; Chicago, IL 60611; (312) 908-4744; **BDCERT:** PMR 91; **MS:** U Chicago-Pritzker Sch Med 86; **RES:** PMR, Northwestern Mem Hosp, Chicago, IL 87-90; ***SI:*** *Neurorehabilitation; Disabled Women's Health*

Koltun, Douglas (MD) PMR
Christ Hosp & Med Ctr (see page 140)
Christ Hospital, 4440 W 95th St Ste 1042000; Oak Lawn, IL 60453; (708) 346-5428; **BDCERT:** PMR 87; **MS:** Tulane U 83; **RES:** PMR, Rehab Institute of Chicago, Chicago, IL 83-86

Lerner, Ira (MD) PMR
Columbus Hosp
2520 N Lakeview Ave; Chicago, IL 60614; (773) 388-7336; **BDCERT:** PMR 70; **MS:** Univ IL Coll Med 64; **RES:** PMR, Schwab Rehab Hosp and Care Network, Chicago, IL -68; **FAP:** Assoc Prof Northwestern U; ***SI:*** *Rehabilitation; Nerve Conduction Tests*; **HMO:** Blue Cross, American HMO, United Healthcare, Aetna-US Healthcare, Family Med Net
LANG: Sp; Mcr Mcd Immediately

Marciniak, Christina (MD) PMR
Rehab Institute of Chicago
Rehabilitation Institute of Chicago, 345 E Superior St Rm 1126; Chicago, IL 60611; (312) 908-4740; **BDCERT:** PMR 86; **MS:** Univ IL Coll Med 81; **RES:** PMR, Northwestern Mem Hosp, Chicago, IL 82-85; **FAP:** Asst Prof PMR Northwestern U; ***SI:*** *Spinal Cord Injury; Spasticity Management*; **HMO:** Blue Cross, PHS +
A Few Days

Mayer, Robert Samuel (MD) PMR
Rush-Presbyterian-St Luke's Med Ctr
(see page 122)
Rehabilitation Med Clinic, 1725 W Harrison St Ste 1018; Chicago, IL 60612; (312) 942-8905; **BDCERT:** PMR 91; **MS:** Northwestern U 86; **RES:** PMR, Rush Presbyterian-St Luke's Med Ctr, Chicago, IL 86-90; **FAP:** Chrmn Rush Med Coll; **HOSP:** Oak Park Hosp; ***SI:*** *Repetitive Motion Disorder; Low Back Pain*; **HMO:** Blue Cross & Blue Shield, CIGNA, United Healthcare, Aetna Hlth Plan, Rush Prudential +
1 Week VISA

McIlree, Nina (MD) PMR
Rehab Institute of Chicago
Neihoft Pavillion, 800 Biesterfield Rd; Elk Grove Village, IL 60007; (708) 763-6891; **BDCERT:** PMR 97; **MS:** Univ IL Coll Med 92; **RES:** Rehab Institute of Chicago, Chicago, IL 93-96; **FEL:** Rehab Institute of Chicago, Chicago, IL 96-98; **HMO:** Blue Cross & Blue Shield

Press, Joel (MD) PMR
Rehab Institute of Chicago
1030 N Clark Suite 500; Chicago, IL 60610; (312) 908-7767; **BDCERT:** PMR 89; **MS:** Univ IL Coll Med 84; **RES:** PMR, Rehab Institute of Chicago, Chicago, IL 85-88; **FAP:** Asst Prof PMR Northwestern U; ***SI:*** *Sports Medicine; Low Back Pain*
A Few Days VISA

Roth, Elliot (MD) PMR
Rehab Institute of Chicago
Rehabilitation Institute of Chicago, 345 E Superior St; Chicago, IL 60611; (312) 908-4637; **BDCERT:** PMR 87; **MS:** Northwestern U 82; **RES:** PMR, Northwestern Mem Hosp, Chicago, IL 83-85; **FEL:** Rehab Med, Rehab Institute of Chicago, Chicago, IL 86; **FAP:** Prof/Chmn Northwestern U; **HOSP:** Northwestern Mem Hosp; ***SI:*** *Stroke Rehabilitation; Neurologic Rehabilitation*; **HMO:** Blue Cross & Blue Shield, CIGNA, Humana Health Plan, Health First +
A Few Days VISA

Shahani, Bhagwan (MD) PMR
Univ of Illinois at Chicago Med Ctr
PM & R Assoc, 901 S Wolcott Ave W130; Chicago, IL 60612; (312) 996-7210; **BDCERT:** PMR 74; **MS:** India 62; **RES:** PMR, New York University Med Ctr, New York, NY 63-66; **FEL:** N, Oxford Univ, Oxford, UK 66-70; Neur, Mass Gen Hosp, Boston, MA 71-73; **FAP:** Prof Univ IL Coll Med; ***SI:*** *Electromyography; Neurologic Rehabilitation*
LANG: Sp, Hin, Ur;
A Few Days

Sisung, Charles (MD) PMR
Rehab Institute of Chicago
Rehab Institute of Chicago, 345 E Superior S; Chicago, IL 60611; (312) 908-1246; **BDCERT:** PMR 91; Ped 97; **MS:** U Mich Med Sch 81; **RES:** Ped A&I, U Mich Med Ctr, Ann Arbor, MI 81-84; PMR, Schwab Rehab Hosp and Care Network, Chicago, IL 86-89; **FEL:** Ped Rhu, U Chicago Hosp, Chicago, IL 89-91; **FAP:** Asst Prof Ped U Chicago-Pritzker Sch Med

Sliwa, James A (DO) PMR
Rehab Institute of Chicago
345 E Superior St Ste 684; Chicago, IL 60611; (312) 908-4093; **BDCERT:** PMR 85; **MS:** Chicago Coll Osteo Med 80; **RES:** PMR, Rehab Institute of Chicago, Chicago, IL 81-84; **FAP:** Assoc Clin Instr PMR Northwestern U

Thornton, Lisa (MD) PMR
Schwab Rehab Hosp and Care Network
1401 S California Blvd; Chicago, IL 60608; (773) 522-5870; **BDCERT:** PMR 94; Ped 91; **MS:** U Mich Med Sch 87; **RES:** PMR, Rehab Institute of Chicago, Chicago, IL 90-93; Ped A&I, Children's Mem Med Ctr, Chicago, IL 87-90; ***SI:*** *Pediatric Rehabilitation*; **HMO:** +
1 Week

Yee, Martin J (MD) PMR
Grant Hosp
1 Ingalls Dr; Harvey, IL 60426; (708) 915-3112; **BDCERT:** PMR 88; **MS:** Rush Med Coll 84; **RES:** New York University Med Ctr, New York, NY 84; New York University Med Ctr, New York, NY 85-87; **FAP:** Asst Prof Rush Med Coll

PLASTIC SURGERY

Bauer, Bruce (MD) PlS
Children's Mem Med Ctr **(see page 139)**
Childrens Memorial Hospital, 2300 N Childrens Plz Ste 28; Chicago, IL 60614; (773) 880-4000; **BDCERT:** PlS 80; **MS:** Northwestern U 74; **RES:** S, Northwestern Mem Hosp, Chicago, IL 75-77; PlS, Northwestern Mem Hosp, Chicago, IL 77-79; **FAP:** Asst Prof S Northwestern U; **HMO:** Aetna Hlth Plan, Blue Cross & Blue Shield, Chicago HMO, CIGNA, Humana Health Plan

Bittar, Sami (MD) **PlS**
La Grange Mem Hosp **(see page 141)**
5201 S Willow Springs Rd Ste 440; La Grange, IL 60525; (708) 354-4667; **BDCERT:** PlS 92; **MS:** Syria 80; **RES:** S, Western Penn Hosp, Pittsburgh, PA 82-87; **FEL:** PlS, Rush-Presby-St Lukes Hosp, Chicago, IL 87-89; Microsurgery, Southern IL Sch of Med, Springfield, IL 89; **FAP:** Assoc Prof Rush Med Coll; **HOSP:** Rush-Presbyterian-St Luke's Med Ctr; ***SI:*** *Palate Reconstruction; Cosmetic Surgery*; **HMO:** Bc/BS, Rush Health Plans, La Grange IPA, Macneal Hlth
LANG: Fr, Ar; Immediately

Bradley, Craig (MD) **PlS**
Rush-Presbyterian-St Luke's Med Ctr **(see page 122)**
Cosmetic & Reconstructive, 1133 Westgate Fl 1; Oak Park, IL 60301; (708) 848-7607; **BDCERT:** PlS 74; **MS:** U Tenn Ctr Hlth Sci, Memphis 66; **RES:** PlS, Rush Presbyterian-St Luke's Med Ctr, Chicago, IL 71-72; PlS, Illinois Masonic Med Ctr, Chicago, IL 72-73; **FAP:** Asst Prof S Rush Med Coll; **HMO:** Blue Cross & Blue Shield

Burget, Gary C. (MD) **PlS**
St Joseph Hosp-Chicago
2913 N Commonwealth Ave Ste 400; Chicago, IL 60657; (773) 880-0062; **BDCERT:** PlS 80; **MS:** Yale U Sch Med 67; **RES:** S, Jackson Mem Hosp, Miami, FL 69-72; PlS, Jackson Mem Hosp, Miami, FL 73-74; **FEL:** Kleinert-Kutz Hand Clinic, Louisville, KY 72; Ped PlS, Children's Mem Med Ctr, Chicago, IL 85-86; **FAP:** Asst Prof U Chicago-Pritzker Sch Med; **HOSP:** Children's Mem Med Ctr; ***SI:*** *Reconstructive Nose Surgery; Facial Cosmetic Surgery*
LANG: Sp; 1 Week

Caridi, Robert (MD) **PlS**
Good Samaritan Hosp **(see page 274)**
Suburban Plastic Surgery, 810 Beastfield Rd; Elk Grove, IL 60007; (847) 981-3650; **BDCERT:** PlS 94; **MS:** Univ Texas, Houston 85; **RES:** Mount Sinai Med Ctr, New York, NY 86-90; **FEL:** Mount Sinai Med Ctr, New York, NY 90-91

Casas, Laurie (MD) **PlS**
Glenbrook Hosp
2050 Pfingsten Rd Ste 365; Glenview, IL 60025; (847) 657-7550; **BDCERT:** PlS 92; **MS:** Northwestern U 82; **RES:** S, Northwestern Mem Hosp, Chicago, IL 82-85; PlS, Northwestern Mem Hosp, Chicago, IL 85-88; **FEL:** Aesthetic Surgery, Manhattan Eye, Ear & Throat Hosp, New York, NY 88-89; Breast Surg, St Joseph Hosp, Atlanta, GA 89-90; **FAP:** Asst Prof Northwestern U; **HOSP:** Evanston Hosp; ***SI:*** *Cosmetic Surgery; Breast Surgery*; **HMO:** Blue Cross & Blue Shield, Aetna Hlth Plan, CIGNA, Preferred Plan, Rush Prudential
2-4 Weeks VISA

Cohen, Mimis (MD) **PlS**
Univ of Illinois at Chicago Med Ctr
Division of Plastic Surgery-Univ of Illinois Med Ctr, 820 S Wood St Ste 515CSN; Chicago, IL 60612; (312) 996-9313; **BDCERT:** PlS 83; **MS:** Greece 70; **RES:** S, Aretaeion Hosp, Athens, Greece 63-71; U Chicago Hosp, Chicago, IL 73-77; **FEL:** CCM, U IL Med Ctr, Chicago, IL 80; **HOSP:** Michael Reese Hosp & Med Ctr; ***SI:*** *Cosmetic Surgery; Cleft Lip And Palate*; **HMO:** Blue Cross & Blue Shield, United Healthcare, Oxford, NY Life
LANG: Sp, Fr, Grk, Itl;
1 Week VISA

Cook, John Q (MD) **PlS**
Swedish Covenant Hosp
12 E Delaware Pl Fl 1; Chicago, IL 60611; (312) 751-2112; **BDCERT:** PlS 91; S 86; **MS:** Northwestern U 80; **RES:** S, Rush Presby-St Lukes, Chicago, IL 81-85; PlS, Northwestern Mem Hosp, Chicago, IL 85-88; **HOSP:** Rush-Presbyterian-St Luke's Med Ctr; **HMO:** Blue Cross & Blue Shield, Prudential, Travelers

Dolezal, Rudolph (MD) **PlS**
Lutheran Gen Hosp **(see page 143)**
Parkside Building, 1875 Dempster St; Park Ridge, IL 60068; (847) 295-8844; **BDCERT:** PlS 85; Oto 81; **MS:** Rush Med Coll 74; **RES:** S, U IL Med Ctr, Chicago, IL 75-76; Oto, U Mich Med Ctr, Ann Arbor, MI 77-81; **FAP:** Assoc Clin Prof S Univ IL Coll Med; **HOSP:** Univ of Illinois at Chicago Med Ctr; ***SI:*** *Nasal Surgery; Breast Augmentation*
1 Week

Galal, Hatem (MD) **PlS**
Macneal Mem Hosp
28 E Burlington St; Riverside, IL 60546; (630) 572-1477; **BDCERT:** PlS 80; **MS:** Egypt 64; **RES:** Loyola U Med Ctr, Maywood, IL 75-77; Cook Cty Hosp, Chicago, IL 71-74; **FEL:** PlS, Cook Cty Hosp, Chicago, IL 74-75; **FAP:** Asst Clin Prof S Loyola U-Stritch Sch Med, Maywood; ***SI:*** *Hand Surgery*; **HMO:** Aetna Hlth Plan, Blue Cross & Blue Shield, Californiacare, Takecare Health Plan, Travelers

Guide to symbols and abbreviations can be found on pages 110-113.

Geldner, Peter (MD) PlS
Michael Reese Hosp & Med Ctr
New Dimensions Ctr-Cosmetic, 60 E Delaware Pl Fl 15; Chicago, IL 60611; (312) 440-5050; **BDCERT:** PlS 93; **MS:** U Wisc Med Sch 83; **RES:** PlS, Wayne State U, Detroit, MI 87-88; PlS, U TX Med Branch Hosp, Galveston, TX 88-90; **FAP:** Asst Clin Prof Univ IL Coll Med; **HOSP:** Illinois Masonic Med Ctr; ***SI:*** *Cosmetic Surgery; Breast Reconstruction*; **HMO:** Guardian, Aetna Hlth Plan, Humana Health Plan, Principal Health Care
LANG: Pol;
A Few Days VISA

Gottlieb, Lawrence (MD) PlS
U Chicago Hosp (see page 124)
MC6035, 5841 S Maryland Ave RmJ641; Chicago, IL 60637; (773) 702-6302; **BDCERT:** S 83; PlS 86; **MS:** Penn State U-Hershey Med Ctr 77; **RES:** S, Yale-New Haven Hosp, New Haven, CT 78-82; **FEL:** PlS, USC Med Ctr, Los Angeles, CA 82-84; **FAP:** Clin Prof S U Chicago-Pritzker Sch Med

Gress, Damian (MD) PlS
Good Shepherd Hosp
Suburban Plastic Surgery, 1585 Barrington Rd Ste 601; Hoffman Estates, IL 60194; (847) 843-7733; **BDCERT:** PlS 94; **MS:** Cornell U 80; **RES:** S, Montefiore Med Ctr, Bronx, NY 80-84; PlS, Albany Med Ctr, Albany, NY 86-88; **FEL:** CCM, Montefiore Med Ctr, Bronx, NY 84-85; Burns, Westchester County Med Ctr, Valhalla, NY 85-86; **HOSP:** Good Samaritan Hosp; ***SI:*** *Breast Reconstruction; Cosmetic Surgery*; **HMO:** Blue Cross & Blue Shield, HMO Illinois, Travelers, CIGNA +
LANG: Sp;
A Few Days VISA

Johnson, Peter (MD) PlS
Lutheran Gen Hosp (see page 143)
Advocate Medical Group, 8901 Golf Rd Ste 204; Des Plaines, IL 60016; (847) 296-5470; **BDCERT:** PlS 89; **MS:** Northwestern U 79; **RES:** PlS, Northwestern Mem Hosp, Chicago, IL 83-86; S, Northwestern Mem Hosp, Chicago, IL 81-83; **FEL:** PlS, Jackson Mem Hosp, Miami, FL 87; PlS, Children's Mem Med Ctr, Chicago, IL 86

Kalimuthu, Ramasamy (MD) PlS
Little Company of Mary Hosp & Hlth Care Ctrs (see page 142)
Suburban Plastic Surgery, 5346 W 95th St; Oak Lawn, IL 60453; (708) 636-8222; **BDCERT:** PlS 85; HS 93; **MS:** India 70; **RES:** S, Little Company of Mary Hosp & Hlth Care Ctrs, Evergreen Park, IL 75-80; PlS, Loyola U Med Ctr, Maywood, IL 80-83; **FAP:** Asst Prof Rush Med Coll; **HOSP:** Christ Hosp & Med Ctr; ***SI:*** *Hand Surgery*

Kraus, Helen (MD) PlS
Lutheran Gen Hosp (see page 143)
7447 Talcott St Ste 308; Park Ridge, IL 60631; (847) 803-1000; **BDCERT:** PlS 89; **MS:** Northwestern U 80; **RES:** PlS, Northwestern Mem Hosp, Chicago, IL 83-86; S, Northwestern Mem Hosp, Chicago, IL 80-83; **FEL:** Children's Mem Med Ctr, Chicago, IL 86-87; **FAP:** Assoc Clin Prof S Northwestern U

Lease, John (MD) PlS
Columbus Hosp
3000 N Halsted St Ste 506; Chicago, IL 60657; (773) 883-8234; **BDCERT:** PlS 95; **MS:** Duke U 83; **RES:** S, U Chicago Hosp, Chicago, IL 83-88; PlS, U Chicago Hosp, Chicago, IL 88-90; **HOSP:** Illinois Masonic Med Ctr; ***SI:*** *Cosmetic Surgery; Breast Reconstruction*; **HMO:** Blue Cross & Blue Shield, CIGNA
2-4 Weeks VISA

Lewis, Victor (MD) PlS
Northwestern Mem Hosp
707 N Fairbanks Ct Ste 1210; Chicago, IL 60611; (312) 335-9155; **BDCERT:** PlS 78; S 75; **MS:** Northwestern U 68; **RES:** PlS, Northwestern Mem Hosp, Chicago, IL 75-77; S, Charity Hosp, New Orleans, LA 69-73; **FAP:** Clin Prof S Northwestern U

Madda, Frank (MD) PlS
Good Samaritan Hosp (see page 274)
Suburban Plastic Surgery Assoc, 1585 N Barrington Rd Ste 601; Downers Grove, IL 60194; (630) 960-0023; **BDCERT:** PlS 82; **MS:** Rush Med Coll 80

Makhlouf, Mansour V (MD) PlS
Ravenswood Hosp Med Ctr
1945 W Wilson Ave Ste 5110; Chicago, IL 60640; (773) 275-1101; **BDCERT:** PlS 90; HS 92; **MS:** Lebanon 81; **RES:** S, St Joseph's Hosp, Chicago, IL 81-84; PlS, St Louis U Hosp, St Louis, MO; **FEL:** HS, CT Combined HS Program, Hartford, CT 86-87; ***SI:*** *Breast Augmentation; Liposuction*; **HMO:** +
LANG: Ar, Fr; 1 Week

Mc Kinney, Peter (MD) PlS
Northwestern Mem Hosp
60 N Fairbanks Ct Ste 1207; Chicago, IL 60611; (312) 266-0300; **BDCERT:** PlS 68; **MS:** Canada 60; **RES:** PlS, NY Hosp-Cornell Med Ctr, New York, NY 64-67; S, Bellevue Hosp Ctr, New York, NY 61-64; **FAP:** Prof PlS Northwestern U

Mc Nally, Randall (MD) PlS
Rush-Presbyterian-St Luke's Med Ctr (see page 122)
1725 W Harrison St Ste 106; Chicago, IL 60612; (312) 666-2225; **BDCERT:** PlS 62; **MS:** St Louis U 55; **RES:** PlS, Rush Presbyterian-St Luke's Med Ctr, Chicago, IL 58-59; PlS, U IL Rsch - Ed Hosp, Chicago, IL 59-60; **FAP:** Prof PlS Rush Med Coll

Mooney, Gabriel (MD) PlS
Christ Hosp & Med Ctr (see page 140)
4400 W 95th St Ste 303; Oak Lawn, IL 60453; (708) 424-2411; **BDCERT:** PlS 79; **MS:** Ireland 70; **FAP:** Asst Prof PlS Univ IL Coll Med

Mustoe, Thomas (MD) PlS
Northwestern Mem Hosp
NW Med Faculty Foundation-Plastic Surgery, 707 N Fairbanks Ct Ste 812; Chicago, IL 60611; (312) 908-7154; **BDCERT:** PlS 87; **MS:** Harvard Med Sch 78; **RES:** IM, Mass Gen Hosp, Boston, MA 78; S, Brigham & Women's Hosp, Boston, MA 89-90; **FEL:** PlS, Brigham & Women's Hosp, Boston, MA 83; Oto, Mass Eye & Ear Infirmary, Boston, MA 90; **FAP:** Prof S Northwestern U; **HOSP:** Evanston Hosp; ***SI:*** *Facial Aesthetic Surgery; Breast-Plastic Surgery*; **HMO:** Aetna Hlth Plan, Blue Cross & Blue Shield, Californiacare, CIGNA, HealthNet
4+ Weeks VISA

Pelletiere, Vincent (MD) PlS
Northwest Comm Hlthcare
Barrington Plastic Surgery Ltd, 1602 W Colonial Pkwy; Inverness, IL 60067; (847) 358-9444; **BDCERT:** PlS 78; **MS:** Univ IL Coll Med 69; **RES:** S, Loyola U Med Ctr, Maywood, IL 72-75; Loyola U Med Ctr, Maywood, IL 75-78; **HOSP:** Good Shepherd Hosp; **HMO:** Aetna Hlth Plan, Blue Cross & Blue Shield, Californiacare
2-4 Weeks

Pensler, Jay Michael (MD) PlS
Evanston Hosp
680 N Lakeshore Dr; Chicago, IL 60611; (847) 642-7777; **BDCERT:** PlS 90; **MS:** U Chicago-Pritzker Sch Med 80; **RES:** S, New York University, New York, NY 81-83; PlS, U TX Med Branch Hosp, Galveston, TX 83-86; **FEL:** Facial PlS, Brigham & Women's Hosp, Boston, MA 86-87; **FAP:** Assoc Prof S Northwestern U; **HOSP:** Northwestern Mem Hosp

Randolph, David (MD) PlS
Resurrection Med Ctr
7447 W Talcott Ave Ste 451; Chicago, IL 60631; (847) 866-8083; **BDCERT:** PlS 75; S 73; **MS:** Northwestern U 66; **RES:** S, Northwestern Mem Hosp, Chicago, IL 67-71; PlS, Indiana U Med Ctr, Indianapolis, IN 71-73; **FAP:** Assoc Clin Instr Northwestern U; **HMO:** Aetna Hlth Plan, Blue Cross & Blue Shield, Chicago HMO, CIGNA, HealthNet

Schlenker, James (MD) PlS
Christ Hosp & Med Ctr (see page 140)
6311 W 95th St; Oak Lawn, IL 60453; (708) 423-2258; **BDCERT:** PlS 80; HS 90; **MS:** Harvard Med Sch 69; **RES:** S, U Hosp of Cleveland, Cleveland, OH 70-74; PlS, Vanderbilt U Med Ctr, Nashville, TN 76-78; **FEL:** HS, U Louisville Hosp, Louisville, KY 78-79

Shah, Rajendra (MD) PlS
Christ Hosp & Med Ctr (see page 140)
Surgery & Laser Ctr, 4400 W 95th St Ste 312; Oak Lawn, IL 60453; (708) 424-3999; **BDCERT:** PlS 84; S 82; **MS:** India 75; **RES:** S, Christ Hosp & Med Ctr, Oak Lawn, IL 76-79; S, Rush Presbyterian-St Luke's Med Ctr, Chicago, IL 79-81; **FEL:** PlS, Ohio State U Hosp, Columbus, OH 81-83; **FAP:** Asst Prof PlS Univ IL Coll Med

Sperling, Richard (MD) PlS
Rush North Shore Med Ctr
Richard L Sperling M.D. Ltd., 9669 Kenton Ave Ste 604; Skokie, IL 60076; (847) 674-5122; **BDCERT:** PlS 80; **MS:** Univ IL Coll Med 63; **RES:** PlS, Rush Presbyterian-St Luke's Med Ctr, Chicago, IL 68-69; PlS, U Chicago Hosp, Chicago, IL 69-70; **FAP:** Asst Prof Univ IL Coll Med; **HOSP:** Lutheran Gen Hosp; ***SI:*** *Cosmetic Surgery; Breast Reconstruction*; **HMO:** Aetna Hlth Plan, Blue Cross & Blue Shield, Chicago HMO, Choicecare, Principal Health Care
A Few Days VISA

Springer, Harry (MD) PlS
St Francis Hosp
Aesthetic Surgery Ltd, 1000 Skokie Blvd Ste 155; Wilmette, IL 60091; (847) 853-9900; **BDCERT:** PlS 75; **MS:** U Tex SW, Dallas 64; **RES:** S, Cook Cty Hosp, Chicago, IL 65-69; **FEL:** PlS, Northwestrn-Cook Cty Hosp, Chicago, IL 68-71

Tauras, Arvydas P (MD) PlS
Northwest Comm Hlthcare
Northwest Plastic Surgeons, 3 W Central Rd; Mt Prospect, IL 60056; (847) 398-2466; **BDCERT:** PlS 73; **MS:** Univ IL Coll Med 64; **RES:** S, Marquette U Affil Hosp, Milwaukee, WI 65-69; PlS, Med College Wisc Affil Hosp, Milwaukee, WI 69-71

Walton, Robert (MD) PlS
U Chicago Hosp (see page 124)
University of Chicago, 5841 S Maryland Ave MC6035; Chicago, IL 60637; (773) 702-6302; **BDCERT:** PlS 80; HS 90; **MS:** Univ Kans Sch Med 72; **RES:** S, Johns Hopkins Hosp, Baltimore, MD 72-74; PlS, Yale-New Haven Hosp, New Haven, CT 74-78; **FEL:** HS, Hartford Hosp, Hartford, CT 77-78; **FAP:** Professor PlS U Chicago-Pritzker Sch Med; **HOSP:** St Joseph Hosp-Chicago; ***SI:*** *Reconstructive Microsurgery; Aesthetic Surgery*; **HMO:** Aetna Hlth Plan, John Hancock, Medicare, CIGNA
2-4 Weeks VISA

Warpeha, Raymond L (MD) PlS
Loyola U Med Ctr (see page 120)
2160 S 1st Ave; Maywood, IL 60153; (708) 327-2654; **BDCERT:** PlS 73; S 71; **MS:** Northwestern U 65; **RES:** S, Cook Co Hosp, Chicago, IL 66-70; PlS, Northwestern Mem Hosp, Chicago, IL 70-72; **HMO:** +
A Few Days VISA

Guide to symbols and abbreviations can be found on pages 110-113.

Zachary, Lawrence (MD) PlS
Louis A Weiss Mem Hosp
4646 N Marina Dr 7th Fl; Chicago, IL 60640; (773) 564-5166; **BDCERT:** PlS 88; HS 92; **MS:** U Hlth Sci/Chicago Med Sch 78; **RES:** S, U Chicago Hosp, Chicago, IL 79-83; PlS, U Chicago Hosp, Chicago, IL 84-85; **FEL:** HS, Raymond Curtis Hand Ctr, Baltimore, MD 85-86; **FAP:** Asst Prof U Chicago-Pritzker Sch Med; **HOSP:** U Chicago Hosp; ***SI:*** *Body Sculpture*; **HMO:** + **LANG:** Sp, Pol, Rus; Immediately VISA

PSYCHIATRY

Allen, Albert (MD & PhD) Psyc
Univ of Illinois at Chicago Med Ctr
Inst for Juvenile Rsch - UIC Dept of Psych, 907 S Wolcott Ave MC 747; Chicago, IL 60612; (312) 413-9093; **BDCERT:** Psyc 96; ChAP; **MS:** U Iowa Coll Med 88; **RES:** ChAP, U IA Hosp, Iowa City, IA 90-92; Psyc, Nat Inst Mental Health, Bethesda, MD 92-94; **FEL:** ChAP, Nat Inst Mental Health, Bethesda, MD; **FAP:** Asst Prof Univ IL Coll Med; ***SI:*** *Obsessive Compulsive Disorders; Tourette's Syndrome*; **HMO:** Advocate, Blue Cross & Blue Shield, American Health Plan, Magellan, Bc/BS +
Mcr Mcd 4+ Weeks VISA

Altman, David (MD) Psyc
Lutheran Gen Hosp **(see page 143)**
9933 Lawler Ave Ste 444; Skokie, IL 60077; (847) 674-2025; **BDCERT:** Psyc 78; AdP 94; **MS:** U Chicago-Pritzker Sch Med 71; **RES:** Michael Reese Hosp Med Ctr, Chicago, IL 72-75

Anzia, Daniel (MD) Psyc
Lutheran Gen Hosp **(see page 143)**
Out Patient Mental Health, 1700 Luther Ln; Park Ridge, IL 60068; (847) 696-5885; **BDCERT:** Psyc 79; **MS:** Stanford U 73; **RES:** Psyc, Loyola U Med Ctr, Maywood, IL 74-77; **FAP:** Assoc Clin Prof U Chicago-Pritzker Sch Med

Astrachan, Boris (MD) Psyc
Univ of Illinois at Chicago Med Ctr
912 S Wood St Ste 709G; Chicago, IL 60612; (312) 996-3580; **BDCERT:** Psyc 66; **MS:** Albany Med Coll 56; **RES:** Psyc, US Naval Hosp, Philadelphia, PA 57-58; Psyc, Yale-New Haven Hosp, New Haven, CT 61-63; **FAP:** Prof Psyc Univ IL Coll Med
Mcr Mcd

Berent, Philip (MD) Psyc
Lutheran Gen Hosp **(see page 143)**
3375 N Arlington Heights Rd; Arlington Hts, IL 60004; (847) 398-5600; **BDCERT:** Psyc 74; ChAP 76; **MS:** Univ IL Coll Med 66; **RES:** Psyc, Rush Presbyterian-St Luke's Med Ctr, Chicago, IL 67-68; Psyc, U IL Med Ctr, Chicago, IL 70-71; **FEL:** ChAP, Inst Juvenile Rsch, Chicago, IL 71-73; **HOSP:** Forest Hosp
1 Week

Bloom, Robert (MD) Psyc
Rush-Presbyterian-St Luke's Med Ctr **(see page 122)**
Neuro-Psychiatric Evaluation, 3633 W Lake Ave Ste 404; Glenview, IL 60025; (847) 657-6007; **BDCERT:** Psyc 89; **MS:** Rush Med Coll 83; **RES:** Psyc, Rush Presbyterian-St Luke's Med Ctr, Chicago, IL 83-87; **FAP:** Asst Prof Rush Med Coll; **HMO:** Blue Cross & Blue Shield
VISA

Burton, Robert (MD) Psyc
Northwestern Mem Hosp
405 N Wabash Ave Ste 4605; Chicago, IL 60611; (312) 642-3482; **BDCERT:** Psyc 91; AdP 94; **MS:** Mich St U 84; **RES:** Psyc, Northwestern Mem Hosp, Chicago, IL 84-88; **FAP:** Asst Prof of Clin Psyc Northwestern U; **HOSP:** Rehab Institute of Chicago; ***SI:*** *Sports Medicine Related Psychiatry*

Canelas, Elizabeth W (MD) Psyc
Mount Sinai Hosp Med Ctr
6425 Cermak Rd; Berwyn, IL 60402; (708) 484-9903; **BDCERT:** Psyc 95; **MS:** Bolivia 88; **RES:** Michael Reese Hosp, Chicago, IL 90-92; Loyola U Med Ctr, Maywood, IL 92-94; **FAP:** Asst Prof Rush Med Coll

Cavanaugh, James (MD) Psyc
Rush-Presbyterian-St Luke's Med Ctr **(see page 122)**
Isaac Ray Ctr Inc, 1725 W Harrison St Ste 110; Chicago, IL 60612; (312) 829-1463; **BDCERT:** Psyc 74; **MS:** Univ Penn 67; **RES:** Psyc, Hosp of U Penn, Philadelphia, PA 68-71; **FAP:** Prof Psyc Rush Med Coll

Chor, Philip (MD) Psyc
Rush-Presbyterian-St Luke's Med Ctr **(see page 122)**
1725 W Harrison St Ste 964; Chicago, IL 60612; (312) 243-8277; **BDCERT:** Psyc 78; **MS:** U Cincinnati 72; **RES:** Psyc, Loyola U Med Ctr, Maywood, IL 73-76; **FAP:** Asst Prof Rush Med Coll

Davis, Gilla (MD) Psyc
Evanston Hosp
2650 Ridge Ave; Evanston, IL 60201; (847) 570-2692; **BDCERT:** Psyc 80; **MS:** Northwestern U 75; **RES:** Psyc, UCLA Med Ctr, Los Angeles, CA 76-79; **FAP:** Asst Prof Northwestern U; ***SI:*** *Women's Mental Health*; **HMO:** Blue Cross & Blue Shield, Humana Health Plan
Mcr A Few Days VISA

Douglas, Zachariah (MD) Psyc
Rush North Shore Med Ctr
1725 W Harrison St Ste 744; Chicago, IL 60612; (312) 942-8084; **BDCERT:** Psyc 91; **MS:** Med Coll Wisc 84; **RES:** Psyc, Michael Reese Hospital 84-88; **FAP:** Asst Prof Psyc Rush Med Coll

Dunkas, Nicholas (MD) **Psyc**
Columbus Hosp
Nicholas Dunkas & Assoc, 708 Church St Ste 215; Evanston, IL 60201; (847) 864-4744; **BDCERT:** Psyc 66; **MS:** Italy 53; **RES:** Psyc, Il State Psych Inst, Chicago, IL 57-62; **FAP:** Asst Clin Prof Psyc Northwestern U

Durburg, John R (MD) **Psyc**
Evanston Hosp
1565 Maple Ave Ste 310; Evanston, IL 60201; (847) 570-0973; **BDCERT:** Psyc 76; AdP 93; **MS:** Loyola U-Stritch Sch Med, Maywood 64; **RES:** West Side VA Hosp, Chicago, IL 65-68; Northwestern Mem Hosp, Chicago, IL 71-74; **HOSP:** Northwestern Mem Hosp; ***SI:*** *Addictive Dependency*

Earley, Willie R (MD) **Psyc**
Tinley Park Mental Hlth Ctr
7400 W 183rd St; Tinley Park, IL 60477; (708) 614-4015; **BDCERT:** Psyc 89; **MS:** Univ IL Coll Med 89; **RES:** Psyc, U IL Med Ctr, Chicago, IL 89-93; **FAP:** Asst Clin Prof Psyc Univ IL Coll Med; ***SI:*** *Emergency Psychiatric Treatment*

Ebenhoeh, Patrick (MD) **Psyc**
Rush North Shore Med Ctr
9700 North Kenton Ave K; Skokie, IL 60076; (847) 674-9100; **BDCERT:** Psyc 68; **MS:** Loyola U-Stritch Sch Med, Maywood 61; **RES:** Univ of Illinois at Chicago Psyciatric Institute, Chicago, IL 62-65; **FAP:** Asst Prof Rush Med Coll; **HOSP:** Rush-Presbyterian-St Luke's Med Ctr; **HMO:** Blue Cross & Blue Shield, Compare Health Service, Health Options, Metlife, Principal Health Care
VISA

Edger, Robert (MD) **Psyc**
Northwestern Mem Hosp
Lavoll & Edger, 645 N Michigan Ave Ste 820; Chicago, IL 60611; (312) 988-7180; **BDCERT:** Psyc 82; ChAP 86; **MS:** Ky Med Sch, Louisville 76; **RES:** EM, U Louisville Hosp, Louisville, KY 77-78; Psyc, U Louisville Hosp, Louisville, KY 78-80; **FEL:** ChAP, U Louisville Hosp, Louisville, KY 80-82; ***SI:*** *Adult Psychiatry; Child Psychiatry*

Egan, William (MD) **Psyc**
Macneal Mem Hosp
3231 Euclid Ave Fl 4; Berwyn, IL 60402; (708) 484-0515; **BDCERT:** Psyc 73; **MS:** Loyola U-Stritch Sch Med, Maywood 67; **RES:** Psyc, Cincinnati Med Ctr, Cincinnati, OH 68-71; **FAP:** Assoc Clin Prof Loyola U-Stritch Sch Med, Maywood

Eisenstein, Richard (MD) **Psyc**
Evanston Hosp
2530 Ridge Ave; Evanston, IL 60201; (847) 869-2252; **BDCERT:** Psyc 67; **MS:** Case West Res U 60; **RES:** Psyc, U Chicago Hosp, Chicago, IL 61-64; **FAP:** Assoc Prof of Clin Psyc Northwestern U; ***SI:*** *Depressive Disorders; Anxiety Disorders*; **HMO:** Blue Cross & Blue Shield
2-4 Weeks

Fawcett, Jan A. (MD) **Psyc**
Rush-Presbyterian-St Luke's Med Ctr
(see page 122)
Dept of Psych-Rush Presbyterian, 1653 W Congress Pkwy; Chicago, IL 60612; (312) 942-5372; **BDCERT:** Psyc 67; **MS:** Yale U Sch Med 60; **RES:** Langley Porter Psych Inst, San Francisco, CA 61-63; Rochester Gen Hosp, Rochester, NY 63-64; ***SI:*** *Depression*; **HMO:** Aetna Hlth Plan, Blue Cross & Blue Shield +

Finkel, Sanford (MD) **Psyc**
Northwestern Mem Hosp
303 E Ohio St Ste 550; Chicago, IL 60611; (312) 263-0139; **BDCERT:** Psyc 76; **MS:** U Mich Med Sch 67; **RES:** Psyc, Michael Reese Hosp Med Ctr, Chicago, IL 68-71; **FAP:** Prof Northwestern U; ***SI:*** *Depression; Alzheimer's Disease*; **HMO:** United Healthcare, Magellan
2-4 Weeks

Flaherty, Joseph (MD) **Psyc**
Univ of Illinois at Chicago Psyciatric Institute
Dept of Psychiatry, 912 S Wood St M/C-913; Chicago, IL 60612; (312) 996-7383; **BDCERT:** Psyc 76; GerPsy 92; **MS:** Univ IL Coll Med 71; **RES:** Psyc, U IL Med Ctr, Chicago, IL 72-75; **FAP:** Prof Univ IL Coll Med; **HMO:** American Health Plan, Blue Cross & Blue Shield, Aetna-US Healthcare, Prudential +
LANG: Sp, Hin; 1 Week **VISA**

Gaviria, Moises (MD) **Psyc**
Univ of Illinois at Chicago Psyciatric Institute
912 S Wood St; Chicago, IL 60612; (312) 996-6139; **BDCERT:** Psyc 77; **MS:** Peru 66; **RES:** Psyc, U Conn Hlth Ctr, Farmington, CT 72-75; **FEL:** Soc/Comm, Univ of Illinois at Chicago Psyciatric Institute, Chicago, IL 75-76; **FAP:** Prof Psyc Univ IL Coll Med; **HOSP:** Ravenswood Hosp Med Ctr; ***SI:*** *Neuropsychiatry - Post Operative; Dementia from Strokes*; **HMO:** +
LANG: Sp, Prt; 1 Week **VISA**

Gehlhoff, David A (MD) **Psyc**
St Joseph Hosp-Chicago
2900 N Lake Shore Dr; Chicago, IL 60657; (773) 348-3535; **BDCERT:** Psyc 76; **MS:** U Minn 64; **RES:** Psyc, U Chicago Hosp, Chicago, IL 67-70; ***SI:*** *Marital Therapy; Anxiety Disorders*

Guide to symbols and abbreviations can be found on pages 110-113.

Gilmer, William (MD) **Psyc**
Northwestern Mem Hosp
Northwestern Medical Faculty Fdtn., 303 E Ohio St Ste 550; Chicago, IL 60611; (312) 908-3511; **BDCERT:** Psyc 93; **MS:** U Iowa Coll Med 86; **RES:** Psyc, Rush Presbyterian-St Luke's Med Ctr, Chicago, IL; **FAP:** Asst Prof Psyc Northwestern U; ***SI:*** *Mood Disorders*
2-4 Weeks VISA

Gojkovich, Dusan (MD) **Psyc**
Ingalls Mem Hosp
Olympia Fields Psychiatry, 2555 Lincoln Hwy Ste 209; Olympia Fields, IL 60461; (708) 747-0810; **BDCERT:** Psyc 78; **MS:** Yugoslavia 60; **RES:** Cook Cty Hosp, Chicago, IL 63-64; Univ of Illinois at Chicago Psyciatric Institute, Chicago, IL 64-67; **FAP:** Assoc Prof Psyc Loyola U-Stritch Sch Med, Maywood

Greenberg, Sheldon (MD) **Psyc**
Louis A Weiss Mem Hosp
Louis A Weiss Memorial Hospital, 4646 N Marine Dr; Chicago, IL 60640; (773) 561-3365; **BDCERT:** Psyc 74; AdP 93; **MS:** Loyola U-Stritch Sch Med, Maywood 68; **RES:** Psyc, Northwestern Mem Hosp, Chicago, IL 69-72

Halderman, John (MD) **Psyc**
Evanston Hosp
444 Skokie Blvd Ste 340; Wilmette, IL 60091; (847) 853-0077; **BDCERT:** Psyc 85; GerPsy 92; **MS:** Med Coll Va 73; **RES:** Psyc, Evanston Hosp, Evanston, IL 73-76; ***SI:*** *Psychotherapy; Geriatric Psychiatry*
A Few Days

Hoag, Emily (MD) **Psyc**
Illinois Masonic Med Ctr
(see page 118)
122 S Michigan Ste 1406; Chicago, IL 60613; (312) 587-7716; **BDCERT:** Psyc 93; **MS:** Univ IL Coll Med 86; **RES:** Psyc, Loyola U Med Ctr, Maywood, IL 89-92

Jacobs, Leo (MD) **Psyc**
Good Shepherd Hosp
450 W Highway 22 Ste 2210; Barrington, IL 60010; (847) 382-5015; **BDCERT:** Psyc 66; **MS:** Belgium 60; **RES:** Univ of Illinois at Chicago Psyciatric Institute, Chicago, IL 61-63; **HMO:** Blue Cross & Blue Shield, Travelers

Kapoor, Deepak (MD) **Psyc**
Cook Cty Hosp
Cook County Hospital, 1900 W Polk St Fl 8; Chicago, IL 60612; (312) 633-7766; **BDCERT:** Psyc 80; AdP 94; **MS:** India 73; **RES:** NS, Chicago Hosp, Chicago, IL 67-68; NS, Chicago Hosp, Chicago, IL 70-73; **HMO:** Aetna Hlth Plan, Blue Cross & Blue Shield, Californiacare, CIGNA, Compare Health Service

Kayton, Lawrence (MD) **Psyc**
Hinsdale Hosp **(see page 275)**
120 Oakbrook Ctr Rm 720; Oak Brook, IL 60523; (630) 990-1532; **BDCERT:** Psyc 72; **MS:** Univ IL Coll Med 63; **RES:** Psyc, Michael Reese Hosp Med Ctr, Chicago, IL 64-67; **FAP:** Clin Prof Loyola U-Stritch Sch Med, Maywood; **HOSP:** Loyola U Med Ctr; ***SI:*** *Psychotherapy; Psychopharmacology*; **HMO:** Blue Cross
1 Week VISA

Kelly, Jonathan (MD) **Psyc**
Rush-Presbyterian-St Luke's Med Ctr
(see page 122)
1720 W Polk St; Chicago, IL 60612; (312) 942-2832; **BDCERT:** Psyc 81; FPsy 94; **MS:** SUNY Syracuse 75; **RES:** Psyc, Strong Mem Hosp, Rochester, NY 75-79; **FEL:** FPsy, Rush Presbyterian-St Luke's Med Ctr, Chicago, IL 79-80; **FAP:** Asst Prof Rush Med Coll; ***SI:*** *Depression, Forensic Psychiatry; Sexual Disorders*; **HMO:** Blue Cross & Blue Shield, Prudential, Travelers
A Few Days

Kraus, Louis (MD) **Psyc**
Evanston Hosp
2650 Ridge Ave; Evanston, IL 60201; (847) 570-2037; **BDCERT:** Psyc 93; ChAP 95; **MS:** U Hlth Sci/Chicago Med Sch 87; **RES:** Psyc, Northwestern U, Chicago, IL 88-92; **FEL:** ChAP, U Chicago Hosp, Chicago, IL 92-94; **HOSP:** Glenbrook Hosp

Kuhs, Leon (MD) **Psyc**
Illinois Masonic Med Ctr
(see page 118)
Il Masonic Med Ctr, 919 W Wellington Ave; Chicago, IL 60657; (773) 296-5868; **BDCERT:** Psyc 75; **MS:** Univ IL Coll Med 60; **RES:** Psyc, Northwestern Mem Hosp, Chicago, IL 61-64; ***SI:*** *Substance Abuse*
4+ Weeks VISA

Kurland, Howard D (MD) **Psyc**
Evanston Hosp
500 Green Bay Rd; Kenilworth, IL 60043; (847) 251-0065; **BDCERT:** Psyc 66; **MS:** Northwestern U 59; **RES:** Psyc, Northwestern Mem Hosp, Chicago, IL 60-61; US Naval Hosp, Oakland, CO 61-63; **FEL:** Research, Clinical Investigation Center, Oakland, CA 61-65; **FAP:** Assoc Prof Northwestern U; ***SI:*** *Neuropsychiatric Treatments; Holistic Pain Relief-Laser*

Lavoll, Gunnbjorg (MD) **Psyc**
Northwestern Mem Hosp
645 N Michigan Ave Ste 820; Chicago, IL 60611; (312) 988-7877; **BDCERT:** Psyc 80; ChAP 81; **MS:** Ireland 71; **RES:** Psyc, Northwestern Mem Hosp, Chicago, IL 73-76; **FEL:** ChAP, Michael Reese Hosp Med Ctr, Chicago, IL 76-78; **FAP:** Assoc Prof Northwestern U; ***SI:*** *Psychoanalysis*

Leff, Joel (MD) **Psyc**
Christ Hosp & Med Ctr **(see page 140)**
7350 W College Dr Ste 106; Palos Heights, IL 60463; (708) 361-5110; **BDCERT:** Psyc 80; **MS:** Univ IL Coll Med 72; **RES:** Psyc, Univ of Illinois at Chicago Psyciatric Institute, Chicago, IL 72-75; **FAP:** Clin Instr Psyc Univ IL Coll Med

Leventhal, Bennett (MD) Psyc
U Chicago Hosp (see page 124)
University of Chicago Psychiatry-MC 3077, 5841 S Maryland Ave W304; Chicago, IL 60637; (773) 702-3858; **BDCERT:** Psyc 79; ChAP 80; **MS:** LSU Sch Med, New Orleans 74; **RES:** Psyc, Duke U Med Ctr, Durham, NC 74-78; **FEL:** ChAP, Duke U Med Ctr, Durham, NC 76-77; **FAP:** Prof U Chicago-Pritzker Sch Med; ***SI:*** *Developmental Disorders; Psychopharmacology*
4+ Weeks VISA

Martini, D Richard (MD) Psyc
Children's Mem Med Ctr (see page 139)
Child Psychiatry Dept - Children's Mem Hosp, 530 Wisner St; Park Ridge, IL 60068; (773) 880-4000; **BDCERT:** Psyc 87; ChAP 90; **MS:** Univ Nebr Coll Med 82; **RES:** Psyc, Pittsburgh Med Ctr, Pittsburgh, PA 83-85; ChAP, Pittsburgh Med Ctr, Pittsburgh, PA 85-87; **FEL:** Pittsburgh Med Ctr, Pittsburgh, PA 82-83; **FAP:** Asst Prof Psyc; ***SI:*** *Medically Ill Children; Brain Injury;* **HMO:** Bronx Health, Greenspring, Magellan, Northwestern POS, VBH
LANG: Sp; 2-4 Weeks
VISA

Martorana, Andrew (MD) Psyc
Michael Reese Hosp & Med Ctr
1945 W Wilson Ave Ste 1117; Chicago, IL 60640; (773) 346-9595; **BDCERT:** Psyc 87; **MS:** Univ IL Coll Med 81; **RES:** Psyc, U IL Med Ctr, Chicago, IL 82-85; **FAP:** Asst Clin Prof Univ IL Coll Med; **HOSP:** Chicago Lakeshore Hosp; ***SI:*** *Depression; Anxiety*

Mc Kenna, Kathleen (MD) Psyc
Children's Mem Med Ctr (see page 139)
Children's Memorial Hospital, 2300 Children's Plaza Ste 10; Chicago, IL 60614; (773) 880-8391; **BDCERT:** Psyc 91; ChAP 92; **MS:** Baylor 85; **RES:** Psyc, Mass Mental Hlth Ctr, Boston, MA 86-88; **FEL:** ChAP, Nat Inst Mental Health, Bethesda, MD 91-94; ChAP, McLean Hosp, Belmont, MA 88-90; **FAP:** Asst Prof Northwestern U; **HOSP:** Northwestern Mem Hosp; ***SI:*** *Children Psychosis*
2-4 Weeks VISA

Mc Kinney, William (MD) Psyc
Northwestern Mem Hosp
Northwestern Univ Med Sch/Dept of Psych, 303 E Chicago Ave Ste 9-176; Chicago, IL 60611; (312) 908-9380; **BDCERT:** Psyc 70; **MS:** Vanderbilt U Sch Med 63; **RES:** Stanford Med Ctr, Stanford, CA 66-67; U NC Hosp, Chapel Hill, NC 64-66; ***SI:*** *Depression; Manic Depression;* **HMO:** +
2-4 Weeks VISA

Mehta, Harshad M (MD) Psyc
Little Company of Mary Hosp & Hlth Care Ctrs (see page 142)
4700 W 95th St Ste 308; Oak Lawn, IL 60453; (708) 425-8900; **BDCERT:** Psyc 80; **MS:** India 71; **RES:** Univ of Illinois at Chicago Psyciatric Institute, Chicago, IL 74-77

Menezes, Ralph (MD) Psyc
Forest Hosp
555 Wilson Ln; Des Plaines, IL 60016; (847) 635-4100; **BDCERT:** Psyc 85; **MS:** Sri Lanka 73; **RES:** Psyc, U Chicago Hosp, Chicago, IL 75-78; **HMO:** Aetna Hlth Plan, Blue Cross & Blue Shield, Chicago HMO, CIGNA, HealthNet

Meredith, Heidi (MD) Psyc
Lutheran Gen Hosp (see page 143)
Associates In Psychiatric Med, 1500 Waukegan Rd Ste 213; Glenview, IL 60025; (847) 998-5556; **BDCERT:** Psyc 93; GerPsy 96; **MS:** Northwestern U 88; **RES:** Psyc, U Chicago Hosp, Chicago, IL 89-92

Meyer, James (MD) Psyc
St Mary's of Nazareth Hosp Ctr
Dept of Psychiatry -Floor 14, 2233 W Division St 14th Flr; Chicago, IL 60622; (312) 770-2000; **BDCERT:** Psyc 82; **MS:** Loyola U-Stritch Sch Med, Maywood 74

Miller, Frederick E (MD) Psyc
Evanston Hosp
Evanston Hospital - Psychiatry, 2650 Ridge Ave; Evanston, IL 60201; (847) 570-1247; **BDCERT:** Psyc 89; **MS:** U Chicago-Pritzker Sch Med 83; **RES:** Psyc, U IL Med Ctr, Chicago, IL 83-87; **FAP:** Asst Prof Psyc Northwestern U

Miller, Laura Jo (MD) Psyc
Univ of Illinois at Chicago Psyciatric Institute
University of Illinois - Dept Psych, 912 Southwood St M/C-913; Chicago, IL 60612; (312) 355-1223; **BDCERT:** Psyc 88; **MS:** Harvard Med Sch 82; **RES:** Psyc, U Chicago Hosp, Chicago, IL 83-86; **FAP:** Assoc Prof Univ IL Coll Med; ***SI:*** *Pregnancy-Psychiatric Disorders; Women's Mental Health;* **HMO:** Blue Cross & Blue Shield, Aetna-US Healthcare, Prudential +
LANG: Sp; A Few Days

Miller, Sheldon (MD) **Psyc**
Northwestern Mem Hosp
Northwest Univ Medical - Passavant 561, 303 E Superior St; Chicago, IL 60611; (312) 908-2323; **BDCERT:** Psyc 72; AdP 93; **MS:** Tufts U 64; **RES:** U Hosp of Cleveland, Cleveland, OH 65-68; **FAP:** Prof Psyc Northwestern U; **HMO:** +

Pedemonte, Walter (MD) **Psyc**
St Mary's of Nazareth Hosp Ctr
Latino Family Institute, 6551 W North Ave; Oak Park, IL 60302; (708) 445-0480; **BDCERT:** Psyc 82; **MS:** Argentina 71; **RES:** Psyc, ISPI, Chicago, IL 71-75; **FEL:** Psyc, U Chicago Hosp, Chicago, IL 75-78

Perri, John (MD) **Psyc**
Michael Reese Hosp & Med Ctr
111 N Wabash Ave; Chicago, IL 60602; (312) 443-8970; **BDCERT:** Psyc 91; **MS:** Loyola U-Stritch Sch Med, Maywood 85; **RES:** Psyc, U IL Med Ctr, Chicago, IL 85-89; **FAP:** Asst Prof Univ IL Coll Med

Reeves, Robert (MD) **Psyc**
Swedish Covenant Hosp
Dixon F Spivy MD, Ltd, 1011 W Wellington Ave Fl 1; Chicago, IL 60657; (773) 883-0200; **BDCERT:** Psyc 91; **MS:** St Louis U 78; **RES:** FP, Lutheran Gen Hosp, Park Ridge, IL 78-79; Psyc, Loyola U Med Ctr, Maywood, IL 79-82; **HOSP:** Chicago Lakeshore Hosp

Renshaw, Domeena (MD) **Psyc**
Loyola U Med Ctr **(see page 120)**
Dept Psyc Loyola U Hosp, 2160 S 1st Ave; Maywood, IL 60153; (708) 821-3752; **BDCERT:** Psyc 72; **MS:** South Africa 60; **RES:** Ped, Children's Hosp, Boston, MA 62-63; Psyc, Loyola U Med Ctr, Maywood, IL 65-68; **FAP:** Prof Loyola U-Stritch Sch Med, Maywood; ***SI:** Sexual Problems-Adults & Seniors; Sexual Problems-Children*; **HMO:** Blue Cross & Blue Shield, HMO Illinois

Ripeckyj, Andrew (MD) **Psyc**
Rush-Presbyterian-St Luke's Med Ctr
(see page 122)
Midwest Neuropsychiatric Assoc, 1725 W Harrison St Ste 744; Chicago, IL 60612; (312) 942-0118; **BDCERT:** Psyc 82; **MS:** Northwestern U 76; **RES:** Psyc, U UT Hosp, Salt Lake City, UT 76-79; **FEL:** GerPsy, Rush Presbyterian-St Luke's Med Ctr, Chicago, IL 79-80; **FAP:** Asst Prof Rush Med Coll; ***SI:** Geriatric Psychiatry*; **HMO:** None
LANG: Ukr; A Few Days
VISA

Schwartz, Lee (MD) **Psyc**
Rehab Institute of Chicago
150 E Huron St; Chicago, IL 60611; (847) 256-0576; **BDCERT:** Psyc 84; GerPsy 91; **MS:** Univ IL Coll Med 79; **RES:** Psyc, U IL Med Ctr, Chicago, IL 80-83; **FAP:** Assoc Prof Psyc Northwestern U; **HOSP:** Northwestern Mem Hosp; **HMO:** +

Seidenberg, Henry (MD) **Psyc**
Michael Reese Hosp & Med Ctr
122 S Michigan Ave Ste 1037; Chicago, IL 60603; (312) 922-6988; **BDCERT:** Psyc 55; **MS:** Jefferson Med Coll 46; **RES:** N, Montefiore Med Ctr, Bronx, NY 49-50; Psyc, Michael Reese Hosp Med Ctr, Chicago, IL 50-53; **FAP:** Assoc Clin Prof Univ IL Coll Med; ***SI:** Parent Loss; Anxiety and Depression*
1 Week

Shapiro, Daniel (MD) **Psyc**
Michael Reese Hosp & Med Ctr
111 N Wabash Ave Ste 1319; Chicago, IL 60602; (312) 346-8569; **BDCERT:** Psyc 65; **MS:** Univ IL Coll Med 53; **RES:** Psyc, Michael Reese Hosp Med Ctr, Chicago, IL 55-58; **FAP:** Asst Clin Prof Psyc Univ IL Coll Med; **HOSP:** Hines VA Hosp; ***SI:** Psychotherapy*; **HMO:** Michael Reese Phys Grp +
1 Week

Shaw, Geoffrey (MD) **Psyc**
Lutheran Gen Hosp **(see page 143)**
1500 Waukegan Rd Ste 213; Glenview, IL 60025; **BDCERT:** Psyc 95; GerPsy 96; **MS:** Northern Ireland 88; **RES:** Psyc, Belfast City Hosp, Belfast, Northern Ireland 88-91; Psyc, Northwestern Mem Hosp, Chicago, IL 91-94; **HOSP:** Evanston Hosp; ***SI:** Geriatrics; Electroconvulsive Therapy*
LANG: Sp; 2-4 Weeks **VISA**

Teas, Gregory (MD) **Psyc**
Alexian Brothers Med Ctr
(see page 138)
A B B H R, 25 E Schaumburg Rd Ste 101; Schaumburg, IL 60194; (847) 352-4540; **BDCERT:** Psyc 79; AdP 93; **MS:** Loyola U-Stritch Sch Med, Maywood 74; **RES:** Psyc, Loyola U Med Ctr, Maywood, IL 74-77; **FAP:** Asst Clin Prof Loyola U-Stritch Sch Med, Maywood; ***SI:** Mood Disorders; Addictions*; **HMO:** CIGNA, United Healthcare, Aetna Hlth Plan, Blue Cross & Blue Shield, First Health +
2-4 Weeks **VISA**

Terman, David (MD) **Psyc**
122 S Michigan Ave Ste 1307; Chicago, IL 60603; (312) 431-9694; **BDCERT:** Psyc 68; **MS:** U Chicago-Pritzker Sch Med 59; **RES:** Psyc, Michael Reese Hosp Med Ctr, Chicago, IL 60-63; **FEL:** Psychoanalysis, Univ of Illinois at Chicago Psyciatric Institute, Chicago, IL 65-72; ***SI:** Psychoanalysis; Psychoanalytic Psychotherapy*
LANG: Fr; A Few Days

Trager, Eugene (MD) **Psyc**
Lutheran Gen Hosp **(see page 143)**
1775 Dempster St Ste 8S; Park Ridge, IL 60068; (847) 696-5887; **BDCERT:** Psyc 75; **MS:** Univ IL Coll Med 59; **RES:** Psyc, Univ Hosp SUNY Syracuse, Syracuse, NY 60-63; **FAP:** Asst Clin Prof Psyc Rush Med Coll; **HMO:** Blue Cross & Blue Shield, Chicago HMO, CIGNA, Compare Health Service, Humana Health Plan

Visotsky, Harold (MD) **Psyc**
Northwestern Mem Hosp
Dept of Psychiatry, 303 E Ohio St Ste 550; Chicago, IL 60611; (312) 908-8049; **BDCERT:** Psyc 59; **MS:** Univ IL Coll Med 51; **RES:** Psyc, Neuropsychiatric Inst - U IL, Chicago, IL 52-55; **FAP:** Prof/Chrmn Psyc Northwestern U; ***SI:*** *Depression and Mood Disorder; Stress Disorders*; **HMO:** Private Healthcare, Magnacare +

Wolpert, Edward (MD) **Psyc**
Rush-Presbyterian-St Luke's Med Ctr **(see page 122)**
1725 W Harrison Ste 955; Chicago, IL 60612; (312) 256-2204; **BDCERT:** Psyc 70; **MS:** U Chicago-Pritzker Sch Med 60; **RES:** Psyc, Michael Reese Hosp Med Ctr, Chicago, IL 61-64; **FAP:** Prof Psyc Rush Med Coll; ***SI:*** *Manic-Depressive Illness & Psychoanalysis; Bipolar Disorder*
A Few Days

Zajecka, John (MD) **Psyc**
Rush-Presbyterian-St Luke's Med Ctr **(see page 122)**
1725 W Harrison St Ste 956; Chicago, IL 60612; (312) 942-5592; **BDCERT:** Psyc 91; **MS:** Loyola U-Stritch Sch Med, Maywood 84; **RES:** Psyc, Rush Presby-St Lukes MC, Chicago, IL 84-88

PULMONARY DISEASE

Ahmad, Zubair (MD) **Pul**
Good Shepherd Hosp
450 W Highway 22 Ste 250; Barrington, IL 60010; (847) 381-4491; **BDCERT:** PPul 82; CCM 89; **MS:** Pakistan 77; **HOSP:** Sherman Hosp
1 Week ***VISA***

Akhter, Javeed (MD) **Pul**
Christ Hosp & Med Ctr **(see page 140)**
4440 W 95th St; Oak Lawn, IL 60453; (708) 346-5810; **BDCERT:** PPul 86; A&I 81; **MS:** India 68; **RES:** Ped, Niloufer Hospital 70-73; Ped, Cook Cty Hosp, Chicago, IL 75-77; **FEL:** A&I, U Chicago Hosp, Chicago, IL 77-79; **FAP:** Assoc Prof PPul U Chicago-Pritzker Sch Med; **HOSP:** Good Samaritan Hosp

Alderman, Sarah (MD) **Pul**
Our Lady Of the Resurrection Med Ctr
Midwest Pulmonary Consultants & Sleep Consultants, 5600 W Addison St Ste 304; Chicago, IL 60634; (773) 481-1570; **BDCERT:** Pul 88; IM 86; **MS:** Univ Mo-Columbia Sch Med 83

Arias, Ada (MD) **Pul**
St Elizabeth's Hosp
1431 N Clairmont Ave; Chicago, IL 60622; (312) 633-5857; **BDCERT:** Pul 86; CCM 89; **MS:** Peru 81; **RES:** IM, Cook Cty Hosp, Chicago, IL 82-84; **FEL:** Pul, U WI Sch Med, Milwaukee, WI 84-86; **FAP:** Assoc Prof CCM Univ IL Coll Med; **HOSP:** St Mary's of Nazareth Hosp Ctr; ***SI:*** *Asthma; Pneumonia*; **HMO:** Aetna Hlth Plan, United Healthcare, Rush Health Plans
LANG: Sp; A Few Days

Balk, Robert (MD) **Pul**
Rush-Presbyterian-St Luke's Med Ctr **(see page 122)**
1653 W Congress Pkwy; Chicago, IL 60612; (312) 942-5873; **BDCERT:** Pul 86; CCM 87; **MS:** U MO-Kansas City Sch Med 78; **RES:** IM, U MO Kansas City Sch Med, Kansas City, MO 78-81; **FEL:** Pul Intensive Care, U Arkansas, Little Rock, AR 81-83; **FAP:** Assoc Prof Med Rush Med Coll; ***SI:*** *Respiratory Failure*; **HMO:** +
2-4 Weeks

Barr, Lewis (MD) **Pul**
Resurrection Med Ctr
Northwest Pulmonary, 7447 W Talcott Ave Ste 542; Chicago, IL 60631; (773) 631-2180; **BDCERT:** IM 76; Pul 86; **MS:** U Hlth Sci/Chicago Med Sch 71

Budinger, G R Scott (MD) **Pul**
Loyola U Med Ctr **(see page 120)**
Loyola University Med Ctr, 2160 S First Ave; Maywood, IL 60153; (708) 216-5402; **BDCERT:** Pul 96; CCM 97; **MS:** Univ IL Coll Med 89; **RES:** IM, U Chicago Hosp, Chicago, IL 90-92; **FEL:** Pul/CCM, U Chicago Hosp, Chicago, IL 92-96; **FAP:** Asst Prof Pul Loyola U-Stritch Sch Med, Maywood; ***SI:*** *Pulmonary Embolism; Thrombosis-Deep Vein*

Cromydas, George (MD) **Pul**
Northwest Comm Hlthcare
North Shore Lung Specialist, 1614 W Central Rd Ste 205; Arlington Hts, IL 60005; (847) 818-1184; **BDCERT:** IM 80; CCM 89; **MS:** Univ IL Coll Med 77; **RES:** U IL Med Ctr, Chicago, IL 77-82

Diamond, Terrence (MD) **Pul**
Christ Hosp & Med Ctr **(see page 140)**
Pulmonary & Critical Care, 9907 Southwest Highway; Oak Lawn, IL 60453; (708) 636-3113; **BDCERT:** PPul 88; CCM 91; **MS:** Loyola U-Stritch Sch Med, Maywood 81; **RES:** IM, Hines VA Hosp, Hines, IL 82-84; IM, Loyola U Med Ctr, Maywood, IL 84-85; **FEL:** Pul, Loyola U Med Ctr, Maywood, IL 85-87

Guide to symbols and abbreviations can be found on pages 110-113.

Fahey, Patrick J (MD) Pul
Loyola U Med Ctr (see page 120)
Loyal Medical Center, 2160 S 1st Ave; Elmhurst, IL 60153; (708) 216-6046; **BDCERT:** Pul 78; CCM 89; **MS:** U Wisc Med Sch 73; **RES:** IM, St Elizabeth's Med Ctr, Boston, MA 73-76; **FEL:** Pul, St Elizabeth's Med Ctr, Boston, MA 76-77; Pul, Strong Mem Hosp, Rochester, NY 77; **FAP:** Professor Pul Loyola U-Stritch Sch Med, Maywood; **HOSP:** Hines VA Hosp; ***SI:*** *Asthma; Pulmonary Fibrosis*
2-4 Weeks

Geppert, Eugene (MD) Pul
U Chicago Hosp (see page 124)
5758 S Maryland; Chicago, IL 60637; (773) 702-9660; **BDCERT:** Pul 78; CCM 87; **MS:** Yale U Sch Med 74; **RES:** IM, U Chicago Hosp, Chicago, IL 75-76; **FEL:** Pul, UC San Francisco Med Ctr, San Francisco, CA 76-79; **FAP:** Asst Prof Med U Chicago-Pritzker Sch Med

Gupta, Raj G (MD) Pul
South Suburban Hosp
17850 Kedzie Ave Ste 2250; Hazel Crest, IL 60429; (708) 799-5677; **BDCERT:** Pul 76; IM 74; **MS:** India 70; **RES:** IM, Michael Reese Hosp Med Ctr, Chicago, IL 72-73; **FEL:** Pul, U IL Med Ctr, Chicago, IL 73-74; Pul, Boston U Med Ctr, Boston, MA 74-75; ***SI:*** *Chronic Obstructive Lung Disease; Asthma-Bronchitis*; **HMO:** Blue Cross & Blue Shield, CIGNA
A Few Days

Hart, Robert W (MD) Pul
Alexian Brothers Med Ctr
(see page 138)
Suburban Lung Assoc, 810 W Biesterfield Ste 404; Elk Grove Village, IL 60007; (847) 981-3660; **BDCERT:** Pul 84; CCM 87; **MS:** Univ IL Coll Med 79; **RES:** IM, U IL Med Ctr, Chicago, IL 80-82; **FEL:** Pul, U IL Med Ctr, Chicago, IL 82-84; **FAP:** Asst Clin Prof Univ IL Coll Med; **HOSP:** Central DuPage Hosp; ***SI:*** *Sleep Medicine; Sleep Apnea*; **HMO:** Aetna Hlth Plan, CIGNA, Bc/BS, Medicare +
Immediately ***VISA***

Herena, Juan (MD) Pul
West Suburban Hosp Med Ctr
1 Erie Ct Ste 3000; Oak Park, IL 60302; (708) 383-1619; **BDCERT:** Pul 96; CCM 97; **MS:** McGill U 88; **RES:** IM, Michael Reese Hosp Med Ctr, Chicago, IL 88-91; **FEL:** Pul & CCM, NY Hosp-Cornell Med Ctr, New York, NY 92-95; ***SI:*** *Sarcoidosis; Pulmonary Fibrosis*
LANG: Sp; A Few Days

Itkonen, Jerry (MD) Pul
Ingalls Mem Hosp
71 W 156th St Ste 203; Harvey, IL 60426; (708) 331-0405; **BDCERT:** IM 81; Pul 84; **MS:** Southern IL U 78; **RES:** IM, SIU Hosp, Springfield, IL 79-80; **FEL:** Pul, Northwestern Mem Hosp, Chicago, IL 81-83; **HMO:** Humana Health Plan

Kehoe, Thomas (MD) Pul
Evanston Hosp
Northshore Pulmonary Assoc Ltd, 2100 Pfingston Rd; Glenview, IL 60025; (847) 657-1965; **BDCERT:** Pul 80; IM 75; **MS:** U Wisc Med Sch 68; **RES:** IM, Northwestern Mem Hosp, Chicago, IL 73-75; **FEL:** Pul, Northwestern Mem Hosp, Chicago, IL 75-77; **HMO:** Aetna Hlth Plan, Blue Cross & Blue Shield, Chicago HMO, CIGNA, HealthNet

Kern, Richard (MD) Pul
Little Company of Mary Hosp & Hlth Care Ctrs (see page 142)
Pulmonary Medicine Consultants LTD, 2800 W 95th St; Evergreen Park, IL 60805; (708) 424-9288; **BDCERT:** Pul 86; CCM 91; **MS:** U Tex SW, Dallas 79; **RES:** IM, Michael Reese Hosp Med Ctr, Chicago, IL 80-82; **FEL:** Pul, Northwestern Mem Hosp, Chicago, IL 83-85; ***SI:*** *Asthma; Sleep Disorders*; **HMO:** Aetna Hlth Plan, Blue Cross & Blue Shield, Chicago HMO, CIGNA, Health Alliance Plan
1 Week

Lester, Lucy (MD) Pul
U Chicago Hosp (see page 124)
U Chicago Hosp Ped Pulmonary- MC6057, 5841 S Maryland Ave; Chicago, IL 60637; (773) 702-6178; **BDCERT:** PPul 92; Ped 77; **MS:** U Chicago-Pritzker Sch Med 72; **RES:** Ped A&I, U Chicago Hosp, Chicago, IL 73-74; **FEL:** PCd, U Chicago Hosp, Chicago, IL 74-77; **FAP:** Assoc Prof Ped U Chicago-Pritzker Sch Med

Liao, Thomas E (MD) Pul
Illinois Masonic Med Ctr
(see page 118)
Mid West Pulm & Sleep Consultants, 2800 N Sheridan Rd Ste 510; Chicago, IL 60657; (773) 404-0118; **BDCERT:** IM 84; CCM 91; **MS:** Rush Med Coll 81; **RES:** IM, Rush Presbyterian-St Luke's Med Ctr, Chicago, IL 82-84; **FEL:** Pul, Geo Wash U Med Ctr, Washington, DC 85-87; ***SI:*** *Sleep Disorders*

Mann, Stewart (MD) Pul
Columbus Hosp
Columbus Hospital, 2520 N Lakeview St; Chicago, IL 60614; (773) 388-5801; **BDCERT:** Pul 84; CCM 91; **MS:** Univ IL Coll Med 76; **RES:** IM, Northwestern Mem Hosp, Chicago, IL 77-79; **FEL:** Pul, Northwestern Mem Hosp, Chicago, IL 80-82; **FAP:** Clin Instr Northwestern U

Margolis, Benjamin (MD) Pul
West Suburban Hosp Med Ctr
1 Erie Ct Ste 3000; Oak Park, IL 60302; (708) 383-7899; **BDCERT:** IM 88; Pul 90; **MS:** Rush Med Coll 85; **RES:** IM, Evanston Hosp, Evanston, IL 85-88; **FEL:** Pul & CCM, U IL Med Ctr, Chicago, IL 88-91; Sleep Medicine, U IL Med Ctr, Chicago, IL 90-91; ***SI:*** *Asthma; Sleep Apnea*; **HMO:** +
A Few Days

Marinelli, Anthony (MD) **Pul**
West Suburban Hosp Med Ctr
1 Erie Ct Ste 3000; Oak Park, IL 60302; (708) 848-5353; **BDCERT:** Pul 78; IM 76; **MS:** Northwestern U 73; **RES:** IM, Youngstown Hosp, Youngstown, OH 74-76; **FEL:** Pul, U IL Med Ctr, Chicago, IL 76-78; **FAP:** Asst Prof Med Rush Med Coll

Mc Leod, Evan (MD) **Pul**
Little Company of Mary Hosp & Hlth Care Ctrs **(see page 142)**
Pulmonary Medicine, 2800 W 95th St; Evergreen Park, IL 60805; (708) 424-9288; **BDCERT:** IM 74; Pul 78; **MS:** UC San Francisco 71; **RES:** IM, Hosp of U Penn, Philadelphia, PA 72-73; IM, UC San Francisco, San Francisco, CA 73-74; **FEL:** Pul, UC San Francisco Med Ctr, San Francisco, CA 75-78; ***SI:*** *Asthma; Emphysema*

Muthuswamy, Petham (MD) **Pul**
Jackson Park Hosp & Med Ctr
Pulmonary & Critical Care Medicine Consultant, 7531 S Stony Island Avenue Suite 169; Chicago, IL 60649; (773) 947-7715; **BDCERT:** Pul 76; CCM 89; **MS:** India 69; **RES:** IM, Edgewater Med Ctr, Chicago, IL 71; IM, Cook Cty Hosp, Chicago, IL 72-73; **FEL:** Pul, Cook Cty Hosp, Chicago, IL 74-75; **FAP:** Assoc Professor Pul Univ IL Coll Med; **HOSP:** Cook Cty Hosp; ***SI:*** *Asthma/Respiratory Disease; Sarcoidosis*; **HMO:** Blue Cross & Blue Shield, HMO, Blue Choice PPO
LANG: Tam, Sp; SA SU Mcr Mcd
1 Week

Razma, Antanas (MD) **Pul**
Christ Hosp & Med Ctr **(see page 140)**
Pulmonary & Critical Care, 9907 Southwest Highway; Oak Lawn, IL 60453; (708) 636-3113; **BDCERT:** Pul 84; IM 80; **MS:** Univ IL Coll Med 77; **RES:** IM, U Mich Med Ctr, Ann Arbor, MI 78-80; **FEL:** Pul & CCM, U Mich Med Ctr, Ann Arbor, MI 81-83; **FAP:** Asst Prof IM Univ IL Coll Med

Ries, Michael (MD) **Pul**
St Joseph Hosp-Chicago
Chest Medicine Consultants, 2800 N Sheridan St; Chicago, IL 60657; (847) 679-8470; **BDCERT:** IM 78; **MS:** U Hlth Sci/Chicago Med Sch 75; **RES:** IM, Rush Presbyterian-St Luke's Med Ctr, Chicago, IL 76-78; **FEL:** Pul, Cedars-Sinai Med Ctr, Los Angeles, CA 78-80; **HOSP:** Rush North Shore Med Ctr; **HMO:** Aetna-US Healthcare, Rush Health Plans, HealthStar
LANG: Rus, Sp, Ger; Mcd
1 Week VISA

Rosenberg, Neil (MD) **Pul**
Westlake Comm Hosp
Chest Medicine Consultants, 2800 N Sheridan Rd Ste 301; Chicago, IL 60657; (773) 935-5556; **BDCERT:** Pul 84; CCM 97; **MS:** Med Coll Va 78; **RES:** IM, Rush Presbyterian-St Luke's Med Ctr, Chicago, IL 79-81; **FEL:** Pul, Cedars-Sinai Med Ctr, Los Angeles, CA 82-84; **FAP:** Instr Rush Med Coll; **HOSP:** St Joseph Hosp-Elgin

Silver, Michael (MD) **Pul**
Rush-Presbyterian-St Luke's Med Ctr **(see page 122)**
1725 W Harrison St Ste 54; Chicago, IL 60612; (312) 942-6744; **BDCERT:** PPul 88; IM 84; **MS:** Albany Med Coll 81; **RES:** IM, Rush Presbyterian-St Luke's Med Ctr, Chicago, IL 81-84; Rush Presbyterian-St Luke's Med Ctr, Chicago, IL 84-85; **FEL:** Pul, Rush Presbyterian-St Luke's Med Ctr, Chicago, IL 85-87; **FAP:** Assoc Prof Rush Med Coll; **HOSP:** Elmhurst Mem Hosp; ***SI:*** *Asthma-Emphysema; Lung Problems*; **HMO:** Aetna Hlth Plan, Blue Cross, Travelers, United
Mcr Mcd NFI Immediately

Simpson, Kevin (MD) **Pul**
Loyola U Med Ctr **(see page 120)**
Loyola - Internal Medicine Dept, 2160 S 1st Ave; Maywood, IL 60153; (708) 216-9000; **BDCERT:** Pul 92; CCM 93; **MS:** U Chicago-Pritzker Sch Med 87

Smith, Lewis (MD) **Pul**
Northwestern Mem Hosp
Pulmonary & Critical Care, 303 E Superior St Ste 777; Chicago, IL 60611; (312) 908-8163; **BDCERT:** IM 76; **MS:** U Rochester 73; **RES:** IM, Strong Mem Hosp, Rochester, NY 73-76; **FEL:** Pul, Boston U Med Ctr, Boston, MA 76-79; **FAP:** Prof Northwestern U; ***SI:*** *Asthma; COPD*; **HMO:** +
Mcr Mcd NFI 2-4 Weeks VISA

Sporn, Peter (MD) **Pul**
Northwestern Mem Hosp
Northwestern U MedSch-Passavant 777, 303 E Superior St; Chicago, IL 60611; (312) 908-1800; **BDCERT:** Pul 86; CCM 87; **MS:** Wayne State U Sch Med 80; **RES:** IM, Bronx Muncipal Hosp Ctr, Bronx, NY 81-83; **FEL:** Pul & CCM, U Mich Med Ctr, Ann Arbor, MI 84-87; **FAP:** Asst Prof Med Northwestern U; **HOSP:** VA Hlthcare Systems-Lakeside; ***SI:*** *Asthma; Interstitial Lung Diseases*; **HMO:** +
LANG: Sp; Mcr Mcd NFI
A Few Days VISA

Tepeli, Agop (MD) **Pul**
South Suburban Hosp
Pulmonary Medicine Assoc, 17850 Kedzie Ave Ste 250; Hazel Crest, IL 60429; (708) 799-6055; **BDCERT:** Pul 86; CCM 89; **MS:** Italy 79; **RES:** IM, Louis A Weiss Mem Hosp, Chicago, IL 81-84; **FEL:** Pul, Hines VA Hosp, Chicago, IL 84-86

Upadhyay, Naresh (MD) **Pul**
Trinity Hosp
2315 E 93rd St Ste 340; Chicago, IL 60617; (773) 768-8925; **BDCERT:** Pul 96; CCM 97; **MS:** India 85; **RES:** Trenton Affiliated Hosp, Trenton, NJ 88-91; **FEL:** Pul, Chicago Med Ctr, Chicago, IL 95-96

Guide to symbols and abbreviations can be found on pages 110-113.

West, James (MD) **Pul**
Highland Park Hosp
Northshore Pulmonary Assoc Ltd, 2100 Pfingston Rd; Glenview, IL 60025; (847) 657-1965; **BDCERT:** IM 77; Pul 80; **MS:** U Chicago-Pritzker Sch Med 74; **RES:** IM, Hosp of U Penn, Philadelphia, PA 75-77; **FEL:** Physical Medicine, Hosp of U Penn, Philadelphia, PA 75-79; **FAP:** Asst Clin Prof Northwestern U; **HOSP:** Evanston Hosp

Zanetti, Claude (MD) **Pul**
Edgewater Med Ctr
Edgewater Medical Ctr, 5700 N Ashland Ave; Chicago, IL 60660; (773) 878-3614; **BDCERT:** IM 78; Pul 82; **MS:** Wayne State U Sch Med 75

RADIATION ONCOLOGY

Awan, Azhar (MD) **RadRO**
La Grange Mem Hosp **(see page 141)**
La Grange Memorial Treatment, 1325 Memorial Dr; La Grange, IL 60525; (708) 579-3200; **BDCERT:** RadRO 85; **MS:** Loyola U-Stritch Sch Med, Maywood 81; **RES:** Henry Ford Hosp, Detroit, MI 81-82; RadRO, Rush Presbyterian-St Luke's Med Ctr, Chicago, IL 82-85; **FAP:** Assoc Professo RadRO U Chicago-Pritzker Sch Med; **HOSP:** U Chicago Hosp; ***SI:** Sarcomas; Breast And Prostate Cancer*; **HMO:** Aetna Hlth Plan, Blue Cross & Blue Shield, Californiacare, United Healthcare
LANG: Pol, Swa, Pun, Ur, Hin; Mcr Mcd Immediately VISA

Bloomer, William (MD) **RadRO**
Evanston Hosp
Evanston Northwestern Healthcare, 2650 Ridge Ave; Evanston, IL; (847) 570-2590; **BDCERT:** RadRO 74; **MS:** Jefferson Med Coll 70; **RES:** RadRO, Harvard Med Sch, Cambridge, MA 71-74; **FAP:** Prof Northwestern U; ***SI:** Breast Cancer; Prostate Cancer*; **HMO:** Blue Cross, Aetna-US Healthcare, CIGNA, United, Humana Health Plan +
Mcr Mcd A Few Days VISA

Boyer, Martin (DO) **RadRO**
Lutheran Gen Hosp **(see page 143)**
Alexian Brothers Regional Cancer Care Center, 820 Biesterfield Rd Ste 110; Elk Grove Village, IL 60007; (847) 981-5760; **BDCERT:** RadRO 95; **MS:** Ohio U, Coll Osteo Med 89; **RES:** RadRO, Northwestern Mem Hosp, Chicago, IL 90-93; ***SI:** Brain Tumors; Gynecologic Cancer*; **HMO:** Blue Cross, CIGNA, Bay State Health Plan, Medicare, Humana Health Plan
Mcr Mcd NFI Immediately VISA

Conterato, Dean (MD) **RadRO**
Rush North Shore Med Ctr
9600A Gross Point Rd; Skokie, IL 60076; (847) 673-1338; **BDCERT:** RadRO 90; **MS:** Rush Med Coll 85; ***SI:** Prostate Implants*

Griem, Katherine (MD) **RadRO**
Rush-Presbyterian-St Luke's Med Ctr **(see page 122)**
Women Board Cancer Treatment, 1653 W Congress Pkwy; Chicago, IL 60612; (312) 942-5751; **BDCERT:** RadRO 86; **MS:** Harvard Med Sch 82; **RES:** IM, U Chicago Hosp, Chicago, IL 82-83; RadRO, Harvard Joint Center For Radiation Therapy, Boston, MA 83-86; **FAP:** Assoc Professo RadRO Rush Med Coll; **HOSP:** Macneal Mem Hosp; ***SI:** Breast Cancer; Head And Neck Cancer*; **HMO:** Blue Choice, CIGNA, United Healthcare, Principal Health Care
LANG: Sp, Pol, Fr; Mcr Mcd NFI
A Few Days VISA

Haraf, Daniel (MD) **RadRO**
U Chicago Hosp **(see page 124)**
5758 S Maryland MC9006; Chicago, IL 60637; (773) 702-2630; **BDCERT:** RadRO 90; IM 85; **MS:** U Hlth Sci/Chicago Med Sch 82; **RES:** IM, Michael Reese Hosp Med Ctr, Chicago, IL 83-85; **FEL:** RadRO, Michael Reese Hosp Med Ctr, Chicago, IL 85-88; **FAP:** Asst Prof U Chicago-Pritzker Sch Med; ***SI:** Head and Neck Cancer; Lung Cancer*
Mcr Mcd A Few Days VISA

Kiel, Krystyna D (MD) **RadRO**
Northwestern Mem Hosp
Northwestern Memorial Hospital, 250 E Superior St; Chicago, IL 60611; (312) 908-2520; **BDCERT:** Rad 83; **MS:** Univ Mass Sch Med 77; **RES:** Mass Gen Hosp, Boston, MA 78-82; **FAP:** Asst Prof Northwestern U; ***SI:** Breast Cancer; Gastroesophageal Cancer*
Mcr Mcd A Few Days

Mittal, Bharat (MD) **RadRO**
Northwestern Mem Hosp
Weseley Pavillion-Lower 44, 250 E Superior St; Chicago, IL 60611; (312) 908-2520; **BDCERT:** RadRO 81; **MS:** India 75; **RES:** IM, Christian Medical College & Hosp, Punjab, India 75-76; RadRO, Northwestern Mem Hosp, Chicago, IL 77-80; **FEL:** RadRO, Barnes Hosp, St Louis, MO 80-81; **FAP:** Prof Rad Northwestern U; **HMO:** +
LANG: Sp; Mcr Mcd 1 Week
VISA

Moran, Brian (MD) **RadRO**
Lutheran Gen Hosp **(see page 143)**
West Pavilion, 1700 Luther Ln; Park Ridge, IL 60068; (847) 723-2500; **BDCERT:** RadRO 92; **MS:** Loyola U-Stritch Sch Med, Maywood 87; **RES:** RadRO, Loyola U Med Ctr, Maywood, IL 88-91

Morgan, David (MD) RadRO
Christ Hosp & Med Ctr (see page 140)
4440 W 95th St; Oak Lawn, IL 60453; (708) 346-5475; **BDCERT:** RadRO 95; **MS:** Ohio State U 88; **RES:** IM, Rush Presbyterian-St Luke's Med Ctr, Chicago, IL 88-91; **FEL:** RadRO, Rush Presby-St Lukes Med Ctr, Chicago, IL 91-94; ***SI:*** *Pediatrics; Breast*; **HMO:** Medicare, Humana Health Plan, United Healthcare, Bc/BS, AARP +
A Few Days

Sarin, Pramila (MD) RadRO
Christ Hosp & Med Ctr (see page 140)
4440 W 95th St; Oak Lawn, IL 60453; (708) 346-5475; **BDCERT:** RadRO 75; **MS:** Burma 65; **RES:** RadRO, Rush Presbyterian-St Luke's Med Ctr, Chicago, IL 72-75; **FAP:** Asst Prof Rush Med Coll

Saxena, S V Amod (MD) RadRO
Rush-Presbyterian-St Luke's Med Ctr (see page 122)
Rush-Presbyterian-St Luke's Med Ctr, 1653 West Congress Pkwy; Chicago, IL 60612; (312) 942-5751; **BDCERT:** RadRO 67; Rad 67; **MS:** India 60; **RES:** S, Royal Cornwall Infirmary, Truro, England 62; RadRO, Univ of Bristol, Bristol, England 64; **FEL:** Princess Margaret Rose Hosp, Toronto, Canada 66; **FAP:** Prof & Chrmn Rush Med Coll; **HOSP:** Illinois Masonic Med Ctr; ***SI:*** *Prostate Cancer; Head & Neck Cancers*

Sharma, Madie M. (MD) RadRO
Rush-Presbyterian-St Luke's Med Ctr (see page 122)
901 W Wellington St; Chicago, IL 60657; (773) 296-7076; **BDCERT:** RadRO 93; **MS:** Tufts U 86; **RES:** Rad, Rush Presbyterian-St Luke's Med Ctr, Chicago, IL 87-90; **FEL:** Rad, Med Coll WI, Milwaukee, WI 91-93; **FAP:** Asst Prof Rush Med Coll; **HOSP:** Illinois Masonic Med Ctr; ***SI:*** *Lung Cancer; Breast Cancer*; **HMO:** +
LANG: Sp; A Few Days

Shirazi, S Javed (MD) RadRO
Palos Comm Hosp
Radiation Oncology SC, 2800 W 95th St; Evergreen Park, IL 60805; (708) 857-3723; **BDCERT:** RadRO 74; **MS:** Pakistan 68; **RES:** Christ Hosp & Med Ctr, Oak Lawn, IL 69-70; Rush Presbyterian-St Luke's Med Ctr, Chicago, IL 70-73; **HOSP:** Little Company of Mary Hosp & Hlth Care Ctrs; ***SI:*** *Prostate Cancer; Breast Cancer*; **HMO:** +
LANG: Hin, Ur; Immediately

RADIOLOGY
(See also Diagnostic Radiology)

Behinfar, Mehdi (MD) Rad
Alexian Brothers Med Ctr (see page 138)
Diagnostic Imaging, 800 Biesterfield Rd; Elk Grove, IL 60007; (847) 437-5500; **BDCERT:** Rad 70; **MS:** Iran 60

Espinosa, Gustavo (MD) Rad
2114 W Division St; Chicago, IL 60622; (773) 486-8384; **BDCERT:** Rad 75; VIR 95; **MS:** Colombia 68; **RES:** IM, Doctors Hosp, Washington, DC 70-71; Rad, Cook Cty Hosp, Chicago, IL 71-74; **FAP:** Prof Rad Univ IL Coll Med

Ginde, Jay (MD) Rad
Christ Hosp & Med Ctr (see page 140)
South Suburban Cancer Ctr, 17750 S Kedzie Ave; Hazel Crest, IL 60429; (708) 799-9995; **BDCERT:** Rad 77; **MS:** India 70; **RES:** Rad, Columbus Hosp, Chicago, IL 72-75; Rad, Therpy - Columbus Hosp, Chicago, IL 75-77; **HOSP:** South Suburban Hosp

Hogan, George (MD) Rad
Little Company of Mary Hosp & Hlth Care Ctrs (see page 142)
Radiology Dept,Little Company of Mary Hosp & Hlth Care, 2800 W 95th St; Evergreen Park, IL 60805; (708) 229-5651; **BDCERT:** Rad 70; **MS:** Loyola U-Stritch Sch Med, Maywood 63; **RES:** Rad, Rush Presbyterian-St Luke's Med Ctr, Chicago, IL 66-69
A Few Days

Koch, Donald F (MD) Rad
West Suburban Hosp Med Ctr
807 Keystone Ave; River Forest, IL 60305; (708) 763-6515; **BDCERT:** Rad 69; **MS:** Univ IL Coll Med 62; **RES:** Wesley Meml Hosp, Chicago, IL 65-68; Childrens Meml Hosp, Chicago, IL 68

McFadden, John (MD) Rad
Lutheran Gen Hosp (see page 143)
Radiology Pavillion, 1775 Dempster St; Park Ridge, IL 60068; (847) 723-2210; **BDCERT:** Rad 77; PR 95; **MS:** Loyola U-Stritch Sch Med, Maywood 71; ***SI:*** *Pediatric Radiology*

Messersmith, Richard (MD) Rad
Lutheran Gen Hosp (see page 143)
Assoc Radiologist, 1775 Dempster; ParkRidge, IL 60068; (847) 723-5020; **BDCERT:** DR 85; VIR 95; **MS:** Northwestern U 81; **RES:** RadRO, Rhode Island Hosp, Providence, RI 82-85; **FEL:** UC Irvine Med Ctr, Orange, CA 85; **FAP:** Asst Prof U Chicago-Pritzker Sch Med

Guide to symbols and abbreviations can be found on pages 110-113.

Meyer, Joel (MD) Rad
Evanston Hosp
Evanston Northwestern Healthcare, 2650 Ridge Avenue Radiology; Evanston, IL 60201; (847) 570-1293; **BDCERT:** Rad 90; NRad 95; **MS:** SUNY Syracuse 86; **RES:** DR, U Mich Med Ctr, Ann Arbor, MI 86-90; **FEL:** NRad, U Mich Med Ctr, Ann Arbor, MI 90-92; **FAP:** Assoc Prof Rad Northwestern U; ***SI:*** *Neuroradiology; Head, Neck, Spine Radiology*
LANG: Ger; A Few Days
VISA

Nadimpalli, Surya P R (MD) Rad
Illinois Masonic Med Ctr
(see page 118)
I M M C Radiologists, 836 W Wellington Ave; Chicago, IL 60657; (773) 296-7820; **BDCERT:** Rad 80; NRad 95; **MS:** India 75; **RES:** RadRO, Illinois Masonic Med Ctr, Chicago, IL 76-80; **FAP:** Asst Clin Prof Rad Rush Med Coll

Nayden, John (MD) Rad
South Suburban Hosp
17800 S Kedzie Ave; Hazel Crest, IL 60429; (708) 799-8000; **BDCERT:** Rad 72; NuM 75; **MS:** Univ IL Coll Med 64; **RES:** RadRO, U IL Med Ctr, Chicago, IL 68-71; ***SI:*** *Nuclear Medicine*; **HMO:** +
Immediately

Petasnick, Jerry (MD) Rad
Rush-Presbyterian-St Luke's Med Ctr
(see page 122)
Affilated Radiologists, 1653 W Congress Pkwy; Chicago, IL 60612; (312) 942-5779; **BDCERT:** Rad 67; **MS:** U Wisc Med Sch 62; **RES:** Rad, Chicago Clin Hosp, Chicago, IL 63-66; **FAP:** Prof Rad Rush Med Coll; **HMO:** +

Phillips, Richard (MD) Rad
Good Shepherd Hosp
Barrington Cancer Care Ctr, 450 W Highway 22 Ste 650; Barrington, IL 60010; (847) 981-5760; **BDCERT:** Rad 66; **MS:** Univ IL Coll Med 59; **RES:** Rad, Rush Presby-St Lukes Med Ctr, Chicago, IL 62-65; **FAP:** Asst Clin Prof Rad Univ IL Coll Med

Ramsey, Ruth Godwin (MD) Rad
U Chicago Hosp **(see page 124)**
Univ of Chicago-Diag Rad MC-2026, 5841 S Maryland Ave; Chicago, IL 60637; (773) 702-1000; **BDCERT:** Rad 73; NRad 95; **MS:** Univ IL Coll Med 68; **RES:** NRad, Wesley Mem Hosp, Chicago, IL 69-72; **FEL:** NRad, Rush Presbyterian-St Luke's Med Ctr, Chicago, IL 74

Rhee, Chang (MD) Rad
South Shore Hosp
South Shore Hospital, 8012 S Crandon Ave; Chicago, IL 60617; (773) 768-0810; **BDCERT:** Rad 75; **MS:** South Korea 65; **HMO:** Aetna Hlth Plan, Blue Cross & Blue Shield, Chicago HMO, CIGNA

Sunko, Gerald (MD) Rad
St Mary's of Nazareth Hosp Ctr
2233 W Division St; Chicago, IL 60622; (312) 770-2068; **BDCERT:** Rad 76; **MS:** Loyola U-Stritch Sch Med, Maywood 70; **RES:** Radium Therapy, Northwestern Mem Hosp, Chicago, IL 73-76

Wiggins, Henry W Jr (MD) Rad
St Bernard Hosp
326 W 64th St; Chicago, IL 60621; (773) 962-4437; **BDCERT:** Rad 65; **MS:** Howard U 59

Wilczynski, Michael (MD) Rad
Jackson Park Hosp & Med Ctr
7531 Stony Island Ave; Chicago, IL 60649; (773) 947-7870; **BDCERT:** Rad 87; **MS:** U Chicago-Pritzker Sch Med 86
LANG: Sp; 1 Week

REPRODUCTIVE ENDOCRINOLOGY

Confino, Edmund (MD) RE
Northwestern Mem Hosp
680 N Lake Shore Drive Ste 1000; Chicago, IL 60611; (312) 908-7269; **BDCERT:** RE 96; **MS:** Israel 77; **RES:** ObG, Tel-Aviv Med Ctr, Tel-Aviv, Israel 80-83; **FEL:** RE, Mount Sinai Hosp Med Ctr, Chicago, IL 84-85; Rush Presbyterian-St Luke's Med Ctr, Chicago, IL 91-93; **FAP:** Assoc Prof U Chicago-Pritzker Sch Med; ***SI:*** *Infertility*; **HMO:** +
LANG: Bul; 2-4 Weeks
VISA

Hoxsey, Rodney J (MD) RE
Evanston Hosp
3150 Pfiugsten Rd; Glenview, IL 60025; (847) 657-5710; **BDCERT:** ObG 77; **MS:** Northwestern U 71; **RES:** ObG, Northwestern Mem Hosp, Chicago, IL 71-75; **FEL:** RE, Michael Reese Hosp Med Ctr, Chicago, IL 81-83; **FAP:** Asst Prof ObG Northwestern U; **HOSP:** Glenbrook Hosp; ***SI:*** *Infertility; Conservative Pelvic Surgery*; **HMO:** HMO Illinois, Aetna Hlth Plan
A Few Days VISA

Jacobs, Laurence (MD) RE
Lutheran Gen Hosp **(see page 143)**
4019 Brittany Court; NorthBrook, IL 60062; (847) 215-8899; **BDCERT:** ObG 81; **MS:** Northwestern U 75; **RES:** ObG, Northwestern Mem Hosp, Chicago, IL 75-79; **FEL:** RE, Mayo Clinic, Rochester, MN 86-88; **HOSP:** Northwest Comm Hlthcare; ***SI:*** *Laser Surgery IVF; Endometriosis*; **HMO:** Prucare, Blue Cross & Blue Shield, Humana Health Plan, PHCS, Principal Health Care +
2-4 Weeks VISA

Kaplan, Brian (MD) RE
Illinois Masonic Med Ctr
(see page 118)
Illinois Masonic Med Ctr-Fertility, 3000 N Halsted St Ste 509; Chicago, IL 60657; (773) 296-7090; **BDCERT:** ObG 92; **MS:** South Africa 81; **RES:** ObG, Michael Reese Hosp Med Ctr, Chicago, IL 84-88; **FEL:** RE, Michael Reese Hosp Med Ctr, Chicago, IL 88-90; **HOSP:** Highland Park Hosp; ***SI:*** *In Vitro Fertilization; Infertility*; **HMO:** Blue Cross & Blue Shield, United Healthcare, Rush Pru, CIGNA +
LANG: Sp, Rus; 2-4 Weeks VISA

Kazer, Ralph (MD) RE
Northwestern Mem Hosp
680 N Lakeshore Drive Rm 1000; Chicago, IL 60611; (312) 908-7269; **BDCERT:** ObG 96; RE 96; **MS:** Tufts U 79; **RES:** ObG, Tufts U, Boston, MA 79-83; **FEL:** RE, UC San Diego Med Ctr, San Diego, CA 83-86; **FAP:** Assoc Prof Northwestern U; ***SI:*** *General Infertility; Polycsystic Ovarian Syndrome*; **HMO:** +
4+ Weeks VISA

Rinehart, John (MD) RE
Glenbrook Hosp
Center For Human Reproduction, 2150 Pfingsten Rd Ste 3200; Glenview, IL 60025; (847) 657-5710; **BDCERT:** RE 88; ObG 85; **MS:** St Louis U 78; **RES:** ObG, Johns Hopkins Hosp, Baltimore, MD; **FEL:** RE, Brigham Women's Hosp, Boston, MA; **HOSP:** Evanston Hosp

Soltes, Barbara (MD) RE
Rush-Presbyterian-St Luke's Med Ctr
(see page 122)
Center for Womens Care, 1725 W Harrison Suite 842; Chicago, IL 60612; (312) 563-9389; **BDCERT:** ObG 94; **MS:** Mexico 84; **RES:** IM, Mount Sinai Med Ctr, New York, NY; ObG, Univ Hosp SUNY Bklyn, Brooklyn, NY; **FEL:** RE, Rush Presbyterian-St Luke's Med Ctr, Chicago, IL; **FAP:** Asst Prof Rush Med Coll; **HOSP:** Christ Hosp & Med Ctr; ***SI:*** *Endometriosis; Menopausal Syndrome*; **HMO:** Aetna Hlth Plan, United Healthcare, Californiacare, Guardian, Rush Prudential +
LANG: Sp; 2-4 Weeks

Wood-Molo, Mary (MD) RE
Rush-Presbyterian-St Luke's Med Ctr
(see page 122)
Womens Health Consultants, 1725 W Harrison St Ste 408 East; Chicago, IL 60612; (312) 666-0285; **BDCERT:** ObG 91; RE 94; **MS:** Southern IL U 82; **RES:** ObG, SIU Affil Hosps, Springfield, IL 83-84; ObG, Rush Presbyterian-St Luke's Med Ctr, Chicago, IL 84-87; **FEL:** RE, Rush Presbyterian-St Luke's Med Ctr, Chicago, IL 87-89; **FAP:** Asst Prof Rush Med Coll; **HMO:** Aetna Hlth Plan, Blue Cross & Blue Shield, CIGNA, Metlife, Prudential

RHEUMATOLOGY

Adams, Elaine (MD) Rhu
Loyola U Med Ctr (see page 120)
Loyola Medical Center, 2160 S 1st Avenue; Maywood, IL 60153; (708) 216-8563; **BDCERT:** Rhu 84; IM 81; **MS:** Loyola U-Stritch Sch Med, Maywood 78; **RES:** IM, Loyola U Med Ctr, Maywood, IL 79-81; **FEL:** Rhu, U WI Sch Med, Milwaukee, WI 81-83; **FAP:** Assoc Prof Med Loyola U-Stritch Sch Med, Maywood; **HOSP:** Hines VA Hosp; ***SI:*** *Rheumatoid Arthritis; SLE*
2-4 Weeks

Ajmani, Harpinder (MD) Rhu
St Mary's of Nazareth Hosp Ctr
2222 W Division St Ste 310; Chicago, IL 60622; (773) 395-8500; **BDCERT:** Rhu 94; IM 91; **MS:** India 81; **RES:** IM, Cook Cty Hosp, Chicago, IL 88-91; **FEL:** Rhu, U IL Med Ctr, Chicago, IL 91-93; **FAP:** Clin Instr Univ IL Coll Med

Brown, Calvin (MD) Rhu
Rush-Presbyterian-St Luke's Med Ctr
(see page 122)
1725 W Harrison St Ste 1017; Chicago, IL 60612; (312) 829-4349; **BDCERT:** IM 82; Rhu 86; **MS:** Wayne State U Sch Med 79; **RES:** IM, Northwestern Memorial Hospital, Chicago, IL 80-82; **FEL:** Rhu, U Mich Medical Center, Chicago, IL 83-85; **FAP:** Asst Prof IM Rush Med Coll; **HMO:** Aetna Hlth Plan, Blue Cross & Blue Shield, Californiacare, CIGNA, Prudential
LANG: Sp; VISA

Broy, Susan (MD) Rhu
Lutheran Gen Hosp (see page 143)
1875 W Dempster; Park Ridge, IL 60068; (847) 375-3000; **BDCERT:** IM 84; Rhu 86; **MS:** Univ IL Coll Med 81; **RES:** IM, Lutheran Gen Hosp, Park Ridge, IL 82-84; **FEL:** Rhu, Northwestern Mem Hosp, Chicago, IL 84-86; **FAP:** Assoc Prof of Clin Med U Chicago-Pritzker Sch Med; ***SI:*** *Osteoporosis*

Chang, Rowland (MD) Rhu
Northwestern Mem Hosp
345 E Superior St Ste 883; Chilcago, IL 60611; (312) 908-6094; **BDCERT:** Rhu 82; **MS:** Tufts U 76; **RES:** IM, Mt Auburn Hosp, Cambridge, MA 77-79; **FEL:** Rhu, Hammersmith Hosp, London, England 79-80; Rhu, Brigham & Women's Hosp, Boston, MA 80-82; **FAP:** Assoc Prof Med Northwestern U; ***SI:*** *Arthritis*

Cohen, Lewis (MD) Rhu
Lutheran Gen Hosp (see page 143)
Advocate Medical Group, 6000 W Touhy Ave; Chicago, IL 60646; (773) 763-1800; **BDCERT:** IM 78; Rhu 80; **MS:** U Cincinnati 70; **RES:** Michael Reese Hosp Med Ctr, Chicago, IL 72-74; **FEL:** Rhu, Northwestern Mem Hosp, Chicago, IL 74-76; **FAP:** Asst Clin Prof Med Univ IL Coll Med; **HOSP:** Ravenswood Hosp Med Ctr

Crane, Kenneth (MD) Rhu
Lutheran Gen Hosp (see page 143)
150 N River Rd Ste 204; Des Plaines, IL 60016; (847) 298-8470; **BDCERT:** IM 76; Rhu 78; **MS:** Univ IL Coll Med 72; **RES:** IM, U IL Med Ctr, Chicago, IL 74-76; **FEL:** Rhu, U IL Med Ctr, Chicago, IL 76-78; **HOSP:** Northwest Comm Hlthcare; ***SI:*** *Arthritis*
1 Week ***VISA***

Del Busto, Paul (MD) Rhu
Little Company of Mary Hosp & Hlth Care Ctrs (see page 142)
Mary Potter Pavilion, 2850 W 95th St Ste 205; Evergreen, IL 60642; (708) 422-7544; **BDCERT:** IM 92; Rhu 94; **MS:** Univ IL Coll Med 89; **FAP:** Asst Prof Rush Med Coll; **HMO:** +
LANG: Sp;
4+ Weeks

Ellman, Michael H (MD) Rhu
U Chicago Hosp (see page 124)
University of Chicago, 5841 S Maryland Ave MC2050; Chicago, IL 60637; (773) 256-4630; **BDCERT:** Rhu 72; IM 72; **MS:** Univ IL Coll Med 64; **RES:** IM, Michael Reese Hosp Med Ctr, Chicago, IL 68-70; **FEL:** Rhu, U Chicago Hosp, Chicago, IL 70-72; **FAP:** Prof U Chicago-Pritzker Sch Med

Frank, Judith (MD) Rhu
Gottlieb Mem Hosp
Frank & Meisles, 675 W North Ave Ste 305; Melrose Park, IL 60160; (708) 450-5085; **BDCERT:** Rhu 92; IM 89; **MS:** Rush Med Coll 86; **RES:** IM, Rush Presbyterian-St Luke's Med Ctr, Chicago, IL 87-89; **FEL:** Rhu, Rush Presbyterian-St Luke's Med Ctr, Chicago, IL 89-91; ***SI:*** *Rheumatoid Arthritis; Gout*; **HMO:** Medicare, Aetna Hlth Plan, Blue Cross, United Healthcare, Travelers

Froelich, Christopher (MD) Rhu
Evanston Hosp
Arthritis Treatment Ctr, 1000 Central St; Evanston, IL 60201; (847) 570-2503; **BDCERT:** Rhu 82; IM 79; **MS:** Loyola U-Stritch Sch Med, Maywood 76; **RES:** IM, U New Mexico Med Center, Albuquerque, NM 77-79; **FEL:** Rhu, U New Mexico Med Center, Albuquerque, NM 79-80

Glickman, Paul (MD) Rhu
Rush-Presbyterian-St Luke's Med Ctr (see page 122)
University Rheumatologists, 1725 W Harrison St Ste 1017; Chicago, IL 60612; (312) 829-4349; **BDCERT:** IM 61; Rhu 72; **MS:** U Chicago-Pritzker Sch Med 53; **RES:** IM, U Chicago Hosp, Chicago, IL 54-59; **FAP:** Assoc Prof Rush Med Coll; ***SI:*** *Rheumatoid Arthritis; Osteoarthritis*; **HMO:** Rush Prudential
A Few Days ***VISA***

Golbus, Joseph (MD) Rhu
Evanston Hosp
Arthritis Treatment Ctr, 2650 Ridge Ave Ste 800; Evanston, IL 60201; (847) 570-2503; **BDCERT:** Rhu 84; **MS:** Univ IL Coll Med 81; **RES:** IM, Evanston Hosp, Evanston, IL 81-84; **FEL:** Rhu, U Mich Med Ctr, Ann Arbor, MI 84-87; **FAP:** Assoc Prof Med Northwestern U; **HOSP:** Glenbrook Hosp; ***SI:*** *Rheumatoid Arthritis; Systemic Lupus*; **HMO:** United Healthcare, Blue Cross & Blue Shield, HMO Illinois, Humana Health Plan
2-4 Weeks

Grober, James (MD) Rhu
Evanston Hosp
1000 Central St Ste 800; Evanston, IL 60201; (847) 570-2503; **BDCERT:** Rhu 90; **MS:** Yale U Sch Med 83; **RES:** IM, Yale-New Haven Hosp, New Haven, CT 83-86; **FEL:** Rhu, U Mich Med Ctr, Ann Arbor, MI 88-90; **FAP:** Asst Prof Med Northwestern U; **HOSP:** Glenbrook Hosp
2-4 Weeks

Harris, Max (MD) Rhu
West Suburban Hosp Med Ctr
West Suburban Hospital, 1 Erie Ct L500; Oak Park, IL 60302; (708) 763-2537; **BDCERT:** Rhu 82; **MS:** Rush Med Coll 76; **RES:** IM, Rush Presbyterian-St Luke's Med Ctr, Chicago, IL 76-79; **FEL:** Rhu, U Chicago Hosp, Chicago, IL 80-82; **FAP:** Assoc Clin Prof Loyola U-Stritch Sch Med, Maywood; ***SI:*** *Lupus; Rheumatoid Arthritis*; **HMO:** Humana Health Plan, HMO Illinois, Rush Pru
LANG: Sp, Pol;
A Few Days ***VISA***

Katz, Robert (MD) Rhu
Rush-Presbyterian-St Luke's Med Ctr (see page 122)
Rheumatology Associates, 1725 W Harrison St Ste 1039; Chicago, IL 60612; (312) 226-8228; **BDCERT:** Rhu 76; IM 75; **MS:** U Md Sch Med 70; **RES:** IM, Barnes Hosp, St Louis, MO 70-72; **FEL:** Rhu, Johns Hopkins Hosp, Baltimore, MD 74-76; **FAP:** Assoc Prof Med Rush Med Coll; ***SI:*** *Lupus; Fibromyalgia*; **HMO:** Blue Cross & Blue Shield, Aetna Hlth Plan, Prudential, Principal Health Care, HealthStar +
LANG: Sp; 2-4 Weeks
VISA

Kazmar, Raymond E (MD) Rhu
Ingalls Mem Hosp
Olympia Fields Internal Med, 2605 Lincoln Hwy Ste 130; Olympia Fields, IL 60461; (708) 747-9780; **BDCERT:** Rhu 82; IM 78; **MS:** Northwestern U 75; **RES:** IM, Hennepin Cty Med Ctr, Minneapolis, MN 76-79; **FEL:** Rhu, Mayo Clinic, Rochester, MN 79-82; **HOSP:** South Suburban Hosp; ***SI:*** *Rheumatoid Arthritis; Lupus*; **HMO:** Aetna Hlth Plan, Humana Health Plan, United Healthcare, CIGNA PPO
2-4 Weeks VISA

Mael, David (MD) Rhu
Illinois Masonic Med Ctr
(see page 118)
White Crane Medical Svc, 3000 N Halsted St Ste 409; Chicago, IL 60657; (773) 296-3200; **BDCERT:** Rhu 97; IM 88; **MS:** Mexico 84; **RES:** IM, Illinois Masonic Med Ctr, Chicago, IL 86-89; **FEL:** Rhu, U IL Med Ctr, Chicago, IL 92-94; **HMO:** +
LANG: Sp, Heb;
1 Week VISA

Michalska, Margaret (MD) Rhu
Rush-Presbyterian-St Luke's Med Ctr
(see page 122)
White Crane Medical Svc, 3000 N Halsted St Ste 409; Chicago, IL 60657; (773) 296-3200; **BDCERT:** Rhu 90; IM 88; **MS:** Poland 79; **RES:** IM, Hines VA Hosp, Chicago, IL 85-88; **FEL:** Rhu, Rush Presbyterian-St Luke's Med Ctr, Chicago, IL 88-90; Northwestern Mem Hosp, Chicago, IL 80-85; **FAP:** Asst Prof Med Rush Med Coll; **HMO:** Aetna Hlth Plan, Blue Cross & Blue Shield, Chicago HMO, CIGNA, Healthpartners

Pachman, Lauren (MD) Rhu
Children's Mem Med Ctr (see page 139)
Childrens Memorial Hospital, 2300 N Childrens Plz MH 50; Chicago, IL 60614; (773) 880-4360; **BDCERT:** A&I 74; Ped Rhu 92; **MS:** U Chicago-Pritzker Sch Med 61; **RES:** Ped, Columbia-Presbyterian Med Ctr, New York, NY 62-64; **FEL:** Rockefeller Univ Hosp, New York, NY 64-66; **FAP:** Prof Ped Northwestern U

Palella, Thomas Daniel (MD) Rhu
Northwest Comm Hlthcare
150 N River Rd Ste 270; Des Plaines, IL 60016; (847) 298-8470; **BDCERT:** Rhu 86; IM 82; **MS:** Univ IL Coll Med 77; **RES:** IM, U Mich Med Ctr, Ann Arbor, MI 80-82; IM, U Mich Med Ctr, Ann Arbor, MI 82-83; **FEL:** Rhu, U Mich Med Ctr, Ann Arbor, MI 78-80

Pope, Richard Mitchell (MD) Rhu
Northwestern Mem Hosp
303 E Ohio St; Chicago, IL 60611; (312) 908-8688; **BDCERT:** IM 73; Rhu 76; **MS:** Loyola U-Stritch Sch Med, Maywood 70; **RES:** IM, Michael Reese Hosp Med Ctr, Chicago, IL 71-72; **FEL:** Rhu, U WA Med Ctr, Seattle, WA 72-74; **FAP:** Prof Northwestern U; ***SI:*** *Rheumatoid Arthritis; Psoriatic Arthritis*; **HMO:** CIGNA, Aetna Hlth Plan, United Healthcare, Prudential +
1 Week VISA

Schroeder, James (MD) Rhu
Northwestern Mem Hosp
Northwestern Med Fac Found, 303 E Ohio St; Chicago, IL 60611; (312) 908-8628; **BDCERT:** Rhu 84; IM 81; **MS:** U Va Sch Med 78; **RES:** IM, Northwestern Mem Hosp, Chicago, IL 78-79; IM, Northwestern Mem Hosp, Chicago, IL 79-81; **FEL:** Rhu, Barnes Hosp, St Louis, MO 81-83; **FAP:** Asst Prof Northwestern U; ***SI:*** *Rheumatoid Arthritis; Psoriatic Arthritis*
2-4 Weeks

Schuette, Patrick (MD) Rhu
Grant Hosp
Advocate Medical Group - Rheumatology, 6000 W Touhy Ave; Chicago, IL 60646; (773) 763-1800; **BDCERT:** IM 77; Rhu 80; **MS:** Univ SC Sch Med 74; **RES:** IM, U IL Med Ctr, Chicago, IL 75-77; **FEL:** Rhu, Northwestern Mem Hosp, Chicago, IL 77-78; **HOSP:** Lutheran Gen Hosp

Skosey, John (MD) Rhu
Macneal Mem Hosp
Macneal Rheumatology Associates, 3340 S Oak Park Ave Ste 200; Berwyn, IL 60402; (708) 783-0222; **BDCERT:** Rhu 74; IM 74; **MS:** U Chicago-Pritzker Sch Med 61; **RES:** IM, U Chicago Hosp, Chicago, IL 62-63; IM, U Chicago Hosp, Chicago, IL 65-67; **FAP:** Clin Prof Med U Chicago-Pritzker Sch Med

Tartof, David (MD) Rhu
Michael Reese Hosp & Med Ctr
Rothschild Ctr, 2816 S Ellis Ave Room 1200; Chicago, IL 60616; (312) 791-4162; **BDCERT:** IM 76; Rhu 80; **MS:** U Mich Med Sch 70; **RES:** IM, U IL Med Ctr, Chicago, IL 73-75; Path CP, U Chicago Hosp, Chicago, IL 77-78; **FEL:** Rhu, U Chicago Hosp, Chicago, IL 78-80

Weiner, Glenn (MD) Rhu
Alexian Brothers Med Ctr
(see page 138)
Northwest Rheumatology, 850 Biesterfield Rd Ste 3007; Elk Grove Village, IL 60007; (847) 364-0800; **BDCERT:** Rhu 80; **MS:** Chicago Coll Osteo Med 74; **RES:** Rhu, Hines VA Hosp, Chicago, IL 77-79; **FEL:** Rhu, Hines VA Hosp, Chicago, IL 77-79; **HOSP:** Good Shepherd Hosp

Guide to symbols and abbreviations can be found on pages 110-113.

SPORTS MEDICINE

Alleva, Joseph (MD) SM
Highland Park Hosp
Spine Center, 2100 Pfingsten Rd B8; Glenview, IL 60025; (847) 657-5677; **BDCERT:** PMR 95; **MS:** Chicago Coll Osteo Med 90; **RES:** Northwestern Mem Hosp, Chicago, IL 91-94; **FEL:** Buffalo Spine & Sports Medicine, Williamsville, NY 94-95; **FAP:** Asst Prof Northwestern U; **HOSP:** Evanston Hosp; ***SI:*** *Neck and Low Back Pain*; **HMO:** Blue Cross & Blue Shield, Aetna Hlth Plan, CIGNA
1 Week

Briner, William (MD) SM
Lutheran Gen Hosp (see page 143)
1775 Dempster St G10; Park Ridge, IL 60068; (847) 318-6020; **BDCERT:** FP 88; SM 93; **MS:** Ohio State U 85; **RES:** FP, Macneal Mem Hosp, Berwyn, IL 86; **FEL:** SM, Marshall U, Huntington, WV; **HMO:** +
LANG: Sp;
Immediately

Frank, Lawrence W (MD) SM
Glen Oaks Hosp and Med Ctr (see page 273)
Chicago Institute of Neurosurgery, 2515 N Clark St Ste 800; Chicago, IL 60614; (773) 388-7700; **BDCERT:** PMR 96; **MS:** Univ IL Coll Med 91; **RES:** Northwestern Mem Hosp, Chicago, IL 92-95; **FEL:** SM, IL Spine and Sportscare, Bloomingdale, IL 95-96; **FAP:** Asst Clin Prof OrS Loyola U-Stritch Sch Med, Maywood

Ho, Sherwin (MD) SM
U Chicago Hosp (see page 124)
University of Chicago, 4343 Lincoln Hwy Ste 230; Matteson, IL 60443; (708) 748-2310; **BDCERT:** OrS 94; **MS:** U Hawaii JA Burns Sch Med 85; **RES:** IM, Michael Reese Hosp Med Ctr, Chicago, IL 82-84

Schafer, Michael F. (MD) SM
Northwestern Mem Hosp
675 N St Clair St Ste 17-100; Chicago, IL 60611; (312) 695-6800; **BDCERT:** OrS 74; **MS:** U Iowa Coll Med 67; **RES:** OrS, Northwestern Mem Hosp, Chicago, IL 68-72; **FEL:** SM, National Foundation Spine Surgery, Australia 72; **FAP:** Prof & Chrmn OrS Northwestern U; **HOSP:** Children's Mem Med Ctr; ***SI:*** *Scoliosis Surgery; Knee Injuries*; **HMO:** Aetna Hlth Plan, CIGNA, HealthStar, Blue Cross & Blue Shield, PHCS +
LANG: Sp;
A Few Days

Wahi, Sukhveer K (MD) SM
Mount Sinai Hosp Med Ctr
3700 W 26th St; Chicago, IL 60608; (773) 277-6589; **BDCERT:** SM 93; Ger 90; **MS:** India 73

SURGERY

Anderson, Kenneth (MD) S
St Francis Hosp
Anderson Surgical Group, 2310 York St Ste 2B; Blue Island, IL 60406; (708) 389-4701; **BDCERT:** S 85; **MS:** Univ IL Coll Med 78; **RES:** S, U IL Med Ctr, Chicago, IL 79-84; **FEL:** GI Surg, U IL Med Ctr, Chicago, IL 84-85; **FAP:** Asst Prof S Univ IL Coll Med

Aranha, Gerard (MD) S
Loyola U Med Ctr (see page 120)
2160 S 1st Ave; Maywood, IL 60153; (708) 216-4596; **BDCERT:** S 96; **MS:** India 69; **RES:** S, Loyola U Med Ctr, Maywood, IL 71-75; **FEL:** Surg Onc, U MN Med Ctr, Minneapolis, MN 75-77; **FAP:** Prof Loyola U-Stritch Sch Med, Maywood; **HOSP:** Hines VA Hosp; ***SI:*** *Pancreatic Cancer; Stomach Cancer*; **HMO:** Blue Cross & Blue Shield, Aetna Hlth Plan, Humana Health Plan, Accord +
A Few Days

Barrera Jr, Ermilo (MD) S
St Alexius Med Ctr
North Suburban Clinic Ltd, 1786 Moon Lake Blvd; Hoffman Estates, IL 60194; (847) 885-0400; **BDCERT:** S 86; **MS:** Baylor 80; **RES:** Northwestern Mem Hosp, Chicago, IL 80-85; **FEL:** MD Anderson Cancer Ctr, Houston, TX 85-86; **HOSP:** Alexian Brothers Med Ctr; ***SI:*** *Breast Cancer; Melanoma*; **HMO:** United Healthcare, Blue Cross & Blue Shield, CIGNA, Aetna Hlth Plan +
LANG: Sp;
Immediately

Bekele, Alemaychu (MD) S
St Bernard Hosp
3435 W Van Buren St; Chicago, IL 60624; (773) 265-3403; **BDCERT:** S 82; **MS:** Ethiopia 72; **RES:** St Francis Hosp, Pittsburgh, PA 75-77; Chicago Hosp, Chicago, IL 78-81; **HOSP:** Bethany Hosp; ***SI:*** *Abdominal Surgery; Breast Surgery*; **HMO:** +
LANG: Sp;
Immediately

Benvenuto, Riccardo (MD) S
Grant Hosp
3240 N Lake Shore Dr; Chicago, IL 60657; (773) 975-1100; **BDCERT:** S 69; **MS:** Italy 53; **RES:** S, Northwestern Mem Hosp, Chicago, IL 58-62; ***SI:*** *Laser Treatments*; **HMO:** Aetna Hlth Plan, Blue Cross & Blue Shield, Chicago HMO, Humana Health Plan, Principal Health Care
A Few Days

Berk, Richard (MD) S
Evanston Hosp
2500 Ridge Ave Ste 107; Evanston, IL 60201; (847) 328-3500; **BDCERT:** S 90; **MS:** Univ Penn 68; **RES:** S, Michael Reese Hosp Med Ctr, Chicago, IL 69-70; S, Michael Reese Hosp Med Ctr, Chicago, IL 72-75; **FEL:** Surg Onc, Mem Sloan Kettering Cancer Ctr, New York, NY 75-77; **FAP:** Asst Clin Prof S Northwestern U; **HMO:** Aetna Hlth Plan

Bethke, Kevin (MD) S
Northwestern Mem Hosp
Surgery Department, 676 N Saint Clair St Ste 1525; Chicago, IL 60611; (312) 943-2746; **BDCERT:** S 90; **MS:** U Minn 83; **RES:** S, U Wisc Hosp, Madison, WI 83-89; **FEL:** Surg Onc, Med Coll VA Hosp, Richmond, VA 89-91; **FAP:** Prof S Northwestern U; ***SI:*** *Thyroid and Breast Cancers; Lymphoma*
1 Week

Brosnan, Joseph (MD) S
Christ Hosp & Med Ctr **(see page 140)**
Nasralla Klompien Surgical Assoc, 4400 W 95th St Ste 402; Oak Lawn, IL 60453; (708) 346-4057; **BDCERT:** S 93; **MS:** Loyola U-Stritch Sch Med, Maywood 78; ***SI:*** *Breast Surgery; Colon Surgery*; **HMO:** Aetna Hlth Plan, Blue Cross & Blue Shield, Californiacare, CIGNA, Healthpartners
Immediately VISA

Byrne, Mitchel (MD) S
St Francis Hosp
Surgical Associates East Tower, 800 Austin St Ste 563; Evanston, IL 60202; (847) 869-0522; **BDCERT:** S 75; **MS:** Univ IL Coll Med 69; **RES:** S, St Francis Hosp of Evanston, Evanston, IL 70-74; ***SI:*** *Vascular Surgery*; **HMO:** +
LANG: Sp;
A Few Days VISA

Cacioppo, Phillip (MD) S
Alexian Brothers Med Ctr
(see page 138)
810 Biesterfield Rd Ste 202; Elk Grove Vlg, IL 60007; (847) 806-0106; **BDCERT:** S 75; **MS:** Loyola U-Stritch Sch Med, Maywood 67; **RES:** S, St Francis Hosp of Evanston, Evanston, IL 70-74; **FAP:** Asst Clin Prof S Loyola U-Stritch Sch Med, Maywood; ***SI:*** *Peripheral Vascular Disease Surgery; Gallbladder Surgery*
VISA

Cahill, Gerald (MD) S
Little Company of Mary Hosp & Hlth Care Ctrs **(see page 142)**
2850 W 95th St Ste 300; Evergreen Park, IL 60805; (708) 422-5658; **BDCERT:** S 98; **MS:** Univ IL Coll Med 82; **RES:** S, U IL Med Ctr, Chicago, IL 82-87; **FEL:** CRS, Cook Cty Hosp, Chicago, IL 87-88; ***SI:*** *Laparoscopic Surgery*; **HMO:** Humana Health Plan, Blue Cross & Blue Shield, Aetna Hlth Plan
LANG: Sp;
A Few Days

Chhablani, Asha (MD) S
Michael Reese Hosp & Med Ctr
Chhablani & Sheridan, 2800 S Vernon Ave Fl 2; Chicago, IL 60616; (312) 842-1556; **BDCERT:** S 94; **MS:** India 68; **RES:** S, Michael Reese Hosp Med Ctr, Chicago, IL 71-75; **FAP:** Assoc Clin Prof S U Chicago-Pritzker Sch Med; **HOSP:** Rush-Presbyterian-St Luke's Med Ctr; ***SI:*** *Laparoscopic Gallbladder; Breast Surgery*

Connolly, Mark (MD) S
Columbus Hosp
CDN Surgical Assoc, 2515 N Clark St Ste 903; Chicago, IL 60614; (773) 472-3427; **BDCERT:** S 86; **MS:** U Wisc Med Sch 80; **RES:** S, Northwestern Mem Hosp, Chicago, IL 81-85; **FEL:** Surg Onc, U Chicago Hosp, Chicago, IL 85-86; ***SI:*** *Surgical Oncology*

Coyle, John (MD) S
Evanston Hosp
500 Davis St; Evanston, IL 60201; (847) 866-5473; **BDCERT:** S 95; **MS:** Loyola U-Stritch Sch Med, Maywood 70; **RES:** S, U Minn Hosps, Minneapolis, MN 71-77; **FAP:** Assoc Prof S Northwestern U

Cunningham, Myles (MD) S
St Francis Hosp
800 Austin St Ste 501; Evanston, IL 60202; (847) 869-1770; **BDCERT:** S 65; **MS:** Northwestern U 58; **RES:** S, Cook Cty Hosp, Chicago, IL 59-64; **FEL:** Surg Onc, Mem Sloan Kettering Cancer Ctr, New York, NY 64-67; **FAP:** Assoc Prof Univ IL Coll Med; **HOSP:** Evanston Hosp; ***SI:*** *Breast Diseases; Thyroid Cancer*
A Few Days

Dahlinghaus, Daniel (MD) S
Resurrection Med Ctr
Northwestern General Surgeons, 7447 W Talcott Ave Ste 417; Chicago, IL 60631; (773) 631-9699; **BDCERT:** S 90; **MS:** Loyola U-Stritch Sch Med, Maywood 74; **RES:** S, Loyola U Med Ctr, Maywood, IL 75-79; ***SI:*** *Breast Cancer; Thyroid Surgery*

Das Gupta, Tapas (MD) S
Univ of Illinois at Chicago Med Ctr
University of Illinois-Surgical Oncology, 840 S Wood St MC820; Chicago, IL 60612; (312) 996-6667; **BDCERT:** S 61; **MS:** India 53; **RES:** S, Mount Sinai Hosp Med Ctr, Chicago, IL 56-60; S, Memorial Sloan Kettering Hosp, New York, NY 60-63; **FAP:** Prof S Univ IL Coll Med; ***SI:*** *Breast Cancer; Melanoma*
A Few Days

Diettrich, Nancy (MD) S
Illinois Masonic Med Ctr
(see page 118)
3000 N Halsted Ste 305; Chicago, IL 60657; (773) 296-3030; **BDCERT:** S 96; SCC 93; **MS:** Loyola U-Stritch Sch Med, Maywood 81; **RES:** Columbus Hosp, Chicago, IL 82-87; **FAP:** Asst Clin Prof Univ IL Coll Med; **HOSP:** St Joseph Hosp-Chicago; ***SI:*** *Breast Surgery Cancer/Benign; Gall Bladder Surgery*; **HMO:** Blue Cross, PHCS, Aetna Hlth Plan, CIGNA +
LANG: Sp, Pol;

Guide to symbols and abbreviations can be found on pages 110-113.

Donahue, Philip E (MD) S
Cook Cty Hosp
1226 Belleforte Ave; Oak Park, IL 60302; (312) 633-3147; **BDCERT:** S 76; **MS:** Jefferson Med Coll 68; **RES:** SM, U IL Med Ctr, Chicago, IL 71-76; **FAP:** Prof S U Chicago-Pritzker Sch Med; ***SI:*** *Gastro-esophageal Surgery*

Doolas, Alexander (MD) S
Rush-Presbyterian-St Luke's Med Ctr **(see page 122)**
University Surgeons, 1725 W Harrison St Ste 810; Chicago, IL 60612; (312) 738-2743; **BDCERT:** S 68; **MS:** Univ IL Coll Med 60; **RES:** S, Rush Presbyterian-St Luke's Med Ctr, Chicago, IL 61-62; Rush Presbyterian-St Luke's Med Ctr, Chicago, IL 64-67; **FAP:** Assoc Prof Rush Med Coll; ***SI:*** *Esophageal Surgery; Hepatobiliary Surgery*
LANG: Grk, Sp, Ger; Mcr Mcd
1 Week VISA

Franco, Joseph Anthony (MD) S
West Suburban Hosp Med Ctr
West Suburban Hospital-Plastic Surgery, Erie at Austin L-600; Oak Park, IL 60302; (708) 383-6200; **BDCERT:** S 95; **MS:** Loyola U-Stritch Sch Med, Maywood 87; **HOSP:** Loyola U Med Ctr; ***SI:*** *Hand Surgery*

Frank, Angela R (MD) S
St Joseph Hosp-Chicago
Associates & General Surgery, 2800 N Sheridan Rd Ste 600; Chicago, IL 60657; (773) 281-8300; **BDCERT:** S 82; **MS:** Brazil 73; **RES:** S, St Joseph's Hosp, Chicago, IL 77-81; ***SI:*** *Colorectal Surgery; Breast Surgery*; **HMO:** CIGNA, Aetna Hlth Plan, Humana Health Plan, Oxford +
LANG: Sp, Prt, Fr; Mcr Mcd

Gamelli, Richard Louis (MD) S
Loyola U Med Ctr **(see page 120)**
Loyola U-Stritch Sch Med, 2160 S 1st Ave; Maywood, IL 60153; (708) 216-9186; **BDCERT:** S 80; **MS:** Univ Vt Coll Med 74; **RES:** S, Med Ctr Hosp of VT, Burlington, VT 75-79; ***SI:*** *Burns; Bariatric Surgery*; **HMO:** +
Mcr Mcd 2-4 Weeks

Geller, Robert (MD) S
Gottlieb Mem Hosp
Gottlieb Memorial Hospital, 675 W North Ave Ste 416; Melrose Park, IL 60160; (708) 450-0462; **BDCERT:** S 90; **MS:** U Hlth Sci/Chicago Med Sch 76; **RES:** S, Loyola U Med Ctr, Maywood, IL 77-81; **HMO:** Aetna Hlth Plan, Blue Cross & Blue Shield, Chicago HMO, CIGNA, FHP Inc

Hagan, Colleen (MD) S
La Grange Mem Hosp **(see page 141)**
Midwest Surgical Associates, 1323 Memorial Drive; La Grange, IL 60525; (708) 579-9705; **BDCERT:** S 91; **MS:** Loyola U-Stritch Sch Med, Maywood 76; **RES:** S, Cook Cty Hosp, Chicago, IL 81

Hann, Sang (MD) S
Lutheran Gen Hosp **(see page 143)**
Hann-Stoehr Surgical Assoc, 9301 Golf Rd Ste 206; Des Plaines, IL 60016; (847) 824-7740; **BDCERT:** S 73; **MS:** South Korea 64; **RES:** St Vincent Hosp, Worcester, MA 65-69; ***SI:*** *Thyroid Surgery; Breast Surgery*

Harford, Francis (MD) S
Loyola U Med Ctr **(see page 120)**
Building 110, 2160 S 1st Ave Rm3234; Maywood, IL 60153; (708) 327-2647; **BDCERT:** S 89; CRS 77; **MS:** SUNY Buffalo 67; **RES:** S, U Miami Hosp, Miami, FL 72-76; CRS, Cleveland Clin Fdn, Cleveland, OH 76-77; **FAP:** Clin Prof S Loyola U-Stritch Sch Med, Maywood; ***SI:*** *Colon Surgery; Rectal Surgery*

Hartz, Wilson (MD) S
Northwestern Mem Hosp
Northwestern Surgical Assoc, 251 E Chicago Ave Ste 728; Chicago, IL 60611; (312) 787-5323; **BDCERT:** S 87; **MS:** Northwestern U 73; **RES:** S, Northwestern Mem Hosp, Chicago, IL 74-78; **HMO:** Aetna Hlth Plan, Blue Cross & Blue Shield, Californiacare, Compare Health Service, Healthamerica
Mcr

Hopkins, William (MD) S
Christ Hosp & Med Ctr **(see page 140)**
4440 W 95th St; Oak Lawn, IL 60453; (708) 346-4055; **BDCERT:** S 90; **MS:** Loyola U-Stritch Sch Med, Maywood 75; **RES:** S, Loyola U Med Ctr, Maywood, IL 76-81; **FAP:** Asst Prof Univ IL Coll Med; ***SI:*** *Endocrine Surgery; Breast Surgery*; **HMO:** Blue Cross & Blue Shield, Rush Health Plans, United Healthcare +
Mcr Mcd 1 Week VISA

Huq, Zahurul (MD) S
St Mary's of Nazareth Hosp Ctr
1431 N Western Ave Ste 503; Chicago, IL 60622; (773) 252-0777; **BDCERT:** S 71; **MS:** Bangladesh 57; **RES:** S, St Mary's of Nazareth Hosp Ctr, Chicago, IL 60-64; King George Hosp, Essex, England 64-65; **FEL:** Loyola U Med Ctr, Maywood, IL 64; Weiss Meml Hosp, Chicago, IL; **HOSP:** St Elizabeth's Hosp

Jacob, Abraham (MD) S
South Shore Hosp
4315 N Lincoln Ave; Chicago, IL 60618; (773) 404-0405; **BDCERT:** S 83; **MS:** India 67; ***SI:*** *Trauma*; **HMO:** Blue Cross & Blue Shield, Chicago HMO
Mcr Mcd

Joehl, Raymond (MD) S
Northwestern Mem Hosp
NW Med Faculty Foundation - Tarry Bldg, 300 E Superior St Ste 11-703; Chicago, IL 60611; (312) 908-1414; **BDCERT:** S 81; **MS:** St Louis U 74; **RES:** S, Penn State Univ, Hershey, PA 74-79; **FEL:** Ge, Penn State Univ, Hershey, PA 79-80; **FAP:** Prof S Northwestern U; ***SI:*** *Hernia Repair; Laparoscopic Cholecystectomy*; **HMO:** Blue Cross & Blue Shield, HealthStar +
Mcr Mcd VISA

Kane Jr, James M (MD) S
Northwest Comm Hlthcare
601 W Central Rd Ste 10; Mt Prospect, IL 60056; (847) 255-9697; **BDCERT:** S 91; **MS:** Georgetown U 84; **RES:** S, U IL Med Ctr, Chicago, IL 84-90; **FAP:** Instr S Univ IL Coll Med; **HOSP:** Alexian Brothers Med Ctr

Kaplan, Gerald (MD) S
Illinois Masonic Med Ctr (see page 118)
3000 N Halsted St; Chicago, IL 60657; (773) 296-3030; **BDCERT:** S 71; **MS:** Univ IL Coll Med 62; **RES:** S, Hines VA Hosp, Chicago, IL 66-70; **FAP:** Asst Clin Prof S Univ IL Coll Med; ***SI:*** *Breast & Colon Cancer; Laparoscopic Cholecystectomy*; **HMO:** Aetna-US Healthcare, HMO Illinois, Rush Prudential, Humana Health Plan, United Healthcare +
A Few Days

Kaymakcalan, Orhan (MD) S
Mount Sinai Hosp Med Ctr
2755 W 15th St M307; Chicago, IL 60608; (773) 257-4770; **BDCERT:** S 80; HS 89; **MS:** Turkey 72; **RES:** S, U FL Shands Hosp, Gainesville, FL 73-74; S, Mount Sinai Hosp Med Ctr, Chicago, IL 74-78; **FEL:** HS, U Louisville Hosp, Louisville, KY 82-83; **FAP:** Assoc Clin Prof S U Chicago-Pritzker Sch Med; **HOSP:** St Mary's of Nazareth Hosp Ctr

Kennedy, Michael (MD) S
St Alexius Med Ctr
Surgical Specialists Ltd, 1575 Barrington Rd Ste 425; Hoffman Estates, IL 60194; (847) 884-6086; **BDCERT:** S 89; **MS:** Loyola U-Stritch Sch Med, Maywood 74; **RES:** S, St Francis Hosp-Evanston, Evanston, IL 74-77; Loyola U Med Ctr, Maywood, IL 78-79; **HMO:** Blue Cross & Blue Shield, Chicago HMO, CIGNA, Humana Health Plan, Metlife

Khan, A Haye (MD) S
Little Company of Mary Hosp & Hlth Care Ctrs (see page 142)
4700 W 95th St Ste 304; Oak Lawn, IL 60453; (708) 636-4116; **BDCERT:** S 71; **MS:** Pakistan 61; **RES:** S, Little Company of Mary Hosp & Hlth Care Ctrs, Evergreen Park, IL 65-68; **FEL:** Cv S, Baylor Med Ctr, Dallas, TX; ***SI:*** *General Surgery; Vascular Surgery*

Khorsand, Joubin (MD) S
Lutheran Gen Hosp (see page 143)
Golf Western Surgical Specs, 8901 Golf Rd Ste 305; Des Plaines, IL 60016; (847) 299-8844; **BDCERT:** S 92; **MS:** Iran 73; ***SI:*** *Surgical Oncology*

Kinney, Michael R (MD) S
Northwest Comm Hlthcare
Advanced Surgical Assoc, 500 N Hicks Rd Ste 250; Palatine, IL 60067; (847) 705-9500; **BDCERT:** S 87; **MS:** Case West Res U 81; **RES:** Loyola U Med Ctr, Maywood, IL 81-86; **HOSP:** Alexian Brothers Med Ctr; ***SI:*** *Abdominal Surgery*; **HMO:** Aetna Hlth Plan, Blue Cross & Blue Shield, Californiacare, Choicecare, HealthNet
LANG: Sp;

Krause, Lawrence (MD) S
Michael Reese Hosp & Med Ctr
Lake Shore Surgical Assoc Ltd, 111 N Wabash Ave Ste 1501; Chicago, IL 60602; (312) 641-1150; **BDCERT:** S 94; **MS:** Univ IL Coll Med 79; **RES:** S, Michael Reese Hosp Med Ctr, Chicago, IL; **HOSP:** Highland Park Hosp; ***SI:*** *Breast Disorders; Laparoscopic Surgery*; **HMO:** Blue Cross & Blue Shield, Humana Health Plan, United Healthcare +
Mcr Mcd NFI A Few Days VISA

Krinski, Roseanne (MD) S
St James Hosp & Hlth Ctrs
Suburban Heights Medical Ctr, 333 Dixie Hwy; Chicago Heights, IL 60411; (708) 709-6333; **BDCERT:** S 94; **MS:** St Louis U 78; **RES:** S, Rush Presbyterian-St Luke's Med Ctr, Chicago, IL 79-83; **HOSP:** South Suburban Hosp; ***SI:*** *Breast Diseases*; **HMO:** Blue Cross
LANG: Sp; Mcr 1 Week

Kroczek, Bohdan (MD) S
Our Lady Of the Resurrection Med Ctr
Aki & Kroczeck Surgical Assoc, 1400 E Golf Rd Ste 205; Des Plaines, IL 60016; (773) 631-9371; **BDCERT:** S 97; **MS:** Poland 76; **RES:** Brooklyn Jewish Hosp, Brooklyn, NY 82-83; SM, Interfaith Med Ctr Affil SU, Brooklyn, NY 83-87; **HOSP:** Holy Family Med Ctr
LANG: Pol; Mcr Mcd

Krueger, Barbara (MD) S
Christ Hosp & Med Ctr (see page 140)
4400 W 95 St Ste 413; Oak Lawn, IL 60453; (708) 346-4055; **BDCERT:** S 94; **MS:** Emory U Sch Med 88; **RES:** S, Rush Presbyterian-St Luke's Med Ctr, Chicago, IL 90-93; **FAP:** Clin Prof Univ IL Coll Med; ***SI:*** *Breast Evaluation/Treatment*; **HMO:** United Healthcare, CIGNA, Humana Health Plan, Bc/BS +
Mcr Mcd 1 Week VISA

Kumar, Sanath (MD) S
South Suburban Hosp
Clinic For Diseases & Surgery, 9445 W 144th Pl; Orland Park, IL 60462; (708) 429-7100; **BDCERT:** CRS 80; S 89; **MS:** India 71; **RES:** S, Cook Cty Hosp, Chicago, IL 74-78; CRS, Cook Cty Hosp, Chicago, IL 78-79; **FAP:** Assoc Prof S Univ IL Coll Med; ***SI:*** *Pelvic Reconstruction*; **HMO:** +
LANG: Sp; Mcr Mcd

Lubienski, Mark (MD) S
St Francis Hosp
Hert Care Center, 2310 York St 3rd FL; Blue Island, IL 60406; (708) 371-2057; **BDCERT:** S 93; TS 94; **MS:** Wayne State U Sch Med 84; **RES:** S, Univ Hosp SUNY Bklyn, Brooklyn, NY 89-91; S, U Chicago Hosp, Chicago, IL 85-89; **FAP:** Assoc Prof S Univ IL Coll Med

Luck, Susan (MD) S
Children's Mem Med Ctr **(see page 139)**
Children's Surgical Foundation, 2300 Children's Plaza Box 63; Chicago, IL 60614; (773) 880-4422; **BDCERT:** S 74; TS 78; **MS:** U Colo Sch Med 67; **RES:** S, Baltimore City Hosp, Baltimore, MD 69-73; Children's Mem Med Ctr, Chicago, IL 73-75; **FEL:** Loyola U Med Ctr, Maywood, IL 75-77; **FAP:** Prof S Northwestern U; ***SI:*** *Pediatrics*; **HMO:** +
LANG: Sp; 2-4 Weeks

Maker, Vijay (MD) S
Illinois Masonic Med Ctr
(see page 118)
Illinois Masonic Medical Ctr, 836 W Wellington Ave Ste 3516; Chicago, IL 60657; (773) 883-2520; **BDCERT:** S 95; **MS:** India 67; **RES:** Surg Pathology, Mount Sinai Hosp Med Ctr, Chicago, IL 69; S, Mount Sinai Hosp Med Ctr, Chicago, IL 69-73; **FAP:** Assoc Prof S Rush Med Coll; **HMO:** +
Mcr Mcd 1 Week

Marcus, Elizabeth (MD) S
Cook Cty Hosp
Cook County Hospital - Breast Oncology, 1835 W Harrison St; Chicago, IL 60612; (312) 633-6741; **BDCERT:** S 95; **MS:** Univ Pittsburgh 88; **RES:** S, Boston University, Boston, MA 88-93; **FEL:** Roswell Park, Buffalo, NY 94-95; ***SI:*** *Breast Surgery*
LANG: Sp; Mcr Mcd A Few Days

Mc Grail, Michael (MD) S
Little Company of Mary Hosp & Hlth Care Ctrs **(see page 142)**
2850 W 95th St Ste 102; Evergreen Park, IL 60805; (708) 422-1188; **BDCERT:** S 89; **MS:** Loyola U-Stritch Sch Med, Maywood 82; **RES:** S, Michael Reese Hosp & Med Ctr, Chicago, IL 83-87; ***SI:*** *Laparoscopic Surgery*; **HMO:** +
SA SU Mcr Mcd

Mesleh, George (MD) S
Christ Hosp & Med Ctr **(see page 140)**
Hopkins Mesleh & Hopkins, 4400 W 95th St Ste 413; Oak Lawn, IL 60453; (708) 499-0034; **BDCERT:** S 97; **MS:** Egypt 71

Michel, Arthur (MD) S
Highland Park Hosp
Lake Shore Surgical Associates, 111 N Wabash Ave; Highland Park, 60602; (312) 641-1150; **BDCERT:** S 73; **MS:** Case West Res U 67; **RES:** S, Michael Reese Hosp Med Ctr, Chicago, IL 67-72; **FAP:** Clin.Assoc. Pro S Univ IL Coll Med; **HOSP:** Michael Reese Hosp & Med Ctr; ***SI:*** *Limited To Breast Disease*
Mcr Mcd NFI Immediately VISA

Morrow, Monica (MD) S
Northwestern Mem Hosp
Northwestern Memorial Hospital, 201 E Huron St Fl 13; Chicago, IL 60611; (312) 926-9039; **BDCERT:** S 92; **MS:** Jefferson Med Coll 76; **RES:** S, Med Ctr Hosp of VT, Burlington, VT 77-81; **FEL:** S, Mem Sloan Kettering Cancer Ctr, New York, NY 81-83; **FAP:** Prof S Northwestern U; ***SI:*** *Breast Cancer*; **HMO:** Aetna Hlth Plan, First Choice, Blue Choice, CIGNA PPO, Health Preferred
Mcr Mcd 1 Week VISA

Moscoso, Eloy (MD) S
St Anthony Hosp
Central Medical Latino, 3845 W 26th St; Chicago, IL 60623; (773) 277-2387; **BDCERT:** S 74; **MS:** Bolivia 63; **RES:** S, Little Company of Mary Hosp, Chicago, IL 67-70; ***SI:*** *Varicose Veins - Non Invasive Treatment; Breast Surgery*

Nash, Donald (MD) S
Oak Park Hosp
500 S Maple Ave Ste 102; Oak Park, IL 60304; (708) 660-2970; **BDCERT:** S 90; **MS:** Rush Med Coll 76; **RES:** S, Loyola U Med Ctr, Maywood, IL 77-82; **FAP:** Clin Instr Rush Med Coll

O'Donoghue, Michael (MD) S
Little Company of Mary Hosp & Hlth Care Ctrs **(see page 142)**
O'Donoghue & Rosenow, 2850 W 95th St Ste 306; Evergreen Park, IL 60805; (708) 422-8500; **BDCERT:** S 82; **MS:** Univ IL Coll Med 75; **RES:** S, U IL Med Ctr, Chicago, IL 76-81; **HMO:** Aetna Hlth Plan, Blue Cross & Blue Shield, Chicago HMO, Choicecare, CIGNA

Pandit, Jay (MD) S
Thorek Hosp & Med Ctr
Thorek Hosp, 850 W Irving Park Rd Ste 525; Chicago, IL 60613; (773) 525-6970; **BDCERT:** S 68; **MS:** India 56; **RES:** GS, American Hosp, Chicago, IL 59-62

Patel, Ambalal K (MD) S
St James Hosp & Hlth Ctrs
Boulevard Medical Clinic, 30 E 15th St Ste 200; Chicago Heights, IL 60411; (708) 756-4400; **BDCERT:** S 70; **MS:** India 61; **RES:** St Francis Hosp-Roslyn, Roslyn, NY 66-67; VA Hosp Oteen 67-68

Pawlikowski, James (MD) S
St Alexius Med Ctr
Surgical Specialists Ltd, 1575 Barrington Rd Ste 425; Hoffman Estates, IL 60194; (847) 884-6086; **BDCERT:** S 77; **MS:** Loyola U-Stritch Sch Med, Maywood 72; **RES:** S, St. Francis Hospital, Evanston, IL 72-76; **FAP:** Chrmn S; **HMO:** Aetna Hlth Plan, Blue Cross & Blue Shield, Californiacare, CIGNA, Compare Health Service

Peckler, M Scott (MD) S
Lutheran Gen Hosp **(see page 143)**
Advocate Medical Group, 1875 Dempster St Ste 280; Park Ridge, IL 60068; (847) 318-9071; **BDCERT:** S 75; **MS:** Loyola U-Stritch Sch Med, Maywood 69; **RES:** S, Cook Cty Hosp, Chicago, IL 70-71; S, U KS Med Ctr, Kansas City, KS 71-74; **FAP:** Asst Prof U Chicago-Pritzker Sch Med; **HMO:** Blue Cross & Blue Choice, Humana Health Plan
Mcr Med NFI Immediately VISA

Perez-Tamayo, Alejandra (MD) S
Mercy Hosp & Med Ctr
Surgery Department, 2525 S Michigan Ave; Chicago, IL 60616; (312) 567-2074; **BDCERT:** S 87; CCM 92; **MS:** Univ IL Coll Med 81; **RES:** S, Metro General Hospital, Chicago, IL 81-86; **FAP:** Instr S Univ IL Coll Med; **HMO:** Aetna Hlth Plan, AV-MED Health Plan, Blue Choice, Blue Cross & Blue Shield, Care America Health Plan

Pickleman, Jack R (MD) S
Loyola U Med Ctr **(see page 120)**
Loyola U Med Ctr - Dept Surg, 2160 S 1st Ave; Maywood, IL 60153; (708) 327-2670; **BDCERT:** S 89; **MS:** McGill U 64; **RES:** SM, U Chicago Hosp, Chicago, IL 67-73; **FAP:** Prof S Loyola U-Stritch Sch Med, Maywood; ***SI:*** *Gastrointestinal Surgery; Liver and Pancreas Surgery*
1 Week

Prinz, Richard (MD) S
Rush-Presbyterian-St Luke's Med Ctr
(see page 122)
Affiliated Clinical Surgeons, 1725 W Harrison Street Ste 834; Chicago, IL 60612; (312) 942-6511; **BDCERT:** S 95; **MS:** Loyola U-Stritch Sch Med, Maywood 72; **RES:** S, Barnes Hosp, St Louis, MO 72-74; S, Loyola U Med Ctr, Maywood, IL 74-77; **FEL:** EDM, Hammersmith Hosp, London, England 79-80; **FAP:** Professor S Rush Med Coll; **HOSP:** Oak Park Hosp; ***SI:*** *Thyroid-Parathyroid Surgery; Adrenal Pancreatic Surgery*; **HMO:** Blue Cross, Aetna Hlth Plan, Rush Health Plans, HMO
LANG: Grk, Pol, Sp; Mcr Med NFI
Immediately VISA

Przypyszny, John (MD) S
St Mary's of Nazareth Hosp Ctr
2222 W Division St Ste 225; Chicago, IL 60622; (773) 725-0522; **BDCERT:** S 62; **MS:** Univ IL Coll Med 53; **RES:** S, Hines VA Hosp, Chicago, IL 57-61; **HMO:** Blue Cross & Blue Shield, Chicago HMO, Metlife, Travelers

Pucci, Rita (MD) S
Grant Hosp
Columbia Grant Hosp, 550 W Webster Ave Ste 3NW; Chicago, IL 60614; (773) 929-4300; **BDCERT:** S 81; **MS:** Rush Med Coll 74; **RES:** S, Rush Presbyterian-St Luke's Med Ctr, Chicago, IL 75-79; **FAP:** Asst Prof Rush Med Coll; **HOSP:** St Joseph Hosp-Chicago; **HMO:** Prucare, United Healthcare, Blue Cross PPO, CIGNA, Aetna Hlth Plan +
LANG: Sp; Mcr Med NFI
A Few Days

Robin, Arnold (MD) S
Northwest Comm Hlthcare
Surgical Associates, 1430 N Arlington Hts Rd Ste 210; Arlington Hts, IL 60004; (847) 255-3314; **BDCERT:** S 92; **MS:** Rush Med Coll 77; **RES:** S, U IL Med Ctr, Chicago, IL 81-85; **FEL:** Columbia-Presbyterian Med Ctr, New York, NY 79-81; **FAP:** Asst Clin Prof S Univ IL Coll Med; **HMO:** Aetna Hlth Plan, Blue Cross & Blue Shield, Californiacare, CIGNA, Prudential

Rosanova, Albert (MD) S
Thorek Hosp & Med Ctr
Albert R Rosanova & Assoc, 6811 W Raven St; Chicago, IL 60631; (773) 631-8500; **BDCERT:** S 74; **MS:** U Miss Sch Med 68; **RES:** S, Cook Cty Hosp, Chicago, IL 69-73; **HMO:** Blue Cross & Blue Shield, Chicago HMO, Choicecare, Compare Health Service, Healthcare America

Rosen, Barry (MD) S
St Alexius Med Ctr
Surgical Specialists Ltd, 1575 Barrington Rd Ste 425; Hoffman Estates, IL 60194; (847) 884-6086; **BDCERT:** S 93; **MS:** Northwestern U 87; **RES:** S, Michael Reese Hosp/U IL, Chicago, IL 87-92; **HOSP:** Good Shepherd Hosp; ***SI:*** *Breast Cancer; Minimally Invasive Surgery*; **HMO:** Blue Cross & Blue Shield, Humana Health Plan, United Healthcare, CIGNA +
Mcr Med A Few Days VISA

Rosen, Jeffrey (MD) S
Holy Cross Hosp
Holy Cross Hospital, 2701 W 68th St; Chicago, IL 60629; (773) 471-5635; **BDCERT:** S 94; **MS:** Univ IL Coll Med 88; **RES:** U IL Med Ctr, Chicago, IL 89-93; **HOSP:** Good Samaritan Hosp

Rosenow, Mary (MD & PhD) S
Little Company of Mary Hosp & Hlth Care Ctrs (see page 142)
Little Company of Mary Hosp & Hlth Care Ctrs, 2850 W 95th St Ste 306; Evergreen Park, IL 60805; (708) 422-8500; **BDCERT:** S 93; **MS:** U Chicago-Pritzker Sch Med 78; **RES:** S, U Chicago Hosp, Chicago, IL 79-83

Seed, Randolph (MD) S
Grant Hosp
28 N Sheridan Rd Ste 510; Chicago, IL 60646; (312) 280-8960; **BDCERT:** S 68; **MS:** U Chicago-Pritzker Sch Med 60; **RES:** S, Chicago Clin Hosp, Chicago, IL 62-65; S, Northwestern Mem Hosp, Chicago, IL 65-67; **HMO:** +

Sener, Stephen (MD) S
Evanston Hosp
2650 Ridge Ave Burch 106; Evanston, IL 60201; (847) 570-1328; **BDCERT:** S 83; **MS:** Northwestern U 77; **RES:** S, Northwestern Mem Hosp, Chicago, IL 78-82; **FEL:** S, Mem Sloan Kettering Cancer Ctr, New York, NY 82-84; **FAP:** Assoc Prof S Northwestern U

Sethna, Jehangir (MD) S
Holy Cross Hosp
Holy Cross Neighborhood Assoc, 9401 S Pulaski Rd; Evergreen Park, IL 60805; (708) 636-8088; **BDCERT:** S 77; **MS:** India 66

Sheaff, Charles (MD) S
Northwest Comm Hlthcare
Northwest Suburban Surgical, 1430 N Arlington Hts Rd Ste 210; Arlington Hts, IL 60004; (847) 255-3314; **BDCERT:** S 82; **MS:** Rush Med Coll 75; **RES:** S, U IL Med Ctr, Chicago, IL 75-81; **FAP:** Asst Prof Rush Med Coll; **HOSP:** Holy Family Med Ctr; ***SI:*** *Thyroid, Endocrine Surgery; Vein Treatment*
Immediately
VISA

Stryker, Steven J. (MD) S
Northwestern Mem Hosp
Northwestern Surgical Assoc, 676 N Saint Clair St Ste 1525; Chicago, IL 60611; (312) 943-5427; **BDCERT:** S 84; CRS 86; **MS:** Northwestern U 78; **RES:** S, Northwestern Mem Hosp, Chicago, IL 78-83; **FEL:** CRS, Mayo Clinic, Rochester, MN 83-85; **FAP:** Northwestern U; ***SI:*** *Colorectal Cancer & Polyps; Inflammatory Bowel Disease*; **HMO:** +
A Few Days

Talamonti, Mark S (MD) S
Northwestern Mem Hosp
Northwestern Med Faculty Foundation, Dept of Surgery-Tarry 11-703, 300 E Superior St; Chicago, IL 60611; (312) 908-6909; **BDCERT:** S 90; **MS:** Northwestern U 83; **RES:** S, Northwestern Mem Hosp, Chicago, IL 83-89; **FEL:** Surg Onc, MD Anderson Cancer Ctr, Houston, TX 89-91; **FAP:** Dir Onc Northwestern U; ***SI:*** *Gastrointestinal Oncology*

Ujiki, Gerald (MD) S
Northwestern Mem Hosp
Surgery Department, 676 N Saint Clair St Ste 1525; Chicago, IL 60611; (312) 664-8748; **BDCERT:** S 71; **MS:** Northwestern U 62; **RES:** Northwestern Mem Hosp, Chicago, IL 65-70; **FAP:** Assoc Clin Prof S Northwestern U; **HMO:** Aetna Hlth Plan, Blue Cross & Blue Shield, Californiacare, Metlife, Prudential

Unti, James (MD) S
St Joseph Hosp-Chicago
CDN Surgical Assoc, 2515 N Clark St Ste 903; Chicago, IL 60614; (773) 472-3427; **BDCERT:** S 89; CRS 91; **MS:** Northwestern U 82; **RES:** S, Columbus Hosp, Chicago, IL 83-88; **FEL:** CRS, Cook Cty Hosp, Chicago, IL 88-90; **FAP:** Asst Clin Prof S Univ IL Coll Med; **HOSP:** Illinois Masonic Med Ctr; ***SI:*** *Cancer; Rectal Cancer*; **HMO:** +
A Few Days
VISA

Velasco, Jose (MD) S
Rush North Shore Med Ctr
9669 N Kenton Ave Ste 204; Skokie, IL 60076; (847) 982-1095; **BDCERT:** S 89; SCC 97; **MS:** Spain 70; **RES:** S, U IL Med Ctr, Chicago, IL 75-80; S, U Valladolid, Spain 70-73; **FAP:** Prof S Rush Med Coll

Walsh Jr, James J (MD) S
Illinois Masonic Med Ctr
(see page 118)
3000 N Halsted St Ste 507; Chicago, IL 60657; (773) 296-3103; **BDCERT:** S 87; GVS 90; **MS:** Univ IL Coll Med 81; **RES:** U IL Med Ctr, Chicago, IL 81-85; Tampa Genl Hosp, Tampa, FL 87-88; **HOSP:** Elmhurst Mem Hosp

Witt, Thomas (MD) S
Rush-Presbyterian-St Luke's Med Ctr
(see page 122)
S O Group, 1725 W Harrison St Ste 409; Chicago, IL 60612; (312) 942-2302; **BDCERT:** S 81; **MS:** Northwestern U 75; **RES:** S, Rush Presbyterian-St Luke's Med Ctr, Chicago, IL 75-80; **FEL:** S, Mem Sloan Kettering Cancer Ctr, New York, NY 80-82; **FAP:** Assoc Prof Rush Med Coll; **HOSP:** Glenbrook Hosp; ***SI:*** *Breast Diseases; Cancer*; **HMO:** Blue Cross & Blue Shield, Aetna Hlth Plan, United Healthcare, Rush Prudential +
LANG: Sp;
A Few Days

SURGICAL CRITICAL CARE

Fantus, Richard J. (MD) SCC
Illinois Masonic Med Ctr (see page 118)
Illinois Masonic Medical Center/Trauma Dept, 836 W Wellington Ave; Chicago, IL 60657; (773) 296-7033; **BDCERT:** S 87; SCC 88; **MS:** U Hlth Sci/Chicago Med Sch 81; **RES:** Cook Cty Hosp, Chicago, IL 81-86; **FAP:** Asst Prof S Univ IL Coll Med; **HMO:** +
LANG: Sp;

Merlotti, Gary J (MD) SCC
Christ Hosp & Med Ctr (see page 140)
Christ Hospital Med Ctr, 4440 W 95th St; Oak Lawn, IL 60453; **BDCERT:** S 93; SCC 93; **MS:** U Mich Med Sch 78; **RES:** S, Cook Cty Hosp, Chicago, IL 79-83; **FAP:** Asst Prof S Rush Med Coll; **HOSP:** Univ of Illinois at Chicago Med Ctr; **SI:** *Trauma*
Immediately

THORACIC SURGERY

Alshabkhoun, Shakeab (MD) TS
Christ Hosp & Med Ctr (see page 140)
4400 W 95th St Ste 307; Oak Lawn, IL 60453; (708) 346-0077; **BDCERT:** S 67; TS 68; **MS:** Turkey 56; **RES:** Boston Med Ctr, Boston, MA 63-64; **FEL:** TS, Harvard Med Sch, Cambridge, MA 65-66; **FAP:** Assoc Clin Prof S U Chicago-Pritzker Sch Med

Bakhos, Mamdouh (MD) TS
Loyola U Med Ctr (see page 120)
2160 S First Ave Bldg 210; Maywood, IL 60153; (708) 327-2505; **BDCERT:** TS 87; **MS:** Syria 71; **RES:** Huron Road Hosp, Cleveland, OH 72-76; **FEL:** Loyola U Med Ctr, Maywood, IL 76-78; **FAP:** Prof S Loyola U-Stritch Sch Med, Maywood; **SI:** *Heart Port*; **HMO:** +
A Few Days VISA

Blakeman, Bradford (MD) TS
Loyola U Med Ctr (see page 120)
2160 S 1st Ave Ste 6246; Maywood, IL 60153; (708) 327-2521; **BDCERT:** TS 95; **MS:** Univ IL Coll Med 79; **RES:** S, Loyola U Med Ctr, Maywood, IL 79-84; **FEL:** TS/VS, Loyola U Med Ctr, Maywood, IL 84-86; **FAP:** Prof TS Loyola U-Stritch Sch Med, Maywood; **HOSP:** Provena Mercy Ctr; **SI:** *Jehovah's Witness Patients; Marfan's Syndrome*; **HMO:** +
A Few Days VISA

Breyer, Robert (MD) TS
St Joseph Hosp-Chicago
Lincoln Park Cardiovascular, 2800 N Sheridan Rd Ste 209; Chicago, IL 60657; (773) 477-4343; **BDCERT:** TS 91; S 79; **MS:** Univ IL Coll Med 72; **RES:** S, Rush Presbyterian-St Luke's Med Ctr, Chicago, IL 72-74; TS, Rush Presbyterian-St Luke's Med Ctr, Chicago, IL 78-80; **FEL:** TS, Nat Inst Health, Bethesda, MD 74-76; **HOSP:** Columbus Hosp; **SI:** *Coronary Artery Bypass; Valve Replacement*; **HMO:** Aetna Hlth Plan, Blue Cross & Blue Choice, Californiacare, Humana Health Plan, Blue Choice PPO
Immediately

Brown, Charles Marshal (MD) TS
Michael Reese Hosp & Med Ctr
1875 Demster Dr; ParkRidge, IL 60068; (847) 433-0233; **BDCERT:** S 71; TS 75; **MS:** Northwestern U 65; **RES:** Cook Cty Hosp, Chicago, IL 66-71; **FEL:** Rush Presbyterian-St Luke's Med Ctr, Chicago, IL 71-74; **FAP:** Asst Clin Prof S U Chicago-Pritzker Sch Med; **HOSP:** Lake Forest Hosp

Evans, Richard (MD) TS
Michael Reese Hosp & Med Ctr
Advocate Healthcare, 2545 S King Dr; Chicago, IL 60616; (312) 808-3886; **BDCERT:** TS 67; **MS:** U Chicago-Pritzker Sch Med 58; **RES:** S, U Chicago Hosp, Chicago, IL 60-65; TS, U Chicago Hosp, Chicago, IL 67; **FAP:** Clin Prof TS Univ IL Coll Med; **HOSP:** Mercy Hosp & Med Ctr; **SI:** *Lung Cancer; Endocrine Surgery*; **HMO:** CIGNA, Humana Health Plan
Immediately

Faber, L Penfield (MD) TS
Rush-Presbyterian-St Luke's Med Ctr (see page 122)
Thoracic Surgical Assoc, 1725 W Harrison St Rm 218; Chicago, IL 60612; (312) 738-3732; **BDCERT:** TS 63; S 62; **MS:** Northwestern U 56; **RES:** S, Rush Presbyterian-St Luke's Med Ctr, Chicago, IL 57-61; TS, Hines VA Hosp, Hines, IL 61-63; **FAP:** Prof S Rush Med Coll; **SI:** *Lung Cancer; Thoracic Malignancy*; **HMO:** Aetna Hlth Plan, Chicago HMO, Humana Health Plan, United Healthcare, Prudential +
LANG: Sp;
Immediately

Faraci, Philip (MD) TS
Gottlieb Mem Hosp
Cardiothoracic & Vascular Surg, 4400 W 95th St Ste 205; Oak Lawn, IL 60453; (708) 346-4040; **BDCERT:** TS 96; S 74; **MS:** Tufts U 67; **RES:** S, Boston Med Ctr, Boston, MA 67-72; Cv, New England Med Ctr, Boston, MA 75-77; **HOSP:** Christ Hosp & Med Ctr; **HMO:** Aetna Hlth Plan, Bay State Health Plan, Californiacare, Chicago HMO
VISA

Ferguson, Mark (MD) TS
U Chicago Hosp (see page 124)
5841 S Maryland Ave MC5035; Chicago, IL 60637; (773) 702-3551; **BDCERT:** TS 85; **MS:** U Chicago-Pritzker Sch Med 77; **RES:** S, U Chicago Hosp, Chicago, IL 77-81; S, U Chicago Hosp, Chicago, IL 81-82; **FEL:** TS, U Chicago Hosp, Chicago, IL 82-84; **FAP:** Chf TS U Chicago-Pritzker Sch Med

Guide to symbols and abbreviations can be found on pages 110-113.

Fry, Willard (MD) TS
Evanston Hosp
ENH Medical Group, 2500 Ridge Ave Ste 105; Evanston, IL 60201; (847) 328-4484; **BDCERT:** TS 67; S 65; **MS:** Northwestern U 59; **RES:** U Chicago Hosp, Chicago, IL 59-62; TS, Blodgett Memorial, Grand Rapids, MI 62; **FEL:** S, U Chicago Hosp, Chicago, IL 62-64; **FAP:** Clin Prof Northwestern U; **HOSP:** Glenbrook Hosp; ***SI:** Lung Cancer; Clinical Trials for Chest*; **HMO:** Blue Cross & Blue Shield, Aetna Hlth Plan, United Healthcare
LANG: Fr, Grk; A Few Days

Fullerton, David (MD) TS
Northwestern Mem Hosp
Northwestern U Med Sch, 251 E Chicago Ave Ste 1030; Chicago, IL 60611; (312) 908-3121; **BDCERT:** TS 91; SCC 91; **MS:** Univ Mo-Columbia Sch Med 81; **RES:** S, U WA Med Ctr, Seattle, WA 81-82; TS, U CO Hosp, Denver, CO 87-90; **FAP:** Asst Prof S Northwestern U; ***SI:** Mitral Valve Repair; Ross Procedure*; **HMO:** CCN, CIGNA, United Healthcare, Private Healthcare, BC/BS PPO +
A Few Days

Goldin, Marshall D (MD) TS
Rush-Presbyterian-St Luke's Med Ctr (see page 122)
Cardiovascular Surgical Assoc of Rush Hosp, 1725 W Harrison St Ste 1156; Chicago, IL 60612; (312) 829-2540; **BDCERT:** TS 71; GVS 83; **MS:** Univ IL Coll Med 63; **RES:** S, Rush Presbyterian-St Luke's Med Ctr, Chicago, IL 64-68; TS, Rush Presbyterian-St Luke's Med Ctr, Chicago, IL 68-71; **FAP:** Assoc Prof S Rush Med Coll; ***SI:** Coronary Valve Replacement; Coronary Artery Bypass*; **HMO:** +
LANG: Sp; 1 Week

Joob, Axel (MD) TS
Lutheran Gen Hosp (see page 143)
Professional Building, 1875 Dempster St Ste 530; Park Ridge, IL 60068; (847) 696-4220; **BDCERT:** TS 89; S 97; **MS:** U Mich Med Sch 81; **RES:** S, U of VA Health Sci Ctr, Charlottesville, VA 81-86; **FEL:** TS, U of VA Health Sci Ctr, Charlottesville, VA 86-88; **FAP:** Asst Prof S Northwestern U

Kucich, Vincent (MD) TS
St Francis Hosp
Cardiovasc Med Assoc SC, 2310 York St Ste 3A; Blue Island, IL 60406; (708) 371-2057; **BDCERT:** TS 96; S 92; **MS:** SUNY Downstate 77; **RES:** NS, Northwestern Mem Hosp, Chicago, IL 78-79; S, Montefiore Med Ctr, Bronx, NY 79-83; **FEL:** Cv, Northwestern Mem Hosp, Chicago, IL 83-85; **FAP:** Assoc S U Chicago-Pritzker Sch Med; ***SI:** Cardiothoracic Surgery*; **HMO:** +
A Few Days VISA

Lertsburapa, Yukhol (MD) TS
St Mary's of Nazareth Hosp Ctr
2222 W Division St; Chicago, IL 60622; (773) 486-3535; **BDCERT:** S 75; TS 80; **MS:** Thailand 66; **RES:** S, Hines VA Hosp, Chicago, IL 68-72; TS, Loyola U Med Ctr, Maywood, IL 72-74; **FEL:** Cv, Texas Heart Inst, Houston, TX 78-79; **FAP:** Asst Clin Prof S Loyola U-Stritch Sch Med, Maywood; ***SI:** Cardiac Surgery*
Immediately

Liptay, Michael (MD) TS
Evanston Hosp
2650 Ridge Ave; Evanston, IL 60201; (847) 570-2565; **BDCERT:** TS 98; S 95; **MS:** Northwestern U 88; **RES:** S, Barnes Hospital, Washington, DC 89-91; TS, Brigham & Womens Hosp, Boston, MA 91-93; **FEL:** TS, Brigham & Womens Hospital, Boston, MA 93-95
Immediately VISA

Muasher, Issa E (MD) TS
Hinsdale Hosp (see page 275)
CVT Surgs Ltd, 1111 Superior St Ste 503; Melrose Park, IL 60160; (630) 920-8501; **BDCERT:** TS 95; S 77; **MS:** Lebanon 71; **RES:** S, Illinois Masonic Med Ctr, Chicago, IL 71-75; TS, U Miss Med Ctr, Jackson, MS 82-84; **FEL:** Cv/TS, Texas Heart Inst, Houston, TX 81; **HOSP:** Westlake Comm Hosp

Norman, Douglas (MD) TS
Rush North Shore Med Ctr
9669 Kenton Ave Ste 204; Skokie, IL 60076; (847) 982-1095; **BDCERT:** Cv 72; S 68; **MS:** Canada 61; **RES:** S, Bellevue Hosp Ctr, New York, NY 62-67; TS, Geo Wash U Med Ctr, Washington, DC 68-70; **FAP:** Asst Prof S Rush Med Coll; ***SI:** Lung Cancer; Peripheral Vascular Disease*; **HMO:** United Healthcare, Blue Cross & Blue Shield, Aetna Hlth Plan, Humana Health Plan +
A Few Days VISA

Olak, Jemi (MD) TS
Lutheran Gen Hosp (see page 143)
Lutheran Genl Hosp, 1700 Luther Ln; Park Ridge, IL 60068; (847) 723-2500; **BDCERT:** TS 97; **MS:** Canada 82; **RES:** S, Royal Victoria Hosp-McGill, McGill, CN 82-87; TS, Bristol U-Frenchway Hosp, Canada 87-88; **FEL:** TS, Toronto Gen Hosp, Toronto, CN 89-90; ***SI:** Lung Cancer*; **HMO:** +
LANG: Fr, Sp; 1 Week
VISA

Parvathaneni, K (MD) TS
Holy Cross Hosp
6222 S Pulaski Rd; Chicago, IL 60629; (773) 581-3881; **BDCERT:** S 73; TS 75; **MS:** India 64; **RES:** S, Mercy Hosp, Pittsburgh, PA 70-72; TS, Cook Cty Hosp, Chicago, IL 72-74; **FEL:** TS, St Francis Hosp of Evanston, Evanston, IL 74; **HOSP:** Palos Comm Hosp

Polin, Stanton (MD) TS
St Joseph Hosp-Elgin
Center For Vascular Studies, 4801 W Peterson Ave Ste 406; Chicago, IL 60646; (773) 685-0505; **BDCERT:** TS 69; S 63; **MS:** Univ IL Coll Med 57; **RES:** TS, Hines VA Hosp, Chicago, IL 62-63; TS, Baylor Coll Med, Houston, TX 63; **FAP:** Assoc Prof Chicago Coll Osteo Med; **HOSP:** Trinity Hosp; **HMO:** Aetna Hlth Plan, Blue Cross & Blue Shield, Chicago HMO, CIGNA, Takecare Health Plan

Roberts, Jack (MD) TS
Christ Hosp & Med Ctr (see page 140)
Cardiothoracic & Vascular Asso, 4400 W 95th St Ste 205; Oak Lawn, IL 60453; (708) 834-4065; **BDCERT:** TS 79; **MS:** Chicago Coll Osteo Med 67; **RES:** S, Rush Presbyterian-St Luke's Med Ctr, Chicago, IL 68-72; TS, Cook Cty Hosp, Chicago, IL 76-77; **FAP:** Asst Prof TS Rush Med Coll; **HOSP:** Little Company of Mary Hosp & Hlth Care Ctrs; ***SI:** Lung Surgery; Esophageal Surgery*; **HMO:** Aetna Hlth Plan, Blue Cross & Blue Shield, Chicago HMO, Rush Health Plans, Prudential
Mcr Mcd NFI 2-4 Weeks VISA

Somers, Jonathon (MD) TS
Rush-Presbyterian-St Luke's Med Ctr
(see page 122)
Cardiovascular Surgical Assoc, 1725 W Harrison St Ste 1156; Chicago, IL 60612; (312) 829-2540; **BDCERT:** TS 95; S 92; **MS:** Univ Penn 86; **RES:** S, Brown U Hosp, Providence, RI 87-91; **FAP:** Asst Prof S Rush Med Coll

Sullivan, Henry (MD) TS
Provena Mercy Ctr
Wimmer Medical Plaza, 810 Biesterfield Rd Ste 204; Chicago, IL 60007; (847) 981-2055; **BDCERT:** S 75; TS 76; **MS:** Univ IL Coll Med 67; **RES:** Hines VA Hosp, Chicago, IL 70-72; Loyola U Med Ctr, Maywood, IL 72-74; **FEL:** Rush Presbyterian-St Luke's Med Ctr, Chicago, IL 68-70; **HOSP:** Alexian Brothers Med Ctr; **HMO:** +
Mcr Mcd 1 Week

Veeragandham, Ramesh (MD) TS
St Francis Hosp
Heart Care Centers, 2310 York St Ste 3A; Blue Island, IL 60406; (708) 371-2057; **BDCERT:** S 96; **MS:** India 85; **RES:** S, UC San Diego Med Ctr, San Diego, CA 92-95; TS, Rush Presbyterian-St Luke's Med Ctr, Chicago, IL 95-97; **FEL:** Liver Transplant, U Chicago Hosp, Chicago, IL 90-91; ***SI:** Surgery*; **HMO:** +
Mcr Mcd

Votapka, Timothy V. (MD) TS
Evanston Hosp
2650 Ridge Ave; Evanston, IL 60201; (847) 570-2565; **BDCERT:** TS 93; S 89; **MS:** U MO-Kansas City Sch Med 83; **RES:** TS, St Louis U Hosp, St Louis, MO 92-93; Northwestern Mem Hosp, Chicago, IL 88-91; **FEL:** S, U KS Med Ctr, Kansas City, KS 83-88; ***SI:** Heart Transplant; Cardiac Surgery*; **HMO:** +
Mcr Mcd NFI VISA

Warren, William (MD) TS
Rush-Presbyterian-St Luke's Med Ctr
(see page 122)
Thoracic Surgical Assoc Sc, 1725 W Harrison St Ste 218; Chicago, IL 60612; (312) 738-3732; **BDCERT:** TS 95; **MS:** Canada 76; **RES:** S, U Toronto Hosp, Toronto, Canada 77-81; **FEL:** Rush Presbyterian-St Luke's Med Ctr, Chicago, IL 81-82; S, Rush Presbyterian-St Luke's Med Ctr, Chicago, IL 82-85; **FAP:** Prof Rush Med Coll; **HOSP:** West Suburban Hosp Med Ctr; ***SI:** Laser Bronchoscopy; Lung Cancer Surgery*; **HMO:** Aetna-US Healthcare, Blue Cross & Blue Shield, Rush Prudential, Humana Health Plan, United Healthcare
LANG: Sp; Mcr Mcd NFI
A Few Days

Yario, Robert (MD) TS
St Mary's of Nazareth Hosp Ctr
9501 S New England Ave; Oak Lawn, IL 60453; (708) 430-3543; **BDCERT:** TS 76; S 73; **MS:** Univ IL Coll Med 64; **RES:** Cv, Loyola U Med Ctr, Maywood, IL 71-72; PCd, Mayo Clinic, Rochester, MN 73; **FEL:** Cardiothoracic Surg, Cook Cty Hosp, Chicago, IL 73-74; **FAP:** Asst Clin Prof S Univ IL Coll Med

UROLOGY

Acino, Shawn (MD) U
Holy Family Med Ctr
Urocare, 1430 N Arlington Heights Rd ST205; Arlington Hts, IL 60004; (847) 259-2410; **BDCERT:** U 92; **MS:** Loyola U-Stritch Sch Med, Maywood 84; **RES:** U, Case Western Reserve U Hosp, Cleveland, OH 85-90; **HOSP:** Northwest Comm Hlthcare
Mcr Mcd 1 Week VISA

Albala, David Mois (MD) U
Loyola U Med Ctr (see page 120)
2160 S 1st Ave; Maywood, IL 60153; (708) 216-4076; **BDCERT:** U 94; **MS:** Mich St U 83; **RES:** S, Dartmouth Hitchcock Med Ctr, Lebanon, NH 83-85; U, Dartmouth Hitchcock Med Ctr, Lebanon, NH 86-90; **FEL:** Endo-urology, Barnes Hosp, St Louis, MO 90-91; **FAP:** Prof Loyola U-Stritch Sch Med, Maywood; **HOSP:** Hines VA Hosp; ***SI:*** *Kidney Stones; Laparoscopic Surgery*; **HMO:** United Healthcare, Blue Cross & Blue Shield, PHCS, HealthStar, Aetna Hlth Plan +
LANG: Sp, Fr; Immediately VISA

Bormes, Thomas Pat (MD) U
Lake Forest Hosp (see page 309)
Affiliated Urologists Ltd, 1725 W Harrison St Ste 917; Chicago, IL 60612; (312) 829-1820; **BDCERT:** U 91; **MS:** Loyola U-Stritch Sch Med, Maywood 84; **RES:** U, Rush Presbyterian-St Luke's Med Ctr, Chicago, IL 84-89; **FAP:** Asst Prof U Rush Med Coll; **HOSP:** Rush-Presbyterian-St Luke's Med Ctr; ***SI:*** *Prostate and Bladder Cancer; Lower Urinary Tract Syndrome*; **HMO:** +
1 Week VISA

Brendler, Charles B (MD) U
U Chicago Hosp (see page 124)
University of Chicago MC6038 Sect Urol, 5841 Maryland Ave; Chicago, IL 60637; (773) 702-6105; **BDCERT:** U 81; **MS:** U Va Sch Med 74; **RES:** S, Duke U Med Ctr, Durham, NC 75-76; U, Duke U Med Ctr, Durham, NC 76-79; **FEL:** Johns Hopkins Hosp, Baltimore, MD 80-81; **FAP:** Prof & Chf U U Chicago-Pritzker Sch Med; ***SI:*** *Prostate Cancer; Radical Prostatectomy*; **HMO:** Blue Cross & Blue Shield, Humana Health Plan, CIGNA, Rush Pru, Principal Health Care +
LANG: Sp; 2-4 Weeks VISA

Brown, James Louis (MD) U
Resurrection Med Ctr
7447 S Tellcott Suite 263; Chicago, IL 60631; (773) 763-1314; **BDCERT:** U 69; **MS:** Loyola U-Stritch Sch Med, Maywood 59; **RES:** Hines VA Hosp, Chicago, IL 60-61; U, Cook Cty Hosp, Chicago, IL 62-65; **FAP:** Asst Clin Prof U Loyola U-Stritch Sch Med, Maywood

Carter, Michael (MD) U
Northwestern Mem Hosp
201 E Huron St Ste 10200; Chicago, IL 60611; (312) 926-3535; **BDCERT:** U 75; **MS:** Georgetown U 66; **RES:** Los Angeles Co - Harbor, Los Angeles, CA 67-68; Johns Hopkins Hosp, Baltimore, MD 68-72; **FAP:** Clin Prof Northwestern U; ***SI:*** *Prostate Cancer-Prostatectomy; Kidney & Bladder Cancer*; **HMO:** +
4+ Weeks

Chodak, Gerald (MD) U
Louis A Weiss Mem Hosp
Midwest Prostate & Urology Health Center, 4646 N Marine Dr; Chicago, IL 60640; (773) 564-5006; **BDCERT:** U 84; **MS:** SUNY Buffalo 75; **RES:** U, Brigham & Women's Hosp, Boston, MA 77-79; U, U Chicago Hosp, Chicago, IL 79-81; **FEL:** S Rsrch, Children's Hosp, Boston, MA 81-82; **HOSP:** U Chicago Hosp; ***SI:*** *Prostate Cancer*; **HMO:** +
1 Week

De Marco, Carl (MD) U
Christ Hosp & Med Ctr (see page 140)
Gersack De Marco Hoyme & Assoc, 17850 S Kedzie Ave Ste 1100; Hazel Crest, IL 60429; (708) 799-0119; **BDCERT:** U 76; **MS:** Univ IL Coll Med 67

Engel, Geoffery (MD) U
Alexian Brothers Med Ctr (see page 138)
Northwest Suburban Urology, 810 Biesterfield Rd Ste 303; Elk Grove Village, IL 60007; (847) 593-0404; **BDCERT:** U 81; **MS:** Northwestern U 72; **RES:** U, Northwestern Mem Hosp, Chicago, IL 75-79; S, Northwestern Mem Hosp, Chicago, IL 73-74; **FEL:** U, Northwestern Mem Hosp, Chicago, IL 77-78; **FAP:** Asst Clin Prof U Hlth Sci/Chicago Med Sch; **HOSP:** St Alexius Med Ctr; **HMO:** Blue Cross & Blue Shield, Health Direct, Bay State Health Plan, Humana Health Plan, Principal Health Care
VISA

Falkowski, Walter (MD) U
St Francis Hosp
Northwest Metropolitan Urology Assoc., 800 Austin St West Tower 401; Evanston, IL 60202; (847) 491-1755; **BDCERT:** U 84; **MS:** Geo Wash U Sch Med 74; **RES:** U, Northwestern Mem Hosp, Chicago, IL 78-82; S, Northwestern Mem Hosp, Chicago, IL 77-78; **FEL:** Northwestern Mem Hosp, Chicago, IL 80-81; **HOSP:** Resurrection Med Ctr; **HMO:** IPA, HMO Illinois, IPA, MMS
LANG: Pol, Sp; VISA

Firlit, Casimir (MD) U
Children's Mem Med Ctr (see page 139)
707 W Fullerton; Chicago, IL 60614; (773) 880-4428; **BDCERT:** U 75; **MS:** Loyola U-Stritch Sch Med, Maywood 65; **RES:** S, Hines VA Hosp, Hines, IL 68-70; U, Hines VA Hosp, Hines, IL 70-73; **FEL:** Ped U, Children's Mem Med Ctr, Chicago, IL 73-74; **FAP:** Prof U Northwestern U

Garvey, Daniel (MD) U
Alexian Brothers Med Ctr
(see page 138)
Northwest Suburban Urology, 810 Biesterfield Rd Ste 303; Elk Grove Village, IL 60007; (847) 593-0404; **BDCERT:** U 93; **MS:** Loyola U-Stritch Sch Med, Maywood 84
VISA

Gersack, John (MD) U
Christ Hosp & Med Ctr **(see page 140)**
Gersack, De Marco, Hoyme,Nold & Assoc., 10000 W 151st St; Orland Park, IL 60462; (708) 349-6350; **BDCERT:** U 71; **MS:** Ind U Sch Med 59; **RES:** S, VA Hosp, Long Beach, CA 60-61; Cook Cty Hosp, Chicago, IL 61-64

Gluckman, Gordon (MD) U
Lutheran Gen Hosp **(see page 143)**
7447 W Talcott Ave; Chicago, IL 60631; (773) 775-0800; **BDCERT:** U 97; **MS:** Northwestern U 89; **RES:** S, Univ of California, San Francisco, CA 90-91; U, Univ of California, San Francisco, CA 91-95; **HOSP:** Resurrection Med Ctr

Goldrath, David (MD) U
Good Shepherd Hosp
Gott Goldrath & Troy, 450 W Route 22 Ste 26; Barrington, IL 60010; (847) 382-5080; **BDCERT:** U 90; **MS:** U Mich Med Sch 83; **RES:** U, U WI Sch Med, Milwaukee, WI 83-88; **HOSP:** Northern Illinois Med Ctr
VISA

Gott, Laurence (MD) U
Good Shepherd Hosp
Gott Goldrath & Troy, 450 W Il Route 22 Ste 26; Barrington, IL 60010; (847) 382-5080; **BDCERT:** U 78; **MS:** Univ IL Coll Med 68; **RES:** U IL Med Ctr, Chicago, IL 69-70; Indiana U Med Ctr, Indianapolis, IN 73-76; **HOSP:** Northern Illinois Med Ctr

Grayhack, John (MD) U
Northwestern Mem Hosp
675 N St Clair 20th Floor; Chicago, IL 60611; (312) 908-8145; **BDCERT:** U 56; **MS:** U Chicago-Pritzker Sch Med 47; **RES:** U, Johns Hopkins Hosp, Baltimore, MD 47-53; **FAP:** Prof U Northwestern U; ***SI:*** *Benign Prostate Hyperplasia; Carcinoma of Prostate*; **HMO:** Blue Cross & Blue Shield, Aetna Hlth Plan, CIGNA, Preferred Hlth
1 Week

Hoard, Donald (MD) U
Trinity Hosp
2315 E 93rd St Ste 239; Chicago, IL 60617; (773) 731-7400; **BDCERT:** U 78; **MS:** Meharry Med Coll 71; **RES:** Cook Cty Hosp, Chicago, IL 72-76; **FAP:** Asst Clin Prof Univ IL Coll Med; **HOSP:** Bethany Hosp

Hoeksema, Jerome (MD) U
Rush-Presbyterian-St Luke's Med Ctr
(see page 122)
Affiliated Urologists Ltd, 1725 W Harrison St Ste 917; Chicago, IL 60612; (312) 829-1820; **BDCERT:** U 81; **MS:** Wayne State U Sch Med 74; **RES:** S, Rush Presbyterian-St Luke's Med Ctr, Chicago, IL 74-76; U, Rush Presbyterian-St Luke's Med Ctr, Chicago, IL 76-79; **FAP:** Dir U Rush Med Coll; **HOSP:** Lake Forest Hosp; ***SI:*** *Urologic Cancer; Kidney Stones*; **HMO:** United Healthcare, Aetna Hlth Plan, CIGNA, Bc/BS, Guardian +
LANG: Sp; Immediately
VISA

Hoyme, K Dan (MD) U
Christ Hosp & Med Ctr **(see page 140)**
Gersack, De Marco, Hoyme & Assoc, 4400 W 95th St Ste 109; Oak Lawn, IL 60453; (708) 423-8706; **BDCERT:** U 78; **MS:** Univ IL Coll Med 68

Ignatoff, Jeffrey M (MD) U
Evanston Hosp
1000 Central St Ste 720; Evanston, IL 60201; (847) 475-8600; **BDCERT:** U 77; **MS:** Northwestern U 67; **RES:** U, Northwestern Mem Hosp, Chicago, IL 68-69; S, Northwestern Mem Hosp, Chicago, IL 71-75; **FAP:** Assoc Prof U Northwestern U; **HOSP:** Glenbrook Hosp; ***SI:*** *Prostate Cancer; Bladder Cancer*
LANG: Sp; 2-4 Weeks

Keeler, Thomas (MD) U
Evanston Hosp
ENH- Urology, 1000 Central St Ste 720; Evanston, IL 60201; (847) 475-8600; **BDCERT:** U 89; **MS:** Ind U Sch Med 81; **RES:** S, Northwestern Mem Hosp, Chicago, IL 82-83; U, Northwestern Mem Hosp, Chicago, IL 83-87; **FEL:** U, Northwestern Mem Hosp, Chicago, IL 85-86; **FAP:** Asst Prof U Northwestern U

Khandeparker, Vilas (MD) U
Holy Cross Hosp
6084 S Archer Ave Ste 202; Chicago, IL 60638; (773) 581-5888; **BDCERT:** U 77; **MS:** India 68; **RES:** U, Cook Cty Hosp, Chicago, IL 72-75; S, Norwegian-American Hosp, Chicago, IL 71-72; ***SI:*** *Prostate Cancer; Bladder Cancer*; **HMO:** United Healthcare, Humana Health Plan +
LANG: Sp; A Few Days

Levine, Laurence (MD) U
Rush-Presbyterian-St Luke's Med Ctr
(see page 122)
1725 W Harrison St Ste 917; Chicago, IL 60612; (312) 829-1820; **BDCERT:** U 89; **MS:** U Colo Sch Med 80; **RES:** U, Brigham & Women's Hosp, Boston, MA 83-87; S, Tufts U, Boston, MA 80-82; **FAP:** Asst Prof U Rush Med Coll; **HOSP:** Lake Forest Hosp; ***SI:*** *Male Erectile Dysfunction; Male Infertility; Peyronie's Disease*; **HMO:** Blue Cross & Blue Shield, Aetna Hlth Plan, Guardian, Rush Health Plans +
2-4 Weeks VISA

Guide to symbols and abbreviations can be found on pages 110-113.

Malvar, Thomas (MD) U
St Joseph Hosp-Elgin
Urological Surgeons Assoc, 2800 N Sheridan Rd Ste 602; Chicago, IL 60657; (773) 248-2842; **BDCERT:** U 76; S 81; **MS:** Philippines 66; **RES:** S, St Joseph's Hosp, Chicago, IL 68-71; U, U IL Med Ctr, Chicago, IL 71-74

Merrin, Claude (MD) U
Swedish Covenant Hosp
4015 N Pulaski Rd; Chicago, IL 60641; (773) 588-8855; **BDCERT:** U 74; **MS:** Argentina 62; **RES:** S, Cook Cty Hosp, Chicago, IL 67-68; U, Cook Cty Hosp, Chicago, IL 68-71; **FEL:** Roswell Park Cancer Inst, Buffalo, NY 71-79; **FAP:** Asst Clin Prof Loyola U-Stritch Sch Med, Maywood; **HOSP:** Condell Med Ctr; ***SI:*** *Prostate & Bladder Cancer; Testicular & Kidney Cancer*; **HMO:** Aetna Hlth Plan, Blue Cross & Blue Shield, United Healthcare, CIGNA, Humana Health Plan
LANG: Fr; Mcr NFI
A Few Days

Newmark, Jay (MD) U
Columbus Hosp
2800 N Sheridan Rd; Chicago, IL 60657; (773) 929-2386; **BDCERT:** U 96; **MS:** U Mich Med Sch 87; **RES:** James Bucheman Urol Inst, Baltimore, MD 88-93; Johns Hopkins Hosp, Baltimore, MD 87-88; **FEL:** Methodist Hosp, Indianapolis, IN 93-94; **HOSP:** St Joseph Hosp-Chicago

Nold, Stephen (MD) U
Christ Hosp & Med Ctr (see page 140)
Gersack De Marco Hoyme & Assoc, 10000 W 151st St; Orland Park, IL 60462; (708) 349-6350; **BDCERT:** U 96; **MS:** Southern IL U 78; **RES:** U, SIU Hosp, Springfield, IL 79-83; **FEL:** Children's Med Ctr, Dallas, TX 83-84; **FAP:** Clin Instr Ped Univ IL Coll Med

Rogin, Alan (MD) U
Swedish Covenant Hosp
Associated Urologists, 5140 N California Ave Ste 775; Chicago, IL 60625; (773) 387-7555; **BDCERT:** U 76; **MS:** U Hlth Sci/Chicago Med Sch 65; **RES:** Cook Cty Hosp, Chicago, IL 68-72; Mem Sloan Kettering Cancer Ctr, New York, NY 71; **FEL:** 77; **HOSP:** Ravenswood Hosp Med Ctr; ***SI:*** *Stones; Urologic Cancers*; **HMO:** Blue Cross & Blue Shield, Aetna Hlth Plan, Humana Health Plan, American Health Plan +
LANG: Sp; Mcr Mcd A Few Days
VISA

Ross, Lawrence (MD) U
Univ of Illinois at Chicago Med Ctr
University Ctr of Urology, 900 N Michigan Ave Ste 1420; Chicago, IL 60611; (312) 440-5127; **BDCERT:** U 74; **MS:** U Chicago-Pritzker Sch Med 65; **RES:** Michael Reese Hosp Med Ctr, Chicago, IL 66-70; **FAP:** Prof U Univ IL Coll Med

Schaeffer, Anthony (MD) U
Northwestern Mem Hosp
675 N St. Clair Suite 20-150; Chicago, IL 60611; (312) 908-8146; **BDCERT:** U 78; **MS:** Northwestern U 68; **RES:** S, Northwestern Mem Hosp, Chicago, IL 69-70; U, Stanford Med Ctr, Stanford, CA 72-76; **FAP:** Prof U Northwestern U; ***SI:*** *Prostatitis; Urinary Tract Infections*; **HMO:** Blue Cross & Blue Shield, Aetna Hlth Plan, United, Preferred Plan +
LANG: Sp; Mcr Mcd 1 Week
VISA

Sharifi, Roohollah (MD) U
VA Med Ctr
Urology Clinic, 840 S Wood St Ste 132; Chicago, IL 60612; (312) 996-6622; **BDCERT:** U 78; **MS:** Iran 65; **RES:** S, Sina Hosp 67-71; SM, St Francis Med Ctr, Trenton, NJ 72-73; **FEL:** U, Univ Ill Hosp, Chicago, IL 73-76; **FAP:** Prof S Univ IL Coll Med

Sundar, Balakrishna (MD) U
Columbus Hosp
Lakeshore Urology, 3340 Oak Park Ave Ste 201; Berwyn, IL 60402; (708) 788-6400; **BDCERT:** U 82; **MS:** India 70; **RES:** Cook Cty Hosp, Chicago, IL 76-80; **FAP:** Asst Clin Prof U Univ IL Coll Med; **HOSP:** Thorek Hosp & Med Ctr; **HMO:** Aetna Hlth Plan, Blue Cross & Blue Shield, Chicago HMO, CIGNA, Health Options

Sylora, Herme (MD) U
St Francis Hosp
Francisco Medical, 2850 W 95th St Ste 302; Evergreen Park, IL 60805; (708) 422-2242; **BDCERT:** U 76; S 73; **MS:** Philippines 60; **RES:** S, Sisters of Charity Emer Hosp, Buffalo, NY 62-66; U, U Chicago Hosp-Clinics, Chicago, IL 71-74; **HOSP:** Little Company of Mary Hosp & Hlth Care Ctrs; ***SI:*** *Prostectomy*

Villalba, Roger Alfonso (MD) U
St Mary's of Nazareth Hosp Ctr
1810 W Chicago Ave; Chicago, IL 60622; (312) 829-2238; **BDCERT:** U 75; **MS:** Colombia 63; **RES:** U IL Med Ctr, Chicago, IL 69-70; U IL Med Ctr, Chicago, IL 71-72; **FEL:** U IL Med Ctr, Chicago, IL 72-73; **HOSP:** St Elizabeth's Hosp; ***SI:*** *Urinary Incontinence; Prostatic Problems*; **HMO:** Blue Cross & Blue Shield, United Healthcare, St Mary HMO
LANG: Sp; Mcr Mcd NFI

Waters, William Bedford (MD) U
Loyola U Med Ctr (see page 120)
2160 S First Ave; Maywood, IL 60153; (708) 216-4076; **BDCERT:** U 82; **MS:** Vanderbilt U Sch Med 74; **RES:** S, UC San Diego Med Ctr, San Diego, CA 74-76; U, Brigham & Women's Hosp, Boston, MA 76-80; **FAP:** Prof Loyola U-Stritch Sch Med, Maywood; ***SI:*** *Testicular Cancer; Urologic Cancers*; **HMO:** Blue Cross & Blue Shield, CIGNA, CIGNA, UHC-PPO +
LANG: Sp, Pol; Mcr Mcd 2-4 Weeks VISA

Wheeler, John (MD) U
Loyola U Med Ctr (see page 120)
2160 S First Ave; Maywood, IL 60153; (708) 216-4076; **BDCERT:** U 84; **MS:** Georgetown U 77; **RES:** U, Boston U Med Ctr, Boston, MA 79-82; S, Boston U Med Ctr, Boston, MA 78-79; **FEL:** U, Boston U Med Ctr, Boston, MA 82-83; **FAP:** Prof U Loyola U-Stritch Sch Med, Maywood; **HOSP:** Hines VA Hosp; **SI:** *Urinary Incontinence; Neurogenic Bladder*
2-4 Weeks

Wohlberg, Frederick (MD) U
Little Company of Mary Hosp & Hlth Care Ctrs (see page 142)
Southwest Urology Assoc, 9760 S Kedzie Ave; Evergreen Park, IL 60805; (708) 425-0112; **BDCERT:** U 77; **MS:** Univ IL Coll Med 68; **RES:** S, Cook Cty Hosp, Chicago, IL 69-70; U, Hines VA Hosp, Chicago, IL 72-75

Young, Michael (MD) U
St Joseph Hosp-Chicago
2800 N Sheridan Rd Ste 30; Chicago, IL 60657; (773) 929-2386; **BDCERT:** U 93; **MS:** Rush Med Coll 85; **RES:** U, Loyola U Med Ctr, Maywood, IL 85-91; **HOSP:** Illinois Masonic Med Ctr; **SI:** *Urological Cancer*; **HMO:** +
1 Week

VASCULAR SURGERY (GENERAL)

Baker, William (MD) GVS
Loyola U Med Ctr (see page 120)
Loyola University Medical Ctr, 2160 S 1st Ave Fl 3; Maywood, IL 60153; (708) 327-2685; **BDCERT:** S 70; GVS 91; **MS:** U Chicago-Pritzker Sch Med 62; **RES:** S, U IA Hosp, Iowa City, IA 63-64; S, U Chicago Hosp, Chicago, IL 66-69; **FEL:** GVS, UC San Francisco Med Ctr, San Francisco, CA 69-70; **FAP:** Prof GVS Loyola U-Stritch Sch Med, Maywood; **HOSP:** West Suburban Hosp Med Ctr

Baker, William (MD) GVS
Loyola U Med Ctr (see page 120)
Loyola U Med Ctr - Dept Surg, 2160 S First Ave; Maywood, IL 60153; (708) 327-2685; **BDCERT:** S 70; GVS 91; **MS:** U Chicago-Pritzker Sch Med 62; **RES:** S, U IA Hosp, Iowa City, IA 63-64; S, U Chicago Hosp, Chicago, IL 66-69; **FEL:** GVS, UC San Francisco Med Ctr, San Francisco, CA 69-70; **FAP:** Prof GVS Loyola U-Stritch Sch Med, Maywood; **HOSP:** West Suburban Hosp Med Ctr; **HMO:** +
2-4 Weeks

Clark, Elizabeth (MD) GVS
St Joseph Hosp-Chicago
Columbus Hospital, 2520 N Lakeview Ave 2nd Flr; Chicago, IL 60614; (773) 388-6611; **BDCERT:** S 94; GVS 97; **MS:** U NC Sch Med 86; **RES:** S, U Chicago Hosp, Chicago, IL 86-92; **FEL:** GVS, U Chicago Hosp, Chicago, IL 92-95; **FAP:** Instr U Chicago-Pritzker Sch Med; **SI:** *Repair of Blocked Arteries; Varicose and Spider Veins*; **HMO:** Blue Cross & Blue Shield, CIGNA, Compass, United Healthcare +
LANG: Sp;
A Few Days VISA

Golan, John (MD) GVS
Evanston Hosp
2650 Ridge Ave; Evanston, IL 60201; (847) 570-2562; **BDCERT:** GVS 98; **MS:** Loyola U-Stritch Sch Med, Maywood 78; **RES:** S, Loyola U Med Ctr, Maywood, IL 78-83; **FEL:** GVS, Baylor Med Ctr, Dallas, TX 83-84; **FAP:** Asst Prof Northwestern U; **HOSP:** Glenbrook Hosp; **SI:** *Carotid Endarterectomy; Vein Therapy, Surgery & Laser*; **HMO:** Blue Cross & Blue Shield, Aetna Hlth Plan, HMO of IL, Humana Health Plan +
1 Week
VISA

Halstuk, Kevin (MD) GVS
St Francis Hosp
Surgical Associates, 800 Austin St Ste 563; Evanston, IL 60202; (847) 869-0522; **BDCERT:** S 84; GVS 86; **MS:** Northwestern U 78; **RES:** S, Loyola U Med Ctr, Maywood, IL 78-82; **FEL:** VIR, Loyola U Med Ctr, Maywood, IL 82-83; **FAP:** Asst Clin Prof Univ IL Coll Med; **SI:** *Carotid Endarterectomy; Aortic & Femoral Bypass*; **HMO:** +
LANG: Sp;
A Few Days VISA

Kornmesser, Thomas (MD) GVS
Northwest Comm Hlthcare
8780 W Golf Rd Ste 300; Niles, IL 60714; (847) 699-7474; **BDCERT:** S 73; GVS 91; **MS:** Temple U 66; **RES:** S, Northwestern Mem Hosp, Chicago, IL 67-72; **FEL:** GVS, U WA Med Ctr, Seattle, WA 72-73; **HOSP:** Resurrection Med Ctr

Guide to symbols and abbreviations can be found on pages 110-113.

McCarthy III, Walter J (MD) GVS
Rush-Presbyterian-St Luke's Med Ctr (see page 122)
Rush - Presbyterian - St Lukes Medical, 1653 W Congress Pkwy; Chicago, IL 60612; **BDCERT:** GVS 95; **MS:** Wayne State U Sch Med 78; **RES:** S, Northwestern Mem Hosp, Chicago, IL 79-83; **FEL:** GVS, Northwestern Mem Hosp, Chicago, IL 83-85; **FAP:** Assoc Prof S Northwestern U; **HOSP:** Cook Cty Hosp; **SI:** *Endarterectomy; Aortic Aneurysms*
Mcr Mcd 1 Week

Painter, Thomas (MD) GVS
Lutheran Gen Hosp (see page 143)
8780 W Golf Rd Ste 300; Niles, IL 60714; (847) 699-7474; **BDCERT:** S 86; GVS 88; **MS:** Ohio State U 80; **RES:** S, Cleveland Clinic Hosp, Cleveland, OH 81-85; **FEL:** GVS, Cleveland Clinic Hosp, Cleveland, OH 85-86; **FAP:** Assoc S Northwestern U; **HOSP:** Northwest Comm Hlthcare

Pearce, William (MD) GVS
Northwestern Mem Hosp
Northwestern Medical Faculty, 251 E Chicago Ave Ste 628; Chicago, IL 60611; (312) 908-2714; **BDCERT:** S 90; GVS 92; **MS:** U Colo Sch Med 75; **FAP:** Prof Northwestern U
Mcr

Schneider, Joseph (MD) GVS
Evanston Hosp
Burch 1000, 2650 Ridge Ave; Evanston, IL 60201; (847) 570-2565; **BDCERT:** S 88; GVS 90; **MS:** U Minn 79; **RES:** S, U WA Med Ctr, Seattle, WA 79-80; S, U WA Med Ctr, Seattle, WA 80-87; **FEL:** GVS, Stanford Med Ctr, Stanford, CA 87-88; **HOSP:** Glenbrook Hosp; **SI:** *Carotid Endarterectomy; Aortic Aneurysm*
Mcr Mcd 1 Week VISA

Schuler, James (MD) GVS
Michael Reese Hosp & Med Ctr
1740 W Taylor St Ste 2200; Chicago, IL 60612; (312) 996-7595; **BDCERT:** GVS 92; **MS:** Univ IL Coll Med 72; **RES:** S, Illinois Masonic Med Ctr, Chicago, IL 73-79; **FEL:** GVS, Illinois Masonic Med Ctr, Chicago, IL 79-80; **FAP:** Prof S Univ IL Coll Med

Verta, Michael (MD) GVS
Highland Park Hosp
Veincare Limited, 1500 Shermer Rd; Northbrook, IL 60062; (847) 205-0050; **BDCERT:** GVS 93; S 87; **MS:** Northwestern U 71; **RES:** S, Northwestern Mem Hosp, Chicago, IL 72-77; **FEL:** PeripheralVasSurg, Northwestern Mem Hosp, Chicago, IL 75-76

Yao, James (MD) GVS
Northwestern Mem Hosp
Northwestern Vascular Assoc, 251 E Chicago Ave Ste 628; Chicago, IL 60611; (312) 908-2714; **BDCERT:** S 67; GVS 83; **MS:** Taiwan 61; **RES:** S, Cook Cty Hosp, Chicago, IL 62-67; **FEL:** Research, St Mary's Hosp Medical School, London, England 67-68; **FAP:** Prof Northwestern U; **SI:** *Aortic Aneurysm; Carotid Disease*; **HMO:** Aetna Hlth Plan, US Hlthcre, Blue Cross, United Healthcare, Rush Pru +
Mcr Mcd 1 Week VISA

DU PAGE COUNTY

EDWARD HEALTH SERVICES

Edward Health Services

Edward Health Services
801 South Washington Street
Naperville, Illinois 60540
PHONE: (630) 355-0450

Sponsorship	**Independent, not-for-profit**
Beds	**179 beds**
Accreditation	**Joint Commission on Accreditation of Healthcare Organizations; American College of Surgeons; American College of Radiology**

A GROWING PROVIDER

Edward Health Services is a full-service healthcare provider located in the western suburbs of Chicago. Edward facilities include a 179-bed hospital, an outpatient cardiac center, a dedicated women's health center, in- and outpatient oncology services, two ambulatory care centers, two medically based fitness centers, a home health resource, and a psychiatric facility.

Edward Health Services has more than 650 affiliated primary care and specialty physicians who represent 56 medical specialties; 94 percent of Edward doctors are board certified compared to 62 percent nationwide.

A dynamic healthcare resource, Edward Health Services was named number 34 of the 50 fastest growing healthcare providers in the United States in 1998 by Modern Healthcare magazine. Edward is in the midst of completing its most extensive expansion to date, a three-year project that will add space and services to existing facilities and create brand-new centers of excellence, including a state-of-the-art women and children's pavilion.

OVERVIEW OF SERVICES

Edward cardiology services are led by cardiologists and cardiothoracic surgeons who have trained at some of the nation's most prestigious medical centers, including the Mayo Clinic and Loyola University Medical Center. These experts utilize the latest technology to aggressively treat all forms of heart disease.

In addition to advanced inpatient care, the Edward cardiac continuum includes the Edward Cardiovascular Institute (ECI), a leading outpatient resource that is home to the first freestanding cardiac catheterization lab in Illinois. The ECI is also the first provider in the western suburbs to offer Ultra Fast Heart Scan - the non-invasive heart screening that uses electron beam tomography to detect coronary artery calcification at an early, treatable stage.

Edward in- and outpatient oncology services provide patients virtually every screening, diagnostic, and treatment modality. Outpatient care is available at the Edward Cancer Center. Here, patients can access the latest therapies and participate in nationwide clinical trials through Edward's affiliation with the Cardinal Bernardin Cancer Center at Loyola University Medical Center.

Edward women and children's services include state-of-the-art women's imaging capabilities, the first dedicated outpatient women's health center in DuPage County, and a level II neonatal intensive care unit. A new women and children's pavilion is scheduled to open in 2000, which will centralize services and include a free family health information library.

Edward emergency services include a level II trauma center, an adjoining ER Fast Track, and Immediate Care at the Edward Healthcare Center in Bolingbrook.

Physician Referral	Edward physician referral provides information on hundreds of board-certified affiliated physicians. Referral specialists can detail a physician's specialty, office location, hours, accepted health plans, and more. The service is available Monday through Friday, 9 am to 5 pm, at (630) 369-MDMD.

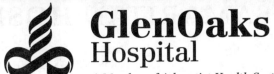

701 Winthrop Avenue,Glendale Heights, IL 60139-9972;PHONE: (630) 545-8000
www.ahsmidwest.org

Sponsorship	Non-profit. A member of Adventist Health System Midwest Region.
Beds	186 licensed beds
Accreditation	JCAHO, CARF

General Description:
The 200 member medical staff and team of professional employees serve more than 36,000 patient visits per year. Services include outpatient and inpatient primary care, the Special Additions Birth Centre, a Level II Trauma Center, occupational health services, outpatient rehabilitation services, outpatient surgery, a full range of diagnostic services including cardiology, sleep lab and radiology, and the most comprehensive behavioral medicine program in the area.

Mission:
A Christian health-care leader committed to a partnering with physicians and community to provide whole-person care and promote wellness.

Dedicated to Primary Care:
GlenOaks emergency department is a certified Level II Trauma Center with board-certified emergency medicine physicians. The hospital is equipped to provide urgent and emergency care. In the event a tertiary level of care is needed, GlenOaks maintains transfer capability to Hinsdale Hospital.

In addition to the trauma center, GlenOaks is the first in DuPage County to dedicate entire obstetric unit to LDRP suites, allowing new mothers to labor, deliver, recover and receive post-partum care in the comfort of one room.

The hospital's community outreach program offers education support classes, screenings, behavior modification programs, health fairs, lectures to the community.

Other Services:

Behavioral Health
The hospital provides inpatient and outpatient behavioral health treatment programs for adolescents, adults and seniors. The goal is to rapidly stabilize the patient and identify the source of their problems.

Special Additions Birth Centre
Offers a full range of services including comprehensive prenatal classes, high risk pregnancy care, Level II nursery, neonatology care for babies in distress, and pain management options.

Physician Referral	Please call (630) 856-7500 for a physician referral (weekdays 8 a.m. - 5 p.m.).

GOOD SAMARITAN HOSPITAL

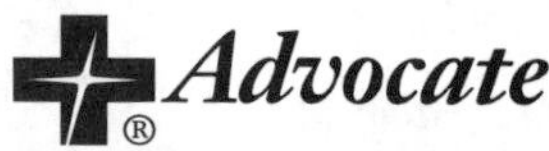

3815 HIGHLAND AVENUE
DOWNERS GROVE, ILLINOIS
630-275-5900

Sponsorship:	Voluntary, not-for-profit
Beds:	316 licensed beds, including 30 transitional care beds and 36 psychiatric beds
Accreditation:	Joint Commission on Accreditation of Healthcare Organizations, American College of Surgeons, American College of Radiology, American College of Pathologists, American Association of Blood Banks, Illinois State Medical Society

Good Samaritan Hospital is a leading provider of health and wellness services in Chicago's western suburbs. The hospital provides one of the most innovative and comprehensive cardiac centers in Illinois, the only Level I Trauma Center between Cook County and the Iowa border, and the highest level of perinatal care in DuPage County. Good Samaritan Hospital's medical staff consists of more than 650 physicians representing 55 specialties.

Good Samaritan Hospital is a member of Advocate Health Care, a non-profit organization of Chicagoland hospitals, health centers, and physician practices. To learn more, visit our web site at advocatehealth.com.

Cardiovascular Services	Good Samaritan Hospital is nationally known as a cardiac care pioneer. With a medical staff of nearly 70 board-certified cardiologists and cardiovascular surgeons, the hospital is a leader in the newest interventional technologies, diagnostics and preventive techniques.
Women's and Children's Services	Good Samaritan and its 40 obstetricians look forward to a renovated obstetrics unit in 1999. The unit's Special Care Nursery provides the highest level of perinatal care in DuPage County, and boasts a perinatologist to care for high-risk moms, and neonatologists on site to care for premature babies and multiple births. A newly renovated pediatric unit is supported by 80 pediatricians, family practitioners and pediatric sub-specialists. Good Samaritan provides mammography at two locations, breast ultrasound, stereotactic breast biopsy and osteoporosis scanning.
Trauma and Emergency Medicine	Good Samaritan Hospital is one of only 18 hospitals in Illinois with a Level I Trauma Center, and one of only two in the state accredited by the American College of Surgeons. The emergency department is staffed with all emergency specialists.
Center for Mental Health	Located on the hospital's campus, this center provides inpatient and outpatient programs and services for children and adolescents, adults and seniors, a chemical dependency program and a Center for Stress Medicine.
Health and Wellness Center	Coming in late 1999, the Good Samaritan Health and Wellness Center will provide equipment and programs to support total health, including fitness, physical rehabilitation, community and employee wellness programs and physician offices.
Good Samaritan Professional Building	Located in Naperville, the Good Samaritan Professional Building houses physician offices, mammography, pharmacy and laboratory services, The Physical Performance Place, a radiology center and a health resource center.
Physician Referral	Good Samaritan Hospital's physician referral line at 1-800-3-ADVOCATE (1-800-323-8622) provides easy access to information about physicians, classes and services at the hospital

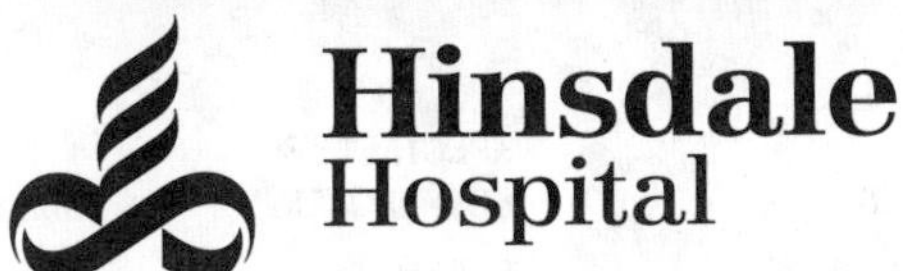

A Member of Adventist Health System

120 N. Oak Street, Hinsdale, IL 60521; PHONE: (630) 856-9000
www.ahsmidwest.org

Sponsorship	Non-profit. A member of Adventist Health System Midwest Region.
Beds	404 licensed beds
Accreditation	JCAHO, CARF

GENERAL DESCRIPTION:

Hinsdale Hospital joined Adventist Health System in May 1997 and is the flagship hospital of the corporation's Midwest Region. Hinsdale Hospital is noted as the second largest hospital within Adventist Health System.

MISSION:

A Christian health-care leader committed to a partnering with physicians and community to provide whole-person care and promote wellness.

Centers of Excellence:

Rooney Heart Institute:

A leading heart care center offering the most advanced method of minimally invasive techniques for bypass surgery, coronary angioplasty, atherectomy and intravascular ultrasound. The Institute provides a comprehensive range of diagnostic, treatment, rehabilitation and educational programs to meet area residents' complete heart care needs.

Opler Cancer Center:

One of the few community hospitals in Illinois to offer tertiary-level cancer services, such as autologous bone marrow transplants, biologic response therapy, prostate seed implants and experimental drugs and treatments.

Birck Family Women's and Children's Center:

From the wide-array of family-centered birthing options to the intensive care neonatal nursery and pediatric intensive care unit, The Birck Family Women's and Children's Center is focused on family health. The center features the first hospital-based Maternal-Fetal Medicine Center in DuPage County for women with high-risk pregnancies, and the Hinsdale Center for Reproduction for couples experiencing infertility problems.

Paulson Rehab Network:

Long recognized as one of the area's leaders in rehabilitation services, Paulson Rehab Network provides comprehensive inpatient and outpatient services at state of the art facilities throughout the area.

Behavioral Health Services/New Day Center:

Comprehensive inpatient and outpatient mental health care and substance abuse treatments are available. Experienced professionals and tailored programs for all ages are helping patients and families change their lives.

Trauma Center/Chest Pain Emergency Center:

In our advanced emergency center, we offer the area's first Chest Pain Emergency Center. This specialized center provides immediate, state of the art treatment such as thrombolitic therapy to persons experiencing chest pain.

The hospital's community outreach program offers education support classes, screenings, health fairs, and lectures to the community.

Physician Referral	Please call (630) 856-7500 for a physician referral (weekdays 8 a.m. - 5 p.m.).

DU PAGE COUNTY

Specialties are indicated in bold-type face. Capital letters indicate Primary Care Specialties. Subspecialties are listed in non-bold type. Listings indicate if a doctor is certified in a subspecialty but predominately practices primary care medicine.

*Oncologists deal with Cancer

ADDICTION PSYCHIATRY

Angres, Dan (MD) AdP
Rush-Presbyterian-St Luke's Med Ctr (see page 122)
2001 Butterfield Rd; Downers Grove, IL 60515; (630) 969-7300; **BDCERT:** AdP 94; Psyc 91; **MS:** Mexico 76; **RES:** N, U IL Med Ctr, Chicago, IL 77-78; Psyc, Rush Presbyterian-St Luke's Med Ctr, Chicago, IL 78-80; **FEL:** Psyc, Rush Presbyterian-St Luke's Med Ctr, Chicago, IL 87-88; **FAP:** Asst Prof Psyc Rush Med Coll; ***SI:** Addiction for Health Care Workers*

ALLERGY & IMMUNOLOGY

Bharani, Sakina N. (MD) A&I
Good Samaritan Hosp (see page 274)
3825 Highland Ave Ste 2B; Downers Grove, IL 60515; (630) 852-4050; **BDCERT:** A&I 75; Ped 75; **MS:** India 67; **RES:** A&I, Rush Presbyterian-St Luke's Med Ctr, Chicago, IL 73-75; Ped A&I, Rush Presbyterian-St Luke's Med Ctr, Chicago, IL 72-73; **FAP:** Asst Prof Ped Rush Med Coll

Chua-Apolinario, Susan (MD) A&I
Christ Hosp & Med Ctr (see page 140)
5423 W 95th St; Oak Lawn, IL 60517; (708) 422-4848; **BDCERT:** A&I 97; Ped 96; **MS:** Philippines 78; **RES:** Ped, Cook Cty Hosp, Chicago, IL 85-88; **FEL:** A&I, Cook Cty Hosp, Chicago, IL 88-90; A&I, Rush Presbyterian-St Luke's Med Ctr, Chicago, IL 94-96; **FAP:** Asst Prof Ped Loyola U-Stritch Sch Med, Maywood; ***SI:** Hives/Eczema*
Immediately VISA

Kelly, Joseph Francis (MD) A&I
Central DuPage Hosp
Allergy & Immunology Dept, 454 Pennsylvania Ave; Glen Ellyn, IL 60137; (630) 469-9200; **BDCERT:** A&I 75; IM 74; **MS:** St Louis U 68; **RES:** IM, St Louis Hosp, St Louis, MO 69-71; **FEL:** A&I, Northwestern Mem Hosp, Chicago, IL 71-73; **FAP:** Asst Prof Med Northwestern U

Ozog, Diane Louise (MD) A&I
Good Samaritan Hosp (see page 274)
3825 Highland Ave Ste 204; Downers Grove, IL 60515; (630) 852-8182; **BDCERT:** A&I 87; Ped 87; **MS:** U Hlth Sci/Chicago Med Sch 82; **RES:** Ped A&I, Cook Cty Hosp, Chicago, IL 83-85; **FEL:** A&I, Children's Mem Med Ctr, Chicago, IL 85-87; **FAP:** Clin Instr Ped Northwestern U; **HOSP:** Hinsdale Hosp

ANESTHESIOLOGY

Agarwal, Suresh (MD) Anes
Ingalls Mem Hosp
5658 S Countryline Rd; Hinsdale, IL 60521; (708) 333-2300; **BDCERT:** Anes 73; **MS:** India 66

Carroll, Gregory (MD) Anes
Hinsdale Hosp (see page 275)
120 North Oak; Hinsdale, IL 60540; (630) 856-6643; **BDCERT:** Anes 88; **MS:** Univ IL Coll Med 84; **RES:** Anes, Children's Mem Med Ctr, Chicago, IL 87-88; Loyola U Med Ctr, Maywood, IL 85-88; **FEL:** Cv,; TS,; ***SI:** Pediatric Anesthesia; Cardiovascular Anesthesia*; **HMO:** +
Mcr Mcd NFI Immediately
VISA

Glaser, Scott (MD) Anes
Hinsdale Hosp (see page 275)
Hinsdale Hosp, 120 N Oak St; Hinsdale, IL 60521; (630) 856-6643; **BDCERT:** Anes 92; PM 96; **MS:** Ind U Sch Med 86; **RES:** Anes, Northwestern Mem Hosp, Chicago, IL 87-90; **HMO:** Aetna Hlth Plan, Blue Cross & Blue Shield

Jain, Neeraj (MD) Anes
Hinsdale Hosp (see page 275)
120 N Oak St; Hinsdale, IL 60521; (630) 856-7246; **BDCERT:** Anes 92; PM 94; **MS:** NE Ohio U 88; **RES:** Anes, Northwestern Mem Hosp, Chicago, IL 89-91; **FEL:** PM, Northwestern Mem Hosp, Chicago, IL 91-92; ***SI:** Pain Management*; **HMO:** Blue Cross & Blue Shield, CIGNA, Aetna Hlth Plan, Prudential, Humana Health Plan +
LANG: Sp; Mcr Mcd NFI 2-4 Weeks

Martucci, John (MD) Anes
Good Samaritan Hosp (see page 274)
Good Samaritan Hosp, 3815 S Highland Ave; Downers Grove, IL 60505; (630) 275-5900; **BDCERT:** Anes 94; **MS:** Ohio State U 89; **RES:** Anes, Loyola U Med Ctr, Maywood, IL 90-93

Wenzel, Dave (MD) Anes
Rush-Copley Med Ctr
Rush-Copley Med Ctr, 2000 Ogden Ave; Aurora, IL 60504; (630) 978-4821; **BDCERT:** Anes 89; **MS:** Jefferson Med Coll 84; **RES:** Anes, Rush Presbyterian-St Luke's Med Ctr, Chicago, IL 85-87; **FEL:** Cv, Rush Presbyterian-St Luke's Med Ctr, Chicago, IL 87-88

Zygmunt, Michael (MD) Anes
Elmhurst Mem Hosp
Anesthesiology Dept, 200 Berteau St; Elmhurst, IL 60126; (630) 832-0050; **BDCERT:** Anes 78; **MS:** Loyola U-Stritch Sch Med, Maywood 72; **RES:** Anes, Loyola U Med Ctr, Maywood, IL 73-75

CARDIOLOGY (CARDIOVASCULAR DISEASE)

Akhtar, Riaz (MD) Cv
Oak Park Hosp
Internal Medical Cardiology, 1 S Summit Ave; Oakbrook Terrace, IL 60181; (708) 386-8118; **BDCERT:** IM 86; Cv 91; **MS:** India 69; **RES:** IM, Cook Cty Hosp, Chicago, IL 74-75; **FEL:** Cv, Lankenau Hosp, Philadelphia, PA 75-77; Cv, Cook Cty Hosp, Chicago, IL 89-90; **HOSP:** Westlake Comm Hosp

Bufalino, Vincent (MD) Cv
Edward Hosp (see page 272)
Midwest Heart Specialists, 120 N Spelding Drive Ste 206; Naperville, IL 60540; (630) 527-2730; **BDCERT:** IM 80; Cv 83; **MS:** Loyola U-Stritch Sch Med, Maywood 77
Mcr Mcd VISA

Cahill, John (MD) Cv
Elmhurst Mem Hosp
386 N York Rd Ste 207; Elmhurst, IL 60126; (630) 782-4050; **BDCERT:** IM 84; Cv 87; **MS:** Loyola U-Stritch Sch Med, Maywood 81; **RES:** IM, Loyola U Med Ctr, Maywood, IL 81-85; **FEL:** Cv, Loyola U Med Ctr, Maywood, IL 85-87; **FAP:** Asst Clin Prof Med Loyola U-Stritch Sch Med, Maywood; ***SI:*** *Cardiac Angiography & Interventions*; **HMO:** +
Mcr Mcd 2-4 Weeks VISA

Clark, James (MD) Cv
Rush-Presbyterian-St Luke's Med Ctr
(see page 122)
Associates In Cardiology Ltd, 3825 Highland Ave Ste 4K; Downers Grove, IL 60515; (312) 243-6800; **BDCERT:** IM 68; Cv 79; **MS:** Univ IL Coll Med 60; **RES:** IM, Rush Presbyterian-St Luke's Med Ctr, Chicago, IL 61-64; **FEL:** Cv, Rush Presbyterian-St Luke's Med Ctr, Chicago, IL 66-68; **HMO:** +
LANG: Sp; Mcr Mcd A Few Days
VISA

Doud, Debra (MD) Cv
Edward Hosp (see page 272)
Midwest Heart Specialists, 120 Spaulding Dr.; Naperville, IL 60540; (630) 527-2730; **BDCERT:** IM 89; Cv 91; **MS:** U Rochester 86; **RES:** IM, Loyola U Med Ctr, Maywood, IL 87-89; **FEL:** Cv, Loyola U Med Ctr, Maywood, IL 89-92

Duerinck, Mark (MD) Cv
Edward Hosp (see page 272)
Cardiovascular Consultants, 100 Spalding Dr Ste 212; Naperville, IL 60540; (630) 357-4111; **BDCERT:** Cv 89; IM 86; **MS:** Univ IL Coll Med 83; **RES:** IM, U IL Med Ctr, Chicago, IL 86-87; IM, U IL Med Ctr, Chicago, IL 83-86; **FEL:** Cv, U Chicago Hosp, Chicago, IL 87-90

Finley, Robert (MD) Cv
Hinsdale Hosp (see page 275)
Suburban Cardiologists, 333 Chestnut St Ste 101; Hinsdale, IL 60521; (630) 325-9010; **BDCERT:** Cv 79; **MS:** Loyola U-Stritch Sch Med, Maywood 76; **HOSP:** Palos Comm Hosp; **HMO:** Rush Prudential
Mcr VISA

Freier, Paul (MD) Cv
Hinsdale Hosp (see page 275)
West Suburban Cardiologists Ltd., 908 N Elm Street Suite 202; Hinsdale, IL 60521; (630) 789-3422; **BDCERT:** IM 83; Cv 85; **MS:** U Chicago-Pritzker Sch Med 80; **RES:** IM, Emory U Hosp, Atlanta, GA 80-83; **FEL:** Cv, U Chicago Hosp, Chicago, IL 83-85; **FAP:** Clinical Asst. Cv U Chicago-Pritzker Sch Med; **HOSP:** La Grange Mem Hosp; ***SI:*** *Non-Invasive Cardiology*
Mcr A Few Days

Giardina, John Joseph (MD) Cv
Central DuPage Hosp
Glen Ellyn Clinic, 25 N Winfield Rd; Winfield, IL 60190; (630) 933-8100; **BDCERT:** Cv 87; IM 85; **MS:** U Hlth Sci/Chicago Med Sch 82; **RES:** IM, U IL Med Ctr, Chicago, IL 83-85; **FEL:** Cv, Loyola U Med Ctr, Maywood, IL 85-87

Hartmann, Joseph (MD) Cv
Good Samaritan Hosp (see page 274)
Midwest Heart Specialist, 3825 Highland Ave Ste 400; Downers Grove, IL 60515; (630) 719-4799; **BDCERT:** Cv 81; IM 76; **MS:** Loyola U-Stritch Sch Med, Maywood 72; **RES:** Loyola U Med Ctr, Maywood, IL 72-74; **FEL:** Cv, Loyola U Med Ctr, Maywood, IL 74-76; **FAP:** Assoc Prof Med Loyola U-Stritch Sch Med, Maywood

Hines, Jerome (MD) Cv
Hinsdale Hosp (see page 275)
West Suburban Cardiologists, 908 N Elm St Ste 202; Hinsdale, IL 60521; (630) 789-3422; **BDCERT:** Cv 87; IM 86; **MS:** Northwestern U 82; **RES:** Northwestern Mem Hosp, Chicago, IL 84-85; **FEL:** Cv, Loyola U Med Ctr, Maywood, IL 85; **FAP:** Asst Prof Loyola U-Stritch Sch Med, Maywood

Kumar, Vijay P (MD) Cv
Glen Oaks Hosp and Med Ctr
(see page 273)
Midwest Cardiac Ctr, 2340 S Highland Ave Ste 160; Lombard, IL 60148; (630) 792-0900; **BDCERT:** Cv 89; IM 83; **MS:** India 74; **RES:** Anes, U IL Med Ctr, Chicago, IL 77-79; IM, VA Hosp Hines/Macneal Hosp, Berwyn, IL 79-82; **FEL:** Cv, Cook Cty Hosp, Chicago, IL 82-84

Malhotra, Rabindra (MD) Cv
Holy Cross Hosp
Midwest Cardiac Consultants, 4121 Fairview Ave Ste 103; Downers Grove, IL 60515; (630) 852-0230; **BDCERT:** IM 78; Cv 81; **MS:** India 71; **RES:** IM, LLRM Med Col, Meerut, India 73-74; IM, Louis A Weiss Mem Hosp, Chicago, IL 75-76; **FEL:** Cv, Michael Reese Hosp Med Ctr, Chicago, IL 78-80; **FAP:** Asst Clin Prof Med Univ IL Coll Med; **HOSP:** Good Samaritan Hosp; ***SI:*** *Interventional Cardiology; Chest Pain - Palpitations*; **HMO:** CIGNA, Aetna Hlth Plan, United Healthcare, Humana Health Plan +
LANG: Hin; Mcr Immediately
VISA

McKeever, Louis (MD) Cv
Elmhurst Mem Hosp
Midwest Heart Specialist, 386 N York; Elmhurst, IL 60126; (630) 782-4050; **BDCERT:** Cv 81; IM 76; **MS:** Loyola U-Stritch Sch Med, Maywood 73; **RES:** IM, Loyola U Med Ctr, Maywood, IL 75-76; **HOSP:** Loyola U Med Ctr

Rauh, R Andrew (MD) Cv
Central DuPage Hosp
Midwest Heart Specialist, 3825 Highland Ave Ste 400; Downers Grove, IL 60515; (630) 719-4799; **BDCERT:** Cv 91; IM 88; **MS:** Loyola U-Stritch Sch Med, Maywood 84; **RES:** Ped, Loyola U Med Ctr, Maywood, IL 84-88; **FEL:** Cv, U Wisc Hosp, Madison, WI 88-91; **FAP:** Asst Prof Loyola U-Stritch Sch Med, Maywood; ***SI:** Congestive Heart Failure*; **HMO:** Blue Cross, CIGNA, United Healthcare +

VISA

Rowley, Stephen (MD) Cv
Good Samaritan Hosp **(see page 274)**
Midwest Heart Specialist, 3825 Highland Ave Ste 400; Downers Grove, IL 60515; (630) 719-4799; **BDCERT:** Cv 89; Ger 94; **MS:** SUNY Syracuse 82; **FEL:** Cv, Loyola U Med Ctr, Maywood, IL 86-89; **FAP:** Assoc Clin Prof Loyola U-Stritch Sch Med, Maywood; **HMO:** Aetna Hlth Plan, Blue Cross & Blue Shield, CIGNA, Metlife, Travelers

CHILD & ADOLESCENT PSYCHIATRY

Belizario, Evangelina (MD) ChAP
Hinsdale Hosp **(see page 275)**
Salt Creek Therapy Ctr, 7 Salt Creek Ln Ste 206; Hinsdale, IL 60521; (630) 850-2120; **BDCERT:** Psyc 81; **MS:** Philippines 72; **RES:** Psyc, EJ Meyer Mem Hosp, Buffalo, NY 74-75; Psyc, Univ of Illinois at Chicago Psychiatric Institute, Chicago, IL 75-77; **FEL:** Univ of Illinois at Chicago Psychiatric Institute, Chicago, IL 77-78; ChAP, Children's Mem Med Ctr, Chicago, IL 84-86; **HMO:** Blue Cross & Blue Shield, HealthNet, Health Options

DERMATOLOGY

Andrews, Thomas (MD) D
Hinsdale Hosp **(see page 275)**
Dermatology Associates, 333 Chestnut Ste 202; Hinsdale, IL 60521; (630) 325-6880; **BDCERT:** D 70; **MS:** U Chicago-Pritzker Sch Med 63; **RES:** Chicago Hosp, Chicago, IL 66-69; **FAP:** Asst Prof D Northwestern U

Ariano, Moira (MD) D
Central DuPage Hosp
7 Blanchard Cir Ste 203; Wheaton, IL 60187; (630) 462-8680; **BDCERT:** D 86; **MS:** Univ IL Coll Med 81; **RES:** D, U IL Med Ctr, Chicago, IL 82-83; **FAP:** Asst Clin Prof Univ IL Coll Med

Davis, James (MD) D
Edward Hosp **(see page 272)**
120 Spalding Dr Ste 307; Naperville, IL 60540; (630) 355-1102; **BDCERT:** D 79; **MS:** Univ IL Coll Med 75; **RES:** Derm, U IL Med Ctr, Chicago, IL 76-79; ***SI:** Acne; Dermatitis*; **HMO:** Blue Cross & Blue Shield, PHCS, Medicare

A Few Days

Ertle, James O (MD) D
Hinsdale Hosp **(see page 275)**
Dermatology Associates, 333 Chestnut St Ste 202; Hinsdale, IL 60521; (630) 325-6880; **BDCERT:** D 73; **MS:** Switzerland 67

Kolbusz, Robert (MD) D
Good Samaritan Hosp **(see page 274)**
Center For Dermatology & Skin Cancer, 3825 Highland Ave Ste 5C; Downers Grove, IL 60515; (630) 964-2000; **BDCERT:** D 93; **MS:** Loyola U-Stritch Sch Med, Maywood 83; **RES:** Path, Loyola U Med Ctr, Maywood, IL 83-87; D, Rush Presbyterian-St Luke's Med Ctr, Chicago, IL 88-92; **FEL:** D, U Chicago Hosp, Chicago, IL 87-88; Moh's Surg, Baylor Coll Med, Houston, TX 92-93; ***SI:** Skin Cancer; Wrinkle Removal*; **HMO:** Blue Cross & Blue Shield, Aetna Hlth Plan, Humana Health Plan, United Healthcare +

A Few Days
VISA

O'Donoghue, Marianne Nelson (MD) D
West Suburban Hosp Med Ctr
120 Oakbrook Ctr Ste 410; Oak Brook, IL 60523; (630) 574-5860; **BDCERT:** D 70; **MS:** Georgetown U 65; **RES:** D, Cincinnati Gen Hosp, Cincinnati, OH 68-69; U Chicago Hosp, Chicago, IL 66-68; **FAP:** Assoc Prof D Rush Med Coll; **HOSP:** Rush-Presbyterian-St Luke's Med Ctr; ***SI:** Acne; Cosmetics*; **HMO:** Blue Cross & Blue Shield, HealthNet, Choicecare, Travelers, Metropolitan

4+ Weeks

DIAGNOSTIC RADIOLOGY

Baker, Dennis (MD) **DR**
Central DuPage Hosp
Central Du Page Hospital-Diagnostic Radiology, 25 N Winfield Rd; Winfield, IL 60190; (630) 682-1600; **BDCERT:** DR 72; **MS:** Loyola U-Stritch Sch Med, Maywood 67; **RES:** DR, Loyola U Med Ctr, Maywood, IL 71-74

Mategrano, Victor (MD) **DR**
Hinsdale Hosp **(see page 275)**
Du Page Radiologist Group, 120 N Oak St; Hinsdale, IL 60521; (630) 856-7400; **BDCERT:** DR 76; **MS:** Univ IL Coll Med 72; **RES:** DR, Rush Presbyterian-St Lukes, Chicago, IL 73-76; **FEL:** Rush Presbyterian-St Lukes, Chicago, IL 76-77; Rush Presbyterian-St Lukes, Chicago, IL 84; **HOSP:** Good Samaritan Hosp; ***SI:*** *CT Scans; MRI*
1 Week VISA

Sullivan, Daniel J (MD) **DR**
Ravenswood Hosp Med Ctr
Midwest Heart Specialists, 2487 W Branch Ct; Naperville, IL 60565; (630) 527-2730; **BDCERT:** NuM 92; DR 92; **MS:** Creighton U 87; **RES:** DR, Illinois Masonic Med Ctr, Chicago, IL 88-91; NuM, Illinois Masonic Med Ctr, Chicago, IL 91-92; **FAP:** Asst Clin Prof Univ IL Coll Med

Wayne, Ralph W. (MD) **DR**
Good Samaritan Hosp **(see page 274)**
3815 Highland Ave; Downers Grove, IL 60521; (630) 275-1154; **BDCERT:** DR 73; **MS:** U Colo Sch Med 66; **RES:** RadRO, Rush Presbyterian-St Luke's Med Ctr, Chicago, IL 69-72

ENDOCRINOLOGY, DIABETES & METABOLISM

Agnoli, Francis (MD) **EDM**
Hinsdale Hosp **(see page 275)**
Mid America Health Partners, 908 N Elm St Ste 301; Hinsdale, IL 60521; (630) 323-3540; **BDCERT:** EDM 73; IM 72; **MS:** U Puerto Rico 65; **RES:** IM, Michael Reese Hosp Med Ctr, Chicago, IL 66-68; **FEL:** EDM, Northwestern Mem Hosp, Chicago, IL 68-70; **HMO:** +
1 Week VISA

Bayer, William (MD) **EDM**
Central DuPage Hosp
Du Page Internal Medicine Ltd, 517 Thornhill Dr; Carol Stream, IL 60188; (630) 668-3210; **BDCERT:** EDM 93; IM 89; **MS:** Loyola U-Stritch Sch Med, Maywood 86; **RES:** IM, Loyola U Med Ctr, Maywood, IL 86-89; **FEL:** Ge, Loyola U Med Ctr, Maywood, IL 89-91; **HMO:** Blue Cross & Blue Shield, Humana Health Plan

Lebbin, Dennis (MD) **EDM**
Hinsdale Hosp **(see page 275)**
333 Chestnut St Rm104; Hinsdale, IL 60521; (630) 323-3191; **BDCERT:** EDM 81; IM 72; **MS:** Duke U 68; **RES:** IM, Rush Presbyterian-St Luke's Med Ctr, Chicago, IL 69-71; **FEL:** EDM, Rush Presbyterian-St Luke's Med Ctr, Chicago, IL 71-73; **HMO:** Aetna Hlth Plan, Blue Cross & Blue Shield, Private Healthcare

Stoller, Walter A (MD) **EDM**
Elmhurst Mem Hosp
242 N York St Ste 208; Elmhurst, IL 60126; (630) 834-4060; **BDCERT:** EDM 83; IM 81; **MS:** U Chicago-Pritzker Sch Med 78; **RES:** IM, Med Coll VA Hosp, Richmond, VA 79-81; **FEL:** EDM, U Mass Med Ctr, Worcester, MA 81-83; **HOSP:** Westlake Comm Hosp

Thein-Wai, Winston (MD) **EDM**
Good Samaritan Hosp **(see page 274)**
3825 Highland Ave Ste 4M; Downers Grove, IL 60515; (630) 960-9693; **BDCERT:** IM 76; **MS:** Burma 70; **RES:** IM, Michael Reese Hosp Med Ctr, Chicago, IL 73-75; **FEL:** EDM, Peter Bent Brigham Hosp, Boston, MA 75-77; **HMO:** Aetna Hlth Plan, Blue Cross & Blue Shield, CIGNA, Prudential

FAMILY PRACTICE

Balodis, Anita (MD) **FP**
PCP
Elmhurst Mem Hosp
103 Haven Rd; Elmhurst, IL 60126; (630) 833-0280; **BDCERT:** FP 96; **MS:** Albany Med Coll 70; **RES:** IM, Northwestern Mem Hosp, Chicago, IL 71-72

Bednar, Patrick (MD) **FP**
PCP
Central DuPage Hosp
Johnson & Bednar, 150 Winfield Rd; Winfield, IL 60190; (630) 665-1550; **BDCERT:** FP 93; **MS:** Rush Med Coll 76

Fortman, Lisa (MD) **FP**
PCP
Hinsdale Hosp **(see page 275)**
Family Practice Assoc, 911 N Elm St Ste 301; Hinsdale, IL 60521; (630) 986-1420; **BDCERT:** FP 92; **MS:** Univ IL Coll Med 89; **RES:** FP, Hinsdale Hosp, Hinsdale, IL 89-92; **HMO:** Aetna Hlth Plan, Blue Cross & Blue Shield, Californiacare +
VISA

Frigo, Judith (MD) **FP**
PCP
Hinsdale Hosp **(see page 275)**
Family Health Care of Hinsdale, 908 N Elm St Ste 207; Hinsdale, IL 60521; (630) 323-1558; **BDCERT:** FP 87; **MS:** Loyola U-Stritch Sch Med, Maywood 84; **RES:** FP, Hinsdale Hosp, Hinsdale, IL 84-87

Guide to symbols and abbreviations can be found on pages 110-113.

Hubbard, Robert (MD) FP
PCP
Edward Hosp (see page 272)
Edward Health Ventures, 720 Brom Ct Ste 203; Naperville, IL 60540; (630) 357-7979; **BDCERT:** FP 84; **MS:** Med Coll Wisc 81; **RES:** FP, Waukesha Mem Hosp, Waukesha, WI; ***SI:*** *Orthopedics; Obstetrics-Gynecology*; **HMO:** +
1 Week VISA

Johnson, Robert (MD) FP
PCP
Glen Oaks Hosp and Med Ctr (see page 273)
501 Thorn Hill Ste 110; Carol Stream, IL 60188; (630) 820-6980; **BDCERT:** FP 94; **MS:** Univ IL Coll Med 78; ***SI:*** *Geriatrics*

Lis, Linda (MD) FP
PCP
Hinsdale Hosp (see page 275)
Burr Ridge Family Practice, 7630 S County Line Rd; Burr Ridge, IL 60521; (630) 655-1177; **BDCERT:** FP 97; **MS:** Georgetown U 88; **RES:** Long Beach Mem Med Ctr, Long Beach, CA 90-91; **FEL:** SM, Macneal Mem Hosp, Berwyn, IL 91-92

Morris, Thomas (DO) FP
PCP
Hinsdale Hosp (see page 275)
Burr Ridge Family Practice, 7630 S County Line Rd; Burr Ridge, IL 60521; (630) 655-1177; **BDCERT:** FP 92; **MS:** Chicago Coll Osteo Med 89

Neumann, Charles (DO) FP
PCP
Good Samaritan Hosp (see page 274)
Adventist Health Partners, 6224 Main St; Downers Grove, IL 60516; (630) 963-1400; **BDCERT:** FP 89; **MS:** Chicago Coll Osteo Med 75; **RES:** Chicago Osteopathic Med Ctr, Chicago, IL 75-76; **HOSP:** Hinsdale Hosp; ***SI:*** *Aviation Medicine*; **HMO:** Blue Cross & Blue Shield, CIGNA, Choicecare
A Few Days

Siebert, Joseph (MD) FP
PCP
Good Samaritan Hosp (see page 274)
Downers Grove Family Practice, 4900 Main St; Downers Grove, IL 60515; (630) 963-5440; **BDCERT:** FP 78; **MS:** Univ IL Coll Med 75; **HMO:** Aetna Hlth Plan, Blue Cross & Blue Shield, Californiacare, Travelers

GASTROENTEROLOGY

Berger, Scott (MD) Ge
Edward Hosp (see page 272)
Suburban Gastroenterology, 640 S Washington St; Naperville, IL 60540; (630) 527-6450; **BDCERT:** Ge 91; IM 87; **MS:** Mt Sinai Sch Med 84; **RES:** IM, U MD Hosp, Baltimore, MD 84-87; **FEL:** Ge, Loyola U Med Ctr, Maywood, IL 88-90; **HMO:** +

Bregman, Andrew (MD) Ge
Central DuPage Hosp
Gastroenterolgy, 100 Spalding; Naperville, IL 60540; (630) 377-6229; **BDCERT:** IM 74; Ge 79; **MS:** Northwestern U 71; **RES:** Rush Presbyterian-St Luke's Med Ctr, Chicago, IL 72-74; **FEL:** Ge, Rush Presbyterian-St Luke's Med Ctr, Chicago, IL 74; **HOSP:** Edward Hosp

Chua, David (MD) Ge
St Mary's of Nazareth Hosp Ctr
1710 Midwest Club Pkwy; Oak Brook, IL 60523; (630) 889-9889; **BDCERT:** Ge 89; IM 87; **MS:** Philippines 80; **RES:** Ge, Rush Presbyterian-St Luke's Med Ctr, Chicago, IL 87-90; **HOSP:** Hinsdale Hosp; ***SI:*** *Hepatitis; Peptic Ulcers*; **HMO:** Blue Cross & Blue Shield, HealthStar, HealthNet, Preferred Plan +

Gerard, David (MD) Ge
Hinsdale Hosp (see page 275)
Gastroenterology Services Ltd, 3825 Highland Ave Ste 203; Downers Grove, IL 60515; (630) 969-1167; **BDCERT:** IM 90; Ge 93; **MS:** U Chicago-Pritzker Sch Med 87; **RES:** IM, Johns Hopkins Hosp, Baltimore, MD 87-90; **FEL:** Ge, Yale-New Haven Hosp, New Haven, CT 90-93; **FAP:** Asst Clin Prof Med U Chicago-Pritzker Sch Med; **HOSP:** Good Samaritan Hosp; ***SI:*** *Hepatitis*; **HMO:** United Healthcare, CIGNA, Prudential, Bc/BS +
LANG: Sp, Ger, Rom;
1 Week VISA

Grill, Stephen (MD) Ge
Elmhurst Mem Hosp
Midwest Digestive Disease Spec, 3825 Highland Ave Ste 307; Downers Grove, IL 60515; (630) 852-1009; **BDCERT:** IM 83; Ge 87; **MS:** Loyola U-Stritch Sch Med, Maywood 77; **FEL:** Ge, Loyola U Med Ctr, Maywood, IL 80-82; IM, Loyola U Med Ctr, Maywood, IL 78-80; **FAP:** Assoc Prof Med Loyola U-Stritch Sch Med, Maywood; **HOSP:** Good Samaritan Hosp; **HMO:** +
1 Week VISA

Holden, John (MD) Ge
La Grange Mem Hosp (see page 141)
Digestive Disease Assoc Ltd, 950 N York Rd Ste 101; Hinsdale, IL 60521; (630) 325-4255; **BDCERT:** IM 78; Ge 81; **MS:** Loyola U-Stritch Sch Med, Maywood 75; **RES:** IM, Hines VA Hosp, Hines, IL 75-78; **FEL:** Ge, Hines VA Hosp, Hines, IL 78-80; **HOSP:** Hinsdale Hosp

Issleib, Stuart (MD) **Ge**
Mercy Hosp & Med Ctr
720 W North St; Hinsdale, IL 60521; (312) 567-5653; **BDCERT:** IM 88; Ge 90; **MS:** Loyola U-Stritch Sch Med, Maywood 85; **RES:** IM, Mercy Hosp & Med Ctr, Chicago, IL 85-88; **FEL:** Ge, U Chicago Hosp, Chicago, IL 88-90; ***SI:*** *Colon Polyps; Colon Cancer*; **HMO:** Aetna Hlth Plan, Blue Cross & Blue Shield, HMO Illinois, Private Healthcare +
A Few Days

Jain, Dinesh (MD) **Ge**
Edward Hosp **(see page 272)**
Suburban Gastroenterology, 640 S Washington St Ste 240; Naperville, IL 60540; (630) 527-6450; **BDCERT:** Ge 85; IM 81; **MS:** India 82; **RES:** Cabrini Med Ctr, New York, NY; **FEL:** U, U Chicago Hosp, Chicago, IL 82-84; **HOSP:** Good Samaritan Hosp
1 Week VISA

Mc Kenna, Michael E (MD) **Ge**
Good Samaritan Hosp **(see page 274)**
Midwest Digestive Disease Spec, 360 W Butterfield Rd Ste 280; Elmhurst, IL 60126; (630) 833-0653; **BDCERT:** IM 81; Ge 83; **MS:** Loyola U-Stritch Sch Med, Maywood 77; **RES:** IM, Loyola U Med Ctr, Maywood, IL 78-80; **FEL:** Ge, Loyola U Med Ctr, Maywood, IL 80-82; **HOSP:** Elmhurst Mem Hosp; ***SI:*** *Colon Cancer Screening; Treatment of Ulcers*; **HMO:** Aetna Hlth Plan, United Healthcare, Healthamerica, CIGNA, Blue Cross & Blue Shield +
2-4 Weeks VISA

Morgan, George (MD) **Ge**
Elmhurst Mem Hosp
Midwest Digestive Disease Spec, 360 W Butterfield Rd Ste 280; Elmhurst, IL 60126; (630) 833-0653; **BDCERT:** IM 87; Ge 91; **MS:** Univ IL Coll Med 84; **RES:** IM, Loyola U Med Ctr, Maywood, IL 86-87; **FEL:** Ge, Loyola U Med Ctr, Maywood, IL 88-90; **HOSP:** Good Samaritan Hosp; ***SI:*** *Ulcer Treatment; Colon Cancer Screening*; **HMO:** Blue Cross & Blue Shield, Humana Health Plan, United Healthcare, Aetna Hlth Plan +
2-4 Weeks VISA

Sublette, Gerard (MD) **Ge**
Gottlieb Mem Hosp
Associates-Digestive Diseases, 2340 S Highland Ave Ste 120; Lombard, IL 60148; (630) 261-7530; **BDCERT:** Ge 83; IM 81; **MS:** Univ IL Coll Med 78; **RES:** IM, Lutheran Gen Hosp, Park Ridge, IL 78-81; **FEL:** Ge, Hines VA Hosp, Chicago, IL 81-83

Sweeney, Philip (MD) **Ge**
Hinsdale Hosp **(see page 275)**
Digestive Disease, 950 N York Rd Ste 101; Hinsdale, IL 60521; (630) 325-4255; **BDCERT:** IM 83; Ge 87; **MS:** Univ IL Coll Med 80; **RES:** IM, Loyola U Med Ctr, Maywood, IL 81-83; **FEL:** Ge, Loyola U Med Ctr, Maywood, IL 84-86

Yapp, Rockford (MD) **Ge**
Good Samaritan Hosp **(see page 274)**
3825 Highland Ave; Downers Grove, IL 60515; (630) 434-9312; **BDCERT:** IM 87; Ge 93; **MS:** Univ Nebr Coll Med 84; **RES:** IM, Northwestern Mem Hosp, Chicago, IL; **FEL:** Ge, Yale-New Haven Hosp, New Haven, CT; **HOSP:** Hinsdale Hosp

GERIATRIC PSYCHIATRY

Wiener, Pauline K (MD) **GerPsy**
Central DuPage Hosp
Central Du Page Hosp, 25 N Winfield Rd; Winfield, IL 60190; (630) 682-2746; **BDCERT:** Psyc 93; GerPsy 95; **MS:** Rush Med Coll 88; **RES:** Psyc, St Vincents Hosp Med Ctr, New York, NY 89-92; **FEL:** GerPsy, NY Hosp-Cornell Med Ctr, White Plains, NY 92-94

HAND SURGERY

Thomas, Richard (MD) **HS**
Central DuPage Hosp
Hand Care Assoc, 511 Thornhill Dr L; Carol Stream, IL 60188; (630) 653-7880; **BDCERT:** OrS 93; HS 94; **MS:** Ind U Sch Med 84; **RES:** U MO Kansas City Sch Med, Kansas City, MO 86-90; **FEL:** Christine Kleinert Inst Hand & Microsurgery, Louisville, KY 90-91

INFECTIOUS DISEASE

Augustinsky, James (MD) **Inf**
Central DuPage Hosp
363 Raymond Dr Ste 200; Naperville, IL 60563; (630) 548-4811; **BDCERT:** Inf 90; IM 88; **MS:** U Chicago-Pritzker Sch Med 85; **HOSP:** Edward Hosp

Dumitru, Rodica (MD) **Inf**
La Grange Mem Hosp **(see page 141)**
Metro-Infectious Disease, 1 Salt Creek Ln Ste 105; Hinsdale, IL 60521; (630) 654-4201; **BDCERT:** IM 88; Inf 90; **MS:** Romania 79; **RES:** IM, Christ Hosp & Med Ctr, Oak Lawn, IL 84-87; **FEL:** Inf, Loyola U Med Ctr, Maywood, IL 87-89

Guide to symbols and abbreviations can be found on pages 110-113.

Manam, Bob (MD) Inf
Rush-Copley Med Ctr
Fox Valley Medical Assoc, 2020 Ogdon Ave. Ste 140; Auroa, IL 60505; (630) 851-1144; **BDCERT:** IM 90; Inf 92; **MS:** India 87

Sherman, Edward (MD) Inf
Hinsdale Hosp (see page 275)
120 N Oak St; Hinsdale, IL 60521; (630) 856-4518; **BDCERT:** IM 85; Inf 88; **MS:** U Hlth Sci/Chicago Med Sch 80; **RES:** IM, Illinois Masonic Med Ctr, Chicago, IL 83-85; **FEL:** Inf, Mount Sinai Med Ctr, New York, NY 86-88; **HOSP:** Good Samaritan Hosp; ***SI:*** *Infectious Disease Problems; Obesity*
A Few Days VISA

Waitley, David (MD) Inf
Good Samaritan Hosp (see page 274)
Metro-Infectious Disease, 1 Salt Creek Ln Ste 105; Hinsdale, IL 60521; (630) 654-4201; **BDCERT:** Inf 90; IM 87; **MS:** U Hlth Sci/Chicago Med Sch 84; **RES:** IM, Loyola U Med Ctr, Maywood, IL 84-87; **FEL:** Inf, Loyola U Med Ctr, Maywood, IL 87-89; **HOSP:** Hinsdale Hosp; ***SI:*** *Wound Care; Travel Medicine*; **HMO:** +
LANG: Sp; Immediately

INTERNAL MEDICINE

Allen, James E (MD & PhD) IM
PCP
Hinsdale Hosp (see page 275)
1 Salt Creek Lane Ste 105; Hinsdale, IL 60521; (630) 654-4201; **BDCERT:** IM 89; Inf 90; **MS:** U Miami Sch Med 73; **RES:** IM, Loyola U Med Ctr, Maywood, IL 73-76; **FEL:** Inf, U CO Hosp, Denver, CO 76-78; **FAP:** Asst Clin Prof Loyola U-Stritch Sch Med, Maywood; **HOSP:** Elmhurst Mem Hosp; ***SI:*** *Infectious Disease*; **HMO:** +
1 Week VISA

Arain, Azizur (MD) IM
PCP
Hinsdale Hosp (see page 275)
4121 Fairview Ave Ste 103; Downers Grove, IL 60515; (630) 971-3323; **BDCERT:** IM 72; Hem 74; **MS:** Pakistan 66; **RES:** IM, Cook Cty Hosp, Chicago, IL 69-72; **FEL:** Hem, Cook Cty Hosp, Chicago, IL 73-74; ***SI:*** *Hematology*
1 Week

Carbone, Robert (MD) IM
PCP
Hinsdale Hosp (see page 275)
Mid America Health Partners, 908 N Elm St Ste 301; Hinsdale, IL 60521; (630) 323-3540; **BDCERT:** IM 79; **MS:** Loyola U-Stritch Sch Med, Maywood 76; **RES:** IM, Northwestern Mem Hosp, Chicago, IL 76-79; **HOSP:** Good Samaritan Hosp; **HMO:** HMO Illinois, Blue Cross & Blue Shield, United Healthcare, Aetna PPO, HMO +
1 Week VISA

Collins, James J (MD) IM
PCP
Edward Hosp (see page 272)
10 Martin Ave Ste 111; Naperville, IL 60540; (630) 355-6200; **BDCERT:** IM 83; **MS:** Rush Med Coll 79; **RES:** IM, Rush Presbyterian-St Luke's Med Ctr, Chicago, IL 80-82

Dunphy, James V (MD) IM
PCP
Edward Hosp (see page 272)
10 W Martin Ave Ste 111; Naperville, IL 60540; (630) 369-2600; **BDCERT:** IM 69; **MS:** Loyola U-Stritch Sch Med, Maywood 58; **RES:** Hines VA Hosp, Chicago, IL 61-63; Cook Cty Hosp, Chicago, IL 59-60; **FEL:** Cook Cty Hosp, Chicago, IL 58-59; ***SI:*** *Hypertension; Sinusitis*; **HMO:** CIGNA
A Few Days VISA

Fearon, Maureen (MD) IM
PCP
Loyola U Med Ctr (see page 120)
Loyola University Medical Ctr, 17 W 740 22nd St; Oak Brook Terrace, IL 60181; (630) 627-7399; **BDCERT:** IM 90; **MS:** Loyola U-Stritch Sch Med, Maywood 87; **RES:** IM, Loyola U Med Ctr, Maywood, IL 87-90; **FEL:** IM, Loyola U Med Ctr, Maywood, IL 90-91; **FAP:** Asst Prof Med Loyola U-Stritch Sch Med, Maywood; **HMO:** Aetna Hlth Plan, Blue Cross & Blue Shield, Chicago HMO, Choicecare, Prudential

Gallagher, Thomas J (MD) IM
PCP
Hinsdale Hosp (see page 275)
Mid America Health Partners, 908 N Elm St Ste 301; Hinsdale, IL 60521; (630) 323-3540; **BDCERT:** IM 81; **MS:** Med Coll Wisc 78; **HOSP:** Good Samaritan Hosp

Klickman, Howard (MD) IM
PCP
Good Samaritan Hosp (see page 274)
Du Page Internists Ltd, 6800 Main St Ste 201; Downers Grove, IL 60516; (630) 434-9700; **BDCERT:** IM 89; Ger 94; **MS:** Loyola U-Stritch Sch Med, Maywood 86; **RES:** IM, Loyola U Med Ctr, Maywood, IL 86-89; ***SI:*** *Geriatrics; Diabetes*; **HMO:** CIGNA, Prucare
A Few Days VISA

Kolbaba, Scott (MD) IM
PCP
Central DuPage Hosp
West Suburban Internist's Ltd, 7 Blanchard Cir Ste 206; Wheaton, IL 60187; (630) 653-0848; **BDCERT:** IM 80; **MS:** Univ IL Coll Med 77; **RES:** IM, Rush-Presy-St Lukes, Chicago, IL 77-78; IM, Mayo Clinic, Rochester, MN 78-80

Krouse, Richard (MD) IM
PCP
Elmhurst Mem Hosp
North Pavillions, 3743 Highland Ave Ste 1001; Downers Grove, IL 60515; (630) 435-9888; **BDCERT:** IM 86; **MS:** Creighton U 83; **RES:** UC Irvine Med Ctr, Irvine, CA 84-86; **HOSP:** Good Samaritan Hosp

Kulczycki, Ted (MD) IM
PCP
Rush-Copley Med Ctr
1315 N Highland Ave Ste 201; Aurora, IL 60504; (630) 264-8000; **BDCERT:** IM 93; **MS:** Wayne State U Sch Med 90; **RES:** IM, Rush Presbyterian-St Luke's Med Ctr, Chicago, IL 90-93; **HOSP:** Provena Mercy Ctr; ***SI:*** *Heart Disease; Osteoporosis*; **HMO:** Blue Cross & Blue Shield, United Healthcare, CIGNA, Rush Prudential, Aetna Hlth Plan +
LANG: Pol; A Few Days

Loeb, Barbara (MD) IM
PCP
Good Samaritan Hosp (see page 274)
3825 Highland Ave Ste 20; Downers Grove, IL 60515; (630) 963-9667; **BDCERT:** IM 83; Ger 90; **MS:** Rush Med Coll 80; **RES:** Loyola U Med Ctr, Maywood, IL 80-83

Nighswander, J Richard (MD) IM
Hinsdale Hosp (see page 275)
Mid America Health Partners, 908 N Elm St Ste 301; Hinsdale, IL 60521; (630) 323-3540; **BDCERT:** IM 67; **MS:** Univ IL Coll Med 61; **RES:** IM, Milwaukee City Hospital, Milwaukee, WS 64-67

O'Leary, Brian (MD) IM
PCP
Edward Hosp (see page 272)
Midwest Internists Inc, 1020 E Ogden Ave Ste 304; Naperville, IL 60563; (630) 717-8707; **BDCERT:** IM 88; **MS:** Northwestern U 85; **RES:** IM, Northwestern Mem Hosp, Chicago, IL 85-88; **FEL:** IM, Northwestern Mem Hosp, Chicago, IL 88-89; **HOSP:** Good Samaritan Hosp
NFI

Sastri, Suriya (MD) IM
Hinsdale Hosp (see page 275)
Midwest Center, 6900 S Madison St Ste 103; Hinsdale, IL 60521; (630) 325-8684; **BDCERT:** IM 86; Ge 91; **MS:** India 78; **RES:** IM, Cook Cty Hosp, Chicago, IL 83-85; **FEL:** Ge, U MO Kansas City Sch Med, Kansas City, MO 86-88

Zimmerman, Richard (MD) IM
PCP
Good Samaritan Hosp (see page 274)
Mid America Health Partners, 3743 Highland Ave Ste 1001; Downers Grove, IL 60515; (630) 435-9888; **BDCERT:** IM 77; **MS:** Germany 63; **RES:** IM, Illinois Masonic Med Ctr, Chicago, IL 64-67; **HMO:** Blue Cross & Blue Shield
VISA

MATERNAL & FETAL MEDICINE

Hussey, Michael (MD) MF
Rush-Presbyterian-St Luke's Med Ctr (see page 122)
Central Du Page Ctr-Womens Hlth, 397 S Schmale Rd; Carol Stream, IL 60188; (630) 221-9663; **BDCERT:** ObG 94; MF 98; **MS:** Univ IL Coll Med 86; **RES:** ObG, Loyola U Med Ctr, Maywood, IL 91-93; **FEL:** MF, Rush Presbyterian-St Luke's Med Ctr, Chicago, IL 93; **FAP:** Asst Prof Rush Med Coll; **HOSP:** Provena Mercy Ctr

MEDICAL GENETICS

Lebel, Robert (MD) MG
Hinsdale Hosp (see page 275)
Genetic Services, 346 Taft Avenue Rd Ste 100; Glen Ellyn, IL 60137; (630) 832-4363; **BDCERT:** CG 90; **MS:** U Wisc Med Sch 82; **RES:** IM, Mt Sinai Med Ctr, Milwaukee, WI 83-85; **FEL:** MG, Mt Sinai Med Ctr, Milwaukee, WI 85-87; **FAP:** Clin Prof Rush Med Coll; **HOSP:** Edward Hosp; ***SI:*** *Genetic Prenatal Diagnosis; Genetic Adult Diagnosis*
VISA

MEDICAL ONCOLOGY

Azuma, Dennis (MD) Onc
Edward Hosp (see page 272)
Hematology-Oncology Consultant, 6800 Main St Ste 102; Downers Grove, IL 60515; (630) 663-1667; **BDCERT:** Onc 88; Hem 87; **MS:** Loyola U-Stritch Sch Med, Maywood 80; **RES:** IM, Nat Naval Med Ctr, Bethesda, MD 82-84; **FEL:** HO, Nat Naval Med Ctr, Bethesda, MD 84; **HOSP:** Good Samaritan Hosp; ***SI:*** *Hematology-Oncology; Breast Cancer*; **HMO:** +
1 Week

Barhamand, Fariborze B (MD) Onc
Edward Hosp (see page 272)
Hematology-Oncology Consultant, 6800 Main St Ste 102; Downers Grove, IL 60515; (630) 663-1667; **BDCERT:** Onc 81; IM 79; **MS:** India 74; **RES:** IM, Louis A Weiss Mem Hosp, Chicago, IL 75-78; **FEL:** HO, Hines VA Hosp, Chicago, IL 78-80; **FAP:** Asst Clin Prof Loyola U-Stritch Sch Med, Maywood; **HOSP:** Good Samaritan Hosp; ***SI:*** *Hematology-Oncology*; **HMO:** +
1 Week

Brandman, James (MD) Onc
Central DuPage Hosp
Glen Ellyn Clinic, 454 Pennsylvania Ave; Glen Ellyn, IL 60137; (630) 790-4209; **BDCERT:** IM 78; Onc 81; **MS:** Boston U 75; **RES:** IM, Cleveland Clinic Hosp, Cleveland, OH 75-78; **FEL:** Onc, Albany Med Ctr, Albany, NY 79-81; **FAP:** Instr Loyola U-Stritch Sch Med, Maywood; ***SI:** Breast Cancer; Palliative Medicine*; **HMO:** Blue Cross, Humana Health Plan, Rush Prudential, CIGNA +
LANG: Fr, Sp; A Few Days

Cohen, Issac (MD) Onc
Central DuPage Hosp
245 S Gary Ave; Bloomingdale, IL 60108; (630) 539-2540; **BDCERT:** Onc 87; IM 85; **MS:** Univ IL Coll Med 81; **HOSP:** Elmhurst Mem Hosp

Evrard, Marilyn (MD) Onc
Elmhurst Mem Hosp
135 Robert T Palmer Dr Ste 200; Elmhurst, IL 60126; (630) 941-8280; **BDCERT:** IM 81; Onc 83; **MS:** Univ IL Coll Med 78; **RES:** IM, U IL Med Ctr, Chicago, IL 78-81; **FEL:** HO, U IL Med Ctr, Chicago, IL 81-84

Hantel, Alexander (MD) Onc
Edward Hosp (see page 272)
Edward Cancer Ctr, 120 Spalding Dr Ste 400; Naperville, IL 60540; (630) 527-3788; **BDCERT:** IM 84; Onc 87; **MS:** Univ IL Coll Med 81; **RES:** IM, U IL Med Ctr, Chicago, IL 81-85; **FEL:** Onc, Johns Hopkins Hosp, Baltimore, MD 85-88; **FAP:** Assoc Professor Onc Loyola U-Stritch Sch Med, Maywood; **HOSP:** Central DuPage Hosp; ***SI:** Breast Cancer; Gastrointestinal Cancer*; **HMO:** Blue Cross & Blue Shield, HealthNet, CIGNA, United Healthcare, HealthNet
LANG: Rus; A Few Days

Kozuh, Gerald (MD) Onc
Elmhurst Mem Hosp
Oncology Joint Practice, 183 N Addison Ave; Elmhurst, IL 60126; (630) 941-8032; **BDCERT:** IM 76; Hem 78; **MS:** Loyola U-Stritch Sch Med, Maywood 73; **HMO:** Aetna Hlth Plan, Blue Cross & Blue Shield, Chicago HMO, CIGNA, HealthNet

Madej, Patricia (MD) Onc
Hinsdale Hosp (see page 275)
Hinsdale Hematology Oncology, 908 N Elm St Ste 210; Hinsdale, IL 60521; (630) 654-1790; **BDCERT:** Hem 82; Onc 83; **MS:** Univ IL Coll Med 77; **RES:** IM, U Ill Hosp, Chicago, IL 78-80; **FEL:** HemOnc, Michael Reese Hosp, Chicago, IL 80; **FAP:** Asst Prof Northwestern U

Patel, Kaushik (MD) Onc
Rush-Copley Med Ctr
Copley Cancer Care Ctr, 2000 W Ogden Ave; Aurora, IL 60504; (630) 978-6252; **BDCERT:** IM 87; Onc 91; **MS:** India 82; **RES:** IM, Christ Hosp & Med Ctr, Oak Lawn, IL 84-87; **FEL:** HO, Univ of Cincinnati, Cincinnati, OH 87; **FAP:** Clin Instr Rush Med Coll

Winter, Christine (MD) Onc
Hinsdale Hosp (see page 275)
Hinsdale Hematology Oncology, 908 N Elm St Ste 210; Hinsdale, IL 60521; (630) 654-1790; **BDCERT:** Hem 80; **MS:** England 72; **RES:** IM, , Canada 74-77; **FEL:** Hem, Mayo Grad Sch Medicine, Rochester, MN 77-80; **FAP:** Asst Prof Northwestern U; **HOSP:** Good Samaritan Hosp; ***SI:** Hematology*

NEONATAL-PERINATAL MEDICINE

Bell, Anthony (MD) NP
Hinsdale Hosp (see page 275)
120 N Oak St; Hinsdale, IL 60521; (847) 991-0440; **BDCERT:** NP 95; Ped 91; **MS:** Rush Med Coll 88; **RES:** U Chicago Hosp, Chicago, IL 89-91; **FEL:** NP, U Chicago Hosp, Chicago, IL 91-94; **HOSP:** Edward Hosp

Covert, Robert (MD) NP
Good Samaritan Hosp (see page 274)
Du Page Neonatology, PO Box 487; Hinsdale, IL 60522; (847) 991-0440; **BDCERT:** NP 87; Ped 87; **MS:** U South Fla Coll Med 82; **RES:** Ped A&I, U NC Hosp, Chapel Hill, NC 82-85; **FEL:** NP, U FL Shands Hosp, Gainesville, FL 85-88; **FAP:** Asst Prof Ped U Chicago-Pritzker Sch Med; **HOSP:** Hinsdale Hosp

Fitzgerald, Michael (MD) NP
Good Samaritan Hosp (see page 274)
PO Box 487 Hinsdale Rd; Hinsdale, IL 60522; (847) 991-0440; **BDCERT:** Ped 90; NP 91; **MS:** U Hlth Sci/Chicago Med Sch 83

Go, Margaret (MD) NP
St Francis Hosp
900 Jorie Blvd Ste 186; OakBrook, IL 60523; (630) 954-6700; **BDCERT:** Ped 84; NP 93; **MS:** Philippines 75; **HOSP:** Alexian Brothers Med Ctr

Reddy, Ravindranath (MD) NP
Alexian Brothers Med Ctr
(see page 138)
A B C Pediatrics, 471 W Army Trail Rd Ste 102; Bloomingdale, IL 60108; (630) 529-6969; **BDCERT:** Ped 77; **MS:** India 73; **RES:** Ped, U IL Med Ctr, Chicago, IL 73-75; **FEL:** NP, Michael Reese Hosp Med Ctr, Chicago, IL 75-77; **FAP:** Asst Clin Prof Ped Loyola U-Stritch Sch Med, Maywood

Suleiman, Khair A (MD) NP
Westlake Comm Hosp
7451 S Woodward Ave Ste 108; Woodridge, IL 60517; (630) 369-9093; **BDCERT:** Ped 83; NP 83; **MS:** Syria 73; **RES:** Ped, St Louis Hosp, St Louis, MO 77-79; **FEL:** NP, St Louis U Hosp, St Louis, MO 80-81; NP, Med Coll of GA Hosp, Augusta, GA 81-82; **FAP:** Asst Prof Rush Med Coll; **HOSP:** La Grange Mem Hosp; **SI:** *Neonatology*; **HMO:** United Healthcare, Blue Cross & Blue Shield, HealthStar, Humana HMO +
LANG: Ar; A Few Days

NEPHROLOGY

Julka, Naresh (MD) Nep
Good Samaritan Hosp (see page 274)
Nephrology Associates, 3825 Highland Ave Ste 4C; Downers Grove, IL 60515; (630) 968-1595; **BDCERT:** IM 77; Nep 78; **MS:** India 69; **RES:** IM, Columbus Hosp, Chicago, IL 75-76; **FEL:** Nep, U IL Med Ctr, Chicago, IL 76-78; **HOSP:** Hinsdale Hosp; **HMO:** Aetna Hlth Plan, Blue Cross & Blue Shield, Californiacare, CIGNA, HealthNet +
4+ Weeks

Kozney, Gregory (MD) Nep
Central DuPage Hosp
Nephrology Assoc. Of Northern Illinois, 120 Spalding Drive Ste 410; Naperville, IL 60540; (630) 690-1220; **BDCERT:** IM 81; Nep 84; **MS:** Loyola U-Stritch Sch Med, Maywood 78; **RES:** IM, Loyola U Med Ctr, Maywood, IL 78-81; **FEL:** Nep, Loyola U Med Ctr, Maywood, IL 81-84; **FAP:** Assoc. Professo Nep Loyola U-Stritch Sch Med, Maywood; **HOSP:** Edward Hosp; **SI:** *Kidney Failure; Hypertension*

NEUROLOGICAL SURGERY

Beatty, Robert (MD) NS
Hinsdale Hosp (see page 275)
333 Chestnut St Ste 203; Hinsdale, IL 60521; (630) 986-8290; **BDCERT:** NS 70; **MS:** U Oreg/Hlth Sci U, Portland 61; **RES:** S, Rush Presbyterian-St Luke's Med Ctr, Chicago, IL 62-63; NS, IL Neuropsy Inst, Chicago, IL 63-66; **FEL:** St George's Med Sch, London, England 66-67; **FAP:** Assoc Clin Prof Univ IL Coll Med; **HMO:** +
A Few Days

Boury, Harb (MD) NS
Central DuPage Hosp
Winfield Neurosurgical Conslnt, 327 Gundersen Dr C; Carol Stream, IL 60188; (630) 653-2599; **BDCERT:** NS 80; **MS:** Lebanon 69; **RES:** N, Strong Mem Hosp, Rochester, NY 70-71; NS, U Wisc Hosp, Madison, WI 71-76; **FAP:** Asst Clin Prof NS Univ IL Coll Med

DiGianflippo, Anthony (MD) NS
La Grange Mem Hosp (see page 141)
West Suburban Neurosurgical, 20 E Ogden Ave; Hinsdale, IL 60521; (630) 655-1229; **BDCERT:** NS 92; **MS:** Univ IL Coll Med 83; **RES:** Rush Presbyterian-St Luke's Med Ctr, Chicago, IL 84-89; **HOSP:** Hinsdale Hosp; **HMO:** Aetna Hlth Plan, Blue Cross & Blue Shield, Californiacare, CIGNA, HealthNet

Fronczak, Stanley (MD) NS
Good Samaritan Hosp (see page 274)
West Suburban Neurosurgical, 20 E Ogden Ave; Hinsdale, IL 60521; (630) 655-1229; **BDCERT:** NS 84; **MS:** Loyola U-Stritch Sch Med, Maywood 73; **RES:** NS, Loyola U Med Ctr, Maywood, IL 73-80; **HOSP:** Hinsdale Hosp; **SI:** *Brain Tumor Surgery; Cranial and Spinal Trauma*; **HMO:** Blue Cross & Blue Shield, PHCS, Aetna Hlth Plan, Preferred Care +
A Few Days

Kazan, Robert (MD) NS
Hinsdale Hosp (see page 275)
West Suburban Neurosurgical, 20 E Ogden Ave; Hinsdale, IL 60521; (630) 655-1229; **BDCERT:** NS 80; **MS:** Loyola U-Stritch Sch Med, Maywood 73; **RES:** Mayo Clinic, Rochester, MN 73-78; **FAP:** Asst Clin Prof Univ IL Coll Med; **SI:** *Spine; Skull Base Tumors*; **HMO:** Blue Cross & Blue Shield, CIGNA, Humana Health Plan
2-4 Weeks **VISA**

Martonffy, Denes (MD) NS
Good Samaritan Hosp (see page 274)
3825 Highland Ave Ste 2L; Downers Grove, IL 60515; (630) 434-0190; **BDCERT:** NS 71; **MS:** Boston U 63; **RES:** NS, Chicago Hosp, Chicago, IL 64-68; **FAP:** Assoc Clin Prof NS Loyola U-Stritch Sch Med, Maywood

Ross, Matthew (MD) NS
Central DuPage Hosp
Neurosurgery Spine & Pain Asso, 150 N Winfield Rd D; Winfield, IL 60190; (630) 690-5990; **BDCERT:** NS 95; **MS:** Univ IL Coll Med 84; **HMO:** Blue Cross & Blue Shield, CIGNA, Humana Health Plan, Metlife, Principal Health Care

NEUROLOGY

Collins, John (MD) N
Central DuPage Hosp
Glen Ellyn Clinic, 231 S Gary Ave Ste 104; Bloomingdale, IL 60108; (630) 671-9800; **BDCERT:** N 84; **MS:** Loyola U-Stritch Sch Med, Maywood 78; **RES:** N, Loyola U Med Ctr, Maywood, IL 79-82; **HMO:** Aetna Hlth Plan, Blue Cross & Blue Shield, CIGNA, Health Options, Humana Health Plan

Guide to symbols and abbreviations can be found on pages 110-113.

Echiverri, Henry C (MD) N
Edward Hosp (see page 272)
Neuromed, 10 E 22nd St Ste 217; Lombard, IL 60148; (630) 792-9504; **BDCERT:** N 90; **MS:** Philippines 81; **RES:** N, Hines VA Hosp, Chicago, IL 81-89; **HOSP:** Good Samaritan Hosp

Frank, Helge (MD) N
Hinsdale Hosp (see page 275)
Medical Neurology Assocs, 20 E Ogden Ave; Hinsdale, IL 60521; (630) 325-8730; **BDCERT:** N 79; **MS:** Loyola U-Stritch Sch Med, Maywood 72

Glista, Glen (MD) N
Good Samaritan Hosp (see page 274)
Medical Neurology Assocs, 20 E Ogden Ave; Hinsdale, IL 60521; (630) 325-8730; **BDCERT:** N 82; **MS:** Northwestern U 71; **RES:** N, Hines VA Hosp, Chicago, IL 76-80; **HMO:** Aetna Hlth Plan, Blue Cross & Blue Shield, Chicago HMO, Healthpartners, Humana Health Plan

Mc Coyd, Kevin (MD) N
Elmhurst Mem Hosp
Rlt Neurologic Assoc, 255 W 1st St; Elmhurst, IL 60126; (630) 530-4449; **BDCERT:** N 76; **MS:** Loyola U-Stritch Sch Med, Maywood 71; **RES:** Albany Med Ctr, Albany, NY 72-75; **FAP:** Asst Clin Prof Rush Med Coll; **HMO:** Aetna Hlth Plan, Blue Cross & Blue Shield, Chicago HMO, CIGNA, HealthNet

Nour, Fred (MD) N
Central DuPage Hosp
Comprehensive Neurological Svc, IN141 County Farm Rd Ste 130; Winfield, IL 60190; (630) 690-3333; **BDCERT:** N 88; **MS:** Egypt 76; **RES:** PMR, LSU Hosp, New Orleans, LO 81-83; N, Baylor Med Ctr, Dallas, TX 83-86; **HOSP:** Delnor Comm Hosp; ***SI:*** *Headaches; Seizures*; **HMO:** Blue Cross & Blue Shield, CIGNA, Blue Choice
A Few Days ***VISA***

OBSTETRICS & GYNECOLOGY

Barbour, Christopher (MD) ObG
PCP
Good Samaritan Hosp (see page 274)
West Suburban Ob & Gyn, 3825 Highland Ave Ste 210; Downers Grove, IL 60515; (630) 960-1310; **BDCERT:** ObG 80; **MS:** Univ IL Coll Med 78; **RES:** ObG, U IL Med Ctr, Chicago, IL 75-78

Cannon, Mary Jean (MD) ObG
Hinsdale Hosp (see page 275)
Women Ob-Gyn Assoc, 4121 Fairview Ave Ste 201; Downers Grove, IL 60515; (630) 719-9229; **BDCERT:** ObG 88; **MS:** Univ IL Coll Med 82; **RES:** ObG, Illinois Masonic Med Ctr, Chicago, IL 83-86

Carroll, John (MD) ObG
Central DuPage Hosp
Du Page Obstetrics, 503 Thornhill Dr; Carol Stream, IL 60188; (630) 653-4200; **BDCERT:** ObG 87; **MS:** Med Coll Wisc 76; **HMO:** Aetna Hlth Plan, Blue Cross & Blue Shield, Californiacare, Chicago HMO, Choicecare

Carver, Thomas Richard (MD) ObG
PCP
Edward Hosp (see page 272)
Terrace Obstetricians, 1 S 132 Summit Ave Ste 305; Oak Brook, IL 60181; (630) 627-4954; **BDCERT:** ObG 86; **MS:** St Louis U 80; **RES:** ObG, McGraw Hosp/Loyola U, Maywood, IL 80-84; **FAP:** Asst Clin Prof Med Loyola U-Stritch Sch Med, Maywood; **HOSP:** Good Samaritan Hosp; **HMO:** +
2-4 Weeks ***VISA***

Chen, Thomas (MD) ObG
PCP
Edward Hosp (see page 272)
Terrace Obstetricians, 132 Summit Ave Ste 105; Oakbrook Terrace, IL 60181; (630) 627-4954; **BDCERT:** ObG 85; **MS:** Geo Wash U Sch Med 76; **RES:** ObG, Northwestern Mem Hosp, Chicago, IL; **FAP:** Asst Clin Prof ObG Loyola U-Stritch Sch Med, Maywood; **HOSP:** Good Samaritan Hosp; **HMO:** Blue Cross & Blue Shield

Cheng, Elaine (MD) ObG
Hinsdale Hosp (see page 275)
Women Ob-Gyn Assoc, 4121 Fairview Ave Ste 201; Downers Grove, IL 60515; (630) 719-9229; **BDCERT:** ObG 91; **MS:** Northwestern U 85; **RES:** ObG, Northwestern Mem Hosp, Chicago, IL 85-89; **HOSP:** Good Samaritan Hosp; ***SI:*** *Abnormal Pap Smears; Endometriosis*; **HMO:** Aetna Hlth Plan, Blue Cross & Blue Shield, Californiacare, United Healthcare, Rush Prudential +
LANG: Ur, Hin;
A Few Days

Druzak, Karen (MD) ObG
Edward Hosp (see page 272)
10 Martin Ave Ste 100; Naperville, IL 60450; (630) 369-7700; **BDCERT:** ObG 91; **MS:** Ky Med Sch, Louisville 88; **RES:** ObG, Good Samaritan Hosp, Cincinnati, OH 85-89

Fitzmaurice, William (MD) ObG
PCP
Elmhurst Mem Hosp
R-P-W Obstetrics & Gynecology, 360 W Butterfield Rd Ste 250; Elmhurst, IL 60126; (630) 832-4210; **BDCERT:** ObG 90; **MS:** Univ IL Coll Med 82; **RES:** ObG, St John's Mercy Med Ctr, St Louis, MO 83-87

Gallo, Martin (MD) **ObG**
Good Samaritan Hosp **(see page 274)**
Tre Medical Ltd, 3825 Highland Ave Ste 3K; Downers Grove, IL 60515; (630) 968-2144; **BDCERT:** ObG 92; **MS:** Northwestern U 86; **RES:** ObG, Northwestern Mem Hosp, Chicago, IL 86-90; **HOSP:** Edward Hosp; ***SI:*** *Endometriosis; Menopause*; **HMO:** CIGNA, Aetna Hlth Plan, Rush Pru, Blue Cross +
1 Week VISA

Gulling, Edward (MD) **ObG**
PCP
Central DuPage Hosp
Glen Ellyn Clinic, 454 Pennsylvania Ave; Glen Ellyn, IL 60137; (630) 858-3200; **BDCERT:** ObG 79; **MS:** Loyola U-Stritch Sch Med, Maywood 73; **RES:** Loyola U Med Ctr, Maywood, IL; **HMO:** Blue Cross & Blue Shield, CIGNA, Bay State Health Plan, Metlife, Principal Health Care
4+ Weeks VISA

Jenks, James (MD) **ObG**
Good Samaritan Hosp **(see page 274)**
Tre Medical Ltd, 3825 Highland Ave Ste 3K; Downers Grove, IL 60515; (630) 968-2144; **BDCERT:** ObG 85; **MS:** Northwestern U 79; **RES:** Northwestern Mem Hosp, Chicago, IL 79-83; **HMO:** HMO Illinois, American Health Plan
4+ Weeks

Kim, Taek (MD) **ObG**
Edward Hosp **(see page 272)**
6800 S Main St; Downess Grove, IL 60516; (630) 971-0335; **BDCERT:** ObG 76; **MS:** South Korea 72; **RES:** ObG, Mercy Hosp & Med Ctr, Chicago, IL 74; **HOSP:** Hinsdale Hosp; ***SI:*** *Infertility*; **HMO:** Aetna Hlth Plan, Blue Cross & Blue Shield +
LANG: Kor; VISA

Kuppuswami, Narmadha (MD) **ObG**
Good Samaritan Hosp **(see page 274)**
Midwest Women Ob/Gyn, 3825 Highland Ave Ste 2F; Downers Grove, IL 60515; (630) 852-3762; **BDCERT:** ObG 82; **MS:** India 71; **RES:** Cook Cty Hosp, Chicago, IL 77-80; **HOSP:** Edward Hosp; **HMO:** Blue Shield, CIGNA, Prucare
4+ Weeks VISA

Shangle, Elizabeth (MD) **ObG**
PCP
Elmhurst Mem Hosp
R-P-W Obstetrics & Gynecology, 815 S Main St; Lombard, IL 60148; (630) 495-2603; **BDCERT:** ObG 90; **MS:** Loyola U-Stritch Sch Med, Maywood 84

Wickman, Doris (MD) **ObG**
Central DuPage Hosp
Female Health Care, 471 W Army Trail Rd Ste 103; Bloomingdale, IL 60108; (630) 980-3366; **BDCERT:** ObG 86; **MS:** Ky Med Sch, Louisville 80; **RES:** ObG, Michael Reese Hosp Med Ctr, Chicago, IL 80-84; **HOSP:** Alexian Brothers Med Ctr; ***SI:*** *Endometriosis; Family Centered Obstetrics*; **HMO:** Blue Cross & Blue Shield, Rush Prudential, PHCS +
VISA

Yu, Mario (MD) **ObG**
PCP
Hinsdale Hosp **(see page 275)**
1919 Midwest Rd; Oak Brook, IL 60523; (630) 629-8282; **BDCERT:** ObG 85; **MS:** Loyola U-Stritch Sch Med, Maywood 79; **RES:** IM, Loyola U Med Ctr, Maywood, IL 79-80; ObG, St Joseph's Hosp, Chicago, IL 80-83; **HOSP:** Glen Oaks Hosp and Med Ctr; ***SI:*** *Infertility; Acupuncture Herbal Therapy*; **HMO:** Blue Cross & Blue Shield, CIGNA, Aetna Hlth Plan, United Healthcare +
LANG: Man, Can, Chi;

OCCUPATIONAL MEDICINE

Shadel, Robert F (MD) **OM**
Good Samaritan Hosp **(see page 274)**
Advocate Occupational Health, 3800 Highland Ave Ste 301; Downers Grove, IL 60515; (630) 969-8558; **BDCERT:** FP 95; OM 95; **MS:** Univ IL Coll Med 71; **FAP:** Adjct Clin Prof Univ IL Coll Med

OPHTHALMOLOGY

Barnes, Robert J (MD) **Oph**
Central DuPage Hosp
Glen Ellyn Ophthalmology Assoc, 45 S Park Blvd Ste 375; Glen Ellyn, IL 60137; (630) 858-4660; **BDCERT:** Oph 90; **MS:** Rush Med Coll 82; **RES:** Oph, Northwestern Mem Hosp, Chicago, IL 83-86; **FEL:** Glaucoma, U IL Med Ctr, Chicago, IL 86-87; **FAP:** Asst Clin Prof Loyola U-Stritch Sch Med, Maywood; **HOSP:** Rush-Copley Med Ctr

Daily, Mark (MD) **Oph**
Central DuPage Hosp
Wheaton Eye Clinic Ltd, 2015 N Main St; Wheaton, IL 60187; (630) 668-8250; **BDCERT:** Oph 78; **MS:** Univ IL Coll Med 73; ***SI:*** *Retina*

Haag, Jeffery (MD) **Oph**
Loyola U Med Ctr **(see page 120)**
Wheaton Eye Clinic Ltd, 2015 N Main St; Wheaton, IL 60187; (630) 668-8250; **BDCERT:** Oph 85; **MS:** Jefferson Med Coll 79; **RES:** Oph, Loyola U Med Ctr, Maywood, IL 80-83; Oph, Bascom Palmer Eye Inst, Miami, FL 83-84; **HOSP:** Central DuPage Hosp

Guide to symbols and abbreviations can be found on pages 110-113.

Larson, Bruce (MD) **Oph**
Hinsdale Hosp (see page 275)
Eye Center, 126 W First St; Hinsdale, IL 60521; (630) 325-5200; **BDCERT:** Oph 84; **MS:** Univ IL Coll Med 79; **RES:** Oph, Wills Eye Hosp, Philadelphia, PA 80-83; **FEL:** Retina, U IL Med Ctr, Chicago, IL 83-84; **FAP:** Assoc Clin Prof Univ IL Coll Med

Nagpal, Krishan (MD) **Oph**
Elmhurst Mem Hosp
135 Robert T Palmer Dr Ste 25; Elmhurst, IL 60126; (630) 832-3055; **BDCERT:** Oph 75; **MS:** India 66; **RES:** Oph, U IL Med Ctr, Chicago, IL 68-70; **HOSP:** Hinsdale Hosp

Wayne, Audrey (MD) **Oph**
Hinsdale Hosp (see page 275)
12 Salt Creek Ln Ste 100; Hinsdale, IL 60521; (630) 654-4551; **BDCERT:** Oph 82; **MS:** Loyola U-Stritch Sch Med, Maywood 76; **RES:** Oph, Barnes Hosp-Walsh U, St Louis, MO 77-80; **HOSP:** La Grange Mem Hosp

Zlioba, Aras (MD) **Oph**
Good Samaritan Hosp (see page 274)
1020 E Ogden Ave Ste 310; Naperville, IL 60563; (630) 527-0090; **BDCERT:** Oph 91; **MS:** Northwestern U 86; **RES:** Oph, Loyola U Med Ctr, Maywood, IL 87-90; **HOSP:** Edward Hosp; **HMO:** Aetna Hlth Plan, Blue Cross & Blue Shield, Californiacare, CIGNA, Metlife +
LANG: Lth; 4+ Weeks
VISA

ORTHOPAEDIC SURGERY

Brash, Richard (MD) **OrS**
Westlake Comm Hosp
Du Page Sports Injury Ctr, 2425 W 22nd St Ste 214; Oak Brook, IL 60523; (630) 954-5906; **MS:** U Chicago-Pritzker Sch Med 76; **RES:** OrS, Loyola Univ, Chicago, IL 76-81; **FEL:** OrS, Univ of California, San Diego, CA 81-82; ***SI:*** *Sports Medicine*; **HMO:** +
Immediately
VISA

Collins, Michael (MD) **OrS**
Hinsdale Hosp (see page 275)
Hinsdale Orthopaedic Assoc, 550 W Ogden Ave; Hinsdale, IL 60521; (630) 323-6116; **BDCERT:** OrS 85; **MS:** Loyola U-Stritch Sch Med, Maywood 78; **RES:** OrS, Mayo Clinic, Rochester, MN 79-83; **HOSP:** Good Samaritan Hosp; ***SI:*** *Arthroscopy; Sports Medicine*; **HMO:** Aetna-US Healthcare, Rush Health Plans, Bc/BS, CIGNA, HMO Illinois +
LANG: Sp; 1 Week
VISA

Gandhi, Vikram (MD) **OrS**
Good Samaritan Hosp (see page 274)
7530 S Woodward Ave A; Woodridge, IL 60517; (630) 910-5933; **BDCERT:** OrS 79; **MS:** India 68; **RES:** OrS, SSG Affiliated Hosp, Baroda, India 69-73; OrS, Loyola U Med Ctr, Maywood, IL 74-77; **FEL:** HS, Loyola U Med Ctr, Maywood, IL 77-78; **HOSP:** St Mary's of Nazareth Hosp Ctr

Gilligan, William (MD) **OrS**
Good Samaritan Hosp (see page 274)
Hinsdale Orthopaedic Assoc, 550 W Ogden Ave; Hinsdale, IL 60521; (630) 323-6116; **BDCERT:** OrS 69; **MS:** Northwestern U 62; **RES:** Northwestern Mem Hosp, Chicago, IL 64-67; **FEL:** HS, Los Angeles Orthopaedic Hosp, Los Angeles, CA 67; **FAP:** Assoc Clin Prof Rush Med Coll; **HOSP:** Hinsdale Hosp

Hadesman, William (MD) **OrS**
Elmhurst Mem Hosp
Elmhurst Clinic, 172 Schiller St; Elmhurst, IL 60126; (630) 941-2630; **BDCERT:** OrS 89; **MS:** Mich St U 82; **HOSP:** Condell Med Ctr

Heim, Stephen (MD) **OrS**
Central DuPage Hosp
Orthopaedic Associates of Du Page Ltd, 515 Thornhill Dr; Carol Stream, IL 60188; (609) 369-3514; **BDCERT:** OrS 89; OrS 89; **MS:** Northwestern U 82; **RES:** OrS, Northwestern Mem Hosp, Chicago, IL 82-87; **FEL:** Spine Trauma, 86-87; ***SI:*** *Disorders of the Back and Cervical Spine*; **HMO:** Aetna Hlth Plan, CIGNA, Blue Cross/Blue Shield, Private Healthcare
2-4 Weeks

Ibrahim, Kamal (MD) **OrS**
Hinsdale Hosp (see page 275)
1 S 224 Summit Ave Ste 203; Oak Brook Terrace, IL 60181; (630) 620-4141; **BDCERT:** OrS 82; **MS:** Egypt 71; **RES:** OrS, McMaster Univ Hosp, Hamilton, Canada 76-79; S, Jewish Gen Hosp, Montreal, Canada 74-75; **FEL:** Ped, Alfred Du Point Inst, Wilmington, DE 80; **FAP:** Assoc Clin Prof Loyola U-Stritch Sch Med, Maywood; **HOSP:** Good Samaritan Hosp; ***SI:*** *Pediatric Orthopaedics*; **HMO:** Aetna Hlth Plan, Blue Choice, Californiacare, Chicago HMO, CIGNA +
LANG: Ar, Fr, Itl, Sp; 1 Week
VISA

Khan, Hamid (MD) **OrS**
Central DuPage Hosp
Glen Ellyn Clinic, 454 Pennsylvania Ave; Glen Ellyn, IL 60137; (630) 790-1872; **BDCERT:** OrS 82; **MS:** Other Foreign Country 60; **RES:** S, Jewish Hosp, Cincinati, OH 64-67; OrS, U Manitoba-Affil Hosps, Winnipeg, CN 68-71; **HMO:** +
A Few Days VISA

Payne, Timothy (MD) **OrS**
Good Samaritan Hosp **(see page 274)**
M & M Orthopaedics Ltd, 4115 Fairview Ave; Downers Grove, IL 60515; (630) 968-1881; **BDCERT:** OrS 85; **MS:** Rush Med Coll 77; **RES:** S, Rush Presbyterian-St Luke's Med Ctr, Chicago, IL 78; OrS, Rush Presbyterian-St Luke's Med Ctr, Chicago, IL 79-82

Rodts, Thomas (MD) **OrS**
Elmhurst Mem Hosp
183 N Addison Ave; Elmhurst, IL 60126; (630) 530-4200; **BDCERT:** OrS 83; **MS:** St Louis U 76; **RES:** OrS, Rush Presbyterian-St Luke's Med Ctr, Chicago, IL 77-81; **FAP:** Instr Rush Med Coll

Schiffman, Kenneth (MD) **OrS**
Good Samaritan Hosp **(see page 274)**
Hinsdale Orthopaedic Assoc, 550 W Ogden Ave; Hinsdale, IL 60521; (630) 323-6116; **BDCERT:** OrS 89; **MS:** U South Fla Coll Med 81; **RES:** OrS, Loyola U Med Ctr, Maywood, IL 82-86; **FEL:** HS, Princess Margaret Rose Hosp, Toronto, Canada 86-87; **FAP:** Asst Prof Loyola U-Stritch Sch Med, Maywood; **HOSP:** Hinsdale Hosp

Velagapudi, Suresh (MD) **OrS**
Rush-Copley Med Ctr
Castle Orthopedics & Sports, 1315 N Highland Pkwy; Aurora, IL 60506; (630) 978-2663; **BDCERT:** OrS 95; **MS:** Univ IL Coll Med 87; **RES:** OrS, U IL Med Ctr, Chicago, IL 88-92

Zindrick, Michael (MD) **OrS**
Hinsdale Hosp **(see page 275)**
Hinsdale Orthopaedic Assoc, 550 W Ogden Ave; Hinsdale, IL 60521; (630) 323-6116; **BDCERT:** OrS 87; **MS:** Loyola U-Stritch Sch Med, Maywood 79; **RES:** OrS, Loyola U Med Ctr, Maywood, IL 79-84; **FEL:** PM, Long Beach Mem Med Ctr, Long Beach, CA 84-85

OTOLARYNGOLOGY

Battista, Robert (MD) **Oto**
Good Samaritan Hosp **(see page 274)**
Associates Head & Neck Surgery, 950 York Rd Ste 102; Hinsdale, IL 60521; (630) 789-3110; **BDCERT:** Oto 92; **MS:** UMDNJ-NJ Med Sch, Newark 86; **RES:** Oto, U Hosp, Newark, NJ 87-91; **FEL:** Oto, Warren Oto Group, Warren, NJ 91-92; **HOSP:** Hinsdale Hosp; ***SI:*** *Dizziness; Acoustic Tumor*; **HMO:** Blue Cross & Blue Shield, Principal Health Care, HealthNet, PHCS +
Mcr Mcd Immediately VISA

Bulger, Richard (MD) **Oto**
Hinsdale Hosp **(see page 275)**
Bulger, Rejowski & Dillon, 950 N York Rd Ste 108; Hinsdale, IL 60521; (630) 654-1391; **BDCERT:** Oto 72; **MS:** Univ IL Coll Med 67; **HMO:** Aetna Hlth Plan, Blue Cross & Blue Shield, Californiacare, Humana Health Plan, Metlife
SA SU $ Mcr Mcd NFI
A Few Days VISA

Bumstead, Robert (MD) **Oto**
Good Samaritan Hosp **(see page 274)**
University Head & Neck Assoc, 120 Oakbrook Ctr Ste 508; Oak Brook, IL 60523; (630) 574-8222; **BDCERT:** Oto 77; **MS:** U Wisc Med Sch 69; **RES:** S, Lutheran Hosp, La Crosse, WI 71; Oto, U IA Hosp, Iowa City, IA 72; **FAP:** Prof Oto Rush Med Coll

Collins, Sharon (MD) **Oto**
Loyola U Med Ctr **(see page 120)**
567 Lake Rd; Glen Ellyn, IL 60137; (708) 216-9000; **BDCERT:** Oto 83; **MS:** U Mich Med Sch 78; **RES:** Barnes Hosp, St Louis, MO 79-83; **FAP:** Assoc Prof Loyola U-Stritch Sch Med, Maywood; ***SI:*** *Head and Neck Cancer*; **HMO:** +
Mcr Mcd 2-4 Weeks VISA

Delicata, Dino S (MD) **Oto**
Good Samaritan Hosp **(see page 274)**
Suburban Practice Management, 3825 Highland Ave Ste 302; Downers Grove, IL 60515; (630) 960-5310; **BDCERT:** Oto 81; **MS:** Rush Med Coll 75; **RES:** Rush Presbyterian-St Luke's Med Ctr, Chicago, IL 76-80; **HMO:** Blue Cross & Blue Shield, Chicago HMO, Bay State Health Plan, Humana Health Plan, Maxicare Health Plan

Hanna, Wafik (MD) **Oto**
Hinsdale Hosp **(see page 275)**
Hanna Facial Cosmetics, 12 Salt Creek Ln Ste 225; Hinsdale, IL 60521; (630) 887-8180; **BDCERT:** Oto 73; **MS:** Egypt 65; **RES:** S, Macneal Mem Hosp, Berwyn, IL 69; Oto, IL Eye & Ear Infirmary, Chicago, IL 70-73; ***SI:*** *Facial Reconstructive Surgery*

Mahoney, Eileen (MD) **Oto**
Good Samaritan Hosp **(see page 274)**
Dr Gergis Associates, 908 N Elm St Ste 306; Hinsdale, IL 60521; (630) 323-5214; **BDCERT:** Oto 93; **MS:** Rush Med Coll 86; **RES:** Oto, Tripler Army Med Ctr 89-92; **FEL:** PedOto, Children's Memorial Hosp, Chicago, IL 95-96; ***SI:*** *Pediatric Otolaryngology*

Rejowski, James (MD) **Oto**
Hinsdale Hosp **(see page 275)**
Bulger Rejowski & Dillon, 950 N York Rd Ste 109; Hinsdale, IL 60521; (630) 654-1391; **BDCERT:** Oto 83; **MS:** Rush Med Coll 78; **RES:** Rush Presby-St Lukes Med Ctr, Chicago, IL 79-83; **FAP:** Instr Rush Med Coll; **HMO:** Aetna Hlth Plan, Blue Cross & Blue Shield, CIGNA, Humana Health Plan, Metlife

Guide to symbols and abbreviations can be found on pages 110-113.

Rubach, Bryan (MD) Oto
Rush-Copley Med Ctr
Cosmetic Surgery Ctr, 4050 Healthway Dr Ste 220; Aurora, IL 60504; (630) 851-3223; **BDCERT:** Oto 95; **MS:** U Wisc Med Sch 85; **RES:** Oto, Milwaukee County Med Complex, Milwaukee, WI 90-94; **FEL:** Facial PlS, UC San Francisco Med Ctr, San Francisco, CA 94-95; **HOSP:** Mercy Hosp & Med Ctr

Stankiewicz, James (MD) Oto
Loyola U Med Ctr (see page 120)
6 Carriage Ln; Lemont, IL 60439; (630) 216-9183; **BDCERT:** Oto 78; **MS:** U Chicago-Pritzker Sch Med 74; **RES:** Oto, U Chicago Hosp, Chicago, IL 74-78; **FAP:** Prof Loyola U-Stritch Sch Med, Maywood; ***SI:*** *Sinus Surgery; Nasal and Sinus Disease*; **HMO:** Blue Cross, Aetna Hlth Plan, NYLCare
4+ Weeks VISA

PAIN MANAGEMENT

Belavic, Andrew (MD) PM
Elmhurst Mem Hosp
200 Berteau Ave; Elmhurst, IL 60126; (630) 782-7836; **BDCERT:** PM 96; Anes 91; **MS:** Dominican Republic 86; **RES:** Anes, Northwestern Mem Hosp, Chicago, IL 87-90; **FEL:** PM, Northwestern Mem Hosp, Chicago, IL 91; ***SI:*** *Pain Management*
1 Week

Hwang, Kwang-Ko (MD) PM
Central DuPage Hosp
25 N Winfield Rd; Winfield, IL 60190; (630) 682-1600; **BDCERT:** Anes 76; PM 94; **MS:** Taiwan 66; **RES:** Anes, Illinois Masonic Med Ctr, Chicago, IL 71-74; **HMO:** Aetna Hlth Plan, Blue Cross & Blue Shield, Californiacare, Chicago HMO, CIGNA

PEDIATRIC ENDOCRINOLOGY

Rich, Barry H (MD) PEn
La Rabida Children's Hosp
908 N Elm St C908; Hinsdale, IL 60521; (773) 363-6700; **BDCERT:** PEn 80; Ped 79; **MS:** U Chicago-Pritzker Sch Med 74; **RES:** Ped, Children's Mem Med Ctr, Chicago, IL 74-76; **FEL:** PEn, U Chicago Hosp, Chicago, IL 76-79; **FAP:** Assoc Prof Ped U Chicago-Pritzker Sch Med; **HOSP:** Hinsdale Hosp; ***SI:*** *Diabetes Mellitus; Growth Disorders*
2-4 Weeks

PEDIATRIC SURGERY

Black, Preston (MD) PdS
Good Samaritan Hosp (see page 274)
1 N 121 County Farm Rd Ste 100; Winfield, IL 60190; (630) 668-0833; **BDCERT:** PdS 87; S 98; **MS:** Harvard Med Sch 75; **RES:** S, Peter Bent Brigham Hosp, Boston, MA 75-80; PdS, Childrens Hosp, Boston, MA 82-83; **HMO:** +
1 Week VISA

PEDIATRICS

Campbell, Daniel (MD) Ped
PCP
Hinsdale Hosp (see page 275)
Hinsdale Pediatric Assoc, 911 N Elm St Ste 115; Hinsdale, IL 60521; (630) 323-0890; **BDCERT:** Ped 85; **MS:** Loyola U-Stritch Sch Med, Maywood 80; **RES:** Ped, U Chicago Hosp, Chicago, IL 81-83; **FEL:** PCd, U Chicago Hosp, Chicago, IL 83-85; **FAP:** Asst Prof U Chicago-Pritzker Sch Med; ***SI:*** *Pediatric Cardiology*

Coufal, Stanislava (MD) Ped
PCP
Good Samaritan Hosp (see page 274)
3825 Highland Ave Ste 2C; Downers Grove, IL 60515; (630) 971-6511; **BDCERT:** Ped 76; **MS:** Czechoslovakia 68; **RES:** U Ill Hosp, Chicago, IL 72-74; **FAP:** Asst Clin Prof Univ IL Coll Med

Coyer, William (MD) Ped
PCP
Central DuPage Hosp
Glen Ellyn Clinic, 1250 N Mill St; Naperville, IL 60563; (630) 961-4166; **BDCERT:** Ped 72; NP 75; **MS:** U Tenn Ctr Hlth Sci, Memphis 67; **RES:** Ped, Tenn-City Memphis Hosps, Memphis, TN 68-69; **FEL:** NP, Colo Med Ctr 69-71

Eckberg, Lorene (MD) Ped
PCP
Rush-Copley Med Ctr
Dreyer Medical Clinic, 4100 Healthway Dr; Aurora, IL 60504; (630) 851-3105; **BDCERT:** Ped 89; **MS:** Loyola U-Stritch Sch Med, Maywood 85; **RES:** Ped, Loyola U Med Ctr, Maywood, IL 85-89; **HOSP:** Provena Mercy Ctr

Grunenwald, Christienne (MD) Ped
PCP
Central DuPage Hosp
Wheaton Pediatrics, 199 Town Sq A; Wheaton, IL 60187; (630) 690-7300; **BDCERT:** Ped 94; **MS:** U Cincinnati 91; **RES:** Ped, Childrens Meml Med Ctr, Chicago, IL 92-94

Han, Sang Jo (MD) Ped
PCP
St Alexius Med Ctr
Neonatal & Pediatric Svc, 471 W Army Trail Ste 102; Bloomingdale, IL 60559; (630) 529-6969; **BDCERT:** Ped 80; **MS:** South Korea 72; **RES:** Ped, Jersey City Med Ctr, Jersey City, NJ 78; **FEL:** N, Newark Beth Israel Med Ctr, Newark, NJ 80; **HOSP:** Glen Oaks Hosp and Med Ctr
LANG: Kor, Sp; 2-4 Weeks

Huang, Pamela Claire (MD) Ped
PCP
Good Samaritan Hosp **(see page 274)**
Du Page Pediatrics, 1306 Plainfield Rd; Darien, IL 60561; (630) 810-0900; **BDCERT:** Ped 83; **MS:** Univ IL Coll Med 78; **RES:** Ped A&I, Cook Cty Hosp, Chicago, IL 79-82; **HOSP:** Hinsdale Hosp

Liber, Peter (MD) Ped
PCP
Central DuPage Hosp
Wheaton Pediatrics, 199 Town Sq A; Wheaton, IL 60187; (630) 690-7300; **BDCERT:** Ped 96; **MS:** Ind U Sch Med 84; **RES:** Ped, Children's Mem Med Ctr, Chicago, IL 84-87; **FAP:** Clin Instr Northwestern U; **HMO:** Blue Cross & Blue Shield, Principal Health Care

Moosabhoy, Nafeesa (MD) Ped
PCP
Hinsdale Hosp **(see page 275)**
Hinsdale Pediatric Assoc, 911 N Elm St Ste 115; Hinsdale, IL 60521; (630) 323-0890; **BDCERT:** Ped 73; **MS:** Pakistan 68; **RES:** Ped, Cook Cty Hosp, Chicago, IL 70-73

Morris, David (MD) Ped
PCP
Central DuPage Hosp
Glen Ellyn Clinic, 1250 N Mill St; Naperville, IL 60563; (630) 961-4166; **BDCERT:** Ped 86; **MS:** Bowman Gray 81; **RES:** Michael Reese Hosp Med Ctr, Chicago, IL 82-84

Veselik, Keith (MD) Ped
PCP
Loyola U Med Ctr **(see page 120)**
Loyola University Medical Ctr, 7511 Lemont Rd Ste 122; Darien, IL 60561; (630) 985-4989; **BDCERT:** Ped 93; **MS:** Univ IL Coll Med 89; **RES:** Ped, Loyola U Med Ctr, Maywood, IL 89-93; IM, Loyola U Med Ctr, Maywood, IL 89-93; **FAP:** Asst Professor Ped Loyola U-Stritch Sch Med, Maywood; **HOSP:** Loyola U Med Ctr; ***SI:** Primary Care; Prevention*; **HMO:** Blue Cross & Blue Shield, CIGNA PPO, Humana Health Plan, Most
2-4 Weeks VISA

PHYSICAL MEDICINE & REHABILITATION

Chaudhuri, Gouri (MD) PMR
Marianjoy Rehab Hosp & Clinics
26 W 171 Roosevelt Rd; Wheaton, IL 60189; (630) 462-4071; **BDCERT:** PMR 77; **MS:** India 67; ***SI:** Stroke*

Eilers, Robert (MD) PMR
Hinsdale Hosp **(see page 275)**
Physical Medicine & Rehab, 619 Plainfield Rd Ste 314C; Willow Brook, IL 60521; (630) 887-7676; **BDCERT:** PMR 83; **MS:** Ky Med Sch, Louisville 79; **RES:** PMR, Rehab Institute of Chicago, Chicago, IL 79-82; **FAP:** Instr Northwestern U

Keane, Dennis (MD) PMR
Rush-Copley Med Ctr
Rehabilitation Medicine Clinic, 2020 Ogden Ave Ste 365; Aurora, IL 60504; (630) 851-0008; **BDCERT:** PMR 94; **MS:** U Mich Med Sch 89; **RES:** PMR, Rush Presbyterian-St Luke's Med Ctr, Chicago, IL 90-93; **HMO:** +
LANG: Sp; A Few Days
VISA

Keen, Mary (MD) PMR
Marianjoy Rehab Hosp & Clinics
Marionjoy Rehab Med Clin, 26 W 171 Roosevelt Rd; Wheaton, IL 60187; (630) 462-4071; **BDCERT:** PMR 84; Ped 90; **MS:** Northwestern U 79; **RES:** PMR, U WA Med Ctr, Seattle, WA 81-83; Ped, Loyola U Med Ctr, Maywood, IL 87-90; **FAP:** Asst Prof Loyola U-Stritch Sch Med, Maywood; **HOSP:** Central DuPage Hosp; ***SI:** Physical Disability in Children; Spasticity*; **HMO:** Blue Cross & Blue Shield, First Health, Naperville Health Care IPA, PPO, Principal Health Care +
1 Week VISA

Krieger, Richard (MD) PMR
Marianjoy Rehab Hosp & Clinics
26 W 171 Roosevelt Rd; Wheaton, IL 60187; (630) 462-4239; **BDCERT:** PMR 95; **MS:** Rush Med Coll 90; **RES:** Macneal Mem Hosp, Berwyn, IL 90-91; PMR, Baylor Coll Med, Houston, TX 91-94; **FAP:** Asst Prof Rush Med Coll; **HOSP:** St Joseph Hosp-Elgin; ***SI:** Neck, Back, and Joint Pain; Stroke and Neurologic Rehab*; **HMO:** Blue Cross & Blue Shield, Aetna Hlth Plan, United Healthcare, Prudential +
A Few Days
VISA

Oken, Jeffrey Edward (MD) PMR
Marianjoy Rehab Hosp & Clinics
PO Box 795, 26 W 171 Roosevent Rd; Wheaton, IL 60189; (708) 462-5581; **BDCERT:** PMR 92; **MS:** Univ IL Coll Med 87; **RES:** Rehab Institute of Chicago, Chicago, IL 88-91; ***SI:** Pain Syndromes; Arthritis*
2-4 Weeks

Rao, Noel (MD) PMR
Marianjoy Rehab Hosp & Clinics
26 W 171 Roosevelt Rd; Wheaton, IL 60187; (630) 462-4070; **BDCERT:** PMR 80; **MS:** India 72; **RES:** PMR, Temple U Hosp, Philadelphia, PA 76-79; **FAP:** Assoc Prof Rush Med Coll

Guide to symbols and abbreviations can be found on pages 110-113.

Smith, Joanne C (MD) PMR
Rehab Institute of Chicago
807 The Pines; Hinsdale, IL 60521; (312) 908-0815; **BDCERT:** PMR 93; **MS:** Mich St U 88; ***SI:*** *Lower Back Pain*; **HMO:** +
2-4 Weeks VISA

Steiner, Monica (MD) PMR
Marianjoy Rehab Hosp & Clinics
Rehabilitation Medicine Clinic, 26 Roosevelt Rd; Wheaton, IL 60187; (630) 345-5151; **BDCERT:** PMR 87; **MS:** U Cincinnati 83; **RES:** Northwestern Mem Hosp, Chicago, IL 83-86; Rush Presbyterian-St Luke's Med Ctr, Chicago, IL 87-90; ***SI:*** *Neuromuscular Rehabilitation*
1 Week

PLASTIC SURGERY

Ferlmann, James (MD) PlS
Rush-Copley Med Ctr
2020 Ogden Ave Ste 210; Aurora, IL 60504; (630) 585-7300; **BDCERT:** PlS 97; **MS:** Univ IL Coll Med 87; **RES:** S, U IL Med Ctr, Chicago, IL 87-91; PlS, Rush-Presby-St Luke's Hosp, Chicago, IL 92-94; **HOSP:** Provena Mercy Ctr; ***SI:*** *Breast Augmentation, Liposuction, Laser Surgery; Breast Reduction, Face Lift*; **HMO:** United Healthcare, Aetna Hlth Plan, Bc/BS, CIGNA, Rush Prudential +
LANG: Ukr, Pol, Rus, Sp; 1 Week VISA

Janevicius, Raymond V (MD) PlS
Elmhurst Mem Hosp
360 W Butterfield Rd Ste 230; Elmhurst, IL 60126; (630) 833-1800; **BDCERT:** PlS 84; **MS:** Univ IL Coll Med 78; **RES:** S, U IL Med Ctr, Chicago, IL 78-81; PlS, Med Coll of Ohio, Toledo, OH 81-83; ***SI:*** *Hand Surgery*; **HMO:** Aetna Hlth Plan, Blue Cross & Blue Shield, Californiacare, Humana Health Plan, Prudential
1 Week VISA

Marschall, Michael (MD) PlS
La Grange Mem Hosp (see page 141)
7 Blanchard Cir Ste 204; Wheaton, IL 60187; (630) 462-6858; **BDCERT:** PlS 89; **MS:** U South Fla Coll Med 82; **RES:** S, U of South Florida, Tampa, FL 83-85; PlS, U of IL, Chicago, IL 85-87; **FAP:** Asst Clin Prof S Univ IL Coll Med

Maximovich, Stanley (MD) PlS
Edward Hosp (see page 272)
Plastic & Reconstructive Surg, 40 S Clay St Ste 237W; Hinsdale, IL 60521; (630) 325-5040; **BDCERT:** PlS 91; **MS:** Rush Med Coll 83; **RES:** S, Loyola U Med Ctr, Maywood, IL 83-86; **FEL:** PlS, Loyola U Med Ctr, Maywood, IL 86-89; **HOSP:** Hinsdale Hosp

Monasterio, Jack (MD) PlS
Central DuPage Hosp
Glen Ellyn Clinic, 454 Pennsylvania Ave; Glen Ellyn, IL 60137; (630) 790-1700; **BDCERT:** PlS 74; **MS:** Philippines 61; **RES:** St Francis Hosp of Evanston, Evanston, IL 66-67; Mount Sinai Hosp Med Ctr, Chicago, IL 64-66; **FAP:** Asst Prof PlS Loyola U-Stritch Sch Med, Maywood

Payne, Deming (MD) PlS
Hinsdale Hosp (see page 275)
20 E Ogden Ave; Hinsdale, IL 60521; (630) 325-9430; **BDCERT:** PlS 79; **MS:** SUNY Buffalo 66; **RES:** S, Med Coll VA Hosp, Richmond, VA 70-73; PlS, Strong Memorial Hospital, Rochester, NY 73-75; ***SI:*** *Cosmetic Surgery*

Raine, Talmage (MD) PlS
Hinsdale Hosp (see page 275)
Plastic Surgeons Assoc, 908 N Elm St Ste 204; Hinsdale, IL 60521; (630) 794-0700; **BDCERT:** PlS 85; **MS:** Med Coll Wisc 77; **RES:** S, Michael Reese Hosp, Chicago, IL 78-82; PlS, Emory U Hosp, Atlanta, GA 82-84; **FAP:** Asst Prof S U Chicago-Pritzker Sch Med; ***SI:*** *Cosmetic Surgery; Reconstructive Surgery*

PSYCHIATRY

Ali, Fatima (MD) Psyc
Linden Oaks Hosp
Du Page Mental Health, 1776 S Naperville Rd B103; Wheaton, IL 60187; (630) 690-2222; **BDCERT:** Psyc 92; **MS:** Pakistan 72; **RES:** Psyc, Loyola U Med Ctr, Maywood, IL 83-87; **FAP:** Asst Prof Psyc Loyola U-Stritch Sch Med, Maywood; **HMO:** +
1 Week VISA

Barnett, Arden (MD) Psyc
Univ of Illinois at Chicago Med Ctr
1112 S Wasington Ste 201; Naperville, IL 60540; (630) 527-4123; **BDCERT:** Psyc 92; ChAP 93; **MS:** U Tenn Ctr Hlth Sci, Memphis 84; **RES:** U Chicago Hosp, Chicago, IL; **FEL:** U Chicago Hosp, Chicago, IL; **FAP:** Asst Clin Prof Loyola U-Stritch Sch Med, Maywood; **HOSP:** Good Samaritan Hosp

Bernardino, Elizabeth (MD) Psyc
Hinsdale Hosp (see page 275)
Salt Creek Therapy Ctr, 7 Salt Creek Ln Ste 206; Hinsdale, IL 60521; (630) 850-2120; **BDCERT:** Psyc 91; ChAP 94; **MS:** Philippines 80; **RES:** Psyc, Loyola U Med Ctr, Maywood, IL 85-88; **FEL:** ChAP, Boston U Med Ctr, Boston, MA 90-92

Chaudhry, Naseem (MD) Psyc
Rock Creek Ctr
Nehal Psychiatric Group Inc, 6800 Main St Ste 214; Downers Grove, IL 60516; (630) 852-8451; **BDCERT:** Psyc 93; **MS:** Pakistan 82; **RES:** Psyc, Northwestern Mem Hosp, Chicago, IL 85-89; **HOSP:** Linden Oaks Hosp; ***SI:*** *Geriatric Mood & Anxiety Disorders; Medication Management*; **HMO:** Blue Cross & Blue Shield, Greenspring, United, Merit Behavioral Health Plans
LANG: Ur; Immediately VISA

Hussain, Ahmed (MD) Psyc
Ravenswood Hosp Med Ctr
40 Timberline Drive; Lemont, IL 60523; (773) 275-4646; **BDCERT:** Psyc 95; **MS:** India 84; **RES:** Psyc, Harvard Med School, Cambridge, MA 90-93; **FEL:** ChAP, Univ of Chicago, Chicago, IL 93-95; **FAP:** Instr Rush Med Coll; **HOSP:** Rock Creek Ctr; ***SI:*** *Depression; Attention Deficit*; **HMO:** United Behavior, Humana Health Plan, Rush Pru, Private Healthcare, Principal Health Care
LANG: Ur, Hin; A Few Days

Sadauskas, J Linas (MD) Psyc
Provena Mercy Ctr
Dreyer Medical Clinic, 1877 W Galena Pl Ste 100; Aurora, IL 60504; (630) 906-5120; **BDCERT:** Psyc 91; **MS:** Univ IL Coll Med 76; **RES:** Psych, Univ of North Carolina NC Meml Hosp, Chapel Hill, NC 84-87

Wyma, Daniel (MD) Psyc
Central DuPage Hosp
1761 S Naperville Rd Ste 200; Wheaton, IL 60187; (630) 260-0606; **BDCERT:** Psyc 85; **MS:** U Iowa Coll Med 80; **RES:** Psyc, U Chicago Hosp, Chicago, IL 81-84; **FEL:** N, Univ of Rochester Medical Center, Rochester, NY 84-85; **HMO:** Blue Cross & Blue Shield
LANG: Sp; 1 Week
VISA

PULMONARY DISEASE

Barsanti, Carl (MD) Pul
Good Samaritan Hosp (see page 274)
Midwest Pulmonary Assoc, 2340 S Highland Ave Ste 230; Lombard, IL 60148; (630) 932-2040; **BDCERT:** Pul 86; CCM 89; **MS:** Loyola U-Stritch Sch Med, Maywood 75; **RES:** IM, Hines VA Hosp, Chicago, IL 80-81; **FEL:** Pul, Rush Presbyterian-St Luke's Med Ctr, Chicago, IL 84; **HOSP:** Gottlieb Mem Hosp; **HMO:** Blue Cross & Blue Shield, Unihealth America, CIGNA, Aetna Hlth Plan +
LANG: Chi, Pol; 1 Week

Freebeck, Peter (MD) Pul
Hinsdale Hosp (see page 275)
Suburban Pulmonary Assoc, 700 E Ogden Ave Ste 202; Westmont, IL 60559; (630) 789-9785; **BDCERT:** IM 89; Pul 92; **MS:** U Chicago-Pritzker Sch Med 86; **RES:** IM, U NC Hosp, Chapel Hill, NC 87-89; **FEL:** Pul, Loyola U Med Ctr, Maywood, IL 89-91

Schupp, Elizabeth (MD) Pul
Alexian Brothers Med Ctr
(see page 138)
1144 Conan Doyle Rd; Naperville, IL 60564; (630) 980-0500; **BDCERT:** IM 90; Pul 98; **MS:** Univ Kans Sch Med 87; **RES:** IM, Rush Presbyterian-St Luke's Med Ctr, Chicago, IL 87-90; IM, Rush Presbyterian-St Luke's Med Ctr, Chicago, IL 90-91; **FEL:** Rhu, Rush Presbyterian-St Luke's Med Ctr, Chicago, IL 91-94; **HOSP:** St Alexius Med Ctr; ***SI:*** *Lung Cancer; Asthma*; **HMO:** Blue Cross & Blue Shield, Aetna Hlth Plan, United Healthcare
A Few Days ***VISA***

Wicks, Mark (MD) Pul
La Grange Mem Hosp (see page 141)
Suburban Pulmonary & Sleep Assoc, 700 E Ogden Ave Ste 202; Westmont, IL 60559; (630) 789-9785; **BDCERT:** Pul 82; CCM 89; **MS:** LSU Med Ctr, Shreveport 73; **RES:** IM, Northwestern Mem Hosp, Chicago, IL 74-75; IM, LSU Hosp, New Orleans, LA 75-76; **FEL:** Pul, Hines VA Hosp, Chicago, IL 76-78; **HOSP:** Hinsdale Hosp; ***SI:*** *Asthma; Emphysema*; **HMO:** Aetna Hlth Plan, Rush Prudential, HMO of IL, CIGNA, UHC +
2-4 Weeks

Zinn, Mary (MD) Pul
Hinsdale Hosp (see page 275)
40 S Chay St Ste 200E; Hinsdale, IL 60521; (630) 734-8550; **BDCERT:** Pul 88; CCM 91; **MS:** Loyola U-Stritch Sch Med, Maywood 82; **RES:** IM, Loyola U Med Ctr, Maywood, IL 83-85; **FEL:** Pul, Northwestern Mem Hosp, Chicago, IL 85-87; **HOSP:** Central DuPage Hosp; **HMO:** +
LANG: Sp;
Immediately ***VISA***

RADIATION ONCOLOGY

Feinstein, Jeffrey M (MD) RadRO
Hinsdale Hosp (see page 275)
120 Oak St; Hinsdale, IL 60521; (630) 856-7350; **BDCERT:** RadRO 76; **MS:** NYU Sch Med 71; **RES:** New York University Med Ctr, New York, NY 72-75; **FAP:** Asst Clin Prof Rad Loyola U-Stritch Sch Med, Maywood; ***SI:*** *Prostate Cancer; Brain Tumors*; **HMO:** Rush Prudential, Blue Cross, CIGNA, Principal Health Care
LANG: Fil, Sp, Hin;
Immediately

Fischer, William (MD) RadRO
Hinsdale Hosp (see page 275)
120 N Oak St; Hinsdale, IL 60521; (630) 856-7350; **BDCERT:** Rad 76; **MS:** Northwestern U 68; **RES:** Rad, Hines VA Hosp, Hines, IL 72-73; RadRO, Therapy - U Chicago, Chicago, IL 73-75

Guide to symbols and abbreviations can be found on pages 110-113.

Galinsky, Dennis (MD) RadRO
Central DuPage Hosp
126 Winfield Rd; Winfield, IL 60190; (847) 781-2300; **BDCERT:** Rad 79; **MS:** U Iowa Coll Med 74; **RES:** RadRO, U Arizona, Tucson, AZ 75-77; RadRO, U MN Med Ctr, Minneapolis, MN 78; **FAP:** Assoc Prof Rush Med Coll; **HOSP:** St Alexius Med Ctr; **HMO:** Aetna Hlth Plan, Blue Cross & Blue Shield, Rush Pru, CIGNA +
LANG: Sp; Immediately VISA

Murthy, Anantha (MD) RadRO
Central DuPage Hosp
Du Page Onc Ctr, 126 Winfield Rd; Winfield, IL 60190; (630) 690-3400; **BDCERT:** Rad 75; **MS:** India 69; **RES:** Harvard Med Sch, Cambridge, MA 72-76; **FAP:** Assoc Prof Rush Med Coll

Sidrys, Jonas (MD) RadRO
Edward Hosp (see page 272)
Intercommunity Cancer Ctr, 3100 Ogden Ave; Lisle, IL 60532; (630) 505-3192; **BDCERT:** RadRO 92; **MS:** Loyola U-Stritch Sch Med, Maywood 86; **RES:** RadRO, UCLA Med Ctr, Los Angeles, CA 87-90; **HOSP:** Hinsdale Hosp; ***SI:*** *Breast Cancer; Prostate Cancer*; **HMO:** Naperville Health Care, CIGNA, Aetna Hlth Plan, Humana Health Plan, PHCS +
LANG: Lth, Sp; Immediately VISA

REPRODUCTIVE ENDOCRINOLOGY

Hickey, Michael (MD) RE
Hinsdale Hosp (see page 275)
Hinsdale Center-Reproduction, 121 N Elm St; Hinsdale, IL 60521; (630) 856-3535; **BDCERT:** ObG 92; **MS:** Loyola U-Stritch Sch Med, Maywood 84; **RES:** ObG, Georgetown U Hosp, Washington, DC 85-88; **FEL:** RE, UCLA Med Ctr, Los Angeles, CA 88-90; ***SI:*** *Ovulation Induction; Endometriosis*; **HMO:** Blue Cross & Blue Shield
2-4 Weeks VISA

Radwanska, Eva (MD) RE
Rush-Presbyterian-St Luke's Med Ctr (see page 122)
Rush-Copley Med Ctr, 2020 Ogden Ave Suite 215; Aurora, IL 60504; (630) 978-6254; **BDCERT:** ObG 81; **MS:** Poland 62; **RES:** ObG, Hillingdon Hosp, London, England 76-77; **FEL:** Univ College, London, England 70-75; Rush Presbyterian-St Luke's Med Ctr, Chicago, IL 83-84; **FAP:** Prof Rush Med Coll; **HOSP:** Rush-Copley Med Ctr; ***SI:*** *Infertility; Endometriosis; Fibroids; Menopause*; **HMO:** UHC, Aetna Hlth Plan, Blue Cross & Blue Shield, Pilgrim Health Care
LANG: Pol, Sp, Rus, Heb;
2-4 Weeks VISA

RHEUMATOLOGY

Graham, Lee D (MD) Rhu
Good Samaritan Hosp (see page 274)
Arthritis Associates Ltd, 1 S 260 Summit Ave Ste 104; Oakbrook, IL 60181; (630) 268-0200; **BDCERT:** IM 87; Rhu 88; **MS:** Stanford U 79; **RES:** Stanford Med Ctr, Stanford, CA 80-83; Oregon Health Sci U Hosp, Portland, OR 85-86; **FEL:** Rhu, Oregon Health Sci U Hosp, Portland, OR 87-89; Ped Rhu, Children's Mem Med Ctr, Chicago, IL 89-90; **HOSP:** Hinsdale Hosp; **HMO:** Aetna Hlth Plan, Blue Cross & Blue Shield, Californiacare, CIGNA, HealthNet

Iammartino, Albert (MD) Rhu
Elmhurst Mem Hosp
Arthritis Associates, 1 Summit Ave Ste 104; Villa Park, IL 60181; (630) 268-0200; **BDCERT:** IM 78; Rhu 80; **MS:** Univ IL Coll Med 75; **RES:** U IL Med Ctr, Chicago, IL 75-78; **FEL:** Northwestern Mem Hosp, Chicago, IL 78-80; **HOSP:** Hinsdale Hosp; ***SI:*** *Arthritis; Osteoporosis*
A Few Days VISA

Lichon, Francis (MD) Rhu
Edward Hosp (see page 272)
511 Thornhill Dr; Carol Stream, IL 60188; (630) 462-7676; **BDCERT:** Rhu 84; IM 81; **MS:** Univ IL Coll Med 78; **RES:** IM, Lutheran Gen Hosp, Park Ridge, IL 79-81; **FEL:** Rhu, U IL Med Ctr, Chicago, IL 81-83; **HMO:** Blue Choice, Blue Cross & Blue Shield, Chicago HMO, CIGNA, Humana Health Plan

SURGERY

Abbasy, Iftikharul (MD) S
Elmhurst Mem Hosp
Villa Medical Arts, 10 E Central Blvd; Villa Park, IL 60181; (630) 832-9000; **BDCERT:** S 74; **MS:** Pakistan 61; **RES:** S, Michael Reese Hosp Med Ctr, Chicago, IL 64-69; **HMO:** Blue Cross & Blue Shield, Humana Health Plan, Aetna Hlth Plan, Private Healthcare, Rush Prudential +
VISA

Airan, Mohan (MD) S
Good Samaritan Hosp (see page 274)
2340 S Highland Ave Ste 250; Lombard, IL 60148; (630) 268-0132; **BDCERT:** S 67; **MS:** India 58; **RES:** S, Mercy Hosp & Med Ctr, Chicago, IL 61-64; S, Mount Sinai Hosp Med Ctr, Chicago, IL 65-66; **FEL:** S, Mount Sinai Hosp Med Ctr, Chicago, IL 67; **FAP:** Clin Prof S U Chicago-Pritzker Sch Med

Altimari, Anthony (MD) S
Central DuPage Hosp
Du Page Surgical Consultants, 1 N 121 County Farm Rd Ste 100; Winfield, IL 60190; (630) 668-0833; **BDCERT:** S 89; **MS:** U Hlth Sci/Chicago Med Sch 83; **RES:** S, Loyola U Med Ctr, Maywood, IL 83-88; ***SI:*** *Laparoscopic Surgery*

Banich, Francis (MD) S
Elmhurst Mem Hosp
Chicago Surgical Society, 340 W Butterfield Rd Ste 1D; Elmhurst, IL 60126; (630) 279-5701; **BDCERT:** S 80; **MS:** Loyola U-Stritch Sch Med, Maywood 57; **RES:** S, Cook Cty Hosp, Chicago, IL 58-63; **FAP:** Assoc Clin Prof S Loyola U-Stritch Sch Med, Maywood; **HOSP:** Good Samaritan Hosp; **HMO:** Aetna Hlth Plan, Blue Cross & Blue Shield, Californiacare, Humana Health Plan, Maxicare Health Plan
1 Week

Belmonte, John (MD) S
Gottlieb Mem Hosp
JVB Medical Ltd, 2340 S Highland Ave Ste 380; Lombard, IL 60148; (630) 261-8111; **BDCERT:** S 72; **MS:** Loyola U-Stritch Sch Med, Maywood 63; **RES:** S, Hines VA Hosp, Chicago, IL 64-68; **HOSP:** Good Samaritan Hosp

Bloom, Allen (MD) S
Rush-Copley Med Ctr
2020 Ogden Ave Ste 210; Aurora, IL 60504; (630) 585-0200; **BDCERT:** S 88; **MS:** Northwestern U 82; **RES:** S, Rush Presbyterian-St Luke's Med Ctr, Chicago, IL 83-87; **FEL:** U Miami Hosp, Miami, FL 87-88; **HOSP:** Provena Mercy Ctr; ***SI:*** *Breast Surgery; Endocrine Surgery*; **HMO:** Blue Cross, CIGNA, Prudential
LANG: Rus, Ukr;
1 Week VISA

Braxton, Jeffrey (MD) S
Delnor Comm Hosp
Brinkman, Spitz & Braxton, 2000 Ogden Ave; Aurora, IL 60504; (630) 820-2727; **BDCERT:** S 95; **MS:** U Mich Med Sch 89; **RES:** S, Rush Presbyterian-St Luke's Med Ctr, Chicago, IL 89-94; **HOSP:** Rush-Copley Med Ctr; ***SI:*** *Hernia Repair; Minimally Invasive Surgery*
Immediately

Broido, Peter (MD) S
Central DuPage Hosp
511 Thornhill Dr; Carol Stream, IL 60188; (630) 665-2101; **BDCERT:** S 74; **MS:** Washington U, St Louis 67; **RES:** S, Barnes Hosp, St Louis, MO 68-69; S, U IL Med Ctr, Chicago, IL 70-71; **FAP:** Asst Clin Prof Univ IL Coll Med; **HMO:** +
Immediately
VISA

Dillon, Bruce C (MD) S
Good Samaritan Hosp (see page 274)
Surgical Consultants-Du Page, 3825 Highland Ave Ste 5H; Downers Grove, IL 60515; (630) 968-4086; **BDCERT:** S 93; **MS:** Eastern VA Med Sch, Norfolk 77; **HOSP:** Hinsdale Hosp

Douglas, Daniel (MD) S
Hinsdale Hosp (see page 275)
Surgical Consultants-Du Page, 3825 Highland Ave Ste 5H; Downers Grove, IL 60515; (630) 325-3310; **BDCERT:** S 96; GVS 93; **MS:** U Hlth Sci/Chicago Med Sch 82; **RES:** S, U IL Med Ctr, Chicago, IL 82-88; **FEL:** GVS, St Louis U Hosp, St Louis, MO 88-89; **HOSP:** Good Samaritan Hosp; **HMO:** Aetna Hlth Plan, Blue Cross & Blue Shield, Californiacare, CIGNA, Healthplus

Gunn, Larry (MD) S
Hinsdale Hosp (see page 275)
Surgical Consultants-Du Page, 3825 Highland Ave Ste 5H; Downers Grove, IL 60515; (630) 968-4086; **BDCERT:** S 69; **MS:** Univ IL Coll Med 63; **RES:** S, U IL Med Ctr, Chicago, IL 64-68; **FAP:** Asst Prof S Univ IL Coll Med; **HOSP:** Good Samaritan Hosp; ***SI:*** *Breast Surgery; Mesh Hernia Repair*; **HMO:** Blue Cross & Blue Choice, HealthNet, Aetna-US Healthcare, Humana Health Plan +
1 Week VISA

Gutta, Gandhi (MD) S
Glen Oaks Hosp and Med Ctr
(see page 273)
Glendale Family Practice, 1919 Midwest Rd; Oak Brook, IL 60523; (630) 351-2021; **BDCERT:** S 81; **MS:** India 64

Hui, Peter (MD) S
Hinsdale Hosp (see page 275)
493 S York St; Elmhurst, IL 60126; (630) 530-0442; **BDCERT:** S 77; HS 90; **MS:** Taiwan 70; **RES:** S, Mount Sinai Hosp Med Ctr, Chicago, IL 72-76; **FEL:** HS, Cook Cty Hosp, Chicago, IL 76-77; **FAP:** Clin Instr Rush Med Coll; **HOSP:** Good Samaritan Hosp; ***SI:*** *Carpal Tunnel Syndrome; Dupuytren's Contracture*; **HMO:** Blue Cross & Blue Shield, Aetna Hlth Plan, Health Options, Prudential
LANG: Chi, Man, Can, Sp;
2-4 Weeks

Indiraraj, Chenni (MD) S
Edward Hosp (see page 272)
6800 S Main St Ste 108; Downers Grove, IL 60516; (630) 852-7575; **BDCERT:** S 96; **MS:** India 65; **RES:** Mount Sinai Hosp Med Ctr, Chicago, IL 70-74; **HMO:** Aetna Hlth Plan, Blue Cross & Blue Shield, Californiacare, CIGNA, Healthcare America

Montana, Louis (MD) S
Edward Hosp (see page 272)
801 S Washington St; Naperville, IL 60566; (630) 961-0423; **BDCERT:** S 94; **MS:** Rush Med Coll 87; **HOSP:** Central DuPage Hosp
VISA

Shayani, Vafa (MD) S
Loyola U Med Ctr (see page 120)
Loyola University MC, 110 N Quincy St; Hinsdale, IL 60521; (708) 327-2899; **BDCERT:** S 96; **MS:** Geo Wash U Sch Med 88; **RES:** S, Geo Wash U Med Ctr, Washington, DC 89-95; **FEL:** S, Geo Wash U Med Ctr, Washington, DC 95-96; **FAP:** Asst Prof S Loyola U-Stritch Sch Med, Maywood; ***SI:*** *Laparoscopic Surgery*

Guide to symbols and abbreviations can be found on pages 110-113.

Tolin, Fredrik (MD) S
Hinsdale Hosp (see page 275)
Surgical Consultants-Du Page, 3825 Highland Ave Ste 5H; Downers Grove, IL 60515; (630) 325-3310; **BDCERT:** S 93; **MS:** Univ Pittsburgh 87; **RES:** LSU Hosp, New Orleans, LA 88-90; U Chicago Hosp, Chicago, IL 91-92; **FAP:** Asst Clin Prof S Univ IL Coll Med; **HOSP:** Good Samaritan Hosp; ***SI:*** *Laparoscopic Surgery*

Wander, John (MD) S
Good Samaritan Hosp (see page 274)
Surgical Consultants-Du Page, 3825 Highland Ave Ste 5H; Downers Grove, IL 60515; (630) 325-3310; **BDCERT:** S 74; **MS:** Univ IL Coll Med 66; **RES:** S, U IL Med Ctr, Chicago, IL 69-73; **FAP:** Asst Clin Prof Univ IL Coll Med; **HOSP:** Hinsdale Hosp; **HMO:** Aetna Hlth Plan, Blue Cross & Blue Shield, CIGNA, Metlife, Principal Health Care

THORACIC SURGERY

Calandra, David (MD) TS
Hinsdale Hosp (see page 275)
Metropolitan Cardiac Surgeons, 111 W Chicago Ave Ste 102; Hinsdale, IL 60521; (630) 655-3031; **BDCERT:** TS 98; S 96; **MS:** Loyola U-Stritch Sch Med, Maywood 80; **RES:** Path CP, Univ of Chicago, Chicago, IL 80-81; S, Loyola U Med Ctr, Maywood, IL 81-86; **FEL:** TS, Loyola U Med Ctr, Maywood, IL 86-88; **FAP:** Asst Prof TS U Chicago-Pritzker Sch Med; ***SI:*** *Cardiovascular Surgery*; **HMO:** +
Mcr Mcd A Few Days

Dieter, Raymond (MD) TS
Central DuPage Hosp
Glen Ellyn Clinic, 454 Pennsylvania Ave; Glen Ellyn, IL 60137; (630) 790-1700; **BDCERT:** TS 69; S 68; **MS:** Loyola U-Stritch Sch Med, Maywood 60; **RES:** S, Hines VA Hosp, Chicago, IL 63-67; TS, Hines VA Hosp, Chicago, IL 67-69; **HOSP:** Elmhurst Mem Hosp; **HMO:** Aetna Hlth Plan

Grieco, John (MD) TS
Good Samaritan Hosp (see page 274)
Cardiac Surgery Assoc, 3825 Highland Ave Ste 310; Downers Grove, IL 60515; (630) 663-1100; **BDCERT:** S 83; TS 85; **MS:** Loyola U-Stritch Sch Med, Maywood 77

Gunnar, William (MD) TS
Hinsdale Hosp (see page 275)
Metropolitan Cardiac Surgeons, 111 W Chicago Ave Ste 102; Hinsdale, IL 60521; (630) 655-3031; **BDCERT:** TS 92; S 91; **MS:** Northwestern U 83; **RES:** S, U IL Med Ctr, Chicago, IL 84-89; **FEL:** TS, Loyola U Med Ctr, Maywood, IL 89-91; **FAP:** Assoc U Chicago-Pritzker Sch Med; **HOSP:** Mercy Hosp & Med Ctr; ***SI:*** *Coronary Artery Disease; Valvular Heart Disease*; **HMO:** Blue Cross & Blue Shield, Aetna Hlth Plan, United Healthcare, Private Healthcare
Mcr Mcd NFI 1 Week

Nigro, Salvatore (MD) TS
Elmhurst Mem Hosp
1 Summit Ave; Oakbrook Terrace, IL 60181; (630) 916-9669; **BDCERT:** TS 61; S 59; **MS:** Univ Nebr Coll Med 52; **RES:** Children's Mem Med Ctr, Chicago, IL 57-58; St Francis Hosp, Blue Island, IL 55-57; **FEL:** TS, U Chicago Hosp, Chicago, IL 59-60; **HOSP:** Edward Hosp

UROLOGY

Bockrath, John M. (MD) U
Edward Hosp (see page 272)
Du Page Urology Assoc, 10 W Martin Ave; Naperville, IL 60540; (630) 369-1572; **BDCERT:** U 84; **MS:** Northwestern U 76; **RES:** S, Northwestern Mem Hosp, Chicago, IL 77-78; U, Northwestern Mem Hosp, Chicago, IL 78-82; **FAP:** Clin Instr Northwestern U; **HOSP:** Good Samaritan Hosp; **HMO:** +
Mcr Mcd 4+ Weeks VISA

Kritsas, John (MD) U
Hinsdale Hosp (see page 275)
York Urologic Assoc, 950 N York Rd Ste 208; Hinsdale, IL 60521; (630) 887-0580; **BDCERT:** U 94; **MS:** Harvard Med Sch 85; **RES:** S, U Chicago Hosp, Chicago, IL 86-88; U, Harvard Med Sch, Cambridge, MA 88-92; **HOSP:** La Grange Mem Hosp; ***SI:*** *Cancer Surgery; Kidney Stone Disease*; **HMO:** Aetna Hlth Plan, Humana Health Plan, Rush Health Plans, Preferred Care +
LANG: Sp, Grk; Mcr Mcd
A Few Days

Merrick, Paul (MD) U
Central DuPage Hosp
Glen Ellyn Clinic, 454 Pennsylvania Ave; Glen Ellyn, IL 60137; (630) 740-1221; **BDCERT:** U 96; **MS:** Rush Med Coll 89

Nuzzarello, Joseph (MD) U
Elmhurst Mem Hosp
Urology Associates of Du Page, 103 Haven Rd; Elmhurst, IL 60126; (630) 833-8525; **BDCERT:** U 93; **MS:** Loyola U-Stritch Sch Med, Maywood 85; **RES:** U, Loyola U Med Ctr, Maywood, IL 87-91; S, Loyola U Med Ctr, Maywood, IL 86-87; **FEL:** Onc, Loyola U Med Ctr, Maywood, IL 90-91; **HMO:** Aetna Hlth Plan, Blue Cross & Blue Shield, Chicago HMO, CIGNA, Humana Health Plan

Sosenko, George (MD) **U**
St Mary's of Nazareth Hosp Ctr
2425 W 22nd St Ste 213; Oak Brook, IL 60523; (630) 574-7770; **BDCERT:** U 84; **MS:** U Hlth Sci/Chicago Med Sch 77; **RES:** U, Rush Presbyterian-St Luke's Med Ctr, Chicago, IL; ***SI:*** *Urinary Incontinence; Prostate & Bladder Cancer*

VASCULAR SURGERY (GENERAL)

Govostis, Dean (MD) **GVS**
Christ Hosp & Med Ctr **(see page 140)**
4400 95th St Ste 205; Oak Lawn, IL 60553; (708) 346-4040; **BDCERT:** GVS 94; S 91; **MS:** Northwestern U 84; **RES:** S, Med Coll WI, Milwaukee, WI 85-90; **FEL:** GVS, U FL Shands Hosp, Gainesville, FL 90-91; **HOSP:** Little Company of Mary Hosp & Hlth Care Ctrs

KANE COUNTY

KANE COUNTY

Specialties are indicated in bold-type face. Capital letters indicate Primary Care Specialties. Subspecialties are listed in non-bold type. Listings indicate if a doctor is certified in a subspecialty but predominately practices primary care medicine.

*Oncologists deal with Cancer

ANESTHESIOLOGY

Cherala, Sundaraj (MD) **Anes**
St Joseph Hosp-Elgin
St Joseph Hosp, 77 N Airlite St; Elgin, IL 60123; (847) 695-3200; **BDCERT:** Anes 88; PM 94; **MS:** India 77; **RES:** S, Interfaith Med Ctr, Brooklyn, NY 83-85; Anes, Maimonides Med Ctr, Brooklyn, NY 85-87; **FEL:** Anes, U of Alabama Hosp, Birmingham, AL 87-88; ***SI:*** *Pain Management*; **HMO:** +
LANG: Sp; A Few Days

Hewell, Charles (MD) **Anes**
Delnor Comm Hosp
300 Randall Rd; Geneva, IL 60134; (630) 208-4060; **BDCERT:** Anes 90; PM 94; **MS:** Loyola U-Stritch Sch Med, Maywood 84; **RES:** Anes, Tulane U Med Ctr, New Orleans, LA 84-87; **HMO:** Blue Cross & Blue Shield

Sison, Jose (MD) **Anes**
Provena Mercy Ctr
Aurora Radiology Consultants, 1325 N Highland Ave; Aurora, IL 60506; (630) 859-2222; **BDCERT:** Anes 78; **MS:** Philippines 71; **RES:** U Wisc Hosp, Madison, WI 73-75; Northwestern Mem Hosp, Chicago, IL 75-76; **HMO:** Blue Cross & Blue Shield, CIGNA

Tsang, Hung-Shing (MD) **Anes**
Provena Mercy Ctr
Aurora Anesthesia, 1325 N Highland Ave; Aurora, IL 60506; (630) 859-2222; **BDCERT:** Anes 72; **MS:** Taiwan 65; **HMO:** Aetna Hlth Plan, Blue Cross & Blue Shield, Chicago HMO, CIGNA, Metlife

CARDIOLOGY (CARDIOVASCULAR DISEASE)

Gill, Santosh (MD) **Cv**
Provena Mercy Ctr
Fox Valley Cardiovascular, 1315 N Highland Ave Ste 204; Aurora, IL 60506; (630) 896-0566; **BDCERT:** IM 82; Cv 89; **MS:** India 76; **RES:** IM, Mount Sinai Hosp Med Ctr, Chicago, IL 79-82; **FEL:** Cv, Michael Reese Hosp Med Ctr, Chicago, IL 82-84; **HOSP:** Grant Hosp

Riaz, Muhamad Khalid (MD) **Cv**
Sherman Hosp
Elgin Cardiology Assoc, 87 N Airlite St; Elgin, IL 60123; (847) 741-6100; **BDCERT:** IM 78; Cv 79; **MS:** Pakistan 71; **RES:** Cv, Cook Cty Hosp, Chicago, IL 73-76; **FEL:** Cv, Cook Cty Hosp, Chicago, IL 76-78

DIAGNOSTIC RADIOLOGY

Kennard, Donald R (MD) **DR**
Sherman Hosp
Sherman Hosp, 934 Centre St; Elgin, IL 60120; (847) 742-9800; **BDCERT:** DR 84; **MS:** Univ IL Coll Med 80

Schwartz, Michael (MD) **DR**
St Joseph Hosp-Elgin
77 N Airlite St; Elgin, IL 60123; (847) 931-5516; **BDCERT:** DR 75; NuM 76; **MS:** Univ IL Coll Med 68; **RES:** Michael Reese Hosp Med Ctr, Chicago, IL 69-70; Michael Reese Hosp Med Ctr, Chicago, IL 72-74; **FEL:** NuM, Michael Reese Hosp Med Ctr, Chicago, IL 74-75; **HMO:** Aetna Hlth Plan, Blue Cross & Blue Shield, CIGNA, Chicago HMO, Metlife

ENDOCRINOLOGY, DIABETES & METABOLISM

Bielski, Steven (MD) **EDM**
Delnor Comm Hosp
Fox Valley Endocrinology, 302 Randall Rd Ste 304; Geneva, IL 60134; (630) 208-6775; **BDCERT:** EDM 92; **MS:** Loyola U-Stritch Sch Med, Maywood 86; **RES:** IM, Loyola U Med Ctr, Maywood, IL 90-92; **FEL:** EDM, Loyola U Med Ctr, Maywood, IL 92-94; **HOSP:** Provena Mercy Ctr; ***SI:*** *Diabetes; Thyroid*; **HMO:** Blue Cross & Blue Shield, Aetna Hlth Plan, PHCS, CIGNA
1 Week

Valika, Karim (MD) **EDM**
Sherman Hosp
1425 N Mclean Blvd Ste 700; Elgin, IL 60123; (847) 697-0770; **BDCERT:** IM 74; EDM 75; **MS:** Pakistan 68; **RES:** IM, Hartford Hosp, Hartford, CT 71-73; **FEL:** EDM, Hartford Hosp, Hartford, CT 73-74

FAMILY PRACTICE

Neubauer, Joseph (MD) **FP**
PCP
Delnor Comm Hosp
Fox Valley Family Physicians, 2425 Fargo Blvd; Geneva, IL 60134; (630) 232-2200; **BDCERT:** FP 94; **MS:** Rush Med Coll 84; **RES:** FP, Lutheran Gen Hosp, Park Ridge, IL 84-87

Poulos, Dorothea (MD) **FP**
PCP
Sherman Hosp
Elgin Family Physicians, 901 Center St Ste 304; Elgin, IL 60120; (847) 888-3661; **BDCERT:** FP 91; **MS:** Harvard Med Sch 82; **RES:** FP, Cook Cty Hosp, Chicago, IL 83-85

FORENSIC PSYCHIATRY

Dinwiddie, Stephen H (MD) FPsy
Elgin Mental Hlth Ctr
Elgin Mental Health Center, 750 S State St; Elgin, IL 60123; (847) 742-1040; **BDCERT:** Psyc 88; FPsy 94; **MS:** Eastern VA Med Sch, Norfolk 82; **RES:** Psyc, Barnes Hosp, St Louis, MO 82-86; **FAP:** Prof FPsy U Hlth Sci/Chicago Med Sch; ***SI:*** *Forensic Psychiatry; Addiction Psychiatry*
♿

GASTROENTEROLOGY

Faulk, David (MD) Ge
Edward Hosp **(see page 272)**
302 Randall Rd; Geneva, IL 60134; (630) 377-6229; **BDCERT:** Ge 79; IM 76; **MS:** U Iowa Coll Med 73; **RES:** IM, Rush Presby-St Lukes Hosp, Chicago, IL 74-76; Ge, U Iowa Hosp, Iowa City, IA 76-78; **HOSP:** Central DuPage Hosp

Gekas, Paul (MD) Ge
Delnor Comm Hosp
Greater Valley Medicine, 302 Randall Rd; Geneva, IL 60134; (630) 208-5959; **BDCERT:** Ge 91; IM 81; **MS:** Loyola U-Stritch Sch Med, Maywood 72; **RES:** IM, Loyola U Med Ctr, Maywood, IL 73-75; **FEL:** Ge, Baltimore City Hosp, Baltimore, MD 76-78

Hossain, Zahur (MD) Ge
Sherman Hosp
Elgin Gastro SC, 1425 N McLean Blvd Ste 600; Elgin, IL 60123; (847) 888-1300; **BDCERT:** Ge 77; IM 73; **MS:** Bangladesh 62; **RES:** IM, Wayne Cnty Gen Hosp, Detroit, MI 65-68; **FEL:** Ge, U UT Hosp, Salt Lake City, UT 68-70; **HOSP:** Good Shepherd Hosp

GERIATRIC MEDICINE

Lewis, Steven (MD) Ger
Delnor Comm Hosp
1725 South St; Geneva, IL 60134; (630) 232-6111; **BDCERT:** Ger 92; IM 80; **MS:** Univ IL Coll Med 77; **RES:** U IL Med Ctr, Chicago, IL; **FEL:** Inf, U IL Med Ctr, Chicago, IL 80-82; **HOSP:** Marianjoy Rehab Hosp & Clinics; **HMO:** Aetna Hlth Plan, Blue Cross & Blue Shield, Chicago HMO, Humana Health Plan, Prudential

Susarla, Visi (MD) Ger
PCP
St Joseph Hosp-Elgin
860 Summit St Ste 123; Elgin, IL 60120; (847) 741-0026; **BDCERT:** Ger 99; IM 77; **MS:** India 69; **RES:** IM, St Francis Hosp of Evanston, Evanston, IL 71-74; **HOSP:** Sherman Hosp; ***SI:*** *Diabetes; Urinary Incontinence*; **HMO:** CIGNA, Aetna Hlth Plan, PHCS, HMO of IL +
LANG: Sp; ♿
A Few Days VISA

INTERNAL MEDICINE

Baley, Richard (MD) IM
PCP
Sherman Hosp
860 Summit St; Elgin, IL 60120; (847) 742-3525; **BDCERT:** IM 88; **MS:** Rush Med Coll 85; **HOSP:** St Joseph Hosp-Elgin

Kerpe, Algimantas Steponas (MD) IM
PCP
Delnor Comm Hosp
Greater Valley Medicine, 302 Randall Rd Ste 20; Geneva, IL 60134; (630) 208-5959; **BDCERT:** IM 83; **MS:** Univ IL Coll Med 80; **RES:** IM, L A Weiss Mem Hosp-U Chicago Hosp, Chicago, IL 81-83; ***SI:*** *Headaches; Women's Health*

Shah, Devendra (MD) IM
PCP
Sherman Hosp
Shah Medical Ctr, 484 Summit St; Elgin, IL 60120; (847) 742-5530; **BDCERT:** IM 90; Ger 92; **MS:** India 72; **RES:** Nep, Westchester County Med Ctr, Valhalla, NY 78-79; IM, Westchester County Med Ctr, Valhalla, NY 77-78; **FEL:** Nep, Bronx Lebanon Hosp Ctr, Bronx, NY 79-80; **HOSP:** St Joseph Hosp-Elgin; **HMO:** Aetna Hlth Plan, Blue Cross & Blue Shield, Principal Health Care, Takecare Health Plan, Travelers

NEPHROLOGY

Ahmad, Nasir (MD) Nep
Sherman Hosp
Elgin Nephrology Assoc, 296 W Spring St; South Elgin, IL 60177; (847) 697-2692; **BDCERT:** Nep 78; IM 74; **MS:** India 68; **RES:** IM, Hines VA Hosp, Chicago, IL 69-71; Nep, Hines VA Hosp, Chicago, IL 71-73

Zahid, Mohammad (MD) Nep
St Joseph Hosp-Elgin
Elgin Clinic, 87 N Airlite St G15; Elgin, IL 60123; (847) 697-6464; **BDCERT:** IM 89; Nep 97; **MS:** Pakistan 78; **RES:** DR, Wayne State U, Detroit, MI 83-84; IM, Wayne State U, Detroit, MI 84-85; **FEL:** Nep, Northwestern Mem Hosp, Chicago, IL 85-87; **HOSP:** Sherman Hosp; **HMO:** +
♿ Mcr Mcd 1 Week

Guide to symbols and abbreviations can be found on pages 110-113.

NEUROLOGICAL SURGERY

Mansfield, James (MD) NS
Sherman Hosp
Neurological & Spinal Surgery, 901 Center St Ste 107; Elgin, IL 60120; (847) 695-6000; **BDCERT:** NS 77; **MS:** Northwestern U 68; **RES:** N, Northwestern Mem Hosp, Chicago, IL 71-72; NS, U IL Med Ctr, Chicago, IL 72-75; **HMO:** Aetna Hlth Plan, Blue Cross & Blue Shield, Californiacare, Chicago HMO, Choicecare
A Few Days

Mazur, John (MD) NS
Provena Mercy Ctr
Premier Healthcare Assoc, 1315 N Highland Rd; Aurora, IL 60506; (630) 262-1210; **BDCERT:** NS 80; **MS:** Northwestern U 72; **RES:** NS, U IL Med Ctr, Chicago, IL 74-78; **FAP:** Asst Clin Instr Univ IL Coll Med; **HMO:** Blue Cross & Blue Shield, Principal Health Care, Prudential, Rush Health Plans, Sanus

NEUROLOGY

Gavino, Wayne (MD) N
Sherman Hosp
Fox Valley Neurology, 860 Summit St Ste 254; Elgin, IL 60120; (847) 695-8721; **BDCERT:** N 86; **MS:** Philippines 73; **RES:** N, Northwestern Mem Hosp, Chicago, IL 75-78; **HMO:** Aetna Hlth Plan
VISA

NUCLEAR MEDICINE

Behal, Rajan (MD) NuM
Sherman Hosp
Nuclear Med Dept - Sherman Hospital, 934 Center St Ext 8220; Elgin, IL 60120; (847) 742-9800; **BDCERT:** NuM 85; DR 84; **MS:** Kenya 76; **RES:** RadRO, Ill Masonic, Chicago, IL 80-83; NuM, Johns Hopkins Hosp, Baltimore, MD 83-85; **FEL:** VIR, U Pittsburgh Hosp, Pittsburgh, PA 85-86

OBSTETRICS & GYNECOLOGY

Epstein, Brad (MD) ObG
PCP
Sherman Hosp
Suburban Women's Health Spclst, 87 N Airlite St Ste 100; Elgin, IL 60123; (847) 931-4747; **BDCERT:** ObG 86; **MS:** U Chicago-Pritzker Sch Med 80; **RES:** ObG, Rush Presbyterian-St Luke's Med Ctr, Chicago, IL 80-84; **HOSP:** St Alexius Med Ctr; ***SI:*** *Menopausal Syndrome; Pelvic Reconstruction*; **HMO:** Blue Cross & Blue Shield, CIGNA, Aetna Hlth Plan, United Healthcare, PHCS +
A Few Days
VISA

Schleifer, Donald (MD) ObG
PCP
Sherman Hosp
374 Summit St; Elgin, IL 60120; (847) 741-5850; **BDCERT:** ObG 62; **MS:** Univ IL Coll Med 53; **RES:** ObG, Cook Cty Hosp, Chicago, IL 54-57; ObG, Northwestern Mem Hosp, Chicago, IL 56; **FAP:** Asst Prof Rush Med Coll; **HOSP:** St Joseph Hosp-Chicago; ***SI:*** *Gynecology; Urinary Incontinence*; **HMO:** Blue Cross & Blue Shield, United Healthcare, Humana Health Plan, CIGNA, Rush Health Plans +
LANG: Sp;
Immediately VISA

West, Ann (MD) ObG
Provena Mercy Ctr
Dreyer Ambulatory Surgery Ctr, 1221 N Highland Ave; Aurora, IL 60506; (630) 264-8840; **BDCERT:** ObG 91; **MS:** U Wisc Med Sch 84; **RES:** ObG, Mount Sinai Hosp Med Ctr, Chicago, IL 84-88

OPHTHALMOLOGY

Bernstein, Sidney (MD) Oph
Sherman Hosp
Simpson Eye Assoc, 650 Springhill Ring Rd Ste 2020; Dundee, IL 60118; (847) 426-0227; **BDCERT:** Oph 75; **MS:** Univ IL Coll Med 65; **RES:** IM, Mayo Clinic, Rochester, MN 68-70; Oph, Mayo Clinic, Rochester, MN 70-73; **HMO:** Blue Cross & Blue Shield, Metropolitan
VISA

Bhatt, Anjali (MD) Oph
St Joseph Hosp-Chicago
Associates Ear Nose & Throat, 2050 Larkin Ave Ste 102; Elgin, IL 60123; (847) 742-7458; **BDCERT:** Oph 77; **MS:** India 68; **RES:** Oph, Irwin Hosp, New Delhi, India 69-71; Oph, Michael Reese Hosp Med Ctr, Chicago, IL 74-77; **FEL:** Retina, Mount Sinai Hosp, Cleveland, OH 73-74
VISA

Foody, Robert (MD) Oph
Provena Mercy Ctr
Aurora Eye Clinic Ltd, 1300 N Highland Ave Ste 1; Aurora, IL 60506; (630) 897-5104; **BDCERT:** Oph 90; **MS:** Loyola U-Stritch Sch Med, Maywood 88; **HOSP:** Rush-Copley Med Ctr; ***SI:*** *Refractive Surgery*
LANG: Sp, Ger;
VISA

Guay-Bhatia, Lise Anne (MD) **Oph**
Central DuPage Hosp
Aurora Eye Clinic Ltd, 1300 N Highland Ave Ste 1; Aurora, IL 60506; (630) 897-5104; **BDCERT:** Ped 91; **MS:** Loyola U-Stritch Sch Med, Maywood 86; **RES:** Oph, Loyola U Med Ctr, Maywood, IL 87-90; Ped, U IL Med Ctr, Chicago, IL 90-92; **HOSP:** Good Samaritan Hosp
1 Week

ORTHOPAEDIC SURGERY

Berkson, Michael (MD) **OrS**
Sherman Hosp
Associates-Orthopaedic Surgery, 380 Summit St; Elgin, IL 60120; (847) 888-0750; **MS:** Loyola U-Stritch Sch Med, Maywood 79; **HOSP:** St Joseph Hosp-Chicago; **HMO:** Aetna Hlth Plan, Blue Cross & Blue Shield

Gitelis, Michael (MD) **OrS**
Good Shepherd Hosp
Orthopedic & Spine Surgery, 75 Market St Ste 4; Elgin, IL 60123; (847) 931-5300; **BDCERT:** OrS 84; **MS:** U Hlth Sci/Chicago Med Sch 76; **RES:** Rush Presbyterian-St Luke's Med Ctr, Chicago, IL 77-80; **FEL:** OrS, Rush Presbyterian-St Luke's Med Ctr, Chicago, IL 80-81; **FAP:** Instr Rush Med Coll; **HMO:** +
VISA

Ketterling, Kevan (MD) **OrS**
Delnor Comm Hosp
Fox Valley Orthopaedic Assoc, 2525 Kaneville Rd; Geneva, IL 60134; (630) 584-1400; **BDCERT:** OrS 93; **MS:** Northwestern U 85; **RES:** OrS, Grand Rapids Res Program, Grand Rapids, MI 86-90; **FEL:** SM, Ortho Cons Cincinnati, Cincinnati, OH 90-91; **HOSP:** St Joseph Hosp-Elgin; ***SI:*** *Knee Reconstruction; Sports Medicine*
LANG: Sp; A Few Days
VISA

O'Connor, Scott (MD) **OrS**
Univ of Illinois at Chicago Med Ctr
Castle Orthopaedics & Sports, 302 Randall Rd Ste 308; Geneva, IL 60134; (630) 208-4600; **BDCERT:** OrS 90; **MS:** Univ IL Coll Med 83

Witt, Paul (MD) **OrS**
Provena Mercy Ctr
Castle Orthopedics, 1315 Highland Avenue; Aurora, IL 60506; (630) 892-4286; **BDCERT:** OrS 83; **MS:** Univ IL Coll Med 76; **RES:** OrS, U IL Med Ctr, Chicago, IL 77-81; **HOSP:** Rush-Copley Med Ctr; ***SI:*** *Arthroscopy; Joint Replacement*; **HMO:** Blue Cross & Blue Shield, Aetna Hlth Plan, Affordable Hlth Plan, Health Direct
A Few Days VISA

OTOLARYNGOLOGY

Bhatt, Nikhil (MD) **Oto**
Sherman Hosp
Associates Ear Nose & Throat, 2050 Larkin Ave Ste 102; Elgin, IL 60123; (847) 742-7458; **BDCERT:** Oto 79; **MS:** India 68

Consiglio, Angelo (MD) **Oto**
Central DuPage Hosp
Otolaryngology Head & Neck Ltd, 2900 Foxfield Rd Ste 202; St Charles, IL 60174; (630) 377-8708; **BDCERT:** Oto 88; **MS:** Univ IL Coll Med 83; **RES:** Oto, Loyola U Med Ctr, Maywood, IL 84-88; S, Loyola U Med Ctr, Maywood, IL 83-84; **FAP:** Asst Prof Loyola U-Stritch Sch Med, Maywood; **HMO:** Aetna Hlth Plan, Blue Cross & Blue Shield, CIGNA, Metlife, Travelers

De Bartolo Jr, Hansel M (MD) **Oto**
Delnor Comm Hosp
11 Debartolo Dr; Sugar Grove, IL 60554; (630) 859-1818; **BDCERT:** Oto 84; **MS:** Loyola U-Stritch Sch Med, Maywood 72; **RES:** Mayo Clinic, Rochester, MN; Geisinger Med Ctr, Danville, PA; ***SI:*** *Laser Skin Resurfacing; Anti-Aging Medicine*
Immediately
VISA

Levine, Toni (MD) **Oto**
Sherman Hosp
1800 McDonough Rd Suite 201; Hoffman Estates, 60192; (847) 741-7300; **BDCERT:** Oto 85; **RES:** S, Cook County 80-82; Oto, Northwestern Mem Med Ctr, Chicago, IL 82-85; **FAP:** Asst Prof Oto Northwestern U

PEDIATRICS

Camras, Louis E (MD) **Ped**
Provena Mercy Ctr
Aurora Pediatric Clinic, 1300 N Highland Ave; Aurora, IL 60506; (630) 896-7788; **BDCERT:** Ped 90; **MS:** Univ IL Coll Med 87; **RES:** Ped, Lutheran Gen Hosp, Park Ridge, IL 88-90

Granger, Sylvia (MD) **Ped**
Provena Mercy Ctr
Aurora Pediatric Clinic, 1300 N Highland Ave; Aurora, IL 60506; (630) 896-7788; **BDCERT:** Ped 72; **MS:** LSU Sch Med, New Orleans 67; **RES:** Tenn Meml Rsch Hosp, Knoxville, TN 68-69; St Paul Childrens Hosp, St Paul, MN 70; **FEL:** U MN Med Ctr, Minneapolis, MN; **HMO:** Aetna Hlth Plan, Blue Cross & Blue Shield, CIGNA, Metlife

Guide to symbols and abbreviations can be found on pages 110-113.

Hao, Crispin (MD) Ped
PCP
Provena Mercy Ctr
Aurora Pediatric Clinic, 1300 N Highland Ave; Aurora, IL 60506; (630) 896-7788; **BDCERT:** Ped 74; **MS:** Philippines 66; **RES:** St Luke's Hosp, Cleveland, OH 68-69; Michael Reese Hosp Med Ctr, Chicago, IL 69-71; **FEL:** Ambulatory Ped, Evanston Hosp, Evanston, IL 71-72; **HMO:** Aetna Hlth Plan, Blue Cross & Blue Shield, Californiacare, Metlife, Travelers

PLASTIC SURGERY

Manus, Dean (MD) PlS
Sherman Hosp
Valley Place Surgical Center, 350 S 8th St; Dundee, IL 60118; (847) 836-3200; **BDCERT:** PlS 97; S 94; **MS:** Rush Med Coll 87; **RES:** S, UC San Francisco Med Ctr, San Francisco, CA 88-92; PlS, Providence Hosp, Southfield, MI 92-94

PSYCHIATRY

Anwar, Syed (MD) Psyc
St Joseph Hosp-Elgin
Associates In Psychiatry, 2050 Larkin Ave Ste 202; Elgin, IL 60123; (847) 697-2400; **BDCERT:** Psyc 93; **MS:** India 78; **RES:** Psyc, Norwich Hosp, Norwich, CT 85-88

Mcr

Hartman, Edith (MD) Psyc
Elgin Mental Hlth Ctr
Elgin Mental Health Ctr, 750 S State St; Elgin, IL 60123; (847) 742-1040; **BDCERT:** Psyc 83; **MS:** Germany 58; **RES:** Psyc, Univ of Illinois at Chicago Psyciatric Institute, Chicago, IL 73-76; **FEL:** Psyc, Univ of Illinois at Chicago Psyciatric Institute, Chicago, IL 76-77; ***SI:*** *Forensic Psychiatry*
LANG: Ger;

PULMONARY DISEASE

Liske, Thomas (MD) Pul
Provena Mercy Ctr
Foxland Respiratory Cnsltnts, 1315 N Highland Ave Ste 204; Aurora, IL 60506; (630) 896-5535; **BDCERT:** Pul 82; IM 77; **MS:** Loyola U-Stritch Sch Med, Maywood 68; **RES:** IM, Hines VA Hosp, Chicago, IL 69-72; **FEL:** Pul, Hines VA Hosp, Chicago, IL 75-77

RADIATION ONCOLOGY

Shafer, Jeff (MD) RadRO
St Joseph Hosp-Elgin
St Joseph Hospital-Elgin, Dept of Radiation, 77 N Airlite St; Elgin, IL 60123; (847) 695-3200; **BDCERT:** RadRO 77; **MS:** UC Irvine 70; **HOSP:** Sherman Hosp

RHEUMATOLOGY

Lichtenberg, Lee (MD) Rhu
Sherman Hosp
1425 N Mclean Blvd Ste 800; Elgin, IL 60123; (847) 931-1988; **BDCERT:** Rhu 80; IM 78; **MS:** Loyola U-Stritch Sch Med, Maywood 75; **RES:** IM, Hines VA Hosp, Chicago, IL 76-78; **FEL:** Rhu, Hines VA Hosp, Chicago, IL 78-80; **FAP:** Asst Clin Prof Med Loyola U-Stritch Sch Med, Maywood; **HOSP:** St Joseph Hosp-Elgin; **HMO:** Blue Cross & Blue Shield, Metropolitan

SURGERY

Aron, Raul (MD) S
Sherman Hosp
General & Vascular Surgery Ltd, 1795 Grandstand Pl; Elgin, IL 60123; (847) 695-6600; **BDCERT:** S 77; **MS:** 71; **RES:** S, Cleveland Clinic Hosp, Cleveland, OH 73-76; **FEL:** GVS, Cleveland Clinic Hosp, Cleveland, OH 76-77; **HOSP:** St Joseph Hosp-Chicago; ***SI:*** *Breast Cancer; Laparoscopic Surgery*; **HMO:** +
LANG: Sp; Mcr
A Few Days

Farbota, Leo (MD) S
Sherman Hosp
General & Vascular Surgery Ltd, 1795 Grandstand Pl; Elgin, IL 60123; (847) 695-6600; **BDCERT:** S 90; **MS:** Univ IL Coll Med 83; **RES:** S, Loyola U Med Ctr, Maywood, IL 83-88; **HOSP:** Provena Mercy Ctr; **HMO:** Health Preferred, Health Direct, Aetna Hlth Plan, Humana Health Plan +

Mcr Mcd

Kim, Chang (MD) S
Delnor Comm Hosp
302 Randall Rd Ste 209; Geneva, IL 60134; (630) 208-1700; **BDCERT:** S 79; **MS:** South Korea 62; **RES:** S, Nassau County Med Ctr, East Meadow, NY 72-76; **FEL:** GVS, Univ Hosp SUNY Stony Brook, Stony Brook, NY 76-77; **HOSP:** Rush-Copley Med Ctr; ***SI:*** *Vascular Surgery*; **HMO:** Aetna Hlth Plan, Blue Cross & Blue Shield, Californiacare, CIGNA, Comprecare Healthcare
LANG: Kor; Mcr Mcd

Michelotti, Joseph (MD) S
Sherman Hosp
Elgin Surgeons Ltd, 1 W American Way; Arlington Hts, IL 60120; (847) 741-3677; **BDCERT:** S 91; **MS:** Northwestern U 76; **RES:** S, Northwestern Mem Hosp, Chicago, IL 76-81

Mcr

Guide to symbols and abbreviations can be found on pages 110-113.

Russ, Joseph (MD) S
Delnor Comm Hosp
Midwest Surgery, S.C., 2210 Dean St Ste B; St Charles, IL 60175; (630) 377-5300; **BDCERT:** S 97; **MS:** Northwestern U 70; **RES:** S, Johns Hopkins Hosp, Baltimore, MD 70-71; S, Northwestern Mem Hosp, Chicago, IL 74-76; **FEL:** Surg Onc, Northwestern Mem Hosp, Chicago, IL 76-77; Surg Onc, MD Anderson Cancer Ctr, Houston, TX 77-78; **HOSP:** Sherman Hosp; ***SI:*** *Laparoscopic Surgery; Cancer Surgery*; **HMO:** Aetna Hlth Plan, Blue Cross & Blue Shield, Californiacare, Principal Health Care +
Immediately VISA

White, John (MD) S
Delnor Comm Hosp
Midwest Surgery, 2210 Dean Street Suite B; St. Charles, IL 60175; (630) 377-5300; **BDCERT:** S 91; **MS:** Ind U Sch Med 84; **RES:** S, Med Coll WI, Milwaukee, WI 85-90; **HOSP:** Sherman Hosp; ***SI:*** *Laparoscopic Surgery; Cancer Surgery*; **HMO:** Aetna Hlth Plan, CIGNA, Medicare, Blue Cross & Blue Shield
Immediately VISA

THORACIC SURGERY

Cavallo, Charles A. (MD) TS
St Joseph Hosp-Elgin
Northwest Cardiothoracic, 87 N Airlite St G16; Elgin, IL 60123; (847) 695-5333; **BDCERT:** TS 97; **MS:** Northwestern U 66; **RES:** Ped, Children's Mem Med Ctr, Chicago, IL 74; Walter Reed Army Med Ctr, Washington, DC; **FEL:** St Francis Hosp of Evanston, Evanston, IL 67-68; **HOSP:** Good Shepherd Hosp; ***SI:*** *Video-Assisted Thoracotomy*; **HMO:** +
Immediately

Steimle, Cynthia (MD) TS
Sherman Hosp
Elgin Cardiac Surgery, 302 Randall Rd; Geneva, IL 60134; (630) 208-7360; **BDCERT:** TS 96; **MS:** U Mich Med Sch 86; **RES:** S, U Mich Med Ctr, Ann Arbor, MI 87-92; TS, U Mich Med Ctr, Ann Arbor, MI 93-95; **FEL:** SCC, U Mich Med Ctr, Ann Arbor, MI 92-93; **FAP:** Asst Clin Prof Univ IL Coll Med

UROLOGY

Banti, Gustavo (MD) U
Delnor Comm Hosp
G M Banti Ltd, 302 Randall Rd Ste 306; Geneva, IL 60134; (630) 377-1368; **BDCERT:** U 84; **MS:** Argentina 72; **RES:** Cook Cty Hosp, Chicago, IL 78-82; **FEL:** Ped U, Montreal Children's Hosp, Montreal, Canada 81; **HMO:** Aetna Hlth Plan, Blue Cross & Blue Shield, Californiacare, CIGNA, Metlife

Guide to symbols and abbreviations can be found on pages 110-113.

LAKE COUNTY

LAKE FOREST HOSPITAL

660 N. WESTMORELAND RD.
LAKE FOREST, IL 60045
PHONE: (847) 234-5600
FAX: (847) 234-6552

www.lakeforesthospital.com

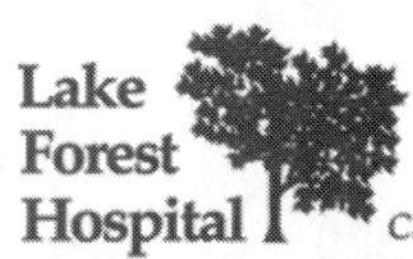

Caring for the Quality of Your Life SM

Sponsorship	Private Not-for-Profit
Beds	204 beds
Accreditation	Joint Commission on Accreditation of Healthcare Organizations (JCAHO), American College of Surgeons, College of American Pathologists, American College of Radiology, Commission on Accreditation of Rehabilitation Facilities, Illinois Department of Public Health.

CARING FOR THE QUALITY OF YOUR LIFE

We want to be the place you think of first in Lake County to get well or stay healthy. To us, that's what "Caring for the Quality of Your Life" means. We strive to achieve this goal through providing comprehensive, state-of-the-art health care in a warm and caring environment.

MEDICAL STAFF

A medical staff of more than 450 dedicated physicians is available to serve you. Nearly all of Lake Forest Hospital's physicians are board certified or pursuing board certification in their specialties - considered the highest standard of physician credentials.

COMPREHENSIVE SERVICES

Lake Forest Hospital's full continuum of services includes:

Maternity Services — More babies are delivered each year at Lake Forest Hospital than at any other hospital in Lake County. Our Level II Perinatal designation allows our on-site perinatologists to care for mothers during high-risk pregnancies and our neonatologists to provide advanced care for newborns. And we offer the services of some of the area's finest pediatricians, so you'll be sure to find just the right one for your baby. Our beautifully decorated birthing suites are designed for patient comfort and include the latest in fetal monitoring equipment.

Oncology Services — Complete cancer care is provided through our Oncology and Radiology departments. A new state-of-the-art linear accelerator enables us to deliver radiation in the most sophisticated way possible. Our comprehensive cancer services include a Breast Center, lead by surgical oncologist Sonya Sharpless, MD. The center focuses on early detection, diagnosis and treatment of breast cancer.

Orthopedic Services — Our wide range of orthopedic services includes sports medicine, physical therapy and the latest surgical techniques.

Other Services

- Level II Trauma Center (24-hour Emergency Department)
- Surgical services
- Cardiac care
- Pediatrics
- Occupational health
- Home care
- Ketogenic Diet Center (for treatment of epilepsy)
- Long-term care
- Magnetic Resonance Imaging (MRI)
- Sleep Disorders Center

CONVENIENTLY LOCATED TO SERVE YOU

Lake Forest Hospital physicians and services are located throughout Lake County. In addition to independent physician offices, Lake Forest Hospital offers services in Lake Bluff, Gurnee, Vernon Hills and Libertyville.

Physician Referral — Lake Forest Hospital's Physician Referral Service is designed to help you select a physician that best suits your needs. Call (847) 234-6171 to gain access to information about each physician's education and experience, insurance plan participation, and more. Physician information is also available via Lake Forest Hospital's website: www.lakeforesthospital.com.

LAKE COUNTY

Specialties are indicated in bold-type face. Capital letters indicate Primary Care Specialties. Subspecialties are listed in non-bold type. Listings indicate if a doctor is certified in a subspecialty but predominately practices primary care medicine.

*Oncologists deal with Cancer

ADDICTION PSYCHIATRY

Cann, Stephen R (MD) **AdP**
Highland Park Hosp
Highland Park Hospital, 718 Glenview Ave; Highland Park, IL 60035; (847) 432-8000; **BDCERT:** Psyc 81; **MS:** U Hlth Sci/Chicago Med Sch 76; **RES:** Psyc, Ill State Psyc Inst, Chicago, IL 76-79

ALLERGY & IMMUNOLOGY

Daddono, Anthony (MD) **A&I**
Condell Med Ctr
Lanoff Daddono Cavanaugh, 2504 Washington St Ste 300; Waukegan, IL 60085; (847) 662-4455; **BDCERT:** A&I 80; Ped 66; **MS:** U Hlth Sci/Chicago Med Sch 61; **RES:** Ped A&I, Children's Mem Hosp, Chicago, IL 62-64; A&I, Michael Reese Hosp Med Ctr, Chicago, IL 68-70; **FAP:** Clin Prof U Chicago-Pritzker Sch Med; **HOSP:** Provena St Therese Med Ctr; ***SI:*** *Asthma; Allergic Rhinitis*; **HMO:** +

Immediately

Gutman, Arnold (MD) **A&I**
Highland Park Hosp
Associated Allergists Ltd, 480 Elm Ste 103; Highland Park, IL 60035; (847) 433-7660; **BDCERT:** A&I 77; IM 74; **MS:** Hahnemann U 55; **RES:** VA Hospital, Philadelphia, PA 56-57; Mayo Foundation, Rochester, MN 59-61; **HMO:** +

2-4 Weeks VISA

Kentor, Paul (MD) **A&I**
Evanston Hosp
1201 B Old Mchenry Rd; Buffalo Grove, IL 60089; (847) 634-1690; **BDCERT:** A&I 77; IM 73; **MS:** Univ IL Coll Med 70; **RES:** IM, U IL Med Ctr, Chicago, IL 70-73; **FEL:** A&I, Grant Hosp, Chicago, IL 75-77; **FAP:** Assoc Prof Med Northwestern U; **HOSP:** Glenbrook Hosp; ***SI:*** *Asthma; Chronic Sinus Problems*; **HMO:** Aetna Hlth Plan, United Healthcare, CIGNA, PHCS, Evanston NW HC +

2-4 Weeks VISA

Klein, Joel (MD) **A&I**
Lake Forest Hosp **(see page 309)**
Deer Path Medical Associates, 71 Waukegen Rd; Lake Forest, IL 60044; (847) 295-1500; **BDCERT:** A&I 95; IM 90; **MS:** U Hlth Sci/Chicago Med Sch 87; **RES:** IM, Rush Presbyterian-St Luke's Med Ctr, Chicago, IL 88-90; **FEL:** A&I, Mayo Clinic, Rochester, MN 92-95; **FAP:** Asst Clin Prof Rush Med Coll

Resnick, Alan (MD) **A&I**
Children's Mem Med Ctr **(see page 139)**
Associated Allergists Ltd, 480 W Elm Pl Ste 103; Highland Park, IL 60035; (773) 883-0274; **BDCERT:** A&I 87; Ped 84; **MS:** Univ IL Coll Med 80; **RES:** Ped A&I, Univ of Iowa Hosp, Iowa City, IA 80-81; Ped A&I, Children's Mem Med Ctr, Chicago, IL 81-83; **FEL:** A&I, Children's Mem Med Ctr, Chicago, IL 83-85; **HMO:** Blue Cross & Blue Shield, CIGNA, HealthNet, Humana Health Plan, Metlife

ANESTHESIOLOGY

Matthew, Edward (MD) **Anes**
Highland Park Hosp
Assoc in Anesthesia-Highland Pk, 718 Glenview Ave; Highland Park, IL 60035; (847) 480-3852; **BDCERT:** Anes 86; **MS:** Univ IL Coll Med 82; **RES:** Anes, Northwestern Mem Hosp, Chicago, IL 82-85; **FEL:** ObG/Anes, Northwestern Mem Hosp, Chicago, IL 86; Cv/Anes, Evanston Hosp, Evanston, IL 86; ***SI:*** *Obstetric Anesthesia; Ambulatory Anesthesia*

Immediately VISA

Shoults, David (MD) **Anes**
Provena St Therese Med Ctr
St Therese Anesthesia Assoc, 2645 Washington St Ste 140; Waukegan, IL 60085; (847) 360-2251; **BDCERT:** Anes 78; **MS:** Univ Mo-Columbia Sch Med 74; **RES:** Anes, Naval Med Ctr, San Diego, CA 75-78; **HMO:** Blue Cross & Blue Shield, Chicago HMO

Wuertz, Peter M. (DO) **Anes**
Good Shepherd Hosp
Dept of Anes-Good Shepherd Hospital, 450 W Highway 22; Barrington, IL 60010; (847) 381-9600; **BDCERT:** Anes 94; **MS:** Chicago Coll Osteo Med 86

CARDIOLOGY (CARDIOVASCULAR DISEASE)

Alexander, Jay (MD) Cv
Lake Forest Hosp **(see page 309)**
Northshore Cardiologists, 900 N Westmoreland Rd Ste 210; Lake Forest, IL 60045; (847) 615-1100; **BDCERT:** Cv 83; IM 79; **MS:** Loyola U-Stritch Sch Med, Maywood 76; **RES:** IM, Northwestern Mem Hosp, Chicago, IL 77-78; N, Bellevue Hosp Ctr, New York, NY 78-79; **FEL:** Cv, Northwestern Mem Hosp, Chicago, IL 80-82; **HOSP:** Highland Park Hosp; **HMO:** Aetna Hlth Plan, Blue Cross & Blue Shield, Californiacare, Choicecare, CIGNA

Campbell, David (MD) Cv
Highland Park Hosp
Cardiology Associates Ltd, 1160 Park Ave W Ste 4S; Highland Park, IL 60035; (847) 432-4844; **BDCERT:** IM 87; Cv 91; **MS:** Cornell U 84; **RES:** IM, Rush Presbyterian-St Luke's Med Ctr, Chicago, IL 84-87; **FEL:** Cv, Rush Presbyterian-St Luke's Med Ctr, Chicago, IL 88; **HMO:** Aetna Hlth Plan, Blue Cross & Blue Shield, Californiacare, CIGNA, Healthcare America
Mcr

Jajeh, Fahd (MD) Cv
Condell Med Ctr
2645 Washington St Ste 245; Waukegan, IL 60085; (847) 360-8440; **BDCERT:** Cv 84; CCM 89; **MS:** Syria 80; **RES:** IM, Cook Cty Hosp, Chicago, IL 82-84; **FEL:** Cv, Cook Cty Hosp, Chicago, IL 84-86; **HOSP:** Provena St Therese Med Ctr; **HMO:** +
Mcr Mcd NFI 1 Week

Mayer, Thomas (MD) Cv
Highland Park Hosp
North Shore Cardiologists, 750 Homewood Ave Ste 340; Highland Park, IL 60035; (847) 432-1580; **BDCERT:** Cv 86; IM 86; **MS:** Rush Med Coll 83; **RES:** IM, U Chicago Hosp, Chicago, IL 83-86; **FEL:** Cv, U Chicago Hosp, Chicago, IL 86-89; **FAP:** Clin Instr U Chicago-Pritzker Sch Med; **HOSP:** Evanston Hosp; ***SI:*** *Catheter Based Treatments for Coronary Artery Disease*; **HMO:** Aetna Hlth Plan, Blue Cross & Blue Shield, Chicago HMO, CIGNA, Humana Health Plan +
Mcr Mcd NFI 2-4 Weeks

Monahan, James (MD) Cv
Victory Mem Hosp
Northern Lake Medical, 103 S Greenleaf Ave J; Gurnee, IL 60031; (847) 623-3200; **BDCERT:** IM 78; Cv 79; **MS:** Univ IL Coll Med 74; **RES:** IM, U IL Med Ctr, Chicago, IL 74-77; **FEL:** Cv, U IL Med Ctr, Chicago, IL 77-79; **HOSP:** Provena St Therese Med Ctr; ***SI:*** *Cholesterol Reduction*; **HMO:** Blue Cross & Blue Shield, Humana Health Plan
SA SU Mcr 2-4 Weeks VISA MasterCard

Pineless, Gary (MD) Cv
Highland Park Hosp
Cardiology Associates Ltd, 1160 Park Ave W Ste 4S; Highland Park, IL 60035; (847) 432-4844; **BDCERT:** IM 84; Cv 87; **MS:** U Chicago-Pritzker Sch Med 81; **RES:** IM, Mayo Clinic, Rochester, MN 82-84; **FEL:** Cv, Rush Presby-St Lukes Med Ctr, Chicago, IL 84-87; **HMO:** Aetna Hlth Plan, Blue Cross & Blue Shield, Chicago HMO, CIGNA, Humana Health Plan

Stern, Mark (MD) Cv
Highland Park Hosp
North Shore Cardiologists, 750 Homewood Ave Ste 340; Highland Park, IL 60035; (847) 432-1580; **BDCERT:** IM 75; Cv 81; **MS:** Univ IL Coll Med 70; **RES:** IM, Evanston Hosp, Evanston, IL 71-74; **FEL:** Cv, Loyola U Med Ctr, Maywood, IL 74-76; **HOSP:** Lake Forest Hosp; **HMO:** Aetna Hlth Plan, Blue Cross of IL, United Healthcare, CIGNA, Humana Health Plan +
Mcr 1 Week

COLON & RECTAL SURGERY

Andrews, Robert (MD) CRS
Lake Forest Hosp **(see page 309)**
Surgeons Group, 800 N Westmoreland Rd Ste 205; Lake Forest, IL 60045; (847) 234-4310; **BDCERT:** S 92; CRS 93; **MS:** Univ IL Coll Med 85; **RES:** S, Illinois Med Ctr, Chicago, IL 85-91; **FEL:** CRS, Cook Cty Hosp, Chicago, IL 91-92; **HMO:** Aetna Hlth Plan, Blue Cross & Blue Shield, Californiacare, CIGNA, Healthplus

DERMATOLOGY

Bronson, Darryl (MD) D
Highland Park Hosp
750 Homewood Ave Ste 310; Highland Park, IL 60035; (847) 432-4650; **BDCERT:** D 80; DP 82; **MS:** Univ IL Coll Med 76; **RES:** D, Cook Cty Hosp, Chicago, IL 77-80; **FEL:** DP, U Chicago Hosp, Chicago, IL 81-82; **FAP:** Prof Rush Med Coll; **HOSP:** Lake Forest Hosp; ***SI:*** *Pediatric Dermatology*

Dworin, Aaron (MD) D
Lake Forest Hosp (see page 309)
900 N Westmoreland Rd; Lake Forest, IL 60045; (847) 234-9200; **BDCERT:** D 86; Rhu 80; **MS:** U Mich Med Sch 73; **RES:** IM, U Mich Med Ctr, Ann Arbor, MI 73-76; D, Harvard Med Sch, Cambridge, MA 76-77; **FEL:** U IL Med Ctr, Chicago, IL 79-80; Rhu, U Mich Med Ctr, Ann Arbor, MI 77-79; **FAP:** Asst Prof Univ IL Coll Med; **HOSP:** Highland Park Hosp

Lazar, Andrew (MD) D
Highland Park Hosp
750 Homewood Ave Ste 130; Highland Park, IL 60035; (847) 433-1501; **BDCERT:** D 87; **MS:** Northwestern U 82; **RES:** D, Northwestern Mem Hosp, Chicago, IL 84-87; **FAP:** Assoc Prof Northwestern U; **SI:** *General Dermatology; Cosmetic Dermatology*; **HMO:** Aetna Hlth Plan, Blue Cross & Blue Shield, Californiacare, CIGNA, Prudential +
LANG: Fr, Sp; Mcr Immediately

Septon, Robert (MD) D
Condell Med Ctr
Dermatology Treatment Ctr, 755 S Milwaukee Ave Ste 224; Libertyville, IL 60048; (847) 367-5575; **BDCERT:** D 74; **MS:** Univ IL Coll Med 69; **RES:** IM, Michael Reese Hosp Med Ctr, Chicago, IL 70-71; D, Cook Cty Hosp, Chicago, IL 71-74

Solomon, Samuel (MD) D
Victory Mem Hosp
North Suburban Dermatology, 900 N Westmoreland Rd Ste 225; Lake Forest, IL 60045; (847) 234-4511; **BDCERT:** D 70; **MS:** Univ IL Coll Med 63; **RES:** D, Northwestern Mem Hosp, Chicago, IL 66-69; **HOSP:** Lake Forest Hosp; **HMO:** Aetna Hlth Plan, Blue Cross & Blue Shield, Chicago HMO, Health Options, Humana Health Plan

DIAGNOSTIC RADIOLOGY
(See also Radiology)

Goodman, Allan L (MD) DR
Lake Forest Hosp (see page 309)
Lake Forest Hosp, 660 W Westmoreland Rd; Westmoreland, IL 60045; (847) 234-5600; **BDCERT:** DR 81; **MS:** Washington U, St Louis 77; **RES:** IM, Rush Presbyterian-St Luke's Med Ctr, Chicago, IL 77-78; DR, Rush Presbyterian-St Luke's Med Ctr, Chicago, IL 78-81

Mintzer, Richard (MD) DR
Highland Park Hosp
North Suburban Imaging Group, 718 Glenview Ave; Highland Park, IL 60035; (847) 480-3744; **BDCERT:** DR 74; **MS:** Ky Med Sch, Louisville 69; **RES:** DR, U Chicago Hosp, Chicago, IL 70-73; **FAP:** Clin Prof Northwestern U; **SI:** *Mammography; Chest Diseases*
Mcr Mcd NFI Immediately
VISA

Rabin, David (MD) DR
Highland Park Hosp
718 Glenview Ave; Highland Park, IL 60035; (847) 480-3744; **BDCERT:** DR 87; **MS:** Univ IL Coll Med 82; **RES:** Rad, Rush Presbyterian-St Luke's Med Ctr, Chicago, IL 83-87; **FEL:** Barnes Hosp, St Louis, MO 87-88; **FAP:** Asst Clin Prof Rad Northwestern U; **HMO:** Aetna Hlth Plan, Blue Cross & Blue Shield, Californiacare, Humana Health Plan, Prudential

Zarian, Lawrence P (MD) DR
Victory Mem Hosp
Northern Illinois Radiological, 1324 N Sheridan Rd; Waukegan, IL 60085; (847) 360-4187; **BDCERT:** DR 83; **MS:** Columbia P&S 77; **RES:** IM, Univ Hawaii, Honolulu, HI 78-79; DR, NYU Med Ctr, New York, NY 79-81; **FEL:** NRad, New York University Med Ctr, New York, NY 81-83; **HMO:** Humana Health Plan

ENDOCRINOLOGY, DIABETES & METABOLISM

Gilden, Janice Laurie (MD) EDM
VA Med Ctr
Univ of Hlth Sci Med School, 3333 Greenbay Rd; Chicago, IL 60064; (847) 688-1900; **BDCERT:** IM 84; EDM 85; **MS:** SUNY Downstate 78; **RES:** IM, Lutheran Gen Hosp, Park Ridge, IL 79-81; **FEL:** EDM, U Chicago Hosp, Chicago, IL 83-84; **FAP:** Asst Prof Med U Hlth Sci/Chicago Med Sch; **HOSP:** St Mary's of Nazareth Hosp Ctr

Lieblich, Jeffrey (MD) EDM
Highland Park Hosp
1971 2nd St Ste 100; Highland Park, IL 60035; (847) 432-5510; **BDCERT:** EDM 81; IM 79; **MS:** Univ Penn 72; **RES:** IM, U Chicago Hosp, Chicago, IL 73-74; **HOSP:** Lake Forest Hosp

FAMILY PRACTICE

Kurowski, Kurt (MD) FP
PCP
Highland Park Hosp
University Clinics, 3333 Green Bay Rd; North Chicago, IL 60064; (847) 473-4357; **BDCERT:** FP 94; **MS:** U Wisc Med Sch 84; **RES:** FP, Resurrection Med Ctr, Chicago, IL 84-87; **FAP:** Asst Prof U Hlth Sci/Chicago Med Sch; **HOSP:** Swedish Covenant Hosp; **SI:** *Urinary Tract Infections*; **HMO:** Humana Health Plan, HMO Illinois, CIGNA, United Healthcare +
Mcr NFI Immediately VISA

Rudy, David R (MD) FP
PCP
Highland Park Hosp
Dept of Family Med - Chicago Med School, 3338 Greenbay Rd; North Chicago, IL 60064; (847) 578-3338; **BDCERT:** FP 95; PM 99; **MS:** Ohio State U 60; **RES:** IM, /Ped - Ohio State Univ Hosp, Columbus, OH 63-64; **FAP:** Prof/Chrmn FP U Hlth Sci/Chicago Med Sch; **SI:** *Hemochromatosis*

Salazar, Luis (MD) FP
PCP
Condell Med Ctr
1170 E Belvidere Rd Ste 105; Grayslake, IL 60030; (847) 548-2200; **BDCERT:** FP 90; **MS:** Univ IL Coll Med 87; **RES:** FP, St Joseph Hosp-Chicago, Chicago, IL 89-90

Szyman, Edward (MD) FP
PCP
Highland Park Hosp
Lakeland Primary Care Assoc, 831 Deerfield Rd; Deerfield, IL 60015; (847) 945-6400; **BDCERT:** FP 96; **MS:** Northwestern U 51; **RES:** S, West Suburban Hosp Med Ctr, Oak Park, IL 52-53; **HMO:** Aetna Hlth Plan, Blue Cross & Blue Shield, Chicago HMO, CIGNA, Humana Health Plan

Tanney, Robert (DO) FP
PCP
Highland Park Hosp
Route 83 & Robert Parker Ste 209; Long Grove, IL 60047; (847) 913-0333; **BDCERT:** FP 89; **MS:** Kirksville Coll Osteo Med 83; **RES:** Lakeview Hospital, Milwaukee, WS 83-88

Uhler, Jeffrey (MD) FP
PCP
Good Shepherd Hosp
Alpine Family Physicians, 15 S Old Rand Rd; Lake Zurich, IL 60047; (847) 438-2144; **BDCERT:** FP 84; **MS:** Rush Med Coll 81; **RES:** FP, Lutheran Gen Hosp, Park Ridge, IL 82-84; **HMO:** Aetna Hlth Plan, Blue Choice, CIGNA, Principal Health Care, Prudential

GASTROENTEROLOGY

Bawani, Mohammad (MD) Ge
Condell Med Ctr
Gastroenterologists Ltd, 1105 W Park Ave Ste 1; Libertyville, IL 60048; (847) 680-5880; **BDCERT:** Ge 89; IM 86; **MS:** Pakistan 79; **RES:** IM, U Chicago Hosp, Chicago, IL 82-86; **FEL:** Ge, U Chicago Hosp, Chicago, IL 86; **FAP:** Assoc Clin Prof U Chicago-Pritzker Sch Med; **HOSP:** Good Shepherd Hosp; **HMO:** Aetna Hlth Plan, Blue Cross & Blue Shield, Californiacare, Health Alliance Plan, HealthNet
Mcr Mcd 1 Week VISA

Blitstein, Mark D. (MD) Ge
Lake Forest Hosp (see page 309)
Deerpath Medical, 800 N Westmoreland Rd Ste 206; Lake Forest, IL 60045; (847) 295-1300; **BDCERT:** IM 79; Ge 81; **MS:** Loyola U-Stritch Sch Med, Maywood 76; **RES:** Northwestern Mem Hosp, Chicago, IL 77-79; **FEL:** Ge, UC San Francisco Med Ctr, San Francisco, CA 79-81

Kane, Mary (MD) Ge
Alexian Brothers Med Ctr
(see page 138)
33 W Higgins Ste 5000; Barrington, IL 60010; (847) 255-9606; **BDCERT:** IM 81; Ge 83; **MS:** Johns Hopkins U 78; **RES:** IM, Parkland Mem Hosp, Dallas, TX 78-81; **FEL:** Ge, Parkland Mem Hosp, Dallas, TX 81-83; Ge, Barnes Hosp, St Louis, MO 83-84; **HOSP:** Northwest Comm Hlthcare; **SI:** *Colon Cancer Prevention; Inflammatory Bowel Disease*; **HMO:** Blue Cross & Blue Shield, United Healthcare +
Mcr 1 Week VISA

Kirch, E P (MD) Ge
Victory Mem Hosp
20 Tower Court C; Gurnee, IL 60031; (847) 244-2960; **BDCERT:** Ge 83; IM 76; **MS:** Univ IL Coll Med 76

Moller, Neal (MD) Ge
Highland Park Hosp
Ravinia Associates, 625 Roger Williams Ave Ste 101; Highland Park, IL 60035; (847) 433-3460; **BDCERT:** IM 87; Ge 89; **MS:** U Chicago-Pritzker Sch Med 84; **RES:** IM, Stanford Med Ctr, Stanford, CA 84-87; **FEL:** Ge, UCLA Med Ctr, Los Angeles, CA 87; **SI:** *Colon Cancer Screening; Inflammatory Bowel Disease*; **HMO:** +
SA SU Mcr Mcd NFI 1 Week VISA

GERIATRIC MEDICINE

Goldberg, Barry (MD) Ger
PCP
Highland Park Hosp
Ravinia Assocs, 625 Roger Williams Ste 101; Highland Park, IL 60035; (847) 433-3460; **BDCERT:** Ger 90; IM 82; **MS:** UCLA 79

HEMATOLOGY

Ballester, Oscar (MD) Hem
Midwestern Regional Med Ctr
2520 Elisha Ave; Zion, IL 60099; (847) 872-4561; **BDCERT:** Hem 88; Onc 89; **MS:** Spain 71

Haid, Max (MD) Hem
Highland Park Hosp
Hematology/Oncology Assoc, 750 Homewood Ave Ste 260; Highland Park, IL 60035; (847) 480-3980; **BDCERT:** IM 78; Onc 81; **MS:** Univ IL Coll Med 71; **RES:** IM, Evanston Hosp, Evanston, IL 72-74; **FEL:** HO, NC Baptist Hosp, Winston-Salem, NC 74-76; **FAP:** Asst Prof Med Northwestern U

Guide to symbols and abbreviations can be found on pages 110-113.

INFECTIOUS DISEASE

Glick, Ellen (MD) Inf
Rush North Shore Med Ctr
750 Homewood Ave; Highland Park, IL 60035; (847) 433-9805; **BDCERT:** IM 88; Inf 90; **MS:** Rush Med Coll 85; **HOSP:** Highland Park Hosp

Semel, Jeffery (MD) Inf
Highland Park Hosp
750 Homewood Ave; Highland Park, IL 60035; (847) 433-9805; **BDCERT:** Inf 78; IM 76; **MS:** U Chicago-Pritzker Sch Med 73; **RES:** IM, Rush Presbyterian-St Luke's Med Ctr, Chicago, IL 73-76; **FEL:** Inf, Rush Presbyterian-St Luke's Med Ctr, Chicago, IL 76-78; **FAP:** Asst Prof Rush Med Coll; **HOSP:** Rush North Shore Med Ctr; ***SI:*** *Travel Medicine Immunization*; **HMO:** Blue Cross & Blue Shield, United Healthcare, Aetna Hlth Plan, CIGNA
1 Week

INTERNAL MEDICINE

Braunlich, Scott (MD) IM
PCP
Lake Forest Hosp **(see page 309)**
800 N Westmoreland Rd Ste 102; Lake Forest, IL 60045; (847) 234-8866; **BDCERT:** IM 86; **MS:** U Cincinnati 83; **RES:** IM, Northwestern Mem Hosp, Chicago, IL 84-86

Einfalt, Melinda (MD) IM
PCP
Good Shepherd Hosp
Internal Medicine Assoc, 726 S Northwest Hwy; Barrington, IL 60010; (847) 382-7677; **BDCERT:** IM 90; **MS:** Loyola U-Stritch Sch Med, Maywood 87; **RES:** IM, Loyola U Med Ctr, Maywood, IL 87-90; **FEL:** IM, Loyola U Med Ctr, Maywood, IL 90-91; ***SI:*** *Preventative Medicine; Travel Medicine*; **HMO:** United Healthcare, Blue Cross & Blue Shield, CIGNA, PHCS, Bc/BS +
4+ Weeks VISA

Frazin, Bruce (MD) IM
PCP
Victory Mem Hosp
1616 Grand Ave A; Waukegan, IL 60085; (847) 249-0850; **BDCERT:** IM 76; Nep; **MS:** U Mich Med Sch 73; **RES:** Northwestern Mem Hosp, Chicago, IL 74-76; **FEL:** Nep, Northwestern Mem Hosp, Chicago, IL 74-76

Goldberg, Barry (MD) IM
PCP
Highland Park Hosp
Ravinia Associates, 625 Roger Williams Ave Ste 101; Highland Park, IL 60035; (847) 433-3460; **BDCERT:** IM 82; Ger 90; **MS:** UCLA 79

Hadesman, Robert (MD) IM
PCP
Condell Med Ctr
Gastroenterology Consultants, 890 Garfield Ave Ste 210; Libertyville, IL 60048; (847) 680-5858; **BDCERT:** IM 87; Ge 91; **MS:** Washington U, St Louis 84; **RES:** IM, Northwestern Mem Hosp, Chicago, IL 85-87; **HMO:** Aetna Hlth Plan, Blue Cross & Blue Shield, Californiacare, CIGNA, Humana Health Plan

Lowenthal, Mark (MD) IM
Highland Park Hosp
480 Elm Pl Ste 103; Highland Park, IL 60035; (847) 433-7660; **BDCERT:** IM 90; A&I 93; **MS:** Northwestern U 87; **RES:** IM, Northwest Comm Hlthcare, Arlington Heights, IL 87-90; IM, Northwestern Mem Hosp, Chicago, IL 90-91; **FEL:** A&I, Northwestern Mem Hosp, Chicago, IL 91-93; **HOSP:** Northwestern Mem Hosp

Osher, Gerald (MD) IM
PCP
Lake Forest Hosp **(see page 309)**
North Shore Medical, 800 N Westmoreland Rd Ste 102; Lake Forest, IL 60045; (847) 234-4500; **BDCERT:** IM 84; Ger 90; **MS:** U Mich Med Sch 80; **RES:** IM, Michael Reese Hosp Med Ctr, Chicago, IL 82-84; **HMO:** Humana Health Plan

Pickard, Maurice (MD) IM
PCP
Lake Forest Hosp **(see page 309)**
480 Elm Pl; Highland Park, IL 60035; (847) 433-0404; **BDCERT:** IM 77; **MS:** Univ IL Coll Med 61; **RES:** IM, Moffitt Hosp, San Francisco, CA 63-65; IM, U IL Med Ctr, Chicago, IL 62-63; **HMO:** +
A Few Days

Polyak, Valentina (MD) IM
PCP
Victory Mem Hosp
Northern Lake Medical, 103 S Greenleaf Ave J; Gurnee, IL 60031; (847) 623-3200; **BDCERT:** IM 96; **MS:** Ukraine 75

Sultan, John (MD) IM
PCP
Highland Park Hosp
Ravinia Assoc, 625 Roger Williams Ave Ste 101; Highland Park, IL 60035; (847) 433-3460; **BDCERT:** IM 84; Ger 94; **MS:** U Chicago-Pritzker Sch Med 81; **RES:** IM, Michael Reese Hosp Med Ctr, Chicago, IL 82-84; **HMO:** Blue Cross & Blue Shield, CIGNA, Metlife

Tucci, Mark (MD) **IM**
PCP
Provena St Therese Med Ctr
Northern Lake Medical Ltd, 81 E Grand Ave; Fox Lake, IL 60020; (847) 587-0115; **BDCERT:** IM 84; **MS:** Poland 81; **RES:** IM, Ravenswood Hosp Med Ctr, Chicago, IL 81-84; **FAP:** Instr U Hlth Sci/Chicago Med Sch; **HOSP:** Lake Forest Hosp; ***SI:*** *Preventive Medicine*; **HMO:** Aetna Hlth Plan, Blue Cross & Blue Shield, Californiacare, United, Humana Health Plan +
LANG: Pol; SA SU Mcr Mcd NFI
A Few Days

MEDICAL ONCOLOGY

Cochran, Michael (MD) **Onc**
Lake Forest Hosp **(see page 309)**
North Shore Oncology Ltd, 1900 Hollister Dr Ste 220; Libertyville, IL 60048; (847) 367-6781; **BDCERT:** IM 82; Onc 85; **MS:** Rush Med Coll 79; **RES:** IM, Evanston Hosp, Evanston, IL 80-83; **FEL:** Onc, U Mich Med Ctr, Ann Arbor, MI 83-85; **FAP:** Assoc Prof Rush Med Coll; **HMO:** United Healthcare, Blue Cross & Blue Shield, Aetna Hlth Plan, Humana Health Plan, Oxford +
$ Mcr Mcd NFI 1 Week VISA

Kapadia, Naren (MD) **Onc**
Victory Mem Hosp
Oncology-Hematology Assoc, 202 S Greenleaf Ave E; Gurnee, IL 60031; (847) 336-6111; **BDCERT:** IM 80; Onc 83; **MS:** India 73; **RES:** IM, Columbus Hosp, Chicago, IL 78-80; **FEL:** HO, Hines VA Hosp, Hines, IL 80

Wiznitzer, Israel (MD) **Onc**
Highland Park Hosp
Hemotlgy & Onclgy Assoc of Il, 750 Homewood Ave Ste 260; Highland Park, IL 60035; (847) 432-0300; **BDCERT:** IM 81; Onc 83; **MS:** Northwestern U 78; **RES:** Northwestern Mem Hosp, Chicago, IL 78-81; **FEL:** HO, Yale-New Haven Hosp, New Haven, CT 81-84; **FAP:** Clin Instr Med Northwestern U

Wiznitzer, Israel (MD) **Onc**
Highland Park Hosp
Hematology & Oncology Assoc, 750 Homewood Ave Ste 320; Highland Park, IL 60035; (847) 432-0300; **BDCERT:** Onc 83; IM 81; **MS:** Northwestern U 78; **FEL:** Hem, Yale-New Haven Hosp, New Haven, CT 81-84; **FAP:** Clin Instr Northwestern U; **HOSP:** Northwestern Mem Hosp

NEPHROLOGY

Ginsburg, David S (MD) **Nep**
Highland Park Hosp
David Ginsburg Ltd, 750 Homewood Ave Ste 250; Highland Park, IL 60035; (847) 432-7222; **BDCERT:** Nep 78; IM 72; **MS:** Univ IL Coll Med 67; **RES:** U Chicago Hosp, Chicago, IL 70-72; **FEL:** Nep, U Chicago Hosp, Chicago, IL 72-74; **FAP:** Assoc Northwestern U; **HOSP:** Lake Forest Hosp; **HMO:** Aetna Hlth Plan, Blue Cross & Blue Shield, Californiacare, CIGNA, Healthamerica +
Mcr Mcd

Nora, Nancy (MD) **Nep**
Highland Park Hosp
David Ginsburg Ltd, 750 Homewood Ave Ste 250; Highland Park, IL 60035; (847) 432-7222; **BDCERT:** Nep 92; IM 88; **MS:** Ireland 85; **RES:** IM, St Francis Hosp of Evanston, Evanston, IL 85-88; **FEL:** Nep, Northwestern Mem Hosp, Chicago, IL 88-91

NEUROLOGICAL SURGERY

Gamez, Ramon (MD) **NS**
Victory Mem Hosp
Neurological & Neurosurgical, 200 S Greenleaf Ave A; Gurnee, IL 60031; (847) 244-5660; **BDCERT:** NS 69; **MS:** Mexico 53; **RES:** Hines VA Hosp, Chicago, IL 55-61; Mercy Hosp & Med Ctr, Chicago, IL 55-61; **FAP:** Clin Instr Loyola U-Stritch Sch Med, Maywood; **HMO:** Aetna Hlth Plan, Blue Cross & Blue Shield, Californiacare, CIGNA, Health Options
Mcr Mcd VISA

NEUROLOGY

Metrick, Scott (MD) **N**
Lake Forest Hosp **(see page 309)**
Neurology-Neuro Diagnostics, 900 N Westmoreland Rd Ste 220; Lake Forest, IL 60045; (847) 482-0300; **BDCERT:** N 83; C/NPh 94; **MS:** Univ IL Coll Med 77; **RES:** N, Univ of New Mexico, Albuquerque, NM 78-81

Rowley, Wilbur F (MD) **N**
Condell Med Ctr
755 S Milwaukee Ave Ste 169; Libertyville, IL 60048; (847) 549-0232; **BDCERT:** N 82; **MS:** Univ IL Coll Med 59; **RES:** NS, Northwestern Mem Hosp, Chicago, IL 60-62; N, Northwestern Mem Hosp, Chicago, IL 63-64; **HOSP:** Victory Mem Hosp; ***SI:*** *Multiple Sclerosis; Epilepsy*; **HMO:** Humana Health Plan, First Health, CIGNA, Beech Street, Prudential +
$ Mcr 1 Week VISA

Guide to symbols and abbreviations can be found on pages 110-113.

NUCLEAR MEDICINE

De Bruin, Ronald E. (MD) **NuM**
Lake Forest Hosp **(see page 309)**
660 N Westmoreland Rd; Lake Forest, IL 60045; (847) 234-5600; **BDCERT:** NuM 76; DR 72; **MS:** Univ IL Coll Med 67

Kemel, Alexander (MD) **NuM**
Highland Park Hosp
718 Glenview Ave; Highland Park, IL 60035; (847) 480-3782; **BDCERT:** NuM 94; **MS:** Loyola U-Stritch Sch Med, Maywood 90; **RES:** Path, Loyola U Med Ctr, Maywood, IL 90-92; **FEL:** NuM, Loyola U Med Ctr, Maywood, IL 92-94

OBSTETRICS & GYNECOLOGY

Burstein, Harry (MD) **ObG**
Highland Park Hosp
Highland Park Medical Assoc, 750 Homewood Ave Ste 350; Highland Park, IL 60035; (847) 432-0460; **BDCERT:** ObG 97; **MS:** Univ IL Coll Med 81; **RES:** Ob/GYN, U IL Med Ctr, Chicago, IL 81-85; ***SI:*** *High Risk Infertility & Gynecology; General Obstetrics*; **HMO:** +
A Few Days VISA

Hansfield, Scott (MD) **ObG**
Highland Park Hosp
Northshore Women's Health, 750 HomeWood Ave Ste 240; HighLand Park, IL 60035; (847) 634-1116; **BDCERT:** ObG 87; **MS:** Northwestern U 81; **RES:** ObG, Rush Presbyterian-St Luke's Med Ctr, Chicago, IL 81-85; **HMO:** Aetna Hlth Plan, Blue Cross & Blue Shield, Californiacare, CIGNA, HealthNet

Krantz, Heather (MD) **ObG**
Highland Park Hosp
Highland Park Medical Assoc, 750 Homewood Ave Ste 350; Highland Park, IL 60035; (847) 432-0460; **BDCERT:** ObG 95; **MS:** Univ Kans Sch Med 89; **RES:** U KS Med Ctr, Kansas City, KS 90-93

Logan, Scott (MD) **ObG**
PCP
Lake Forest Hosp **(see page 309)**
Westmoreland Obstetric, 900 N Westmoreland Rd Ste 207; Lake Forest, IL 60045; (847) 234-9110; **BDCERT:** ObG 90; **MS:** Univ IL Coll Med 83; **RES:** ObG, Barnes Hosp, St Louis, MO 83-87

Pesavento, Daniel (MD) **ObG**
Good Shepherd Hosp
450 W Il Route 22 Ste 37; Barrington, IL 60010; (847) 382-4406; **BDCERT:** ObG 90; IM 88; **MS:** Northwestern U 81; **RES:** IM, Evanston Hosp, Evanston, IL 85-88; ObG, Northwestern Mem Hosp, Chicago, IL 81-85; **HMO:** Blue Cross & Blue Shield, CIGNA, Metlife, Principal Health Care, Prudential

Schewitz, David (MD) **ObG**
Lake Forest Hosp **(see page 309)**
Lake Forest Obstetrics, 900 N Westmoreland Rd Ste 228; Lake Forest, IL 60045; (847) 234-3860; **BDCERT:** ObG 85; **MS:** Rush Med Coll 79; **RES:** ObG, Michael Reese Hosp Med Ctr, Chicago, IL 80-83

Strohmayer, Eileen T (MD) **ObG**
Condell Med Ctr
Obstetrics & Gynecology Assoc, 890 Garfield Ave Ste 200; Libertyville, IL 60048; (847) 680-3400; **BDCERT:** ObG 95; **MS:** U Chicago-Pritzker Sch Med 89

Thaker, Pankaj (MD) **ObG**
Victory Mem Hosp
Greenleaf Ob Gyn Assoc, 401 Greenleaf Ave Ste 1; Mc Gaw Park, IL 60085; (847) 623-5445; **BDCERT:** ObG 81; **MS:** India 69; **RES:** ObG, Christ Comm Hosp, Oak Lawn, IL 74-77; **FEL:** GO, Cook Cty Hosp, Chicago, IL 77-78; **HOSP:** Condell Med Ctr

Woods, William (MD) **ObG**
4343 E Grand Ave; Lindenhurst, IL 60046; (847) 356-2156; **BDCERT:** ObG 82; **MS:** Meharry Med Coll 72; **RES:** ObG, Mount Sinai Hosp Med Ctr, Chicago, IL 77-80; **HMO:** Blue Cross & Blue Shield, Chicago HMO, HealthNet, Health Options, Humana Health Plan

OCCUPATIONAL MEDICINE

Sturm, Richard E (MD) **OM**
Highland Park Hosp
Healthworks of Highland Park Hosp, 718 Glenview Ave; Highland Park, IL 60035; (847) 480-2685; **BDCERT:** OM 84; IM 82; **MS:** Mich St U 78; **RES:** IM, Cook Cty Hosp, Chicago, IL 78-81; U IL Med Ctr, Chicago, IL 81-82; **FEL:** Northwestern Mem Hosp, Chicago, IL 97-99; **HOSP:** Lutheran Gen Hosp; ***SI:*** *Work Injuries*
Immediately VISA

OPHTHALMOLOGY

Green, Daniel (MD & PhD) **Oph**
Victory Mem Hosp
Medical Eye Svc Ltd, 48 s GreenLeaf Dr; Gurnee, IL 60048; (847) 664-4016; **BDCERT:** Oph 94; **MS:** Univ IL Coll Med 88; **RES:** IL Eye & Ear Infirmary, Chicago, IL 89-92; **HOSP:** Lake Forest Hosp

Ruff, Bradley (MD) Oph
Lake Forest Hosp (see page 309)
Deerpath Medical Assoc, 750 Homewood Ave Ste 120; Highland Park, IL 60035; (847) 432-7799; **BDCERT:** Oph 88; **MS:** U Hlth Sci/Chicago Med Sch 80; **RES:** Oph, Michael Reese Hosp Med Ctr, Chicago, IL 81-84

ORTHOPAEDIC SURGERY

Becker, Thomas Ray (MD) OrS
Victory Mem Hosp
1 S Greenleaf Ave L; Gurnee, IL 60031; (847) 263-0300; **BDCERT:** OrS 88; **MS:** Univ IL Coll Med 78; **RES:** S, U Chicago Hosp, Chicago, IL 79-80; OrS, U Chicago Hosp, Chicago, IL 80-84; **FAP:** Assoc Prof U Chicago-Pritzker Sch Med; **HMO:** Blue Cross & Blue Shield, Health Options, Metlife
A Few Days VISA

Brna, John (MD) OrS
Lake Forest Hosp (see page 309)
Lake Forest Orthopedic Assoc, 1200 N Westmoreland Rd Ste 100; Lake Forest, IL 60045; (847) 234-2710; **BDCERT:** OrS 89; **MS:** Univ IL Coll Med 80; **RES:** Cook Cty Hosp, Chicago, IL 81-85; **FEL:** SM, USC Med Ctr, Los Angeles, CA 85-86; **HOSP:** Condell Med Ctr; ***SI:*** *Shoulder*; **HMO:** +
A Few Days VISA

Cohn, Arnold (MD) OrS
Highland Park Hosp
Highland Park Orthopedic, 695 Roger Williams Ave; Highland Park, IL 60035; (847) 432-7522; **BDCERT:** OrS 81; **MS:** U Hlth Sci/Chicago Med Sch 75; **RES:** OrS, Loyola U Med Ctr, Maywood, IL 76-80; **FAP:** Assoc Prof OrS Loyola U-Stritch Sch Med, Maywood

Collins, Roger (MD) OrS
Condell Med Ctr
Greenleaf Orthopaedic Assoc, 1900 Hollister Dr Ste 330; Libertyville, IL 60048; (847) 680-4765; **BDCERT:** OrS 89; **MS:** Loyola U-Stritch Sch Med, Maywood 82; **RES:** OrS, Tripler AMC, Honolulu, HI 83-87; **FEL:** SM, U Miami Hosp, Miami, FL 89-90
VISA

Dugan, Robert (MD) OrS
Victory Mem Hosp
Lake Shore Orthopaedics, 202 S Greenleaf Ave A; Gurnee, IL 60031; (847) 336-3335; **BDCERT:** OrS 90; **MS:** LSU Sch Med, New Orleans 83

Hamming, Bruce (MD) OrS
Midwestern Regional Med Ctr
Lake Shore Orthopaedics, 202 S Greenleaf Ave A; Gurnee, IL 60031; (847) 336-3335; **BDCERT:** OrS 97; **MS:** Univ IL Coll Med 79; **RES:** OrS, Northwestern Mem Hosp, Chicago, IL 80-84

Mayer, John (MD) OrS
Condell Med Ctr
Greenleaf Orthopaedic Assoc, 105 N Greenleaf Ave; Gurnee, IL 60031; (847) 623-3090; **BDCERT:** OrS 89; **MS:** U Hlth Sci/Chicago Med Sch 81; **RES:** OrS, Michael Reese Hosp Med Ctr, Chicago, IL 82-86; **FEL:** 86-87; **HOSP:** Victory Mem Hosp

Sherman, Richard (MD) OrS
Highland Park Hosp
Highland Park Orthopedic, 695 Roger Williams Ave; Highland Park, IL 60035; (847) 432-7522; **BDCERT:** OrS 89; **MS:** U Chicago-Pritzker Sch Med 81; **RES:** OrS, Loyola U Med Ctr, Maywood, IL 82-86; **FEL:** SM, Mass Gen Hosp, Boston, MA 86-87; Total Joint Replacement, Brigham & Women's Hosp, Boston, MA 86-87; **FAP:** Asst Clin Prof Loyola U-Stritch Sch Med, Maywood

OTOLARYNGOLOGY

Block, Leslie (MD) Oto
Lake Forest Hosp (see page 309)
Lake Forest Ear Nose & Throat, 700 N Westmoreland Rd F; Lake Forest, IL 60045; (847) 295-1114; **BDCERT:** Oto 77; **MS:** U Chicago-Pritzker Sch Med 72; **RES:** S, Rush Presbyterian-St Luke's Med Ctr, Chicago, IL 73-74; Oto, Rush Presbyterian-St Luke's Med Ctr, Chicago, IL 74-77

Freint, Alan (MD) Oto
Highland Park Hosp
Highland Park Hosp, 1160 E Park Ave Ste 4N; Highland Park, IL 60035; (847) 367-5555; **BDCERT:** Oto 85; **MS:** Univ IL Coll Med 80; **RES:** Oto, IL Eye & Ear Infirmary, Chicago, IL 81-84; **HMO:** Aetna Hlth Plan, Blue Cross & Blue Shield, Californiacare, Choicecare, CIGNA

Mishell, Joseph (MD) Oto
Highland Park Hosp
Northshore ENT, 1160 Park Ave W Ste 4N; Highland Park, IL 60035; (847) 433-5555; **BDCERT:** Oto 90; **MS:** Univ IL Coll Med 85; **RES:** Oto, U IL Med Ctr, Chicago, IL 85-90; **FAP:** Asst Prof Univ IL Coll Med; **HOSP:** Lake Forest Hosp; ***SI:*** *Sinusitis; Otitis*
2-4 Weeks VISA

Nelson, Erik George (MD) Oto
Victory Mem Hosp
Lake County Head & Neck, 100 N Atkinson Rd Ste 201; Grayslake, IL 60030; (847) 548-4442; **BDCERT:** Oto 88; **MS:** Med Coll PA 83; **RES:** Oto, U Chicago Hosp, Chicago, IL 84-88; **HOSP:** Condell Med Ctr; ***SI:*** *Allergy; Hearing Loss*; **HMO:** Humana Health Plan, Principal Health Care, CIGNA, Bc/BS +
A Few Days VISA

Guide to symbols and abbreviations can be found on pages 110-113.

PEDIATRIC HEMATOLOGY-ONCOLOGY

Goodell, William (MD) PHO
Lutheran Gen Hosp (see page 143)
1675 W Dempster St; Lincolnshire, IL 60069; (847) 696-7682; **BDCERT:** PHO 89; **MS:** Wayne State U Sch Med 86; **RES:** Ped, U Chicago Hosp, Chicago, IL 86-89; **FEL:** PHO, U Chicago Hosp, Chicago, IL 89-92

PEDIATRIC NEPHROLOGY

Libit, Sherwood (MD) PNep
Lake Forest Hosp (see page 309)
Vernon Hills Pediatric Assoc, 36100 Brookside Dr Ste 101; Gurnee, IL 60031; (847) 249-5400; **BDCERT:** PNep 74; Ped 72; **MS:** Univ IL Coll Med 67; **RES:** Ped, Rush Presby-St Lukes Med Ctr, Chicago, IL 68-70; **FEL:** PNep, U MN Med Ctr, Minneapolis, MN 70-73; **HMO:** Blue Cross & Blue Shield, Chicago HMO, Humana Health Plan, Metlife, Prudential

PEDIATRICS

Bismonte, Albino (MD) Ped
PCP
Victory Mem Hosp
200 S Greenleaf Ave E; Gurnee, IL 60031; (847) 336-0770; **BDCERT:** Ped 71; **MS:** Philippines 65; **RES:** Grant Hosp, Chicago, IL 67-68; Cook Cty Hosp, Chicago, IL 68-71; **HOSP:** Provena St Therese Med Ctr; ***SI:*** *Allergies*; **HMO:** +
LANG: Fil, Sp; A Few Days

Fondriest, Diane (MD) Ped
PCP
Good Shepherd Hosp
Lake Shore Pediatrics Ltd, 900 N Westmoreland Rd Ste 106; Lake Forest, IL 60045; (847) 615-0700; **BDCERT:** Ped 86; **MS:** U Mich Med Sch 81; **RES:** Ped, Children's Mem Med Ctr, Chicago, IL 82-84; **HOSP:** Lake Forest Hosp; **HMO:** Blue Cross & Blue Shield, Humana Health Plan, Rush Prudential, CIGNA +
Mcr Mcd VISA

Goldman, Barry (MD) Ped
PCP
Provena St Therese Med Ctr
Children's Health Ctr, 95 W Grand Ave Ste 120; Lake Villa, IL 60046; (847) 356-6505; **BDCERT:** Ped 70; **MS:** Univ IL Coll Med 64; **RES:** Boston Fltg Hosp, Boston, MA 68; **FAP:** Asst Prof U Hlth Sci/Chicago Med Sch; **HMO:** Aetna Hlth Plan, Blue Cross & Blue Shield, Californiacare, Choicecare, CIGNA
A Few Days VISA

Goldstein, Arnold (MD) Ped
PCP
Highland Park Hosp
Highland Park Pediatric Assoc, 1160 Park Ave W Ste 3E; Highland Park, IL 60035; (847) 432-8422; **BDCERT:** Ped 71; **MS:** Univ IL Coll Med 66; **RES:** Ped, New York University Med Ctr, New York, NY 67-69; **FEL:** NP, Stanford Med Ctr, Stanford, CA 71-73; **FAP:** Asst Clin Prof Ped Northwestern U
VISA

Lasin, Gerald (MD) Ped
PCP
Lake Forest Hosp (see page 309)
Lake Forest Pediatric Assoc, 900 N Westmoreland Rd Ste 110; Lake Forest, IL 60045; (847) 295-1220; **BDCERT:** Ped 66; **MS:** Univ IL Coll Med 61; **RES:** Ped, Children's Mem Med Ctr, Chicago, IL 62-64; **FAP:** Instr Ped Northwestern U

Levy, Barbara (MD) Ped
PCP
Highland Park Hosp
Levy & O'Brien, 400 Lake Cook Rd Ste 119; Deerfield, IL 60015; (847) 945-3850; **BDCERT:** Ped 79; **MS:** Loyola U-Stritch Sch Med, Maywood 74; **RES:** Ped, MD Inst Emer Med Svcs, Baltimore, MD 76-78; **FEL:** Hem, MD Inst Emer Med Svcs, Baltimore, MD 78-80

Levy, Robert L (MD) Ped
PCP
Highland Park Hosp
Levy & O'Brien, 400 Lake Cook Rd Ste 119; Deerfield, IL 60015; (847) 945-3850; **BDCERT:** Ped 82; PA&I 75; **MS:** Northwestern U 67; **RES:** Ped, Children's Mem Med Ctr, Chicago, IL 67-70; **FEL:** Ped A&I, U WI Sch Med, Milwaukee, WI 70-73; **FAP:** Asst Prof Ped Northwestern U; **HOSP:** Evanston Hosp; ***SI:*** *Asthma; Allergy-Immunology*; **HMO:** Blue Cross & Blue Shield, PHCS, United Healthcare, Humana Health Plan +
A Few Days VISA

O'Brien, Charles (MD) Ped
PCP
Evanston Hosp
Levy & O'Brien, 400 Lake Cook Rd Ste 119; Deerfield, IL 60015; (847) 945-3850; **BDCERT:** Ped 81; **MS:** Tulane U 77; **RES:** Ped, Children's Mem Med Ctr, Chicago, IL 77-80; **HOSP:** Highland Park Hosp; ***SI:*** *Attention Deficit Disorder; Child Development*; **HMO:** Blue Cross & Blue Shield, Principal Health Care, United Healthcare +
A Few Days

Zwirn, Marilyn (DO) Ped
PCP
Highland Park Hosp
Preferred Pediatrics, 1900 Hollister Dr Ste 250; Libertyville, IL 60048; (847) 680-8066; **BDCERT:** Ped 89; **MS:** Chicago Coll Osteo Med 85; **RES:** Ped, Loyola U Med Ctr, Maywood, IL 86-89; **HOSP:** Lutheran Gen Hosp; **HMO:** Aetna Hlth Plan, Blue Cross & Blue Shield, Chicago HMO, CIGNA, Principal Health Care +
LANG: Sp; 1 Week
VISA

PHYSICAL MEDICINE & REHABILITATION

Lanoff, Martin (MD) PMR
Condell Med Ctr
Adult & Pediatric Orthopaedics, 555 Corporate Woods Pkwy; Vernon Hills, IL 60061; (847) 821-7070; **BDCERT:** PMR 91; **MS:** U Hlth Sci/Chicago Med Sch 85; **RES:** Chicago Hosp, Chicago, IL 86-87; **FEL:** PMR, Hines VA Hosp, Chicago, IL 87-90; **FAP:** Asst Prof U Hlth Sci/Chicago Med Sch; **HOSP:** Evanston Hosp; ***SI:*** *Back Pain; Muscular Pain*

PLASTIC SURGERY

Atzeff, Luben (MD) PlS
Provena St Therese Med Ctr
1900 Hollister Dr Ste 190; Libertyville, IL 60048; (847) 623-3299; **BDCERT:** PlS 72; **MS:** Tulane U 65; **RES:** U Wisc Hosp, Madison, WI 66-67; Highland Gen Hosp, Oakland, CA 67-69
1 Week

Bloch, Steven (MD) PlS
Highland Park Hosp
1160 Park Ave W Ste 2E; Highland Park, IL 60035; (847) 432-0840; **BDCERT:** PlS 80; **MS:** SUNY Downstate 73; **RES:** PlS, U Wisc Hosp, Madison, WI 76-77

Kontrick, Andrew (MD) PlS
Victory Mem Hosp
900 N Westmoreland Rd Ste 107; Lake Forest, IL 60045; (847) 234-3284; **BDCERT:** PlS 85; **MS:** Jefferson Med Coll 71; **RES:** S, Cook Co Hosp, Chicago, IL 77-79; PlS, Loyola U Med Ctr, Maywood, IL 79-82

Markus, Norman (MD) PlS
Highland Park Hosp
750 Homewood Ave Ste 180; Highland Park, IL 60035; (847) 432-8180; **BDCERT:** PlS 81; **MS:** Northwestern U 69; **RES:** PlS, U Chicago Hosp, Chicago, IL 73-76; Northwestern Mem Hosp, Chicago, IL 77-79; **FAP:** Asst Clin Prof S Univ IL Coll Med

Steinwald, Osmar (MD) PlS
Lake Forest Hosp (see page 309)
700 N Westmoreland Rd A; Lake Forest, IL 60045; (847) 234-8330; **BDCERT:** PlS 73; **MS:** U Md Sch Med 62; **RES:** S, Rush Presbyterian-St Luke's Med Ctr, Chicago, IL 62-69; PlS, Rush Presbyterian-St Luke's Med Ctr, Chicago, IL 69-71; ***SI:*** *Breast Reduction/Augmentation; Aesthetic Surgery*; **HMO:** Blue Shield, Aetna Hlth Plan, PHCS, Prudential +
1 Week VISA

PSYCHIATRY

Galston, Stephen Al (MD) Psyc
Highland Park Hosp
Women's Circle of Health, 935 Lakeview Pkwy Ste 110; Vernon Hills, IL 60061; (847) 367-1029; **BDCERT:** Psyc 82; **MS:** U Hlth Sci/Chicago Med Sch 77; **RES:** Psyc, Northwestern Mem Hosp, Chicago, IL 78-81; **HOSP:** Lake Forest Hosp
VISA

Greendale, Robert (MD) Psyc
Highland Park Hosp
1803 Saint Johns Ave; Highland Park, IL 60035; (847) 432-1280; **BDCERT:** Psyc 77; **MS:** Univ IL Coll Med 68; **RES:** Psyc, Michael Reese Hosp Med Ctr, Chicago, IL 69-72; **FAP:** Asst Prof Chicago Coll Osteo Med; ***SI:*** *Affective Disorders*; **HMO:** PHCS, Blue Cross & Blue Shield, Aetna Hlth Plan, CIGNA +
A Few Days

Greenspan, Brad (MD) Psyc
Highland Park Hosp
Highland Pk Hosp, 718 Glenview Ave Ste 4NW; Highland Park, IL 60035; (847) 433-0199; **BDCERT:** Psyc 96; **MS:** U Chicago-Pritzker Sch Med 77; **RES:** Psyc, Evanston Hosp, Evanston, IL 77-81; **FAP:** Assoc Prof U Chicago-Pritzker Sch Med; ***SI:*** *Treatment of Mood Disorders*

Miller, Alan (MD) Psyc
Condell Med Ctr
Neuropsych, 935 Lakeview Pkwy Ste 110; Vernon Hills, IL 60061; (847) 367-1611; **BDCERT:** Psyc 90; **MS:** Univ IL Coll Med 84; **RES:** Psyc, U IL Med Ctr, Chicago, IL 84-88; **HMO:** Aetna Hlth Plan, Blue Cross & Blue Shield, Californiacare, HealthNet, Health Options

Guide to symbols and abbreviations can be found on pages 110-113.

PULMONARY DISEASE

Agarwal, Mahesh (MD) Pul
Provena St Therese Med Ctr
2645 Washington St Ste 240; Waukegan, IL 60085; (847) 662-5100; **BDCERT:** Pul 76; IM 72; **MS:** India 63; **RES:** IM, Lucknow Hosp, Lucknow, India 64-67; IM, Cook Cty Hosp, Chicago, IL 67-71; **FEL:** Pul, Cook Cty Hosp, Chicago, IL 71-73; **HMO:** Aetna Hlth Plan, Blue Cross & Blue Shield, Californiacare, CIGNA, Health Options
1 Week

Ankin, Michael (MD) Pul
Lake Forest Hosp (see page 309)
Pulmonary Physicians, 900 N Westmoreland Rd Ste 210; Lake Forest, IL 60045; (847) 234-9340; **BDCERT:** Pul 80; IM 78; **MS:** Northwestern U 75; **RES:** IM, Northwestern Mem Hosp, Chicago, IL 76; **FEL:** Pul, Northwestern Mem Hosp, Chicago, IL 77; **HOSP:** Highland Park Hosp; **HMO:** Aetna Hlth Plan, Chicago HMO, Health Options, Humana Health Plan, Metlife

Katz, Howard (MD) Pul
Highland Park Hosp
900 N Westmoreland Road Ste 210; Lake Forest, IL 60045; (847) 234-9340; **BDCERT:** Pul 82; CCM 87; **MS:** U Hlth Sci/Chicago Med Sch 76; **RES:** IM, Michael Reese Hosp Med Ctr, Chicago, IL 77-79; **FEL:** Pul, Northwestern Mem Hosp, Chicago, IL 79-81; **HOSP:** Lake Forest Hosp; ***SI:*** *Asthma; Emphysema*; **HMO:** Most
A Few Days VISA

Khurana, Anil (MD) Pul
Victory Mem Hosp
2645 Washington St Ste 234; Waukegan, IL 60085; (847) 360-9800; **BDCERT:** Pul 88; IM 85; **MS:** India 74; **RES:** IM, Cook Cty Hosp, Chicago, IL 83-85; **FEL:** Pul, Cook Cty Hosp, Chicago, IL 85-86

RADIATION ONCOLOGY

Mehta, Yashbir (MD) RadRO
Victory Mem Hosp
Radiation Therapy Ctr, 1605 Garden Pl; Waukegan, IL 60085; (847) 244-4115; **BDCERT:** Rad 72; **MS:** India 63; **RES:** Rush Presbyterian-St Luke's Med Ctr, Chicago, IL 70-71; Rush Presbyterian-St Luke's Med Ctr, Chicago, IL 71-73; **HOSP:** Condell Med Ctr; ***SI:*** *Prostate Seed Implants; Cancer treatments*; **HMO:** Aetna Hlth Plan, Blue Cross & Blue Shield, CIGNA +
LANG: Hin;
Immediately

RADIOLOGY
(See also Diagnostic Radiology)

Greenberg, Mark (MD) Rad
Lake Forest Hosp (see page 309)
Greenberg Radiology, 1535 Park Ave W; Highland Park, IL 60035; (847) 831-0500; **BDCERT:** DR 80; **MS:** Northwestern U 76; **RES:** DR, UCLA Med Ctr, Los Angeles, CA 77-80; **FEL:** CT, Northwestern Mem Hosp, Chicago, IL 80-81; **FAP:** Asst Clin Prof Rad U Chicago-Pritzker Sch Med

Stipisic, Ana (MD) Rad
St Mary's of Nazareth Hosp Ctr
1804 Eastwood Ave; Highland Park, IL 60035; (312) 770-2180; **BDCERT:** Rad 78; **MS:** Yugoslavia 67; **RES:** St Francis Hosp of Evanston, Evanston, IL 73-76

REPRODUCTIVE ENDOCRINOLOGY

Marut, Edward (MD) RE
Highland Park Hosp
750 Helmwood Ave Ste 190; Highland Park, IL 60035; (847) 433-4400; **BDCERT:** ObG 80; RE 83; **MS:** Yale U Sch Med 74; **RES:** ObG, UC San Francisco Med Ctr, San Francisco, CA 75-78; **FEL:** RE, Nat Inst Health, Bethesda, MD 79-81; **HOSP:** Michael Reese Hosp & Med Ctr; **HMO:** Aetna Hlth Plan, Blue Cross & Blue Shield, Chicago HMO, Choicecare, CIGNA

Valle, Jorge (MD) RE
Highland Park Hosp
Fertility Centers of Illinois, 750 Homewood Ave Ste 190; Highland Park, IL 60035; (847) 433-4400; **BDCERT:** ObG 74; **MS:** Mexico 67; **RES:** ObG, Michael Reese Hosp Med Ctr, Chicago, IL 69-72; **FEL:** RE, Inst Reproductive Med, Chicago, IL 73-76; **FAP:** Asst Clin Prof Univ IL Coll Med; **HOSP:** Illinois Masonic Med Ctr; ***SI:*** *Infertility; Reproductive Surgery*; **HMO:** United Healthcare, Humana Health Plan, Prudential, CIGNA
LANG: Sp, Rus, Itl; 2-4 Weeks
VISA

RHEUMATOLOGY

Capezio, Jennifer (MD) Rhu
Lake Forest Hosp (see page 309)
Deerpath Medical Assoc, 900 N Westmoreland; Lake Forest, IL 60045; (847) 234-6121; **BDCERT:** Rhu 92; IM 87; **MS:** U Tex SW, Dallas 83; **RES:** IM, Parkland Mem Hosp, Dallas, TX 83-86; **FEL:** Rhu, Northwestern Mem Hosp, Chicago, IL 89-92; ***SI:*** *Arthritis; Osteoporosis*
LANG: Sp;
1 Week VISA

Gall, Eric P (MD) Rhu
Highland Park Hosp
Chicago Med Sch - Dept Med, 3333 Green Bay Rd; North Chicago, IL 60064; (847) 578-1019; **BDCERT:** Rhu 74; IM 72; **MS:** Univ Penn 66; **RES:** IM, Cincinnati Gen Hosp, Cincinnati, OH 67-68; IM, Hosp of U Penn, Philadelphia, PA 70-71; **FEL:** Rhu, Hosp of U Penn, Philadelphia, PA 71-73; **FAP:** Prof, Chrmn Med U Hlth Sci/Chicago Med Sch; **HOSP:** Mount Sinai Hosp Med Ctr; ***SI:*** *Osteo- and Rheumatoid Arthritis; Osteoporosis*; **HMO:** Highland Park IPA, Humana Health Plan
Mcr Mcd NFI 2-4 Weeks VISA

Hozman, Robert (MD) Rhu
Lutheran Gen Hosp **(see page 143)**
900 N Westmoreland Rd Ste 210; Lake Forest, IL 60045; (847) 735-8473; **BDCERT:** IM 85; Rhu 88; **MS:** U Chicago-Pritzker Sch Med 82; **RES:** IM, Lutheran Gen Hosp, Park Ridge, IL 82-85; **FEL:** Rhu, U IL Med Ctr, Chicago, IL 85-87; **FAP:** Asst Prof Univ IL Coll Med; **HOSP:** Highland Park Hosp; ***SI:*** *Fibromyalgia; Rheumatoid Arthritis*; **HMO:** Blue Cross, Humana Health Plan, Aetna Hlth Plan, CIGNA +
SA SU Mcr Immediately VISA

SPORTS MEDICINE

Pavlatos, Christ (MD) SM
Lake Forest Hosp **(see page 309)**
Lake Forest Orthopedic Assoc, 1200 N Westmoreland Rd Ste 100; Lake Forest, IL 60045; (847) 234-2710; **BDCERT:** OrS 92; **MS:** Univ IL Coll Med 82; **RES:** IM, U IL Med Ctr, Chicago, IL 83-85; OrS, U Wisc Med Ctr, Madison, WI 85-89

SURGERY

Berger, David (MD) S
Lake Forest Hosp **(see page 309)**
800 N Westmoreland Rd Ste 204; Lake Forest, IL 60045; (847) 234-5995; **BDCERT:** S 69; **MS:** U Chicago-Pritzker Sch Med 63; **RES:** S, Cook Cty Hosp, Chicago, IL 64-68; **FEL:** S, Mem Sloan Kettering Cancer Ctr, New York, NY 69-70; **FAP:** Assoc Clin Prof S U Chicago-Pritzker Sch Med; **HMO:** Aetna Hlth Plan, Blue Cross & Blue Shield, Californiacare, HealthNet, Humana Health Plan

Furman, Richard (MD) S
Victory Mem Hosp
Furman & Scheer Surgical Associates SC, 10 Tower Ct Ste A; Gurnee, IL 60031; (847) 244-3525; **BDCERT:** S 96; **MS:** Univ IL Coll Med 78; **RES:** S, Nat Naval Med Ctr, Bethesda, MD 82-86; **HOSP:** Lake Forest Hosp; ***SI:*** *Laparoscopic Surgery; Breast Surgery*
LANG: Sp; Mcr Mcd
A Few Days VISA

Ganshirt, Stephen (MD) S
Lake Forest Hosp **(see page 309)**
Surgeons Group, 800 Westmoreland Rd; Lake Forest, IL 60045; (847) 234-4310; **BDCERT:** S 95; **MS:** Loyola U-Stritch Sch Med, Maywood 89; **RES:** S, Providence, Southfield, MI 89-94; **HOSP:** Highland Park Hosp; ***SI:*** *Laparoscopic Hernia; Laparoscopic Nissen*
Mcr 1 Week VISA

Kraft, Avram R (MD) S
Highland Park Hosp
750 Homewood Ave; Highland Park, IL 60035; (847) 433-1060; **BDCERT:** S 72; **MS:** Univ Vt Coll Med 64.; **RES:** S, Ohio State U Hosp, Columbus, OH 65-70; S, Beth Israel Med Ctr, Boston, MA 70-71; **FEL:** S, Ohio State U Hosp, Columbus, OH 67-68
A Few Days

Romeiser Jr, Adam (MD) S
Lake Forest Hosp **(see page 309)**
Surgeons Group, 800 N Westmoreland Rd Ste 205; Lake Forest, IL 60045; (847) 234-4310; **BDCERT:** S 97; **MS:** Northwestern U 71; **RES:** S, Rush Presbyterian-St Luke's Med Ctr, Chicago, IL 71-73; **FAP:** Asst Clin Prof Rush Med Coll; **HOSP:** Highland Park Hosp; ***SI:*** *Vascular Surgery*; **HMO:** Aetna Hlth Plan, United Healthcare, Preferred Care
Mcr A Few Days VISA

Scheer, Michael (MD) S
Victory Mem Hosp
20 Tower Ct Ste A; Gurnee, IL 60031; (847) 244-3525; **BDCERT:** S 97; **MS:** Creighton U 89; **RES:** S, U MO Kansas City Sch Med, Kansas City, MO 90-95; **FEL:** CCM, U MO Kansas City Sch Med, Kansas City, MO 93-94; **HOSP:** Condell Med Ctr; ***SI:*** *Laparoscopic Surgery; Pancreatic Surgery*
LANG: Sp; Mcr Mcd NFI VISA

Sobinsky, Kim (MD) S
Highland Park Hosp
Surgeons Group, 900 N Westmoreland Rd Ste 105; Lake Forest, IL 60045; (847) 234-4310; **BDCERT:** S 87; **MS:** Univ IL Coll Med 80; **RES:** S, U IL Med Ctr, Chicago, IL 80-86; **FAP:** Asst Clin Prof Univ IL Coll Med; **HOSP:** Lake Forest Hosp; ***SI:*** *Gall Bladder-Thyroid; Breast Disease*; **HMO:** Aetna Hlth Plan, Blue Cross, Humana Health Plan, Rush Prudential, CIGNA +
SA SU Mcr Mcd NFI
A Few Days VISA

Strohmayer, Paul (MD) S
Condell Med Ctr
2645 Washington St Ste 405; Waukegan, IL 60085; (847) 249-2525; **BDCERT:** S 92; **MS:** Jefferson Med Coll 84; **RES:** S, U Chicago Hosp, Chicago, IL; **HOSP:** Provena St Therese Med Ctr; ***SI:*** *Breast Lumps; Hernias*; **HMO:** Blue Cross & Blue Shield, Rush Prudential, Aetna Hlth Plan, CIGNA +
Mcr Mcd Immediately

UROLOGY

Friedman, Neil R (MD) U
Rush North Shore Med Ctr
71 S Waukegan Rd Ste 1000; Lake Bluff, IL 60044; (847) 735-0430; **BDCERT:** U 81; **MS:** U Mich Med Sch 74; **RES:** Dartmouth Hitchcock Med Ctr, Lebanon, NH 75-76; Barnes Hosp, St Louis, MO 76-79

Janson, Kenneth (MD) U
Lake Forest Hosp **(see page 309)**
900 N Westmoreland Rd Ste 125; Lake Forest, IL 60045; (847) 295-0010; **BDCERT:** U 79; **MS:** Tulane U 69; **RES:** S, Rush Presbyterian-St Luke's Med Ctr, Chicago, IL; U, Tulane U Med Ctr, New Orleans, LA 73-77; **FEL:** Inf, Tulane U Med Ctr, New Orleans, LA 74-75; ***SI:** Prostate Cancer; Benign Prostatic Hyperplasia*; **HMO:** Principal Health Care, Blue Cross & Blue Shield, Californiacare, CIGNA, United Healthcare +

A Few Days **VISA**

Mutchnik, David (MD) U
Highland Park Hosp
North Urology, 750 Homewood Ave Ste 220; Highland Park, IL 60035; (847) 480-3993; **BDCERT:** U 70; **MS:** Univ IL Coll Med 60; **RES:** U, Baylor Med Ctr, Dallas, TX 63-66; S, Baylor Med Ctr, Dallas, TX 62-63; **HMO:** Aetna Hlth Plan, Blue Cross & Blue Shield, Californiacare, Choicecare, CIGNA

Pessis, Dennis (MD) U
Lake Forest Hosp **(see page 309)**
Affiliated Urologists Ltd, 900 N Westmoreland Rd Ste 128; Lake Forest, IL 60045; (847) 234-3300; **BDCERT:** U 80; **MS:** U Hlth Sci/Chicago Med Sch 73; **RES:** U, Rush Presbyterian-St Luke's Med Ctr, Chicago, IL 74-78; **FAP:** Assoc Prof U Rush Med Coll; **HOSP:** Rush-Presbyterian-St Luke's Med Ctr

MCHENRY
COUNTY

MCHENRY COUNTY

Specialties are indicated in bold-type face. Capital letters indicate Primary Care Specialties. Subspecialties are listed in non-bold type. Listings indicate if a doctor is certified in a subspecialty but predominately practices primary care medicine.

*Oncologists deal with Cancer

CHILD & ADOLESCENT PSYCHIATRY

Madamala, Thakshaka Mani (MD) ChAP
Mem Med Ctr
Horizons, 970 Mchenry Ave; Crystal Lake, IL 60014; (815) 455-7100; **BDCERT:** Psyc 80; ChAP 83; **MS:** England 69; **RES:** ChAP, U IA Hosp, Iowa City, IA 74-76; Psyc, U IA Hosp, Iowa City, IA 76-78; **HOSP:** Northern Illinois Med Ctr; **HMO:** First Health, Blue Cross, CCN, Affordable Hlth Plan +
LANG: Hin, Tel;

CRITICAL CARE MEDICINE

Dellinger, Richard (MD) CCM
Rush-Presbyterian-St Luke's Med Ctr
(see page 122)
1653 W Congress Pkwy Ste 979; Chicago, IL 60012; (312) 942-5020; **BDCERT:** Pul 80; CCM 96; **MS:** Med U SC, Charleston 75; **RES:** IM, Wilford Hall USAF Med Ctr, San Antonio, TX 75-78; **FEL:** Pul, Wilford Hall USAF Med Ctr, San Antonio, TX 78-80; **FAP:** Prof Rush Med Coll; ***SI:*** *Intensive Care*

DERMATOLOGY

Chyu, Juliana (MD) D
Mem Med Ctr
278 Memorial Dr; Crystal Lake, IL 60014; (815) 477-9858; **BDCERT:** D 84; **MS:** Johns Hopkins U 80; **RES:** D, U Chicago Hosp, Chicago, IL 81-84

DIAGNOSTIC RADIOLOGY

(See also Radiology)

Gerolimatos, Spiridon G (MD) DR
Northern Illinois Med Ctr
4201 Medical Center Dr; McHenry, IL 60050; (815) 759-4300; **BDCERT:** DR 81; **MS:** Univ IL Coll Med 77
LANG: Grk;

FAMILY PRACTICE

Bruah, David (MD) FP
PCP
Mem Med Ctr
Family Medicine For McHenry, 3703 Doty Rd Ste 1; Woodstock, IL 60098; (815) 338-3627; **BDCERT:** FP 96; **MS:** Univ IL Coll Med 81; **RES:** FP, Southern IL U Hosp, Decatur, IL 81-84

GASTROENTEROLOGY

Khurana, Deepak (MD) Ge
Sherman Hosp
Specialists-Gastroenterology, 4900 S Il Route 31 Ste 118; Crystal Lake, IL 60012; (815) 477-7550; **BDCERT:** Ge 83; IM 80; **MS:** India 77; **RES:** IM, Cook Cty Hosp, Chicago, IL 77-80; **FEL:** Ge, Cook Cty Hosp, Chicago, IL 80-82; **HOSP:** Good Shepherd Hosp; **HMO:** Aetna Hlth Plan, Blue Cross & Blue Shield, Care America Health Plan, Chicago HMO, Choicecare

INTERNAL MEDICINE

Hernandez, Michael (MD) IM
PCP
Sherman Hosp
Signature Medical Grp, 2320 Royal Blvd; Elgin, IL 60123; (847) 458-4305; **BDCERT:** IM 97; **MS:** Univ IL Coll Med 84

Lipov, Sergei (MD) IM
PCP
St Joseph Hosp-Elgin
Key Medical Group Ltd, 2250 W Algonquin Rd Ste 105; Lake in the Hills, IL 60102; (847) 854-7711; **BDCERT:** IM 85; Ger 92; **MS:** Loyola U-Stritch Sch Med, Maywood 81; **RES:** IM, Evanston Hosp, Evanston, IL 82-84

NEUROLOGICAL SURGERY

Yuk, Antonio (MD) NS
Mem Med Ctr
285 Memorial Dr; Crystal Lake, IL 60014; (815) 356-5577; **BDCERT:** NS 93; **MS:** Univ Penn 82

OBSTETRICS & GYNECOLOGY

Warren, Ann (MD) ObG
PCP
Good Shepherd Hosp
Barrington Obstetrics & Gynecology, 450 W Hwy 22 Ste 32; Barrington, IL 60010; (847) 381-8181; **BDCERT:** ObG 91; **MS:** Northwestern U 85; **RES:** ObG, Rush Presbyterian-St Luke's Med Ctr, Chicago, IL 85-89; **FAP:** Clin Instr Northwestern U

Zaino, Ricca Yao (MD) **ObG**
Mem Med Ctr
Woodstock Medical Assoc, 666 W Jackson St; Woodstock, IL 60098; (815) 338-2210; **BDCERT:** ObG 96; **MS:** Creighton U 89; **RES:** ObG, U NE Med Ctr, Omaha, NE 90-93

PAIN MANAGEMENT

Prunskis, John (MD) **PM**
Northern Illinois Med Ctr
Illinois Pain Treatment Inst, 4309 W Medical Center Dr b103; Mc Henry, IL 60050; (815) 363-9595; **BDCERT:** Anes 92; PM 93; **MS:** Rush Med Coll 82; **RES:** S, U IL Med Ctr, Chicago, IL 82-83; Anes, U Chicago Hosp, Chicago, IL 83-87; **FEL:** PM for Ambulatory Surg, U Chicago Hosp, Chicago, IL 87; **HOSP:** St Joseph Hosp-Elgin; ***SI:** Spine Pain-Neck & Back; Generalized Pain*; **HMO:** Blue Cross, United Healthcare +
LANG: Sp, Fr, Lth; Mcr
A Few Days VISA

PEDIATRIC CARDIOLOGY

Halstead, R David (MD) **PCd**
Northern Illinois Med Ctr
Northern Illinois Pedtrc Assoc, 1110 N Green St H; McHenry, IL 60050; (815) 344-0090; **BDCERT:** PCd 76; **MS:** U Utah 71

PEDIATRICS

Braverman, Charles (MD) **Ped**
PCP
Good Shepherd Hosp
Pediatric Specialists, 475 W Terra Cotta Ave D1; Crystal Lake, IL 60014; (815) 455-2100; **BDCERT:** Ped 90; **MS:** Univ IL Coll Med 87; **RES:** Ped, Lutheran Gen Hosp, Park Ridge, IL 87-90; **HMO:** Aetna Hlth Plan, Blue Cross & Blue Shield, Californiacare, Travelers

Collins, Merry (MD) **Ped**
PCP
Good Shepherd Hosp
Pediatric Specialists, 475 W Terra Cotta Ave D1; Crystal Lake, IL 60014; (815) 455-2100; **BDCERT:** Ped 85; **MS:** Univ IL Coll Med 81; **HMO:** IVPA
VISA

Giese, Todd (MD) **Ped**
PCP
Northern Illinois Med Ctr
Caring Family, 2114 W Algonquin Rd; Lake In the Hls, IL 60102; (847) 658-1221; **BDCERT:** Ped 97; IM 89; **MS:** Univ IL Coll Med 84; **RES:** IM, Brookdale Univ Hosp Med Ctr, Brooklyn, NY 84-88; **HMO:** Aetna Hlth Plan, Blue Cross & Blue Shield, CIGNA, Health Alliance Plan, HealthNet +
Mcr Mcd VISA

RADIOLOGY
(See also Diagnostic Radiology)

Horan, Daniel (MD) **Rad**
St Alexius Med Ctr
Radiological Consultants, 521 Devonshire Ln; Crystal Lake, IL 60014; (815) 459-0820; **BDCERT:** Rad 72; **MS:** St Louis U 67; **RES:** Rad, St Louis City Hosp, St Louis, MO 68-71

SPORTS MEDICINE

Daniels, John (MD) **SM**
Northern Illinois Med Ctr
Crystal Lake Orthopedic Surgery, 700 E Terra Cotta Ave Ste 1; Crystal Lake, IL 60014; (815) 455-0800; **BDCERT:** OrS 96; **MS:** Southern IL U 89
Mcr VISA

SURGERY

Kessler, Robert (MD) **S**
Northern Illinois Med Ctr
1110 N Green St K; Mc Henry, IL 60050; (815) 344-2060; **BDCERT:** S 71; **MS:** Univ IL Coll Med 64; **RES:** U, U IL Med Ctr, Chicago, IL 65-70; **HMO:** Blue Cross & Blue Shield
Mcr Mcd

Lind, Richard (MD) **S**
Mem Med Ctr
Surgical Associates, 690 E Terra Cotta Ave A; Crystal Lake, IL 60014; (815) 455-2752; **BDCERT:** S 90; **MS:** Univ IL Coll Med 77; **RES:** S, U IA Hosp, Iowa City, IA 77-82; **FEL:** GVS, U IA Hosp, Iowa City, IA 82-83; **HOSP:** Good Shepherd Hosp
Mcr Mcd 1 Week

UROLOGY

Bielinski, Roger (MD) **U**
Sherman Hosp
Urology Limited, 4900 S Il Route 31; Crystal Lake, IL 60012; (815) 455-3750; **BDCERT:** U 82; **MS:** Ireland 68; **RES:** S, St Francis Hosp of Evanston, Evanston, IL 71; U, Rush Presbyterian-St Luke's Med Ctr, Chicago, IL 72-75; **HOSP:** St Joseph Hosp-Elgin
Mcr VISA

Guide to symbols and abbreviations can be found on pages 110-113.

WILL COUNTY

WILL COUNTY

Specialties are indicated in bold-type face. Capital letters indicate Primary Care Specialties. Subspecialties are listed in non-bold type. Listings indicate if a doctor is certified in a subspecialty but predominately practices primary care medicine.

*Oncologists deal with Cancer

ANESTHESIOLOGY

Gorski, Daniel W (MD) **Anes**
Silver Cross Hosp
1200 Maple Rd; Joliet, IL 60432; (815) 740-1234; **BDCERT:** Anes 82; PM 94; **MS:** Loyola U-Stritch Sch Med, Maywood 77; **RES:** Anes, Loyola U Hosp, Maywood, IL 80; ***SI:*** *Pain Management*; **HMO:** +

Kao, Cheng Fu (MD) **Anes**
St Joseph Med Ctr-Joliet
Associated Anesthesiologists, 333 N Madison St; Joliet, IL 60435; (815) 725-6331; **BDCERT:** Anes 76; **MS:** China 67; **RES:** St Joseph Med Ctr-Joliet, Joliet, IL 72-74

Mathew, Moly (MD) **Anes**
Silver Cross Hosp
Anes Providers Prof Svcs-Silver Cross Hosp, 1100 Maple Rd; Joliet, IL 60432; (815) 740-1100; **BDCERT:** Anes 91; **MS:** India 83; **RES:** Cook Cty Hosp, Chicago, IL 87-90

Myers, Phil (MD) **Anes**
St Joseph Med Ctr-Joliet
Provena St Joseph Hospital-Anesthesiology, 333 N Madison St; Joliet, IL 60435; (815) 725-6331; **BDCERT:** Anes 95; **MS:** Northwestern U 86; **HOSP:** Silver Cross Hosp

CARDIOLOGY (CARDIOVASCULAR DISEASE)

De Girolami, Daniele (MD) **Cv**
St Joseph Med Ctr-Joliet
Cardiology Associates, 2121 Oneida St Ste 202; Joliet, IL 60435; (815) 741-4278; **BDCERT:** IM 87; Cv 93; **MS:** Mexico 81; **RES:** IM, Mercy Hosp & Med Ctr, Chicago, IL 83-86; **FEL:** Cv, Mercy Hospital, Miami, FL 86-88; Cv, S Miami Hosp, Miami, FL 88-89

Dongas, John F (MD) **Cv**
St Joseph Hosp-Chicago
Cardiology Associates, 2121 Oneida St Ste 202; Joliet, IL 60435; (815) 741-4278; **BDCERT:** IM 82; Cv 85; **MS:** Rush Med Coll 79; **RES:** IM, Cleveland Metro Genl Hosp, Cleveland, OH 79-80; IM, Mt Sinai Med Ctr, Milwaukee, WI 82-85; **FEL:** Cv, Mt Sinai Med Ctr, Milwaukee, WI 81-82

Killian, Dennis (MD) **Cv**
St Joseph Med Ctr-Joliet
Cardiology Assoc-N Illinois/Heartland Cardio Ctr, 210 N Hammes Ave Ste 210; Joliet, IL 60435; (815) 729-3280; **BDCERT:** Cv 89; IM 86; **MS:** Northwestern U 83; **RES:** IM, Loyola U Med Ctr, Maywood, IL 83-86; **FEL:** Cv, Loyola U Med Ctr, Maywood, IL 86-89; **FAP:** Asst Prof Med Loyola U-Stritch Sch Med, Maywood

Martini, Seif (MD) **Cv**
Silver Cross Hosp
Cardiology Assoc-N Illinois, 210 N Hammes Ave Ste 210; Joliet, IL 60435; (815) 729-3280; **BDCERT:** Cv 91; IM 88; **MS:** Syria 82; **RES:** IM, Mercy Hosp & Med Ctr, Chicago, IL 85-88; **FEL:** Cv, Loyola U Med Ctr, Maywood, IL 88-91; **HOSP:** St Joseph Hosp-Elgin

Sumida, Colin (MD) **Cv**
Silver Cross Hosp
Cardiology Associates of North Illinois, 210 N Hammes Ave Ste 210; Joliet, IL 60435; (815) 729-3280; **BDCERT:** IM 84; Cv 91; **MS:** Northwestern U 81; **HOSP:** St Joseph Hosp-Chicago

COLON & RECTAL SURGERY

Bass, Eric (MD) **CRS**
St Joseph Med Ctr-Joliet
Joliet Surgery & Health Care, 2 Uno Cir; Joliet, IL 60435; (815) 725-2277; **BDCERT:** CRS 98; S 96; **MS:** USC Sch Med 89; **RES:** S, U IL Med Ctr, Chicago, IL 89-95; **FEL:** CRS, Cook Cty Hosp, Chicago, IL 95-96; **FAP:** Instr S Univ IL Coll Med; ***SI:*** *Rectal Cancer; Anorectal Problems*; **HMO:** Blue Shield, CIGNA, Humana Health Plan, United Mineworkers +
Immediately **VISA**

Nicosia, Jon (MD) **CRS**
St Joseph Med Ctr-Joliet
Joliet Surgery & Health Care, 2 Uno Cir; Joliet, IL 60435; (815) 725-2277; **BDCERT:** CRS 91; S 73; **MS:** Ind U Sch Med 65; **RES:** Lahey Clinic, Burlington, MA 73; Cook Cty Hosp, Chicago, IL 68-72; **FAP:** Clin Prof Univ IL Coll Med; ***SI:*** *Rectal Cancer; Colonoscopy*; **HMO:** +
Immediately **VISA**

DERMATOLOGY

Barnett, Morton (MD) **D**
St Joseph Med Ctr-Joliet
Dermatology Limited, 2400 Glenwood Ave Ste 126; Joliet, IL 60435; (815) 741-4343; **BDCERT:** D 78; **MS:** Loyola U-Stritch Sch Med, Maywood 63; **RES:** D, Cook Cty Hosp, Chicago, IL 66-69

DIAGNOSTIC RADIOLOGY
(See also Radiology)

Bruno, Edward (MD) **DR**
St Joseph Med Ctr-Joliet
333 Madison St; Joliet, IL 60435; (815) 741-7200; **BDCERT:** DR 84; **MS:** U Hlth Sci/Chicago Med Sch 80

FAMILY PRACTICE

Canaday, Lucy (MD) **FP**
PCP
St Joseph Med Ctr-Joliet
Family Health Ctr, 305 Vine St; New Lenox, IL 60451; (815) 485-2541; **BDCERT:** FP 92; **MS:** U Wisc Med Sch 89; **RES:** FP, U Mich Med Ctr, Ann Arbor, MI 89-92

Prajka, Valerie (DO) **FP**
PCP
South Suburban Hosp
Valerie Prajka Assoc, 9475 Bormet Rd; Mokena, IL 60448; (708) 478-0500; **BDCERT:** FP 92; **MS:** Univ Osteo Med & Hlth Sci 89; **HMO:** Aetna Hlth Plan, Blue Cross & Blue Shield, Chicago HMO, CIGNA, Maxicare Health Plan

GASTROENTEROLOGY

Bhalla, Suresh (MD) **Ge**
St Joseph Med Ctr-Joliet
210 N Hammes Ave Ste 205; Joliet, IL 60435; (815) 744-2123; **BDCERT:** Ge 87; IM 84; **MS:** India 77; **RES:** IM, Christ Hosp & Med Ctr, Oak Lawn, IL 82-84; **FEL:** Ge, Henry Ford Hosp, Detroit, MI 84-86

HEMATOLOGY

Pundaleeka, Sarode (MD) **Hem**
Silver Cross Hosp
Joliet Oncology & Hematology, 2420 Glenwood Ave; Joliet, IL 60435; (815) 725-1355; **BDCERT:** IM 78; Onc 81; **MS:** India 72; **RES:** IM, Louis A Weiss Mem Hosp, Chicago, IL 75-78; **FEL:** Onc, Rush Presbyterian-St Luke's Med Ctr, Chicago, IL 78-80; Hem, Rush Presbyterian-St Luke's Med Ctr, Chicago, IL 80-81

INFECTIOUS DISEASE

Alexander, Frederick S (MD) **Inf**
Silver Cross Hosp
Southwest Infectious Disease, 1301 Copperfield Ave Ste 103; Joliet, IL 60432; (815) 726-1818; **BDCERT:** Inf 92; IM 85; **MS:** Univ IL Coll Med 82; **RES:** IM, Lutheran Gen Hosp, Park Ridge, IL 82-85; **FEL:** Inf, Loyola U Med Ctr, Maywood, IL 85-87; **HOSP:** St Joseph Med Ctr-Joliet; **HMO:** Blue Cross & Blue Shield, Chicago HMO, HealthNet
LANG: Sp;

INTERNAL MEDICINE

Schubert, Robert (MD) **IM**
PCP
St Joseph Med Ctr-Joliet
Optima Medical Assoc, 1050 Essington Rd Ste 200; Joliet, IL 60435; (815) 729-0129; **BDCERT:** IM 91; **MS:** Univ IL Coll Med 88; **RES:** IM, Lutheran Gen Hosp, Park Ridge, IL 89-91; ***SI:*** *Asthma; Headache*; **HMO:** United Healthcare, Aetna Hlth Plan, Caterpillar +
Mcr NFI A Few Days VISA

MEDICAL ONCOLOGY

Peterson, Carol (MD) **Onc**
St Joseph Med Ctr-Joliet
Joliet Oncology Hematology, 2420 Glenwood Ave; Joliet, IL 60435; (815) 725-1355; **BDCERT:** Onc 85; IM 83; **MS:** U Mich Med Sch 79; **RES:** Northwestern Mem Hosp, Chicago, IL 80-82; **FEL:** Onc, Northwestern Mem Hosp, Chicago, IL 83-85

NEPHROLOGY

Chawla, Bhuvan (MD) **Nep**
St Joseph Med Ctr-Joliet
Joliet Kidney Ctr, 2121 Oneida St Ste 303; Joliet, IL 60435; (815) 741-8480; **BDCERT:** IM 80; Nep 82; **MS:** India 75; **RES:** RenlDis, Baylor Coll Med, Houston, TX 79-80; **FEL:** Renal Disease, U IL Med Ctr, Chicago, IL 80-81; **HMO:** +
Mcr Mcd 2-4 Weeks

Kathpalia, Satish (MD) **Nep**
Michael Reese Hosp & Med Ctr
Northeast Nephrology Inc, 815 N Larkin Ave Ste 205; Joliet, IL 60435; (815) 744-5550; **BDCERT:** Nep 80; IM 78; **MS:** India 65; **RES:** St Raphael Hosp-Yale Affil, New Haven, CT 74-75; **FEL:** Nep, Michael Reese Hosp Med Ctr, Chicago, IL 75-77; **FAP:** Assoc Clin Prof Med Univ IL Coll Med

NEUROLOGY

Analytis, Peter (MD) **N**
St Joseph Med Ctr-Joliet
Joliet Headache & Neuro Ctr, 801 N Larkin Ave Ste 103; Joliet, IL 60435; (815) 744-6460; **BDCERT:** N 95; **MS:** Univ IL Coll Med 80; **RES:** N, U IL Med Ctr, Chicago, IL -88; ***SI:*** *Neurology Stroke-Adult; Sleep Medicine*; **HMO:** +
SA SU Mcr NFI 1 Week

Guide to symbols and abbreviations can be found on pages 110-113.

Gulati, Surendra (MD) **N**
St Joseph Med Ctr-Joliet
2121 Oneida St Ste 303; Joliet, IL 60435; (815) 741-3942; **BDCERT:** N 82; **MS:** India 72; **RES:** IM, Long Island Jewish Med Ctr, New Hyde Park, NY 75-77; U Mich Med Ctr, Ann Arbor, MI 77-80; **HMO:** Blue Cross & Blue Shield, Travelers

Mc Cahill, Kathleen (MD) **N**
Silver Cross Hosp
1301 Copperfield Ave Ste 212; Joliet, IL 60432; (815) 722-7379; **BDCERT:** N 90; **MS:** Mexico 81; **RES:** N, Northwestern Mem Hosp, Chicago, IL 83-87; ***SI:*** *Parkinson's Disease; Epilepsy*; **HMO:** Blue Cross, United Healthcare, Caterpillar, Fortis +
LANG: Sp; 1 Week

OBSTETRICS & GYNECOLOGY

Al-Khudari, Mohammad A (MD) **ObG**
PCP
Silver Cross Hosp
1301 Copperfield Ave Ste 214; Joliet, IL 60432; (815) 727-6555; **BDCERT:** ObG 82; **MS:** Syria 71; **HMO:** +
LANG: Sp;

Beck, Daniel Lee (MD) **ObG**
St Joseph Med Ctr-Joliet
310 N Hammes Ave Ste 201; Joliet, IL 60435; (815) 741-0070; **BDCERT:** ObG 94; **MS:** Northwestern U 84; **RES:** ObG, Northwestern Mem Hosp, Chicago, IL 84-88; ***SI:*** *Incontinence Therapy; Laparoscopic Surgery*; **HMO:** Blue Cross & Blue Shield, John Deere Health Plan
4+ Weeks

Kent, Vernon (MD) **ObG**
Silver Cross Hosp
Joliet Women's Laser Ctr, 1301 Copperfield Ave Ste 206; Joliet, IL 60432; (815) 723-4551; **BDCERT:** ObG 86; **MS:** Univ IL Coll Med 60; **RES:** Ohio State U Hosp, Columbus, OH 63-64; Cook Cty Hosp, Chicago, IL 71-73; **HOSP:** St Joseph Hosp-Chicago; **HMO:** Aetna Hlth Plan, Blue Cross & Blue Shield, Chicago HMO, Metlife, Prudential

Lopez, Ramon (MD) **ObG**
St Joseph Med Ctr-Joliet
Womens Clinic of Joliet, 2121 Oneida St Ste 305; Joliet, IL 60435; (815) 729-0180; **BDCERT:** ObG 95; **MS:** Philippines 66; **RES:** ObG, Hahnemann U Hosp, Philadelphia, PA 68-71; ObG, U Santo Tomas Hosp, Philippines 66-67; **FEL:** GO, Roswell Park Cancer Inst, Buffalo, NY 71-73

Wrona, Leo A (MD) **ObG**
St Joseph Med Ctr-Joliet
Associated Obstetricians Ltd, 801 N Larkin Ave Ste 101; Joliet, IL 60435; (815) 741-1028; **BDCERT:** ObG 72; **MS:** Loyola U-Stritch Sch Med, Maywood 66; **RES:** ObG, St Joseph's Hosp, Chicago, IL 67-70; **HOSP:** Silver Cross Hosp
2-4 Weeks VISA

OPHTHALMOLOGY

Morimoto, David (MD) **Oph**
St Joseph Med Ctr-Joliet
Associated Ophthalmologists, 219 N Hammes Rd; Joliet, IL 60435; (815) 741-3220; **BDCERT:** Oph 91; **MS:** Northwestern U 86; **RES:** Illinois Eye & Ear Infirmary, Chicago, IL 87-90

Morimoto, Paul (MD) **Oph**
St Joseph Med Ctr-Joliet
Associated Ophthalmologists, 219 N Hammes Ave; Joliet, IL 60435; (815) 741-3220; **BDCERT:** Oph 62; **MS:** Univ IL Coll Med 56; **RES:** Cook Cty Hosp, Chicago, IL 57-60

ORTHOPAEDIC SURGERY

Dhiman, Surender (MD) **OrS**
St Joseph Med Ctr-Joliet
2201 Glenwood Ave; Joliet, IL 60435; (815) 744-4552; **BDCERT:** OrS 93; **MS:** Canada 74; **RES:** U Ottawa, Canada 79-83

Hopkins, Gail (MD) **OrS**
Hinsdale Hosp (see page 275)
Orthopaedic Surgeons of Joliet, 2121 Oneida St Ste 304; Joliet, IL 60435; (815) 744-4551; **BDCERT:** OrS 88; **MS:** Rush Med Coll 81; **RES:** S, Loyola U Affil Hosps, Maywood, IL 81-82; OrS, Loyola U Med Ctr, Maywood, IL 82-86

OTOLARYNGOLOGY

Gartlan, Michael (MD) **Oto**
St Joseph Med Ctr-Joliet
2201 Glenwood Ave; Joliet, IL 60435; (815) 725-1191; **BDCERT:** Oto 94; **MS:** Univ IL Coll Med 88; **RES:** Oto&HNS, U IA Hosp, Iowa City, IA 89-93; **FEL:** PedOto, Children's Mem Med Ctr, Chicago, IL 94-95

PEDIATRIC NEPHROLOGY

Cabana, Emilio C (MD) **PNep**
Good Samaritan Hosp (see page 274)
Downers Grove Pediatrics Ltd, 402 W Boughton Rd F; Bolingbrook, IL 60439; (630) 759-9230; **BDCERT:** Ped 69; **MS:** Philippines 63; **RES:** Ped, Michael Reese Hosp Med Ctr, Chicago, IL 65-67; **FEL:** PNep, Michael Reese Hosp Med Ctr, Chicago, IL 67-69; **HMO:** Aetna Hlth Plan, Blue Cross & Blue Shield, CIGNA, HealthNet, Prudential

PEDIATRICS

Alcala, Gilda (MD) **Ped**
PCP
St Joseph Med Ctr-Joliet
Moore & Alcala, 700 W Jefferson St; Shorewood, IL 60431; (815) 741-2888; **BDCERT:** Ped 73; **MS:** Philippines 67; **RES:** Mount Sinai Hosp Med Ctr, Chicago, IL 69-72; **HMO:** +
2-4 Weeks

Giroux, John (MD) **Ped**
PCP
Silver Cross Hosp
Silver Cross Medical Ctr-Homer, 12701 W 143rd St; Lockport, IL 60441; (815) 726-1164; **BDCERT:** Ped 97; **MS:** U Hlth Sci/Chicago Med Sch 85; **RES:** Ped, Michael Reese Hosp Med Ctr, Chicago, IL 86-88; **FAP:** Instr Ped Rush Med Coll; **HMO:** Blue Cross & Blue Shield, Chicago HMO, Humana Health Plan, Metlife, Prudential

Moore, Thomas (MD) **Ped**
PCP
St Joseph Med Ctr-Joliet
Moore & Alcala, 700 W Jefferson St; Shorewood, IL 60435; (815) 741-2888; **BDCERT:** Ped 81; **MS:** Univ IL Coll Med 77; **RES:** Cook Cty Hosp, Chicago, IL 79-80; Cook Cty Hosp, Chicago, IL 78-79

PHYSICAL MEDICINE & REHABILITATION

Deppe, Frances (MD) **PMR**
St Joseph Med Ctr-Joliet
Midwest Rehabilitation Assoc, 2400 Glenwood Ave Ste 120; Joliet, IL 60435; (815) 741-2201; **BDCERT:** PMR 85; **MS:** Rush Med Coll 80; **RES:** PMR, Rehab Institute of Chicago, Chicago, IL 81-83; ***SI:*** *Low Back Pain; Stroke Rehab*; **HMO:** Humana Health Plan, NYLCare, Aetna Hlth Plan, Blue Cross & Blue Shield
NFI

PSYCHIATRY

Sinibaldi, Mark (MD) **Psyc**
St Joseph Med Ctr-Joliet
Professional Health Assoc Ltd, 12255 S 80th Ave Ste 202; Palos Heights, IL 60463; (815) 744-8253; **BDCERT:** Psyc 78; **MS:** Loyola U-Stritch Sch Med, Maywood 73; **RES:** Psyc, Loyola U Med Ctr, Maywood, IL 73-76; **FAP:** Asst Clin Prof Loyola U-Stritch Sch Med, Maywood; **HOSP:** Linden Oaks Hosp

RADIATION ONCOLOGY

Mc Call, Anne (MD) **RadRO**
St Joseph Med Ctr-Joliet
Sister Theresa Cancer Care Center, 333 N Madison Avenue; Joliet, IL 60435; (815) 741-7560; **BDCERT:** RadRO 90; **MS:** Rush Med Coll 83; **RES:** S, Loyola U Med Ctr, Maywood, IL 84-86; RadRO, Loyola U Med Ctr, Maywood, IL 86-89; **FAP:** Asst Prof Loyola U-Stritch Sch Med, Maywood; ***SI:*** *Breast Cancer; Gynecologic Cancer*

RADIOLOGY

(See also Diagnostic Radiology)

Gagnon, James D (MD) **Rad**
St Joseph Med Ctr-Joliet
333 Madison St; Joliet, IL 60435; (515) 741-7560; **BDCERT:** Rad 76; **MS:** Loyola U-Stritch Sch Med, Maywood 69; **RES:** Rad, Northwestern Mem Hosp, Chicago, IL 73-74; Rad, Oregon Health Sci U Hosp, Portland, OR 74-76

RHEUMATOLOGY

Sosenko, Maria (MD) **Rhu**
St Joseph Med Ctr-Joliet
2121 Oneida St Ste 301; Joliet, IL 60435; (815) 744-7246; **BDCERT:** IM 84; Rhu 86; **MS:** Univ IL Coll Med 81; **RES:** IM, Lutheran Gen Hosp, Park Ridge, IL 81-82; **FEL:** Rhu, U IL Med Ctr, Chicago, IL 84-86; **HOSP:** Silver Cross Hosp; **HMO:** Aetna Hlth Plan, Blue Cross & Blue Shield, CIGNA, Healthamerica, Healthpartners

SURGERY

Anderson, Allan (MD) **S**
St Joseph Med Ctr-Joliet
Joliet Medical Group Ltd, 2100 Glenwood Ave; Joliet, IL 60435; (815) 725-2121; **BDCERT:** S 93; **MS:** Washington U, St Louis 86; **RES:** S, Michael Reese Hosp Med Ctr, Chicago, IL 86-91; ***SI:*** *Breast-Vascular Surgery; Laparoscopy*

Danielson, Mark (MD) **S**
Silver Cross Hosp
1301 Copperfield Ave Ste 103; Joliet, IL 60432; (815) 726-0220; **BDCERT:** S 87; **MS:** Northwestern U 81; **RES:** S, Med Coll WI, Milwaukee, WI 81-86; **HOSP:** St Joseph Med Ctr-Joliet; ***SI:*** *Laparoscopic Surgery*; **HMO:** Blue Cross & Blue Shield, Chicago HMO, CIGNA, Maxicare Health Plan, Metlife +
A Few Days VISA

Gunderson, Holly (MD) **S**
St Joseph Med Ctr-Joliet
Family Medical Group, 330 Madison St; Joliet, IL 60435; (815) 725-3440; **BDCERT:** S 87; **MS:** Southern IL U 80; **RES:** S, Michael Reese Hosp Med Ctr, Chicago, IL 80-85

Guide to symbols and abbreviations can be found on pages 110-113.

Marshall, Wendy (MD) S
St Joseph Hosp-Chicago
Provena St Joseph's Medical Center, 333 N Madison; Joliet, IL 60435; (815) 773-7080; **BDCERT:** S 89; **MS:** Univ Vt Coll Med 78; **RES:** S, Med Ctr Hosp of VT, Burlington, VT 79-83; **FEL:** CCM, MIEMSS, Baltimore, MD 83-84; **FAP:** Assoc Prof S Loyola U-Stritch Sch Med, Maywood; ***SI:*** *Breast Diseases; Trauma/Critical Care*; **HMO:** Blue Cross & Blue Shield, CIGNA, Humana Health Plan, Private Healthcare
A Few Days VISA

Marvin, Joy (MD) S
Silver Cross Hosp
1301 Copperfield Ave Ste 103; Joliet, IL 60432; (815) 726-0220; **BDCERT:** S 96; **MS:** U Chicago-Pritzker Sch Med 89; **RES:** S, U IL - Cook Co Hosp, Chicago, IL 89-94; **HOSP:** St Joseph Med Ctr-Joliet; ***SI:*** *Breast Surgery; Hernia Surgery*; **HMO:** +
A Few Days VISA

Natesha, Ramanathapur K. (MD) S
St Joseph Hosp-Chicago
302 N Hammes Ave; Joliet, IL 60435; (815) 725-2600; **BDCERT:** S 92; **MS:** India 81; **RES:** S, Vanderbilt U Med Ctr, Nashville, TN 87-90; S, Univ Hosp SUNY Buffalo, Buffalo, NY 91-92; **HOSP:** Silver Cross Hosp; ***SI:*** *Laparoscopic Surgery; Vascular Surgery*; **HMO:** HMO Illinois, Blue Cross & Blue Shield
LANG: Hin, Sp; A Few Days

THORACIC SURGERY

Altergott, Rudolph (MD) TS
St Joseph Med Ctr-Joliet
Cardiac Surgery Assoc, 333 N Hammes Ave Ste 107; Joliet, IL 60435; (815) 741-2626; **BDCERT:** TS 97; S 94; **MS:** Loyola U-Stritch Sch Med, Maywood 80; **RES:** S, Loyola U Med Ctr, Maywood, IL 80-85; **FEL:** TS, Loyola U Med Ctr, Maywood, IL 85-87; **FAP:** Assoc Clin Prof Loyola U-Stritch Sch Med, Maywood; ***SI:*** *Thoracic Surgery; Vascular Surgery*

Foy, Bryan (MD) TS
St Joseph Med Ctr-Joliet
333 N Hammes Ave Ste 107; Joliet, IL 60435; (815) 741-2626; **BDCERT:** TS 96; S 92; **MS:** Loyola U-Stritch Sch Med, Maywood 78; **RES:** S, Loyola U Med Ctr, Maywood, IL 79-83; **FEL:** Cv, Loyola U Med Ctr, Maywood, IL 83-85; **FAP:** Assoc Clin Prof TS Loyola U-Stritch Sch Med, Maywood; **HOSP:** Good Samaritan Hosp; ***SI:*** *Cardiac Transplantation; Assist Devices*

UROLOGY

Jones, George (MD) U
St Joseph Med Ctr-Joliet
2112 W Jefferson St Ste 222; Joliet, IL 60435; (815) 725-4566; **BDCERT:** U 78; **MS:** U Iowa Coll Med 71; **RES:** U IA Hosp, Iowa City, IA 72-76

Lewis, Gregory (MD) U
St Joseph Med Ctr-Joliet
Schuster & Lewis, 330 Madison St Ste 303; Joliet, IL 60435; (815) 741-3825; **BDCERT:** U 84; **MS:** Loyola U-Stritch Sch Med, Maywood 77; **RES:** U, Hines VA Hosp, Chicago, IL 77-82; **HOSP:** Silver Cross Hosp; ***SI:*** *Urological Cancers; Urinary Stones*; **HMO:** Blue Cross & Blue Choice, HealthStar
1 Week

Schuster, George (MD) U
St Joseph Med Ctr-Joliet
Schuster & Lewis, 330 Madison St Ste 303; Joliet, IL 60435; (815) 741-3825; **BDCERT:** U 77; **MS:** Univ IL Coll Med 69; **RES:** U, Hines VA Hosp, Chicago, IL 71-75; **FEL:** Nep, Northwestern Mem Hosp, Chicago, IL 70-71; **HOSP:** Silver Cross Hosp; ***SI:*** *Incontinence; Prostatitis*; **HMO:** Blue Cross & Blue Shield, Accord, Health Options, John Deere Health Plan, Joliet PPO
2-4 Weeks

SECTION THREE

CENTERS OF EXCELLENCE

CENTERS OF EXCELLENCE

Health care consumers are not only interested in information on hospitals; they also want to know in which hospitals are leaders or have special programs dealing with a specific disease or health issue. Many hospitals in the region have devoted significant resources to developing superior programs of patient care in these areas. We have invited those institutions selected for inclusion in the Castle Connolly Guide to present information on programs they believe would be of interest to, and meet the special needs of, our readers.

CANCER

Alexian Brothers Regional Cancer Care Center

820 BIESTERFIELD ROAD, SUITE 110
ELK GROVE VILLAGE, IL 60007-3397
PHONE: (847) 981-5760
WEB SITE: WWW.ALEXIAN.ORG

Advanced Technology, Supportive Care

At Alexian Brothers Regional Cancer Care Center, an expert staff practices state-of-the art medicine in a caring and supportive environment, combining the latest in technology with a compassionate, individualized approach to patient care.

The Center's efforts are directed by the team of eleven radiation oncologists - each certified by the American Board of Radiology, with a particular expertise in the treatment of specific malignancies. Collectively, the center's physicians have more than 125 years of clinical experience in treating tumors with radiation therapy.

The Center's staff takes time to evaluate each patient's unique needs and discuss treatment options with the patient, his or her primary care physician and other medical specialists. If radiation therapy is indicated, the staff develops an individualized plan of care in consultation with the patient.

The advanced technology used by the Center to treat patients includes two linear accelerators with multi-leaf collimation, as well as a 3-D planning system to target radiation treatment more precisely thus protecting healthy tissue. The Center participates in several national cooperative group trials allowing patients access to the latest in experimental clinical medicine.

External and internal radiation treatments

The Center's radiation therapists use the linear accelerators to target tumors directly with external beam radiation treatments. Patients also can receive internal radiation therapy, or brachytherapy, which involves the placement of a radioactive source inside the body near the tumor. The 3-D planning system maximizes treatment effectiveness for both external beam radiation and brachytherapy.

To ensure that the staff is providing up-to-date care as cancer treatment techniques continue to evolve, the radiation oncologists, radiation therapists and registered nurses regularly participate in continuing education programs.

When radiation therapy comprises only part of a patient's treatment, the Center's oncologists work with the patient's primary care physician, surgeon, medical oncologist and other specialists to coordinate the best possible care.

BREAST CANCER CLINIC

Alexian Brothers Regional Cancer Care Center offers breast cancer patients the opportunity to meet with a variety of specialists during a single visit to the multidisciplinary clinic.

Patients can consult with a surgeon, medical oncologist and radiation oncologist at one appointment, avoiding multiple trips to see individual doctors.

The doctors discuss the patient's condition, collaborate on the best course of treatment, counsel the patient about their findings and recommendations, and forward their report to the patient's primary care physician.

MAKING PATIENTS FEEL COMFORTABLE

Reflecting the Alexian Brothers' 700 year tradition of treating individuals with the utmost care and concern, the staff of Alexian Brothers Regional Cancer Care Center strives to serve each patient with compassion and respect for their unique needs.

Staff members make every effort to ensure that each patient and his or her family feel supported, well educated, comfortable and in control. Rather than rushing through appointments, they get to know patients and help them understand every aspect of their treatment. They also provide financial counseling and help connect patients with other resources, such as home care and support groups.

The staff is happy to answer any questions and can schedule an initial visit within 48 hours. Please call (847) 981-5760.

Hinsdale Hospital
Opler Cancer Center

120 N. OAK STREET • HINSDALE, IL 60521
PHONE (630) 856-9000 WWW.AHSMIDWEST.ORG

Advanced Technology and Quality Care in a Community Setting

The scope of Opler Cancer Center reaches well beyond the walls of Hinsdale Hospital and physicians' offices. The Center is made up of a dedicated, multidisciplinary team of health care professionals who, with a high degree of skill and compassion, deliver medically advanced inpatient and outpatient care in a community setting, close to patients' home and families.

Since 1982, Hinsdale Hospital's Opler Cancer Center has continually proven itself by providing the most up-to-date care. For instance, Opler specialists have been successfully performing bone marrow transplants since 1985, offering advanced treatment at less cost than most university research medical centers. As a result, people in the community have gained the advantage of being among the first to benefit from state-of-the-art cancer treatment.

As medical science continues to take quantum leaps in preventing and treating cancer, Opler Cancer Center specialists make those advances readily available. With access to more than 100 research protocols usually found only in the university or research setting, the Opler Cancer Center offers the most technologically advanced services, including:

- Bone Marrow/Stem Cell Technology
- Radiation Oncology
- Stereotactic Radiosurgery
- Brachytherapy
- Biologic Response Modifier Therapy (Immunotherapy)
- Stereoscopic Biopsies and Surgery
- Gynecologic Oncology Services
- Clinical Research Protocols, including the latest in chemotherapeutic agents
- Support Groups for Adults and Children
- Blood Component Collection Center
- Pain Management Center

Opler Cancer Center provides comprehensive services, from diagnosis through treatment, to more than 800 individuals a year, with continuity of care that makes patients confident and hopeful. Our commitment also extends to the emotional well being of patients and their families in the form of support groups. And hundreds of men and women take advantage of annual screenings for skin, prostate, breast and colon cancer. It is no accident that Opler Cancer Center is one of the most well respected cancer treatment centers in the region.

CANCER RESOURCE LINE

Cancer Resource Line nurses provide general information about cancer and its treatment, hospitals and community support programs and physician referral. It is also a resource for information about our affiliated services, Health Care at Home and St. Thomas Hospice. Call (630) 856-7526.

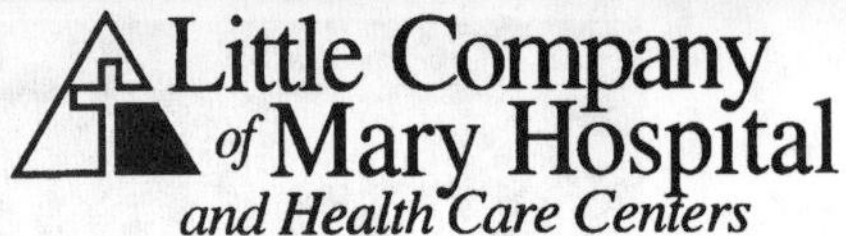

The Cancer Center

2800 W. 95TH STREET
EVERGREEN PARK, ILLINOIS 60805
PHONE (708) 229-5560

Comprehensive Cancer Care

Accredited by the American College of Surgeons, Little Company's Oncology program combines excellence in medical and radiation oncology with a tradition of caring for the whole person, body and spirit. Medical and surgical programs are integrated with a full range of support services ranging from physical therapy to pastoral care services.

A brand new Cancer Center now offers patients a chemotherapy treatment area, new radiation support facilities, a learning resource center, meeting rooms for support groups, play space for children, and other amenities all under one roof. Oncology patients will now have access to the protocols, drugs and therapies generally only provided by a university-based cancer program. State-of-the-art radiation technology is also available.

Integrated support for the Oncology program includes services such as diagnostic services, case management, home care, and hospice. Cancer patients are also invited to join a variety of support groups including Humor Outreach, I Can Cope, C.H.E.E.R., Cancer Closet, and Reach for Recovery.

Little Company of Mary Hospital and Health Care Centers is owned and operated by the Sisters of the Little Company of Mary. They are an international congregation of women founded by Venerable Mary Potter in 1877 in Nottingham England, to provide health care to the communities they serve. Since 1930, Little Company has been a community-based hospital that provides advanced medical technologies in a friendly, compassionate environment. With the power of prayer as a foundation for all of its efforts, Little Company is committed to being a healing presence in this community. For more information about the Cancer Center at Little Company, please call (708)229-5560.

MEDICAL ONCOLOGY AFFILIATION

Little Company of Mary Hospital and Health Care Centers is proud to announce our new affiliation with the Medical Oncology Group of the University of Chicago Hospitals. For years, Little Company has been a leader in cancer care on Chicago's south side. Now, our premier cancer treatment is even better.

With medical oncologists from the University of Chicago Hospitals on staff at Little Company, south side residents will now have access to the best in cancer research, diagnosis and treatment through one of the most prominent cancer care and research organizations in the United States.

Plans are now underway to renovate and expand Little Company's Cancer Center, further enhancing this exciting partnership to provide unmatched cancer treatment close to home. To find out more about Little Company's Cancer Center, please call 708/229-6001 or 708/229-6002.

Lutheran General Hospital

1775 DEMPSTER STREET • PARK RIDGE, ILLINOIS 60068

Lutheran General Cancer Care Center

Scope of Care

In 1995, Lutheran General Hospital opened the most comprehensive Cancer Care Center in the northwest suburban corridor. The center brings a full range of Lutheran General's oncology services together in a convenient, central location. It provides a multidisciplinary approach to prevention, evaluation, diagnosis, treatment and follow-up.

The Cancer Care Center offers the latest technology, featuring an entire range of radiation oncology services, steriotactic radiosurgery and radiotherapy for adults and children, state-of-the-art imaging, and chemotherapy. Other services include autologous bone marrow transplantation, biologics, chemo-prevention in high-risk individuals, lymphoma and multiple myeloma specialty programs. Research activities focus on more than 100 clinical trials and participation in pioneering studies of potential cancer prevention and treatment drugs, as well as new treatment techniques in radiology oncology.

Special Programs

The Lutheran General Cancer Care Center hosts a number of special programs, including:

- The Midwest Children's Brain Tumor Clinic
- The Lutheran General Breast Center
- The Multidisciplinary Head and Neck Tumor Clinic
- Prostate Seed Implantation
- The Pigmented Lesion Clinic

CANCER CARE CENTER

The Cancer Care Center's multidisciplinary team includes:

- *Primary care physicians*
- *Surgeons*
- *Hematologist/oncologists*
- *Radiation oncologists*
- *Gynecological oncologists*
- *Diagnostic radiologists*
- *Nuclear medicine physicians*
- *Pathologists*
- *Otolaryngologists*
- *Dentists*
- *Thoracic surgeons*

The team also features specially trained and dedicated nurse specialists, pharmacists, social workers, pastoral care counselors, therapists and dietitians.

To learn more about the Cancer Care Center at Lutheran General Hospital, it's physicians, programs and support groups... call 1-800-3-ADVOCATE (1-800-323-8622).

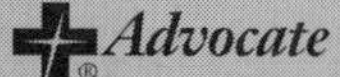

Rush-Presbyterian-St. Luke's Medical Center

Rush Cancer Institute

1725 W. HARRISON STREET, SUITE 809 • Chicago, IL 60612
PHONE (800) CA4-RUSH FAX (312) 455-9635

Research Drives Cancer Care at Rush

Rush-Presbyterian-St. Luke's Medical Center has developed a national reputation for its multidisciplinary cancer treatment and research. This tradition continues through the Rush Cancer Institute.

Physicians at Rush pioneered the concept of a **multidisciplinary breast cancer clinic** where a woman is seen by a team of experts, including a surgeon, radiation therapist and medical oncologist, during the same visit. Patients receive comprehensive treatment plans based on their cancer, age, health and other factors. In addition to its Comprehensive Breast Center, Rush offers other multidisciplinary centers to treat **prostate cancer**; **leukemia** and **lymphoma**; **chest**, **head** and **neck cancers**; **bone** and **soft tissue cancers**; **bone marrow cancers**, including **multiple myeloma**; **skin cancer**; **cervical**, **uterine**, **ovarian and related cancers**; and **brain cancer**.

Patients benefit from continuous research at the Institute — clinical trials of new therapies and surgeries, and basic research exploring the molecular biology of tumor cells, the regulation of tumor growth, the reversal of drug resistance and the use of antitumor vaccines. Through this work, Rush patients benefit from the latest advances in prevention, diagnosis and treatment.

In 1997, Rush received nearly $10 million from the National Cancer Institute of the National Institutes of Health to study acute leukemia and myelodysplasia, a blood disorder that is often fatal.

Rush researchers are studying new biological therapies that combine vitamins and other natural disease-fighters with chemotherapy and radiation therapy. These therapies alter the behavior of malignant cells to make them more responsive to treatment.

The Rush Cancer Institute also offers psychological counseling and support groups aimed at serving the emotional and spiritual needs of patients and their families.

FOCUS ON TREATMENT

Rush was one of only 50 sites where patients participated in the groundbreaking studies of the monoclonal antibody Herceptin, one of the newest anti-cancer drugs to successfully treat metastatic breast cancer.

Positron emission tomography (PET) can detect cancer spread months before standard imaging tests, allowing for early treatment. Rush's PET scanner was the first in Chicago to be used for patient care.

Research in the uses of bone marrow and stem cell transplant offers new hope for people with leukemia and lymphoma, as well as advanced cancers of the breast, ovaries and brain.

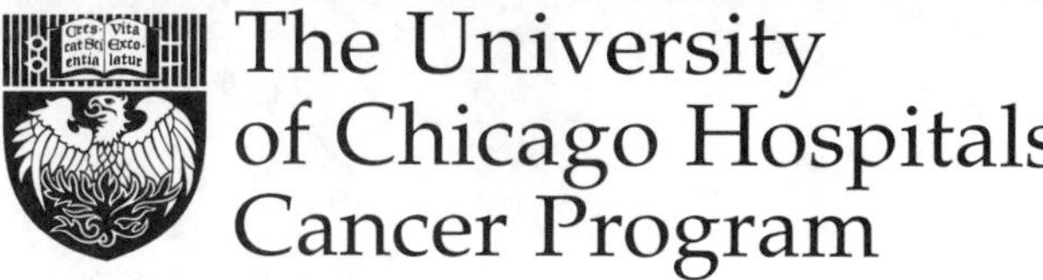

5841 S. MARYLAND AVENUE
CHICAGO, IL 60637-1470
FOR HELP FINDING A PHYSICIAN: 1-888-UCH-0200

At The Forefront of Cancer Care

The University of Chicago Hospitals' cancer program ranks ninth in the nation and first in Illinois, according to *U.S. News and World Report*. More than 500 scientists, physicians, and other professionals from 20 different academic and clinical departments fight cancer here. Their work encompasses all aspects of the disease: prevention, detection, diagnosis, and treatment.

Designated by the National Cancer Institute (NCI) as a Comprehensive Cancer Center, the University of Chicago Hospitals are currently working with more than $30 million in cancer research grants — more funding than any other hospital in the state. We are one of only a few centers in the United States selected by the NCI for Phase I and II clinical trials on new cancer-fighting drugs. Our cancer experts — among the most renowned in the world — can quickly translate new knowledge from the scientific lab to the patient's bedside, providing innovative treatments long before they are available at most other hospitals.

New, Effective Treatments and Clinical Trials

- Sophisticated diagnostics, including a computerized system that combines an MRI, PET scan, and CT scan to produce a three-dimensional image of the brain. This detailed image allows doctors to pinpoint tumor location before radiation therapy or surgery.
- Advanced techniques that preserve organ function and healthy tissue whenever possible, so patients with colon, rectal, head and neck, and other cancers can maintain normal body functioning and appearance.
- Bone marrow transplants for treatment of Hodgkin's and non-Hodgkin's lymphomas, and all types of leukemia in children and adults. Bone marrow transplants are also used to treat solid tumors in the breasts, testicles, and other areas. Stem-cell transplants are provided as well.

To Find a University of Chicago Cancer Specialist,
Call 1-888-UCH-0200
Visit our web site: www.uchospitals.edu

SERVING PATIENTS FROM AROUND THE WORLD

Our cancer program draws patients from throughout the Chicago area, the Midwest, the nation, and even the world. Our patients' problems are diverse, yet they reach for a common goal: to find the most effective solutions to meet their unique needs.

CARDIOVASCULAR

Alexian Brothers Medical Center Cardiology Services

800 BIESTERFIELD ROAD
ELK GROVE VILLAGE, IL 60007-3397
PHONE: (847) 437-5500
WEB SITE: WWW.ALEXIAN.ORG

Diagnostic technology facilitates early detection

Alexian Brothers Medical Center (ABMC) provides a full continuum of cardiology services, beginning with a focus on early detection through sophisticated diagnostic technology.

The Medical Center's diagnostic services include non-invasive and invasive techniques as well as outpatient event monitoring and risk factor analysis.

Non-invasive diagnostic techniques offered by ABMC include echocardiography, stress echocardiography, dobutamine stress echocardiology, transesophageal echocardiology, nuclear cardiology and magnetic resonance imaging.

For invasive diagnostic techniques, the Medical Center features three newly renovated, state-of-the-art cardiac catheterization suites. ABMC's cardiac catheterization program handles more than 2,700 procedures annually.

In addition, the Medical Center's Emergency Department has developed a Chest Pain Evaluation Program to quickly identify and treat heart attack and stroke victims.

Respected surgeons, state-of-the-art facility

ABMC's staff of dedicated physicians demonstrate their commitment to medical advancement through their ongoing involvement in research protocols.

The technologies available at ABMC to treat patients experiencing heart attacks range from various drug therapies to primary angioplasty and stent procedures. Other interventional services offered by ABMC include cardiac atherectomy, cardiac intravascular ultrasound, valvuloplasty, electrophysiology services, peripheral angioplasty, peripheral stenting, peripheral atherectomy and carotid stenting.

ABMC features a state-of-the-art cardiac surgery facility, including open heart operating rooms with sophisticated monitoring systems. The Medical Center's highly skilled and widely respected surgical teams perform a wide range of surgeries, including minimally invasive cardiac surgery, "off-pump" cardiac surgery, cardiac pacemaker implants, cardiac defibrillator implants, and ventricular assist device implants.

RECOVERY, FOLLOW-UP AND PREVENTION

Cardiac surgery patients recover in the Medical Center's specially equipped cardiovascular intensive care units, critical care units, and telemetry units.

ABMC also offers cardiac rehabilitation services, including a collaborative program with William Rainey Harper College in Palatine, IL, under which ABMC physicians refer patients to Harper's extensive rehabilitation facility.

In addition, the Medical Center provides follow-up care for cardiac patients, including pacemaker and defibrillator clinics and home health services.

Other cardiac services offered by ABMC focus on prevention of cardiovascular disease. These services include community and professional education programs and "Fit for a Lifetime", a community based cardiac risk factor reduction program.

A TEAM APPROACH TO HOLISTIC CARE

ABMC is committed to providing the highest quality cardiac care through a team approach that involves not only cardiac surgeons, but also cardiologists, interventional cardiologists, anesthesiologists, medical specialists, nurses, respiratory therapists and other skilled professionals.

All members of the team are dedicated to the Alexian Brothers' Value of Holism, which emphasizes healing of the whole person-body, mind and spirit-through physical, psychological and spiritual care.

Christ Hospital and Medical Center

4440 WEST 95TH STREET • OAK LAWN, ILLINOIS 60453

The #1 Heart Hospital in Northern Illinois

Christ Hospital and Medical Center, recently named one of the Top 100 Cardiovascular Hospitals in the nation by HCIA, Inc. - a leading healthcare information company - treats more heart patients than any other center in Chicagoland. In heart care, higher volumes generally mean a higher quality program. That's because expertise comes with experience — and that extends not just to physicians but to everyone involved in a patient's care. So choosing a team and a facility that has higher volumes for coronary artery bypass, open heart surgery, catheterizations, balloon angioplasties and other interventional procedures is a wise course of action.

Our capabilities include:

Cardiodiagnostics: Christ Hospital maintains comprehensive testing labs that provide a full complement of cardiac procedures to aid physicians in the diagnosis of heart disease. Diagnostic procedures include echocardiograms, stress echocardiograms, EKGs, Holter monitor evaluations, stress tests and thallium stress tests, angiograms and electrophysiology studies — and many are conducted seven days a week.

Interventional Services: Christ Hospital operates four dedicated cardiac catheterization labs. Interventional procedures performed include angioplasty and atherectomy. The hospital's Surgical Pavilion features state-of-the-art capabilities for all cardiac surgical procedures and post-operative monitoring. The intensive care unit and surgical heart unit are supported by 24-hour physician coverage and staffed with nurses specially trained in cardiac care. Christ Hospital also is a leader in management of congestive heart failure.

Continued Care: Cardiac patients can build strength and improve their functional health with the Christ Hospital cardiac and pulmonary rehabilitation services. Patients participate in a four-phase cardiac rehabilitation program that includes telemetry monitoring of patients in a controlled exercise environment, as well as individual instruction on lifestyle modification, diet, medications and continued exercise to ensure long-term health.

CARDIOVASCULAR SERVICES

Healthy Heart Care at Christ Hospital and Medical Center

Christ Hospital believes patient education is the best preventive medicine. The hospital's comprehensive Heart Risk Assessment includes a multi-lead EKG-monitored exercise test, cholesterol screening (including HDL, LDL and Triglycerides), body fat analysis; blood pressure reading; and a personal health questionnaire. Call 1-800-3-ADVOCATE (1-800-323-8622) for an appointment.

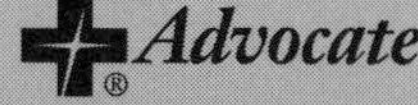

Good Samaritan Hospital

3815 HIGHLAND AVENUE • DOWNERS GROVE, IL 60515

CARDIOVASCULAR SERVICES

The #1 Heart Hospital In DuPage County

In heart care, experience makes a difference. The number of cardiac procedures a hospital performs is a key benchmark for clinical quality. At Good Samaritan Hospital, our experience and expertise span the continuum from cardiac risk prevention to diagnosis and treatment. As a result, Good Samaritan is one of the most innovative and comprehensive cardiac centers in Illinois. For example, each year we:

- perform nearly 500 open heart surgeries, providing post-operative care in our dedicated eight-bed Surgical Heart Unit
- treat more than 1,900 chest pain patients in our Chest Pain Emergency Center
- perform more than 3,500 procedures in our cardiac cath lab, making it one of the busiest in the Midwest

Good Samaritan physicians have pioneered some of cardiac care's newest interventional technologies, diagnostics and pr ventive techniques. For example:

- Our physicians were among the first in Illinois to perform coronary stents
- Good Samaritan was one of the first in the area to perform minimally-invasive surgical procedures including the HeartPort procedure
- Angioplasty has been part of the hospital's repertoire since 1986
- Cardiologists at Good Samaritan were some of the first to master the technique of radiofrequency catheter ablation
- The hospital has a dedicated electrophysiology lab

Call 1-800-3-ADVOCATE (1-800-323-8622) for a referral to nearly 70 board-certified cardiologists and cardiovascular surgeons.

Preventive Care at Good Samaritan Hospital

Preventive care is at the heart of Good Samaritan's cardiovascular program. The hospital's comprehensive Heart Risk Assessment includes a multi-lead EKG monitored exercise test; cholesterol, glucose, triglyceride, and blood pressure screenings; body fat analysis; and detailed results and recommendations for follow-up. Call 1-800-3-ADVOCATE for an appointment.

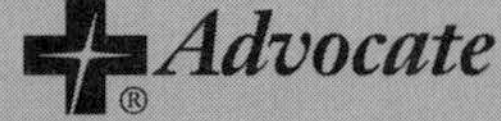

Hinsdale Hospital
Rooney Heart Institute

120 N. OAK STREET • HINSDALE, IL 60521
PHONE (630) 856-9000 WWW.AHSMIDWEST.ORG

The Institute's full range of heart care services span from diagnosis to treatment and rehabilitation. Sophisticated diagnostics and treatments include:

Open Heart Surgery

- Coronary Bypass
- Valve Repair/Replacement
- Adult Congenital
- Treatment of Thoracic Aortic Disease
- Surgical Treatment of Arrhythmia

Non-invasive Cardiac Procedures

- Stress Test
- Stress Echocardiogram
- Thallium/Cardiolite Stress Test
- Treatment of Thoracic Aortic Disease
- Transesophageal Echocardiogram
- Tilt Table

Cardiac Catheterization

- Angiogram*
- Angioplasty*
- Atherectomy*
- Stent Replacement
- EPS
- Pacemaker/Defibrillator

Cardiac Rehab Phases I, II, and III

HeartScore - Cardiac Risk Assessment

Chest Pain Emergency Department

Vascular Lab Testing

Clot-dissolving Medication (TPA, Streptokinases)

Stress Management Classes

Smoking Cessation Classes

**Peripheral and Cardiac*

Physician Referral:

Please call (630) 856-7500 for a physician referral (weekdays 8 a.m. - 5 p.m.).

COMPREHENSIVE CARDIAC CARE

The Rooney Heart Institute is one of the most sophisticated community heart care centers in Illinois, providing advanced expertise and total heart care. In one easily accessible setting, the Institute blends the resources of leading-edge technology with the specialized care and convenience of a community hospital.

The cardiac catheterization lab has marked more than 15 years of advanced care. Since 1984, cardiologists have performed more than 10,000 catheterization procedures, maintaining a success rate above the national average. The cath lab has also grown and expanded in step with the latest medical technology. Hinsdale Hospital has two state of the art cath labs which enable specialists to handle an emergency catheterization procedure even when another procedure is scheduled or in process.

Rush-Presbyterian-St. Luke's Medical Center

Rush Heart Institute

1725 W. HARRISON STREET, SUITE 1159 • Chicago, IL 60612
PHONE (312) 563-2230 FAX (312) 733-1221

A Leader in the Midwest

Staffed by world-renowned physicians, scientists and other health professionals, the Rush Heart Institute is ranked among the country's top medical centers for heart disease prevention, treatment and research.

The patient care provided at the Rush Heart Institute is based on cutting-edge research into the underlying causes of heart disease. The Institute offers the most advanced and comprehensive cardiovascular care for adults and children in Chicago. This includes advanced diagnostic tools such as the Rush Heart Scan, which uses electron-beam tomography to detect disease in the coronary arteries before it causes illness. This scanning device can be used to screen people at high risk of developing blocked arteries.

Cardiovascular surgeons at the Rush Heart Institute are experts in performing all types of cardiac surgery, such as bypass operations and valve repairs, as well as minimal access heart surgery, when appropriate. For patients with chest pain who have not been helped by other treatments, the Rush Heart Institute offers a revolutionary new procedure known as transmyocardial laser revascularization that restores blood flow to damaged areas of the heart. Only two medical centers in the Chicago area provide this technology, and only a few nationwide.

Physicians and scientists at the Institute have received numerous research grants from the National Institutes of Health for pioneering work into the causes and treatment of heart disease. About 40 clinical trials are under way at the Institute to evaluate drugs, devices and technical advances in cardiac care.

Rush also offers preventive health services, including cholesterol-lowering programs, high blood pressure treatments, personalized nutrition counseling, stress management and counseling to quit smoking.

CUTTING-EDGE TECHNIQUES

The Rush Heart Institute is the only medical center in Chicago with advanced, state-of-the-art diagnostic imaging equipment called ***positron emission tomography.*** *This enables physicians to identify damaged, nonfunctioning heart muscle that can be saved, and has allowed patients who had no hope without a heart transplant to receive less drastic treatment and live productive lives.*

The Heart Failure and Cardiac Transplant Program *provides innovative medical and surgical treatment, including transplantation, for patients with advanced heart disease or heart failure.*

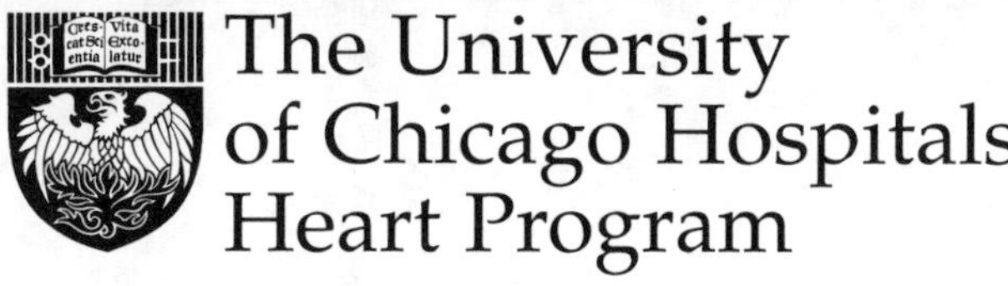

5841 S. MARYLAND AVENUE
CHICAGO, IL 60637-1470
FOR HELP FINDING A PHYSICIAN: 1-888-UCH-0200

At The Forefront Of Cardiac Care

The University of Chicago Hospitals' cardiac center ranks 14th in the nation and first in Illinois, according to *U.S. News and World Report.* Our team of cardiologists and cardiac surgeons at the University of Chicago Hospitals have two goals: to provide state-of-the-art, high quality care to all patients, and to develop new therapies that improve health and prolong lives.

Our team of clinicians, scientists, and medical staff work in the most modern facilities to provide patients with up-to-date treatments often before they are generally available in the community. The new 525,000-square-foot Center for Advanced Medicine houses our outpatient cardiovascular center and offers patients numerous efficiencies, including easier scheduling. And, with all cardiology and related clinics on one floor, multiple tests and procedures can often be performed on the same day.

New and Effective Treatments

Our physicians are at the forefront of exciting advances in clinical cardiology:

- New three-dimensional, non-invasive imaging techniques, which enable physicians to better diagnose, evaluate, and treat cardiac conditions.
- Enhanced electrophysiology capabilities for the treatment of abnormal heart rhythms, including the non-surgical implantation of smart defibrillators.
- The use of newly developed interventional techniques to revascularize patients with severe three-vessel coronary artery disease without open-heart surgery.
- Innovative medical and surgical therapies for patients with severe ventricular dysfunction and congestive heart failure.

As part of the oldest and most successful National Institutes of Health-funded cardiovascular research program in the country, our physician-scientists benefit from millions of dollars in annual research support to study and cure heart disease. Spanning molecular biology, physiology, pharmacology, and biochemistry of the cardiovascular system, this research helps to develop novel therapies for hyperlipidemias, atherosclerosis, cardiac arrhythmias, and heart failure.

To Find a University of Chicago Heart Specialist,
Call 1-888-UCH-0200
Visit our web site: www.uchospitals.edu

FINDING NEW THERAPIES FOR HEART DISEASES

University of Chicago experts are unraveling the genetic basis of heart diseases such as hyperlipidemias, artherosclerosis, and congestive heart failure and are devising new genetic and pharmacological therapies for these disorders.

GASTROENTEROLOGY

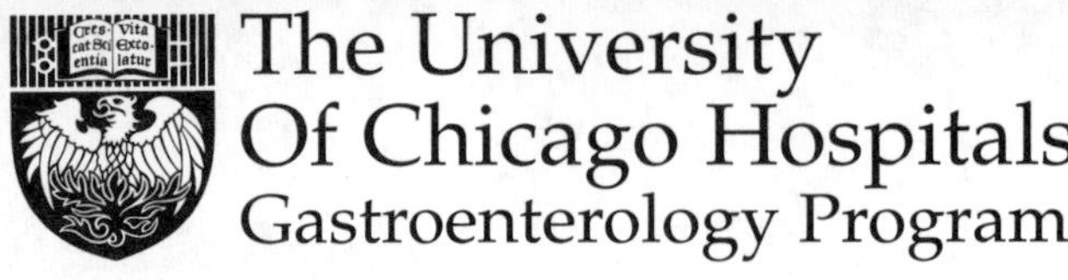

5841 S. MARYLAND AVENUE
CHICAGO, IL 60637-1470
FOR HELP FINDING A PHYSICIAN: 1-888-UCH-0200

At the Forefront of Gastroenterology

The University of Chicago Hospitals' gastroenterology program ranks sixth in the nation and first in Illinois, according to *U.S. News and World Report.* With more than 25 GI specialists on staff, the program plays a leading role in the understanding of digestive diseases and in developing innovative and successful treatments.

Since forming the nation's first full-time department of gastroenterology in 1927, University of Chicago physicians have continually improved treatments for digestive tract and related disorders, including inflammatory bowel disease, hepatitis and other liver diseases, pancreatic disease, and nutrition disorders.

Inflammatory Bowel Disease

The University of Chicago Hospitals have an international reputation in the diagnosis and treatment of inflammatory bowel diseases: Crohn's disease and ulcerative colitis. Because physicians here study the causes of these diseases and continually evaluate new therapies, patients often have access to new medications before they are available elsewhere. Surgery, when necessary, is performed by specialists in complex gastro-intestinal surgery and who work closely with their colleagues on the GI team.

Hepatitis, Other Liver Diseases, and Pancreatic Disease

Here, our primary focus is to develop new therapies for fulminant and chronic hepatitis B and C, as well as for cirrhosis and pancreatic disease. When appropriate, specialists can call upon the University of Chicago's Liver Transplant Program, established in 1984 and the oldest in the Midwest. More than 1,000 liver transplants have been successfully performed in adult patients.

Nutrition Disorders

The Clinical Nutrition Support Team has extensive experience in the treatment of complicated nutritional problems, including obesity disorders. It is one of just eight in the country supported by the National Institutes of Health.

Call 1-888-UCH-0200 To Find A University of Chicago Gastroenterology Specialist

Visit our web site: www.uchospitals.edu

SCREENINGS AND PROCEDURES

The Center for Advanced Medicine offers colorectal cancer screenings, as well as diagnostic tests for an entire range of gastrointestinal disorders. Therapies include removal of polyps, esophageal dilation, gallstone extraction, and infrared coagulation of hemorrhoids.

GERIATRICS

Rush-Presbyterian-St. Luke's Medical Center

Rush Institute for Healthy Aging

710 S. PAULINA, 4TH FLOOR • Chicago, IL 60612
PHONE (312) 942-3600 FAX (312) 492-6019

Facing the Challenge of Aging

As the population ages, physicians, scientists and other health care professionals at the Rush Institute for Healthy Aging are developing innovative approaches to helping older adults remain healthy, active and independent as long as possible.

The Institute provides primary and consultative care for older adults, both in the inpatient and outpatient settings. Under the medical direction of physicians specializing in geriatric medicine, the Institute offers medical, psychiatric and rehabilitative care for people over age 55 through the **Johnston R. Bowman Health Center for the Elderly**. Facilities include subacute and skilled nursing units, where elderly patients recovering from acute illness can continue their recovery.

The **Center for Rehabilitation Services** at the Bowman Center offers physical, occupational and recreational therapy to older adults. Diagnostic and treatment services are offered for patients with back, neck or shoulder pain, reflex sympathetic dystrophy, Parkinson's disease, multiple sclerosis, strokes and amputations.

The **Rush Alzheimer's Disease Center** at Bowman is one of the nation's largest programs providing diagnostic and treatment services for people with signs and symptoms of dementia, such as memory loss and confusion. Counseling and education are available for patients and their families. The Alzheimer's Family Care Center on Chicago's North Side offers adult daycare.

The Bowman Center also offers one- and two-bedroom apartments in a community setting for people aged 60 and over.

The **Rush Home Care Network** serves patients throughout Chicago and in neighboring suburbs. Services available through referral include in-home nursing care; postsurgical care; chemotherapy and other forms of IV therapy; psychosocial support; occupational, physical and speech therapy; and housekeeping support. Comprehensive, compassionate hospice care is also available through **Rush Hospice Partners**.

The Rush Institute for Healthy Aging strives to give older patients the best chance to recover after illness or injury, so they can maintain maximum independence. Its programs emphasize extensive rehabilitation services, care in the home when possible, preventive and diagnostic services, and family involvement with the care team and the care plan.

The Institute is also developing a resource center for older adults and their families that will provide information on physicians, health care services, long-term care and housing options, and community resources.

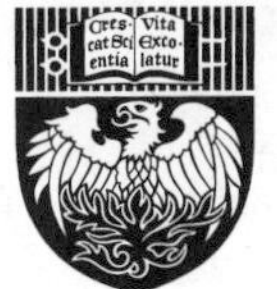

The University of Chicago Hospitals Geriatrics Program

5841 S. MARYLAND AVENUE
CHICAGO, IL 60637-1470
FOR HELP FINDING A PHYSICIAN: 1-888-UCH-0200

Outstanding Care for Older Adults

The University of Chicago Hospitals' geriatrics program ranks 12th in the nation and first in Illinois, according to *U.S. News and World Report.* We have one of the nation's largest groups of physicians who are fellowship-trained and board-certified in geriatric medicine. Called "geriatricians," these specialists focus on health issues facing men and women in their 60s and beyond.

University of Chicago geriatricians see patients at our main campus, as well as at the Windermere Health Center, located near the Museum of Science and Industry. This center offers medical and support services exclusively for older patients. Another center will soon open in Chicago's South Shore neighborhood.

Team of Experts Close At Hand

Our geriatricians have expertise in dealing with conditions common to older adults, such as incontinence, depression, and dementia. They also work in tandem with some of the nation's leading experts in cancer, gastroenterology, neurology, orthopaedics, and urology. For example:

- Physicians here are experts in disorders of memory, cognition, and emotion which can strike older adults. The multidisciplinary approach at the new Memory Disorders Center will enable more precise diagnoses and offer the latest innovations in coordinated patient care.
- Their keen attention to detail and their comprehensive diagnostic procedures aid in identifying dementias including Alzheimer's disease. Sometimes, close scrutiny reveals good news: symptoms which suggest dementia may be caused by a vitamin deficiency.
- Because arthritis is so common among older people, the multidisciplinary Geriatric Arthritis and Musculoskeletal Center at the Windermere focuses specifically on this con dition.

To Find A University Of Chicago Specialist in Geriatrics,
Call 1-888-UCH-0200
Visit our web site: www.uchospitals.edu

KEEPING OLDER ADULTS HEALTHY AND ACTIVE

These specialists understand the needs of older adults. Their mission is to keep them healthy, active, and independent as long as possible. These physicians manage common and chronic disorders including arthritis, diabetes, heart disease, and memory disorders, including Alzheimer's disease. Eye and dental care are also available.

MATERNAL-CHILD HEALTH

Alexian Brothers Medical Center Mother and Child Center

800 BIESTERFIELD ROAD
ELK GROVE VILLAGE, IL 60007-3397
PHONE: (847) 437-5500
WEB SITE: WWW.ALEXIAN.ORG

Personalized care, high-tech support

With a comfortable, homelike environment, an experienced and dedicated staff and advanced medical technology, the Mother and Child Center at Alexian Brothers Medical Center helps patients and their families feel supported, secure and special.

The facility exudes warmth, featuring beautifully decorated rooms and a highly qualified nursing staff that provides compassionate, one-on-one support. Many of the facility's nurses are certified in the specialized field of inpatient obstetrics.

As a state-designated Level II-plus perinatal center, the facility offers 24 hour coverage by a board-certified neonatologist, a pediatrician with special training in the care of healthy newborns and those with special needs. A staff perinatologist meets the special needs of mothers whose pregnancies are considered high risk, and an anesthesiologist is in the hospital around the clock to respond to patient requests for pain relief.

The Mother and Child Center's sophisticated technology is kept behind the scenes to foster a homelike atmosphere, but is available at a moment's notice if needed by a mother or her baby.

Reflecting the staff's commitment to individual needs, the facility has one of the lowest Caesarean section rates among hospitals in Chicago's northwest suburbs. The facility also has a high number of successful vaginal births after Caesarean sections.

Labor, delivery, recovery in one room

The Mother and Child Center helps to prepare patients and their families for the arrival of a new baby by offering a full array of cihldbirth classes, ranging from pre-pregnancy planning to Lamaze training.

When the time comes for the baby's arrival, patients in labor are escorted directly to one of the facility's 10 labor/delivery/recovery rooms, where the entire birthing process occurs. Patients who are scheduled to have a Caesarean section or outpatient testing are evaluated in a specially equipped three-bed assessment and testing area.

After giving birth, patients spend the rest of their hospital stay in a room in the facility's 36-bed post-partum unit. Patients can choose to room in with their baby or to have their baby spend part of the day in the facility's 32-bed nursery. The Mother and Child Center also has a six-bed Level II-plus nursery with a specialized staff and technology to care for babies with special needs.

EASING THE TRANSITION TO LIFE WITH A NEW BABY

The first days at home with a new baby are a period of adjustment for everyone in a family. To ease the transition, the Mother and Child Center offers a special program enabling most parents to receive a home visit from a Center nurse after mother and baby are back home.

The nurse can answer questions about baby care and family life. She also will check the health of the mother and baby and perform any basic necessary testing.

The nurse also will do her best to address any special needs a new mother might have. For example, the nurse can help a mother who chooses to breast feed her baby by putting her in touch with lactation educators available through the Mother and Child Center. These specialists help new mothers learn how to breast feed, providing encouragement and guidance along the way.

TOURS, PHYSICIAN REFERRALS AVAILABLE

To obtain more information about the Mother and Child Center at Alexian Brothers Medical Center, or to schedule a tour, please call 1-888-394-9400.

If you are looking for a physician, ask for the Medical Center's physician referral service which can help you find the right doctor for you.

Hinsdale Hospital Birck Family Women's and Children's Center

120 N. OAK STREET • HINSDALE, IL 60521
PHONE (630) 856-9000 WWW.AHSMIDWEST.ORG

The Birthing Center You Always Wanted Has Arrived

Hinsdale Hospital has been a leader in maternity care since the turn of the century with the delivery of the area's first baby in a hospital setting. Other firsts include birthing rooms, Lamaze classes, nurse midwives, and lactation consultants. Expectant mothers can choose from a wide array of birthing options and a support team of nurses and clinical educators offer new moms baby care education. The Birck Family Women's and Children's Center comes equipped with a Level II with exception Special Care Nursery to stabilize and provide intense medical care for critically ill newborns.

On-Site Maternal-Fetal Medicine Center

For high-risk pregnancies, we have a dedicated Maternal-Fetal Medicine Center that is staffed by a full-time perinatologist. This center, in turn, is backed by the full perinatology staff and capabilities of the University of Chicago Hospitals.

Hinsdale Center for Reproduction

If becoming pregnant is a problem, The Hinsdale Center for Reproduction, located on the campus of Hinsdale Hospital, offers advanced reproductive assistance that has produced one of the highest success rates in the Chicago area.

State-of-the-art Neonatology

For newborns that are at high-risk, our 3,500 square foot neonatal unit, with 13 intensive care stations, is the latest in neonatal medicine. This enables us to care for nearly all of our at-risk newborns at Hinsdale Hospital, instead of transferring them to downtown medical centers.

On-unit Cesarean Delivery

If you should require a Cesarean delivery, we have two surgical rooms right in our birthing center. Both are totally equipped to handle any Cesarean procedure, whether planned or unplanned.

Home at Last

For first-time parents, parents of multiples, and even experienced parents, being at home with the newborn is a little overwhelming. That's why we offer a free, 24-hour parent hot line at (630) 856-6431.

Physician Referral: Please call (630) 856-7500 for a physician referral (weekdays 8 a.m. - 5 p.m.).

MATERNAL CARE

At Hinsdale Hospital, we have always believed in family centered births, backed by the latest medical technology and physician specialists. After nearly 100 years of continually refining this philosophy, we have now taken it to the next level and created the Birck Family Women's & Children's Center. Here, everything is centered on you and your birth experience. From comfortable suites to caring and experienced professionals to the most innovative fetal and neonatal medicine, The Birck Family Women's & Children's Center reflects the newest and best thinking in medicine, birthing and amenities.

Lake Forest Hospital Obstetrics & Gynecology

660 N. WESTMORELAND RD.
LAKE FOREST, IL 60045
PHONE: (847) 234-5600 FAX: (847) 234-6552

A Focus on You and Your Family

Every step of the way, Lake Forest Hospital (LFH) helps you plan and achieve the birth you want. Our beautiful birthing suites are individually decorated to accommodate you, your baby and your family with soothing comfort, plus the latest in fetal monitoring equipment.

From preconception to postpartum education, LFH's "Great Beginnings" maternity classes are dedicated to family health. Our Lactation Center, Newborn Hotline, Universal Hearing Screening and Maternity Home Visit are unique among Lake County hospitals; we go the extra mile to ensure the success of your new family.

With a full staff of quality pediatricians and a variety of pediatric services, you are sure to find the right care for your child.

Clinical Expertise and Support Every Step of the Way

You'll feel secure in the care of some of the area's most distinguished obstetricians/gynecologists who meet the highest standards and are acclaimed for their bedside manner as well as their clinical excellence. Our Level II Perinatal designation allows our on-site perinatologists to care for mothers during high-risk pregnancies and our neonatologists to provide advanced care for newborns.

Our nurses believe that helping you give birth is much more than a job. It's their passion. They provide encouragement and support and they are continually advancing their training, including certification in inpatient obstetrics and fetal monitoring.

Once your baby is born, our nurses provide lactation counseling, newborn care and much more. And help is never more than a phone call away through our 24-hour Newborn Hotline.

Physician Referral

On staff at LFH are over 35 of the most distinguished OB/GYNs in the area. These physicians participate in most major health care programs. To learn more, call our Physician Referral Service at (847) 234-6171. The service operates Monday through Friday from 7 a.m. to 3:15 p.m.

THE LEADER IN MATERNITY SERVICES

The special environment at Lake Forest Hospital surrounds you with everything that's important. You'll feel pampered by our highly skilled, caring professionals and you'll experience an atmosphere of joyful celebration not found anywhere else. That's why over 2,000 babies are born each year at Lake Forest Hospital; that's more than any other hospital in Lake County.

PEDIATRICS

Hope Children's Hospital

4440 WEST 95TH STREET • OAK LAWN, ILLINOIS 60453

Pediatric Services

Chicagoland's Newest Children's Hospital

Hope Children's Hospital, the four-story children's hospital which opened in 1996 on the campus of Christ Hospital and Medical Center, is a specialty hospital that combines extraordinary medical expertise with a child-centered environment. Staffed by more than 120 pediatricians representing more than 30 specialties, Hope Children's Hospital is a premier provider of treatment for children throughout the Midwest.

Hope Children's Hospital is one of the leading providers of pediatric services in the areas of pediatric cardiology, oncology, critical care, perinatology, neonatology, neurology, gastroenterology and rehabilitation and development.

Hope Children's Hospital also houses The Heart Institute for Children, a regional center of excellence in the care of newborns and children with heart disease. The medical staff is internationally recognized for diagnostic, surgical and critical care capabilities. Along with providing superior cardiac care, The Heart Institute for Children is a national center for research and development, pioneering advances in the diagnosis and treatment of heart disease.

The hospital treats nearly 5,000 pediatric patients annually, and has approximately 65,000 outpatient visits. The facility includes: 45 private inpatient rooms with sleeping and bath accommodations for parents, and a 15-bed pediatric intensive care unit.

Separate treatment and recreation rooms preserve the child's perception of safe-haven sleeping and play areas.

At Hope Children's Hospital, every staff member works to minimize children's fear of treatment, to modify the hospitalization experience for maximum comfort, and to view the nature of treatment through the eyes of a child.

PEDIATRIC SERVICES

Pediatric Emergency Center

The Pediatric Emergency Center of Christ Hospital and Medical Center is available to fill urgent care and emergency needs. One of Illinois' first emergency departments approved for pediatric care, this facility has an experienced staff of emergency medicine and pediatric physicians and nurses who specialize in caring for children. The center has a child-friendly environment that makes your experience as easy as possible. For more information call 1-800-3-ADVOCATE (1-800-323-8622).

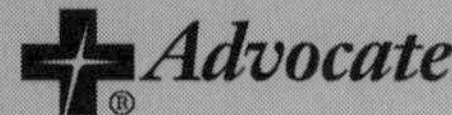

Lutheran General Children's Hospital

1775 DEMPSTER STREET • PARK RIDGE, ILLINOIS 60068

Scope of Care

Lutheran General Children's Hospital is one of the largest and most comprehensive children's hospitals in Illinois. It is the leading resource in the northwest suburban corridor for children and their families, and is a major referral center for a broad range of pediatric services, especially for children with complex illnesses and chronic conditions. The medical staff consists of over 185 pediatricians and pediatric subspecialists that provide primary and tertiary care in every major subspecialty caring for more than 3,500 pediatric inpatients and handling 100,000 outpatient visits annually.

Special Programs

The Victor Yacktman Children's Pavilion is one of the largest and most comprehensive facilities for pediatric outpatient services in the Chicago area. It consolidates under one roof pediatric primary care, subspecialties, diagnostics and therapies, along with specialty clinics for children with complex illnesses and chronic conditions, and one of the largest centers in the state for children with developmental disabilities or delays.

The Midwest Children's Brain Tumor Center is one of the few centers in the nation and the only facility in a five-state area with a comprehensive range of neurological services, clinical expertise and technology.

The Advanced Level III Perinatal Center (the highest designation possible) is one of the most technologically advanced facilities of its type in the Chicago region. Our experienced medical staff deliver nearly 5,000 babies each year — more than any other private hospital in the area.

The Pediatric Emergency and Trauma Services at Lutheran General Children's Hospital is one of only five Pediatric Trauma Centers certified at the highest level (Level I) in the Chicago area, the Children's Hospital is fully staffed 24 hours a day with pediatricians, trauma surgeons and specially trained support staff.

PEDIATRICS

To Access Lutheran General Hospital Children's Hospital...

The first step in accessing the full range of services offered by Lutheran General Children's Hospital is developing a healthy relationship with an affiliated pediatrician or family practice physician. Our physicians will serve as your first and best resource for health care information and treatment guidance. For more information on our affiliated physicians and health care services, or to make an appointment...call 1-3-800-3-ADVOCATE (1-800-232-8622).

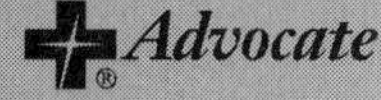

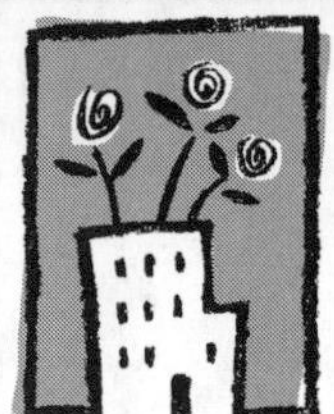

THE UNIVERSITY OF CHICAGO CHILDREN'S HOSPITAL

WYLER HOSPITAL PAVILION
5839 S. MARYLAND AVENUE CHICAGO, IL 60637
FOR HELP FINDING A PHYSICIAN: 1-888-UCH-0200

At The Forefront Of Kids' Medicine

Staffed by more than 100 faculty physicians, the University of Chicago Children's Hospital is dedicated to helping children with medical problems ranging from the routine to the complex. It is a place where patient care, teaching, and research come together to find cures for childhood illnesses.

At the hospital and through its outpatient clinics, pediatricians provide advanced therapies to children and teens in virtually all clinical areas, including allergy, arthritis, asthma, cancer, cardiology, child development, diabetes, ear/nose/throat, emergency medicine, gastroenterology, genetics, gynecology, infectious disease, neonatology, neurology, orthopaedics, psychiatry, and surgery.

World Renowned Specialty Expertise

Critically ill or injured children are cared for in the state-of-the-art Frankel Pediatric Intensive Care Unit. This 22-bed facility treats children with multiple traumas; complex medical problems; major surgery, including cardiac and neurosurgery; renal failure; and transplants. In addition, a 53-bassinet neonatal intensive care unit provides premature and critically ill infants with the most advanced medical care and life support systems available.

Our pediatric liver transplantation program is one of the largest in the country and was the first living-donor program in the world. In 1989, we performed the first successful liver transplant from a living donor.

Our pediatric cancer program offers virtually every available form of therapy, both conventional and investigational, for a child afflicted with cancer. The program is a principal member of the Children's Cancer Study Group, an international consortium of cancer research hospitals that participate in trials and exchange information on the latest advances in diagnosis and treatment. We also perform bone marrow transplants for virtually all indications, from leukemia and solid tumors to inborn errors of metabolism

To Find A University Of Chicago Pediatrician, Call 1-888-UCH-0200
Visit our web site: www.uchospitals.edu

TAILORED TO THE NEEDS OF CHILDREN

Our physicians are particularly sensitive to the special physical and emotional needs of children and their families. Our staff is dedicated to teaching children about their illnesses and medical procedures, as well as helping children and families to cope with the stress of a child's illness.

REHABILITATION

The Rehabilitation Institute of Chicago

At Alexian Brothers Medical Center

955 BEISNER ROAD
ELK GROVE VILLAGE, IL 60007-3397
PHONE: (847) 981-3582
WEB SITE: WWW.ALEXIAN.ORG

Comprehensive care from a team that cares

The Rehabilitation Institute of Chicago at Alexian Brothers Medical Center (RIC at ABMC) offers a comprehensive, results-oriented rehabilitation program featuring a team of specialists that delivers individualized, compassionate care.

RIC at ABMC provides intensive acute rehabilitation through a 40-bed inpatient center and an outpatient department that serve patients with a variety of illnesses and physical disabilities. These include amputation, arthritis, brain injury, burns, cancer, cardiac disorders, chronic pain, deconditioning, incontinence, industrial injury, multiple trauma, musculo-skeletal and soft-tissue injury, neurologic and neuromuscular disorders, organ transplants, orthopedic injury, osteoporosis, spinal cord injury, speech and swallowing disorders, sports injuries, strokes and wound care.

The RIC at ABMC team takes an interdisciplinary approach to evaluating each patient's individual needs and then develops a customized treatment plan for each patient. The patient's family members and personal physician play a key role in developing the treatment plan. Individual plans focus on patient-centered goals, such as optimizing a patient's mobility or improving the patient's communication abilities, cognitive skills or daily living skills.

When a patient completes his or her treatment at RIC at ABMC, the care does not end. RIC at ABMC offers ongoing support through services that provide recreational, social, educational and networking opportunities for patients and other physically challenged individuals.

Special services for special needs

RIC at ABMC understands that some patients might require special assistance beyond intensive acute rehabilitation.

To meet their needs, RIC at ABMC offers a variety of additional programs and services. These include an evaluation of home and mobility equipment needs, low-vision clinic, neonatal swallowing evaluation, neuromuscular rehabilitation program, neuropsychological testing, pediatric rehabilitation outpatient program, driving evaluation/education with adaptive equipment, occupational therapy hands program, and a continence biofeedback program.

ADVANCED, DYNAMIC CARE

RIC at ABMC combines the expertise and resources of the Rehabilitation Institute of Chicago (RIC) and Alexian Brothers Medical Center (ABMC) to provide advanced and dynamic care.

Physicians surveyed by U.S. News and World Report have rated RIC as the nation's top rehabilitation institution for the last eight years.

In addition, the rehabilitation programs at RIC and ABMC are accredited by the Joint Commission of Accreditation of Healthcare Organizations and are licensed by the Illinois Department of Public Health.

BROAD SPECTRUM OF EXPERTISE

A board-certified physiatrist (a physician specializing in rehabilitation medicine) leads the RIC at ABMC team and can tap into a complete array of staff specialists, depending on a patient's needs.

These specialists include physical therapists, occupational therapists, speech and language pathologists, certified rehabilitation nurses, chaplains, dietitians, social workers, recreational therapists, neuropsychologists / rehabilitation psychologists, vocational counselors, orthotists and prosthetists. Additional specialists are available as needed.

WOMEN'S HEALTH

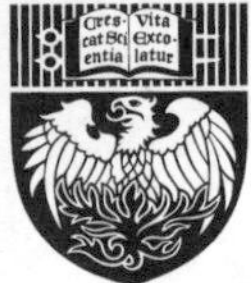

The University of Chicago Hospitals Women's Programs

5841 S. MARYLAND AVENUE, CHICAGO, IL 60637-1470
FOR HELP FINDING A PHYSICIAN: 1-888-UCH-0200

The Breast Center

The University of Chicago Hospitals' new Breast Center, with its own information resource library and boutique, is dedicated to all aspects of breast health, including screening mammograms. If breast cancer is suspected, women are evaluated by specialists in diagnostic mammography and breast surgery. A treatment plan is then individually tailored to the woman's specific needs after discussion with our panel of experts, which includes oncologists, radiation oncologists, and plastic surgeons. A woman coming to the center for a second opinion can have her mammogram results, biopsies, and the full range of treatment options discussed with her during a single visit.

Obstetrics and Gynecology – From Routine to the Most Complex

Our physicians and nurse-midwives manage women's care during normal and high-risk pregnancies, counsel their patients on family planning and contraception, and provide genetic counseling and testing. Eight community hospitals depend on our regional perinatal center to supervise the care during high-risk pregnancies for both mothers and newborns. In addition to routine gynecologic care, our specialists treat endometriosis, uterine fibroids, sexually-transmitted diseases, pelvic pain, recurrent miscarriage, menstrual abnormalities, polycystic ovary syndrome, delayed puberty, pelvic organ prolapse, urinary incontinence, and all menopausal disorders.

Infertility and Reproductive Expertise

Our team of specialists have one of Chicago's highest success rates in solving reproductive system problems and infertility. They provide a full range of treatments for male and female infertility problems, from drug therapy and artificial insemination to donor egg programs, introcytoplasmic sperm injection (ICSI) and in vitro fertilization.

Gynecological Cancers

Our world-renowned multidisciplinary team develops treatment options which may include surgery, radiation, chemotherapy, or a combination of these therapies. Our gynecologic oncologists have special expertise in ovarian, cervical, and DES-related cancers; gynecologic surgery; and human papilloma virus (HPV).

To Find A University Of Chicago Physician
Call 1-888-UCH-0200
Visit our web site: www.uchospitals.edu

AT THE FOREFRONT OF WOMEN'S CARE

The University of Chicago Hospitals provide health care for women during every stage of life, from adolescence through menopause and beyond. According to U.S. News and World Report, the University of Chicago Hospitals' obstetrics and gynecology program ranks 13th in the nation.

SECTION FOUR

APPENDICES

APPENDIX A

AMERICAN BOARD OF MEDICAL SPECIALTIES

PURPOSE OF THE AMERICAN BOARD OF MEDICAL SPECIALTIES

THE STATEMENT OF PURPOSE INCLUDED IN THE ARTICLES OF INCORPORATION IS:

- *To improve the standards of medical care.*
- *To act as spokesman for all approved specialty boards, as a group.*
- *To resolve problems encountered among and between specialty boards.*
- *To deal with the applications for approval of proposed new specialty boards, new types of certification, modification of existing types of certification, and related matters.*
- *To endeavor to avoid duplication of effort by specialty boards.*
- *To establish and maintain standards of organization and operation of specialty boards.*

Following is a list of the addresses of the medical specialty boards approved by the ABMS. Note that there are 24 board organizations for 25 medical specialties. Psychiatry and Neurology share the same board.

To find out if a physician is certified, consumers can call the individual boards which will provide information for a fee, or they can call the ABMS at (800) 776-2378. (No fee)

BOARD SPECIALTIES

- **American Board of Allergy and Immunology**
  510 Walnut Street, Suite 1701
  Philadelphia, PA 19106-3694
  (215) 592-9466
  General Certification in Allergy and Immunology; with Added Qualification in Diagnostic Laboratory Immunology. Certifications awarded since 1989 are valid for 10 years. For those certified prior to 1989 there is no recertification requirement.

- **American Board of Anesthesiology**
  4101 Lake Boone Trail
  The Summit Suite 510
  Raleigh, NC 27607-7506
  (919) 881-2570
  General Certification in Anesthesiology; with Added Qualifications in Critical Care Medicine and Pain Management. In the subspecialty of Pain Management certifications awarded as of 1993 are valid for 10 years.

- **American Board of Colon and Rectal Surgery**
  20600 Eureka Road, Suite 713
  Taylor, MI 48108
  (313) 282-9400
  General Certification is in Colon and Rectal Surgery. Certifications awarded since 1991 are valid for 8 years.

- **American Board of Dermatology**
  Henry Ford Hospital
  One Ford Place
  Detroit, MI 48202
  (313) 874-1088
  General Certification in Dermatology; with Special Qualifications in Dermatopathology, Dermatological Immunology/Diagnostic and Laboratory Immunology. Certifications awarded since 1991 are valid for 10 years. For those certified prior to 1991, there is no recertification requirement.

- **American Board of Emergency Medicine**
  3000 Coolidge Road
  East Lansing, MI 48823
  (517) 332-4800
  General Certification in Emergency Medicine; with Special and Added Qualifications in Pediatric Emergency Medicine and Sports Medicine. Certifications are valid for a 10-year period.

- **American Board of Family Practice**
2228 Young Drive
Lexington, KY 40505
(606) 269-5626
General Certification in Family Practice; with Added Qualifications in Geriatric Medicine and Sports Medicine. Certifications are valid for a 7-year period.

- **American Board of Internal Medicine**
510 Walnut Street, Suite 1701
Philadelphia, PA 19106-3694
(215) 446-3500, (800) 441-ABIM
General Certification in Internal Medicine; with Special Qualifications in Cardiovascular Disease, Critical Care Medicine, Endocrinology, Diabetes and Metabolism, Gastroenterology, Hematology, Infectious Disease, Medical Oncology, Nephrology, Pulmonary Disease, and Rheumatology; and Added Qualifications in Adolescent Medicine, Cardiac Electrophysiology, Diagnostic Laboratory Immunology, Geriatric Medicine, and Sports Medicine. Certifications awarded since 1990 are valid for 10 years. For those certified prior to 1990 there is no recertification requirement.

- **American Board of Medical Genetics**
9650 Rockville Pike
Bethesda, MD 20814
(301) 571-1825
General Certification in Clinical Genetics, Medical Genetics, Clinical Biochemical Genetics, Clinical Cytogenetics, Clinical Biochemical/Molecular Genetics and Clinical Molecular Genetics. Certifications are valid for a 10-year period.

- **American Board of Neurological Surgery**
Smith Tower, Suite 2139
6550 Fannin Street
Houston, TX 77030-2701
(713) 790-6015
General Certification in Neurological Surgery. Presently, there is no recertification requirement.

- **American Board of Nuclear Medicine**
900 Veteran Avenue, Room 12-200
Los Angeles, CA 90024-1786
(310) 825-6787
General Certification in Nuclear Medicine. Certifications awarded since 1992 are valid for 10 years. For those certified prior to 1992, there is no recertification requirement.

- **American Board of Obstetrics and Gynecology**
  2915 Vine Street
  Dallas, TX 75204
  (214) 871-1619
  General Certification in Obstetrics and Gynecology; with Special Qualifications in Gynecologic Oncology, Maternal and Fetal Medicine, Reproductive Endocrinology and Added Qualification in Critical Care. Certifications awarded since 1986 are valid for 10 years. For those certified prior to 1986, there is no recertification requirement.

- **American Board of Ophthalmology**
  111 Presidential Boulevard, Suite 241
  Bala Cynwyd, PA 19004
  (610) 664-1175
  Certifications awarded since 1992 are valid for 10 years. For those certified prior to 1992, there is no recertification requirement.

- **American Board of Orthopaedic Surgery**
  400 Silver Cedar Court
  Chapel Hill, NC 27514
  (919) 929-7103
  General Certification in Orthopaedic Surgery; with Added Qualification in Hand Surgery. Certifications awarded since 1986 are valid for 10 years. For those certified prior to 1986, there is no recertification requirement.

- **American Board of Otolaryngology**
  2211 Norfolk, Suite 800
  Houston, TX 77098-4044
  (713) 528-6200
  General Certification in Otolaryngology; with Added Qualification in Otology/Neurotology and Pediatric Otolaryngology. Presently, there is no recertification requirement.

- **American Board of Pathology**
  P.O. Box 25915
  Tampa, FL 33622-5915
  (813) 286-2444
  General Certification in Anatomic and Clinical Pathology, Anatomic Pathology and Clinical Pathology; with Special Qualifications in Blood Banking/Transfusion Medicine, Chemical Pathology, Dermatopathology, Forensic Pathology, Hematology, Immunopathology, Medical Microbiology, Neuropathology and Pediatric Pathology and Added Qualification in Cytopathology. Presently, there is no recertification requirement.

American Board of Pediatrics

111 Silver Cedar Court
Chapel Hill, NC 27514-1651
(919) 929-0461

General Certification in Pediatrics; with Special Qualifications in Adolescent Medicine, Allergy & Immunology, Pediatric Cardiology, Pediatric Critical Care Medicine, Pediatric Emergency Medicine, Pediatric Endocrinology, Pediatric Gastroenterology, Pediatric Hematology-Oncology, Pediatric Infectious Diseases, Pediatric Nephrology, Pediatric Pulmonology, Neonatal-Perinatal Medicine and Pediatric Rheumatology. Added Qualifications in Diagnostic Laboratory Immunology, Medical Toxicology and Sports Medicine. Certifications valid for 7 years.

American Board of Physical Medicine and Rehabilitation

Norwest Center, Suite 674
21 First Street, S.W.
Rochester, MN 55902
(507) 282-1776

General Certification in Physical Medicine and Rehabilitation; with Added Qualifications in Spinal Cord Injury Medicine. Certifications awarded since 1993 are valid for 10 years.

American Board of Plastic Surgery

Seven Penn Center, Suite 400
1635 Market Street
Philadelphia, PA 19103-2204
(215) 587-9322

General Certification in Plastic Surgery; with Added Qualification in Hand Surgery. Certifications are valid for a 10-year period.

American Board of Preventive Medicine

9950 W. Lawrence Avenue, Suite 106
Schiller Park, IL 60176
(847) 671-1750

General Certification in Aerospace Medicine, Occupational Medicine and Public Health and General Preventive Medicine; with Added Qualification in Underseas Medicine and Medical Toxicology. In the subspecialty of Underseas Medicine and Medical Toxicology certifications are valid for a 10-year period.

American Board of Psychiatry & Neurology

500 Lake Cook Road, Suite 335
Deerfield, IL 60015
(847) 945-7900

General Certification in Psychiatry, Neurology and Neurology with Special Qualification in Child Neurology; with Special Qualification in Child and Adolescent Psychiatry and Added Qualification in Addiction Psychiatry, Clinical Neurophysiology, Forensic Psychiatry and Geriatric Psychiatry. Certifications are valid for a 10-year period.

- **American Board of Radiology**
  5255 E. Williams Circle, Suite 3200
  Tucson, AZ 85711
  (520) 790-2900
  General Certification in Diagnostic Radiology or Radiation Oncology; with Special/Competency in Nuclear Radiology and Added Qualifications in Neuroradiology, Pediatric Radiology and Vasular and Interventional Radiology. Radiation Physics is a non clinical certification. Certificates are valid for a 10-year period.

- **American Board of Surgery**
  1617 John F. Kennedy Boulevard, Suite 860
  Philadelphia, PA 19103-1847
  (215) 568-4000
  General Certification in Surgery; with Special Qualifications in Pediatric Surgery and General Vascular Surgery and Added Qualifications in Surgery of the Hand, Surgical Critical Care and General Vascular Surgery. Certifications are valid for a 10-year period.

- **American Board of Thoracic Surgery**
  One Rotary Center, Suite 803
  1560 Sherman Avenue
  Evanston, IL 60201
  (847) 475-1520
  General Certification in Thoracic Surgery. Certifications awarded since 1976 are valid for 10 years. For those certified prior to 1976, there is no recertification requirement.

- **American Board of Urology**
  2216 Ivy Road, Suite 210
  Charlottesville, VA 22903
  (248) 646-9720
  General Certification in Urology. Certifications awarded as of 1985 are valid for 10 years. For those certified prior to 1985, there is no recertification requirement.

APPENDIX B
OSTEOPATHIC BOARDS

American Osteopathic Association
142 E Ontario Street
Chicago, IL 60611
(800) 621-1773

GENERAL CERTIFICATION

- **American Osteopathic Board of Anesthesiology**
  Anesthesiology
  - No time-limited certificates

- **American Osteopathic Board of Dermatology**
  Dermatology
  - No time-limited certificates

- **American Osteopathic Board of Emergency Medicine**
  Emergency Medicine
  - Beginning 1/1/94, 10-year certificates

- **American Osteopathic Board of Family Physicians**
  Family Practice
  - No time-limited certificates

- **American Osteopathic Board of Internal Medicine**
  Internal Medicine
  - Beginning 1/1/93, 10-year certificates

- **American Osteopathic Board of Neurology and Psychiatry**
  - Neurology
  - Psychiatry
  - • Beginning 1/1/96, 10-year certificates

- **American Osteopathic Board of Obstetrics and Gynecology**
  - Obstetrics and Gynecology
  - • No time-limited certificates

- **American Osteopathic Board of Ophthalmology and Otorhinolaryngology**
  - Ophthalmology
  - • No time-limited certificates
  - Otorhinolaryngology
  - Facial Plastic Surgery
  - Otorhinolaryngology and Facial Plastic Surgery
  - • No time-limited certificates

- **American Osteopathic Board of Orthopaedic Surgery**
  - Orthopaedic Surgery
  - • Beginning 1/1/94, 10-year certificates

- **American Osteopathic Board of Pathology**
  - Laboratory Medicine
  - Anatomic Pathology
  - Anatomic Pathology and Laboratory Medicine
  - • Beginning 1/1/95, 10-year certificates

- **American Osteopathic Board of Pediatrics**
  - Pediatrics
  - • Beginning 1/1/95, 7-year certificates

- **American Osteopathic Board of Preventive Medicine**
  - Preventive Medicine/Aerospace Medicine
  - Preventive Medicine/Occupational-Environmental Medicine
  - Preventive Medicine/Public Health
  - • Beginning 1/1/94, 10-year certificates

- **American Osteopathic Board of Proctology**
  - Proctology
  - • No time-limited certificates

- **American Osteopathic Board of Radiology**
  Diagnostic Radiology
  Radiation Oncology
  - No time-limited certificates

- **American Osteopathic Board of Rehabilitation Medicine**
  Rehabilitation Medicine
  - Beginning 6/1/95, 7-year certificates

- **American Osteopathic Board of Special Proficiency in Osteopathic Manipulative Medicine**
  Special Proficiency in Osteopathic Manipulative Medicine
  - Beginning 1/1/95, 10-year certificates

- **American Osteopathic Board of Surgery**
  Surgery (general)
  Plastic and Reconstructive Surgery
  Thoracic Cardiovascular Surgery
  Urological Surgery
  General Vascular Surgery
  - No time-limited certificates

Consumers may call the American Osteopathic Association at (800) 621-1773 for general certification information.

NOTES:

APPENDIX C

DESCRIPTIONS OF SPECIALTIES AND SUBSPECIALTIES

Addiction Psychiatry
A subspecialty certified by the American Board of Psychiatry and Neurology, Addiction Psychiatry deals with habitual psychological and physiological dependence on a substance or practice which is beyond voluntary control.

Adolescent Medicine
A subspecialty certified by both the American Board of Internal Medicine and the American Board of Pediatrics, Adolescent Medicine involves the primary care treatment of adolescents and young adults.

Allergy & Immunology
A specialty certified by the American Board of Allergy and Immunology, an allergist/immunologist diagnoses and treats allergies, asthma, and skin problems such as hives and contact dermatitis.

Cardiac Electrophysiology (Clinical)
A subspecialty certified by the American Board of Internal Medicine, Clinical Cardiac Electrophysiology involves complicated technical procedures to evaluate heart rhythms and determine appropriate treatment for them.

Cardiovascular Medicine
A subspecialty certified by the American Board of Internal Medicine, Cardiovascular Medicine involves the diagnosis and treatment of disorders of the heart, lungs, and blood vessels.

Child & Adolescent Psychiatry
A subspecialty certified by the American Board of Psychiatry and Neurology, Child & Adolescent Psychiatry deals with the diagnosis and treatment of mental diseases in children and adolescents.

Child Neurology
A specialty certification of Neurology. (See Neurology)

Colon and Rectal Surgery
A specialty certified by the American Board of Colon and Rectal Surgery, a colon and rectal surgeon surgically treats diseases of the intestinal tract, colon, and rectum, anal canal, and perianal area.

Critical Care Medicine
A subspecialty certified by the American Boards of Anesthesiology, Internal Medicine, Neurological Surgery, and Obstetrics & Gynecology, Critical Care Medicine involves diagnosing and taking immediate action to prevent death or further injury of a patient. Examples of critical injuries include shock, heart attack, drug overdose, and massive bleeding.

Dermatology
A specialty certified by the American Board of Dermatology, a dermatologist diagnoses and treats benign and malignant disorders of the skin, mouth, external genitalia, hair and nails, as well as a number of sexually transmitted diseases.

Diagnostic Radiology
A specialty certified by the American Board of Radiology, Diagnostic Radiology involves the study of all modalities of radiant energy in medical diagnoses and therapeutic procedures utilizing radiologic guidance.

Emergency Medicine
A specialty certified by the American Board of Emergency Medicine, an emergency physician deals with acute-care problems such as those seen in emergency room situations.

Endocrinology, Diabetes & Metabolism
A subspecialty certified by the American Board of Internal Medicine, Endocrinology, Diabetes & Metabolism involves the study and treatment of patients suffering from hormonal and chemical disorders.

Family Practice
A specialty certified by the American Board of Family Practice, a family practitioner deals with and oversees the total health care of individual patients and their family members. Family practitioners are more common in rural areas and may perform procedures more commonly performed by specialists (e.g., minor surgery).

Forensic Psychiatry

A subspecialty certified by the American Board of Psychiatry, Forensic Psychiatry concerns the evaluation of certain diagnostic groups of patients that include those with sexual disorders, antisocial personality disorders, paranoid disorders, and addictive disorders.

Gastroenterology

A subspecialty certified by the American Board of Internal Medicine, Gastroenterology is the study, diagnosis and treatment of diseases of the digestive organs including the stomach, bowels, liver, and gallbladder.

Geriatric Medicine

A subspecialty certified by the American Boards of Family Practice and Internal Medicine, Geriatric Medicine deals with diseases of the elderly and the problems associated with aging.

Geriatric Psychiatry

A subspecialty certified by the American Board of Psychiatry and Neurology, Geriatric Psychiatry involves the diagnosis, prevention, and treatment of mental illness in the elderly.

Gynecologic Oncology

A subspecialty certified by the American Board of Obstetrics and Gynecology, Gynecologic Oncology deals with cancers of the female genital tract and reproductive systems.

Hand Surgery

A subspecialty certified by the American Boards of Orthopaedic Surgery, Plastic Surgery, and Surgery, Hand Surgery involves the treatment of injury to the hand through surgical techniques.

Hematology

A subspecialty certified by the American Boards of Internal Medicine and Pathology, Hematology involves the diagnosis and treatment of diseases and disorders of the blood, bone marrow, spleen, and lymph glands.

Infectious Disease
A subspecialty certified by the American Board of Internal Medicine, Infectious Disease is the study and treatment of diseases caused by a bacterium, virus, fungus, or animal parasite. AIDS is an infectious disease.

Internal Medicine
A specialty certified by the American Board of Internal Medicine, an internist diagnoses and nonsurgically treats diseases, especially those of adults. Internists may act as primary care specialists, highly trained family doctors, or they may subspecialize in areas such as cardiology or nephrology.

Maternal & Fetal Medicine
A subspecialty certified by the American Board of Obstetrics and Gynecology, Maternal & Fetal Medicine involves the care of women with high-risk pregnancies and their unborn infants.

Medical Genetics
A specialty certified by the American Board of Medical Genetics, a medical geneticist is a physician or scientist who identifies the genetic causes of inherited diseases and ailments and prevents, when possible, their occurrence.

Medical Oncology
A subspecialty certified by the American Board of Internal Medicine, Medical Oncology refers to the study and treatment of tumors and other cancers.

Neonatal-Perinatal Medicine
A subspecialty certified by the American Board of Pediatrics, Neonatal-Perinatal Medicine involves the diagnosis and treatments of infants prior to, during, and one month beyond birth.

Nephrology
A subspecialty certified by the American Board of Internal Medicine, Nephrology is concerned with disorders of the kidneys, high blood pressure, fluid and mineral balance, dialysis of body wastes when the kidneys do not function, and consultation with surgeons about kidney transplantation.

Neurological Surgery
A specialty certified by the American Board of Neurological Surgery, a neurosurgeon performs surgery on the brain, spinal cord, and nervous system.

Neurology
A specialty certified by the American Board of Psychiatry and Neurology, a neurologist diagnoses and medically treats disorders of the brain, spinal cord, and nervous system.

Neurophysiology (Clinical)
A subspecialty certified by the American Board of Psychiatry and Neurology, Clinical Neurophysiology is the study of the makeup and functioning of the nervous system in patients as opposed to in a laboratory.

Neuroradiology
A subspecialty certified by the American Board of Radiology, Neuroradiology involves the utilization of imaging procedures during diagnosis as they relate to the brain, spine and spinal cord, head, neck, and organs of special sense in adults and children.

Nuclear Medicine
A specialty certified by the American Board of Nuclear Medicine, a nuclear medicine specialist, working in either a laboratory or with patients, evaluates the functions of all the organs in the body and treats thyroid disease, benign and malignant tumors, and radiation exposure through the use of radioactive substances.

Nuclear Radiology
A subspecialty certified by the American Boards of Nuclear Medicine and Radiology, Nuclear Radiology involves the use of radioactive substances to diagnose and treat certain functions and diseases of the body.

Obstetrics & Gynecology
A specialty certified by the American Board of Obstetrics & Gynecology, obstetrics deals with the medical aspects of and intervention in pregnancy and labor. Gynecology involves the medical and surgical care of the female reproductive system and associated disorders.

Occupational Medicine
A subspecialty certified by the American Board of Preventive Medicine, Occupational Medicine concentrates on the effects of the work environment on the health of employees.

Ophthalmology
A specialty certified by the American Board of Ophthalmology, an ophthalmologist diagnoses and treats diseases of and injuries to the eye.

Orthopaedic Surgery
A specialty certified by the American Board of Orthopaedic Surgery, an orthopaedic surgeon operates to correct injuries which interfere with the form and function of the extremities, spine, and associated structures.

Otolaryngology
A specialty certified by the American Board of Otolaryngology, an otolaryngologist (also known as ENT specialist) explores and treats diseases in the interrelated areas of the ears, nose and throat.

Otology/Neurotology
A subspecialty certified by the American Board of Otolaryngology, Otology/ Neurotology concentrates on the management, prevention, cure and care of patients with diseases of the ear and temporal bone, including disorders of hearing and balance.

Pain Management
A subspecialty certified by the American Board of Anesthesiology, Pain Management involves providing a high level of care for patients experiencing problems with acute or chronic pain in both hospital and ambulatory settings.

Pediatric Allergy & Immunology
A subspecialty certified by the American Board of Pediatrics, Pediatric Allergy & Immunology involves the diagnosis and treatment of allergies, asthma and skin problems in children.

Pediatric Cardiology
A subspecialty certified by the American Board of Pediatrics, Pediatric Cardiology involves the diagnosis and treatment of heart disease in children.

Pediatric Critical Care Medicine
A subspecialty certified by the American Board of Pediatrics, Pediatric Critical Care Medicine involves the care of children who are victims of life threatening disorders such as severe accidents, shock, and diabetes acidosis.

Pediatric Emergency Medicine
A subspecialty certified by both the American Boards of Emergency Medicine and Pediatrics, Pediatric Emergency Medicine refers to the treatment of children in an acute-care situation.

Pediatric Endocrinology
A subspecialty certified by the American Board of Pediatrics, Pediatric Endocrinology involves the study and treatment of children with hormonal and chemical disorders.

Pediatric Gastroenterology
A subspecialty certified by the American Board of Pediatrics, Pediatric Gastroenterology is the study, diagnosis, and treatment of diseases of the digestive tract in children.

Pediatric Hematology-Oncology
A subspecialty certified by the American Board of Pediatrics, Pediatric Hematology-Oncology is the study and treatment of cancers of the blood and blood-forming parts of the body in children.

Pediatric Infectious Disease
A subspecialty certified by the American Board of Pediatrics, Pediatric Infectious Disease is the study and treatment of diseases caused by a virus, bacterium, fungus, or animal parasite in children.

Pediatric Nephrology
A subspecialty certified by the American Board of Pediatrics, Pediatric Nephrology deals with the diagnosis and treatment of disorders of the kidneys in children.

Pediatric Otolaryngology
A subspecialty certified by the American Board of Otolaryngology, Pediatric Otolaryngology involves the diagnosis and treatment of disorders of the ear, nose, and throat which affect children.

Pediatric Pulmonology
A subspecialty certified by the American Board of Pediatrics, Pediatric Pulmonology involves the diagnosis and treatment of diseases of the chest, lungs, and chest tissue in children.

Pediatric Radiology
A subspecialty certified by the American Board of Radiology, Pediatric Radiology involves diagnostic imaging as it pertains to the newborn, infant, child, and adolescent.

Pediatric Rheumatology
A subspecialty certified by the American Board of Pediatrics, Pediatric Rheumatology involves the treatment of diseases of the joints and connective tissues in children.

Pediatric Sports Medicine
A subspecialty certified by the American Board of Pediatrics, Pediatric Sports Medicine involves the diagnosis and treatment of injuries to the bone or soft tissue (muscles, tendons, ligaments) in children as a result of participation in athletic activity.

Pediatric Surgery
A subspecialty certified by the American Board of Surgery, Pediatric Surgery treats disease, injury, or deformity in children through surgical techniques.

Pediatrics
A specialty certified by the American Board of Pediatrics, a pediatrician diagnoses and treats diseases of childhood and monitors the growth, development, and well-being of preadolescents.

Physical Medicine & Rehabilitation
A specialty certified by the American Board of Physical Medicine & Rehabilitation, a physiatrist uses physical therapy and physical agents such as water, heat, light, electricity, and mechanical manipulations in the diagnosis, treatment, and prevention of disease and body disorders.

Plastic Surgery
A specialty certified by the American Board of Plastic Surgery, a plastic surgeon specializes in reconstructive and cosmetic surgery of the face and other body parts.

Preventive Medicine
A specialty certified by the American Board of Preventive Medicine, a physician who specializes in preventive medicine focuses on health prevention and on the health of groups rather than individuals.

Psychiatry

A specialty certified by the American Board of Psychiatry and Neurology, a psychiatrist examines, treats, and prevents mental illness through the use of psychoanalysis and/or drugs.

Public Health & General Preventive Medicine

A subspecialty certified by the American Board of Preventive Medicine, Public Health and General Preventive Medicine involves the investigation of the causes of epidemic disease and the prevention of a wide variety of acute and chronic illness.

Pulmonary Disease

A subspecialty certified by the American Board of Internal Medicine, Pulmonary Disease involves the diagnosis and treatment of diseases of the chest, lungs, and airways.

Radiation Oncology

A subspecialty certified by the American Board of Radiology, Radiation Oncology involves the use of radiant energy and isotopes in the study and treatment of disease, especially malignant cancer.

Reproductive Endocrinology

A subspecialty certified by the American Board of Obstetrics and Gynecology, Reproductive Endocrinology deals with the endocrine system (including the pituitary, thyroid, parathyroid, adrenal glands, placenta, ovaries, and testes) and how its failure relates to infertility.

Rheumatology

A subspecialty certified by the American Board of Internal Medicine, Rheumatology involves the treatment of diseases of the joint, muscles, bones and associated structures.

Spinal Cord Injury Medicine

A subspecialty certified by the American Board of Physical Medicine & Rehabilitation, Spinal Cord Injury Medicine involves the prevention, diagnosis, treatment and management of traumatic spinal cord injuries.

Sports Medicine

A subspecialty certified by the American Boards of Emergency Medicine, Family Practice, and Internal Medicine, Sports Medicine refers to the practice of an orthopaedist or other physician who specializes in injuries to bone or soft tissue (muscles, tendons, ligaments) caused by participation in athletic activity.

Surgery
A specialty certified by the American Board of Surgery, a surgeon treats disease, injury, and deformity by surgical procedures.

Surgery of the Hand
A subspecialty certified by the American Board of Surgery, Surgery of the Hand involves providing appropriate care for all structures in the upper extremity directly affecting the hand and wrist function.

Surgical Critical Care
A subspecialty certified by the American Board of Surgery, Surgical Critical Care involves the specialized care in the management of the critically ill patient, particularly the trauma victim and postoperative patient in the emergency department, intensive care unit, trauma unit, burn unit, and other similar settings.

Thoracic Surgery
A specialty certified by the American Board of Thoracic Surgery, a thoracic surgeon performs surgery on the heart, lungs, and chest area.

Urology
A specialty certified by the American Board of Urology, a urologist diagnoses and treats diseases of the genitals in men and disorders of the urinary tract and bladder in both men and women.

Vascular & Interventional Radiology
A subspecialty certified by the American Board of Radiology, Vascular & Interventional Radiology involves diagnosing and treating diseases by percutaneous methods guided by various radiologic imaging modalities.

Vascular Surgery (General)
A subspecialty certified by the American Board of Surgery, General Vascular Surgery involves the operative treatment of disorders of the blood vessels excluding those to the heart, lungs, or brain.

APPENDIX D

SELF-DESIGNATED MEDICAL SPECIALTIES

This list of self-designated medical specialty groups was obtained from the American Board of Medical Specialties. However, it is important to point out that these groups are not recognized by the ABMS, the governing board for the recognized twenty-four medical specialty boards (listed in Appendix A).

The organizations listed below range from highly organized groups that are attempting to formalize training and certification in their field to informal groups interested in a particular aspect of medicine.

If you wish to obtain information from any of these groups you will have to do some detective work. Because so many are informal, the location, phone and mailing addresses change frequently, depending upon the person who is functioning as secretary or administrator.

The best way to track down one of these groups is to consult this book's doctor listings to find a doctor who has expressed a special interest in that field, and call his or her office. You might also call a nearby academic health center in the area to see if they have a faculty or staff member known to be involved in that particular medical interest. If that fails, take the same approach with your community hospital.

A

Abdominal Surgeons
Acupuncture Medicine
Addiction Medicine
Addictionology
Adolescent Psychiatry
Aesthetic Plastic Surgery
Alcoholism and Other Drug Dependencies (AMSAODD)
Algology (Chronic Pain)
Alternative Medicine
Ambulatory Anesthesia
Ambulatory Foot Surgery
Anesthesia
Arthroscopic Surgery
Arthroscopy (Board of North America)

B

Bariatric Medicine
Bionic Psychology
Bloodless Medicine & Surgery

C

Chelation Therapy
Chemical Dependence
Clinical Chemistry
Clinical Ecology
Clinical Medicine and Surgery
Clinical Neurology
Clinical Neurophysiology
Clinical Neurosurgery
Clinical Nutrition
Clinical Orthopaedic Surgery
Clinical Pharmacology
Clinical Polysomnography
Clinical Psychiatry
Clinical Psychology
Clinical Toxicology
Cosmetic Plastic Surgery
Cosmetic Surgery
Council of Non-Board Certified Physicians
Critical Care in Medicine & Surgery

D

Dermalogy
Disability Analysis
Disability Evaluating Physicians

E

Electrodiagnostic Medicine
Electroencephalography
Electromyography & Electrodiagnosis
Environmental Medicine
Epidemiology (College)
Eye Surgery

F

Facial Cosmetic Surgery
Facial Plastic & Reconstructive Surgery
Family Practice, Certification
Forensic Examiners
Forensic Psychiatry
Forensic Toxicology

H

Hand Surgery
Head, Facial & Neck Pain & TMJ Orthopaedics
Health Physics
Homeopathic Physicians
Homeotherapeutics
Hypnotic Anesthesiology, National Board for

I

Independent Medical Examiners
Industrial Medicine & Surgery
Insurance Medicine
International Cosmetic & Plastic Facial Reconstructive Standards
Interventional Radiology

L

Laser Surgery
Law in Medicine
Longevity Medicine/Surgery

M

Malpractice Physicians
Maxillofacial Surgeons
Medical Accreditation (American Federation for)
Medical Hypnosis
Medical Laboratory Immunology
Medical-Legal Analysis of Medicine & Surgery
Medical Legal & Workers
Comp. Medicine & Surgery
Medical-Legal Consultants
Medical Management
Medical Microbiology
Medical Preventics (Academy)
Medical Psychotherapists
Medical Toxicology
Microbiology (Medical Microbiology)
Military Medicine
Mohs Micrographic Surgery &
Cutaneous Oncology

N

Neuroimaging
Neurologic & Orthopaedic Dental
Medicine and Surgery
Neurological & Orthopaedic Medicine
Neurological & Orthopaedic Surgery
Neurological Microsurgery
Neurology
Neuromuscular Thermography
Neuro-Orthopaedic Dental Medicine & Surgery
Neuro-Orthopaedic Electrodiagnosis
Neuro-Orthopaedic Laser Surgery
Neuro-Orthopaedic Psychiatry
Neuro-Orthopaedic Thoracic Medicine/Surgery
Neurorehabilitation
Nutrition

O

Orthopaedic Medicine
Orthopaedic Microneurosurgery
Otorhinolaryngology

P

Pain Management (American Academy of)
Pain Management Specialties
Pain Medicine
Palliative Medicine
Percutaneous Diskectomy
Plastic Esthetic Surgeons
Prison Medicine
Professional Disability Consultants
Psychiatric Medicine
Psychiatry (American National Board of)
Psychoanalysis (American Examining
Board in)
Psychological Medicine (International)

Q

Quality Assurance & Utilization Review

R

Radiology & Medical Imaging
Rheumatologic Surgery
Rheumatological & Reconstructive Medicine
Ringside Medicine & Surgery

S

Skin Specialists
Sleep Medicine (Polysomnography)
Spinal Cord Injury
Spinal Surgery
Sports Medicine
Sports Medicine/Surgery

T

Toxicology
Trauma Surgery
Traumatologic Medicine & Surgery
Tropical Medicine

U

Ultrasound Technology
Urologic Allied Health Professionals
Urological Surgery

W

Weight Reduction Medicine

NOTES:

APPENDIX E
HIPPOCRATIC OATH

The Hippocratic Oath is administered to all medical students when they graduate from their respective medical schools. Today, some Deans of Medicine administer it to their students as they enter medical school in order to instill in them a sense of ethics, because even as students they will have contact with patients.

The oath is attributed to Hippocrates, a Greek physician who is often referred to as the Father of Medicine because of the degree to which he advanced medical practice and ethics. He died circa 377 B.C.

The oath has been modified by various medical schools and professional bodies and will be found in a variety of forms that typically embody the same principles.

Dorland's Illustrated Medical Dictionary. 27th ed. (Philadelphia) W.B. Saunders Co., 1988. Hippocratic Oath. [Hippocrates. Greek physician, 460-377 B.C.] An oath setting forward the duties of a physician to his patients as follows:

I swear by Apollo the physician, and Asklepios, and health, and All-Heal and all the gods and goddesses, that, according to my ability and judgement, I will keep this Oath and this stipulation — to reckon him who taught me this Art equally dear to me as my parents, to share my substance with him, and relieve his necessities if required; to look upon his offspring in the same footing as my own brothers, and to teach them this Art, if they should wish to learn it, without fee or stipulation; and that by precept, lecture and every other mode of instruction,

I will impart a knowledge of the Art to my own sons, and those of my teachers, and to disciples bound by a stipulation and oath according to the law of medicine, but to none others.

I will follow that system of regimen which, according to my ability and judgement, I consider for the benefit of my patients, and abstain from whatever is deleterious and mischievous. I will give no deadly medicine to anyone if asked nor suggest any such counsel; and in like manner I will not give to a woman a pessary to produce abortion. With purity and wholeness I will pass my life and practice my Art.

I will not cut persons labouring under the stone, but will leave this to be done by men who are practitioners of this work. Into whatever houses I enter, I will go into them for the benefit of the sick, and will abstain from every voluntary act of mischief and corruption; and, further, from the seduction of females or males, of freemen and slaves. Whatever, in connection with my professional practice, or not in connection with it, I see or hear, in the life of men, which ought not to be spoken of abroad, I will not divulge, as reckoning that all such should be kept secret. While I continue to keep this Oath unviolated, may it be granted to me to enjoy life and the practice of the art, respected by all men, in all times! But should I trespass and violate this Oath, may the reverse be my lot!

APPENDIX F

PATIENT RIGHTS

YOUR RIGHTS IN THE HOSPITAL

Hospitals in Illinois are required to adopt a bill of rights. The following bill of rights is one that has been adopted by the American Hospital Association (AHA) and is in use in many hospitals throughout the nation.

The patient has the right to:

- *Considerate and respectful care.*
- *Complete information about his/her treatment and condition in terms the patient can reasonably understand.*
- *Know the identity of physicians, nurses, and others involved in their care, as well as when those involved are students, residents, or other trainees.*
- *Information necessary to give informed consent prior to the start of any procedure or treatment.*
- *Refuse treatment and be informed of the consequences.*
- *Have an advance directive (such as a living will, health care proxy, or durable power of attorney) for health care.*
- *Privacy concerning his/her treatment.*
- *Have all records and communications regarding medical treatment kept confidential.*
- *Expect the hospital, within the limits of its capabilities, to respond to a request for services.*

- *Obtain information regarding the relationship of the hospital to any other health care institutions.*
- *Be advised if the hospital proposes human experimentation which affects his/her care.*
- *Reasonable continuity of care.*
- *An explanation of the bill, regardless of payment source.*
- *Know what hospital rules and regulations apply to patient contact.*

(Source: American Hospital Association, Chicago, IL)

According to the American Hospital Association, this was last edited in 1992, so this version should be up to date. However, the AHA now has a "Fax on Demand" service at (312) 422-2020 through which consumers can obtain an up-to-date copy, free of charge, by sending their name, fax# and specifying document # 471124.

APPENDIX G

STATE AGENCIES

While there is a wealth of information available through these state agencies, much of it is not user-friendly. Complicated contractual agreements and other legal documents contain information that might prove to be valuable providing a consumer can locate it and then review it with some understanding. Often a department will suggest that a consumer visit the office for guidance in reviewing the documents. However, some of these agencies provide useful information on doctors, hospitals, and HMOs. They may also offer statistical reports and consumer-oriented studies.

STATE AGENCIES

Check www.state.il.us/dpr to find out if any disciplinary action has been taken against a doctor.

ILLINOIS

Doctors

Department of Human Services
100 South Grand East
Springfield, Illinois 62762
(217) 557-1564

Illinois Department of Professional Regulations
320 West Washington Street
Springfield, Illinois 62786
(217) 782-0458

Illinois Department of Public Health
Legal Services
J.R. Thompson Center
100 West Randolph, Suite 6-600
Chicago, Illinois 60601
(312) 814-2793

Hospitals

Division of Health Care Facilities and Programs
525 West Jefferson, 4th Floor
Springfield, Illinois 62761
(217) 782-7412

Health Plans

Bureau of Comprehensive Health
Medical Programs
201 South Grand East
Springfield, Illinois 62763-0001
(217) 782-5565

Illinois State Department of Insurance
100 West Randolph, Suite 15-100
Chicago, Illinois 60601
(312) 814-2427

Illinois Department of Public Health
535 West Jefferson
Springfield, Illinois 62761
(217) 782-4977

Illinois Department of Aging
421 East Capitol
Springfield, Illinois 62701-1789
(217) 785-3356

APPENDIX H

STATE & COUNTY MEDICAL SOCIETIES

Although formed as professional associations of physicians, county medical societies also may be of importance to consumers through their referral services and to assist if a consumer has a complaint against a doctor.

Each county in Illinois has a medical society. Membership is open to licensed physicians and most have medical student chapters (they also have active auxiliaries that raise money for medical student scholarships). The county chapters relate to the state society which, in turn, relates to the American Medical Association. The relationship is conducted in a number of ways, but especially through elected officers serving on councils or boards at other levels (i.e. county to state, state to national).

County medical societies have a number of functions including education, advocacy for medicine and social camaraderie for doctors. (The membership in county medical societies ranges from about 50 percent to about 70 percent of doctors in a county.)

The educational function is usually carried out through an arm of the society, an Academy of Medicine, which offers continuing medical education (CME) programs for doctors in the region.

The county societies are organized by committee and usually include standing committees on legislation, public relations, ethics and peer review among others.

It is in the latter two areas that the public may be directly served and interact with the medical society.

County medical societies will review complaints by patients about doctors. Their review may be through an Ethics Committee in matters related to finance, legal, ethical or social issues; or through the Peer Review Committee in cases involving the quality or appropriateness of medical care.

If a doctor is found deficient in some respect, a medical society may censure the individual or, in more extreme cases, remove them from membership. Patients may contact the local medical society for further information if they have a problem and desire assistance.

Many county medical societies also sponsor physician referral lines for the public. All members of the medical society are eligible to participate in the referral service. Referrals are generally made on the basis of specialty, geographic proximity, languages spoken, house calls, evening hours, etc. Information such as medical school, board certification and status of medical license may also be provided.

The following is a listing of the county medical societies in the metropolitan Chicago area. They may be helpful if an individual needs information on a physician or has a problem with a physician.

STATE AND COUNTY MEDICAL SOCIETIES
STATE MEDICAL ASSOCIATION

ILLINOIS STATE MEDICAL SOCIETY

600 South 2nd Street, Suite 200
Springfield, Illinois 6704
(217) 528 5609

COUNTY MEDICAL SOCIETIES

Cook County Medical Society
515 North Dearborn
Chicago, Illinois 60610
(312) 670 2550

Du Page County Medical Society
498 Hillside Avenue
Glen Ellyn, Illinois 60137
(630) 858-9603

Kane County Medical Society
2600 Keslinger Road
Geneva, Illinois 60134
(630) 262-9884

Lake County Medical Society
850 Milwaukee Avenue, Suite 209
Vernon Hills, Illinois 60061
(847) 816- 8900

McHenry County Medical Society
123 Creekside Trail
McHenry, Illinois 60050
(815) 363-7951

Will-Grundy County Medical Society
3033 West Jefferson Street
Joliet, Illinois 10435
(815) 744-5676

NOTES:

APPENDIX I

HOW TO FILE A COMPLAINT

Filing a complaint against a physician, other health-care practitioner or hospital is a serious matter. It should be undertaken with great thought and consideration, and is justified only if a patient feels seriously aggrieved and believes a law, regulation or professional ethic has been violated.

Before a complaint is filed, it may be helpful to contact the hospital administration if the problem is with a hospital. If it is a problem with a doctor at a hospital, the chief of the service, medical director or vice-president of medical affairs should be notified.

If these efforts fail, one may consider a formal complaint. If you wish to file a formal complaint against a medical practitioner, hospital, health-care facility or insurance company, you must file it with the State, which is the licensing authority. Contact the appropriate state agency and request a complaint form and any special forms that must be filed with your particular case. Include information such as name of offending party and date, place and nature of incident. Save all records and/or receipts relating to the incident (i.e., billing statements and medical and hospital records including lab reports).

APPENDIX I

HOW TO FILE A COMPLAINT

To file a complaint against a doctor, hospital or health plan write or call the following agencies. Written complaints as well as written documentation are the more effective methods.

ILLINOIS

Doctors

Department of Professional Regulations
Complaint Intake Unit
320 West Washington Street
Springfield, Illinois 62786
(312) 814-6910

Hospitals

Illinois Department of Public Health
Division of Health Care Facilities and Programs
525 West Jefferson, 4th Floor
Springfield, Illinois 62761
(800) 252-4343
(217) 782-7412

Health Plans

Illinois State Department of Insurance
100 West Randolph, Suite 15-100
Chicago, Illinois 60601
(312) 814-2427

APPENDIX J

MEDICARE AND MEDICAID STATE AGENCIES

The following phone numbers are those consumers may call to obtain information on Medicare and Medicaid.

ILLINOIS

Medicare (800) 638-6833
Medicaid (217) 782-2570

Cook County
Medicaid (312) 738-5700

Du Page County
Medicaid (630) 530-1120

Kane County
Medicaid (847) 931-2700

Lake County
Medicaid (847) 336-5212

McHenry County
Medicaid (815) 338-0234

Will-Grundy
Medicaid (815) 740-5350

NOTES:

APPENDIX K

SELECTED RESOURCES

American Ambulance Association
1255 23rd Street Northwest, Suite 200
Washington, District of Columbia 20037
(800) 523-4447 phone
(202) 452-0005 fax
The American Ambulance Association can provide general information on EMS services.

American Board of Medical Specialities
1007 Church Street, Suite 404
Evanston, IL 60201
(800) 776-CERT phone
www.abms.org
The American Board of Medical Specialties can provide a yes/no answer regarding board certification on any specific physician in any state.

American Medical Association
515 North State Street
Chicago IL 60610
(312) 464 5000 phone
www.ama-assn.org
The American Medical Association's website contains verified information on physician members. The AMA recommends the general public contact their local medical State Society or consult hospital physician referral services for specific physician information.

Centers for Disease Control and Prevention (CDC)
Fax Information Service for International Travelers
(404) 639-2573 (information)
(404) 332-4565 (to order a document)
The CDC provides free, immediate faxed reports on disease risk and prevention and disease outbreaks in various parts of the world.

Electronic Medical Exchange (EMX)
520 Madison Avenue, 38th Floor
New York, New York 10022
(212) 758-2053 phone
EMX is a company that supplies medical records, provided to it by a member of the service, to medical personnel at times of emergency. The medical information is accessed by a card which the member carries, as well as a pin number for identification and confidentiality.

International Association for Medical Assistance To Travellers (IAMAT)
417 Center Street
Lewiston, New York 14092
(716) 754-4883 phone
IAMAT is a non-profit organization that disseminates information on health and sanitary conditions worldwide. Membership is free but donations are appreciated. Members will receive a membership card making them eligible to access English speaking physicians all over the world. The organization also provides information on immunization requirements, malaria, and other tropical diseases, and sanitary and climactic conditions around the world. For information, send request in writing.

Medic Alert Foundation
2323 Colorado Avenue
Turlock, CA 95382
(800) 432-5378 phone
The Medic Alert Foundation (a non-profit organization) provides an "ID tag" engraved with personal medical facts, as well as a 24-hour emergency response center which can release additional personal medical details. Membership is $15/year (waived for the first year) and members need to purchase the "ID tag" which sells for as low as $35.

National Center for Complementary and Alternative Medicine Clearing House
P.O. Box 8218
Silverspring, MD 20907
(888) 644-6226 phone
(301) 495-4957 fax
The National Center for Complementary and Alternative Medicine Clearing House facilitates the evaluation of alternative medical treatment modalities to help determine their effectiveness and bring alternative medicine into mainstream medicine. This agency does not provide referrals.

National Consumers League (NCL)
1701 K Street, NW, Suite 1200
Washington, DC 20006
(202) 835-3323 phone
NCL is a private, nonprofit consumer advocacy organization. NCL strives to investigate, educate, and advocate on a variety of issues including healthcare. Membership is $20 annually, but individuals can also write to the organization for a list of publications that non-members can purchase.

National Health Care Rescue Network
Post Office Box 1326
Wheaton, Illinois 60189-1326
(800) 627-0552 voice mail
(708) 510-0256 fax
The Health Care Rescue Network is an alliance that educates the public on the benefits of medical savings accounts and the dangers of managed care. They will refer consumers to local organizations.

National Insurance Consumer Helpline (800) 942-4242
The National Insurance Consumer Helpline advises consumers on how to choose an insurance company or broker. It also offers an analysis of life insurance and assists in insurance complaints.

People's Medical Society
462 West Walnut Street
Allentown, PA 18102
(800) 624-8773 phone
The People's Medical Society is a nonprofit organization that educates and informs consumers about the confusing healthcare market. For a $20 fee, members will receive a newsletter as well as discounts on all publications. Non-members may still order publications from the organization directly. The Society publishes a number of excellent books on health care issues.

Physicians Who Care
10615 Perrin Beitel Street, Suite 201
San Antonio, Texas 78217
(800) 545-9305 phone
(210) 656-1545 fax
Physicians Who Care is an organization which serves as an advocate for quality health care. It offers brochures and newsletters for consumers with questions and concerns regarding managed care. Consumers may contact this organization with complaints concerning HMOs and other managed care organizations.

Public Citizen
Health Research Group
1600 20th Street, NW
Washington, DC 20009
(202) 588-1000 phone
The Health Research Group petitions and testifies before Congress and federal agencies on such issues as banning or relabeling of drugs, improved safety standards at work sites and safer medical devices. Their publications provide information on various health topics including quality of care, insurance, questionable doctors and hospitals, managed care and how to obtain medical records.

NOTES:

APPENDIX L
MEDICAL SCHOOLS

The following is a list of U.S. medical schools and the abbreviations used for each in the doctor listings. The abbreviations as they appear in the listings are in italics below.

ALABAMA

University of Alabama School of Medicine University of Alabama at Birmingham
U Ala Sch Med

University of South Alabama College of Medicine
U South Ala Coll Med

ARIZONA

University of Arizona College of Medicine
Arizona Health Sciences Center
U Ariz Coll Med

ARKANSAS

University of Arkansas College of Medicine
U Ark Sch Med

CALIFORNIA

University of California Davis School of Medicine
UC Davis
University of California Irvine College of Medicine
UC Irvine

University of California San Diego School of Medicine
UC San Diego

Loma Linda University School of Medicine
Loma Linda U

University of California Los Angeles UCLA School of Medicine
UCLA

University of Southern California School of Medicine
USC Sch Med

College of Osteopathic Medicine of the Pacific
Coll of Osteo Med-Pacific

University of California San Francisco School of Medicine
UC San Francisco

Stanford University School of Medicine
Stanford U

COLORADO

University of Colorado School of Medicine
U Colo Sch Med

CONNECTICUT

University of Connecticut School of Medicine
U Conn Sch Med

Yale University School of Medicine
Yale U Sch Med

DISTRICT OF COLUMBIA

George Washington University School of Medicine and Health Science
Geo Wash U Sch Med

Georgetown University School of Medicine
Georgetown U

Howard University College of Medicine
Howard U

FLORIDA

University of Florida College of Medicine
U Fla Coll Med

University of Miami School of Medicine
U Miami Sch Med

Nova Southeastern University, College of Osteopathic Medicine
Nova SE Univ, Coll of Osteo Med

University of South Florida College of Medicine
U South Fla Coll Med

Florida College of Osteopathic Medicine
FL Coll of Osteo Med

GEORGIA

Emory University School of Medicine
Emory U Sch Med

Morehouse School of Medicine
Morehouse Sch Med

Medical College of Georgia School of Medicine
Med Coll Ga

Mercer University School of Medicine
Mercer U Sch Med, Macon, GA

HAWAII

University of Hawaii John A. Burns School of Medicine
U Hawaii JA Burns Sch Med

ILLINOIS

Arizona College of Osteopathic Medicine, Midwestern University
Ariz Coll of Osteo Med

Chicago College of Osteopathic Medicine, Midwestern University
Chicago Coll of Osteo Med

Northwestern University Medical School
Northwestern U

Rush Medical College of Rush University
Rush Med Coll

University of Chicago (Div Bio Sci) Pritzker School of Medicine
U Chicago-Pritzker Sch Med

University of Illinois College of Medicine
U Ill Coll Med

Loyola University of Chicago - Stritch School of Medicine
Loyola U-Stritch Sch Med, Maywood

University of Health Sciences Chicago Medical School
U Hlth Sci/Chicago Med Sch

Southern Illinois University School of Medicine

Southern Ill U

INDIANA

Indiana University School of Medicine
Ind U Sch Med

IOWA

University of Osteopathic Medicine
U of Osteo Med-IA

University of Iowa College of Medicine
U Iowa Coll Med

KANSAS

University of Kansas Medical Center School of Medicine
U Kans Sch Med

KENTUCKY

University of Kentucky College of Medicine
U Ky Coll Med

University of Louisville School of Medicine
KY Sch Med, Louisville

LOUISIANA

Louisiana State University School of Medicine New Orleans
LSU Sch Med, New Orleans

Tulane University School of Medicine
Tulane U

Louisiana State University School Of Medicine Shreveport
LSU Med Ctr, Shreveport

MARYLAND

Johns Hopkins University School of Medicine
Johns Hopkins U

University of Maryland School of Medicine
U Md Sch Med

F. Edward A. Hebert School of Medicine Uniformed Services University of Health Sciences
Uniformed Srvs U, Betheseda

MASSACHUSETTS

Boston University School of Medicine
Boston U

Harvard Medical School
Harvard Med Sch

Tufts University School of Medicine
Tufts U

University of Massachusetts Medical School
U Mass Sch Med

MICHIGAN

University of Michigan Medical School
U Mich Med Sch

Wayne State University School of Medicine
Wayne State U

Michigan State University College of Human Medicine
Mich St U

Michigan State University College of Osteopathic Medicine
Mich St Coll of Osteo Med

MINNESOTA

University of Minnesota Duluth School of Medicine
U Minn-Duluth Sch Med

University of Minnesota Medical School
U Minn

Mayo Medical School
Mayo Med Sch

MISSISSIPPI

University of Mississippi School of Medicine
U Miss Sch Med

MISSOURI

University of Missouri Columbia School of Medicine
U Mo-Columbia Sch Med

Kirksville College of Osteopathic Medicine
Kirksville Coll of Osteo Med

University of Health Sciences/College of Osteopathic Medicine
U of Hlth Sci, Coll of Osteo Med

University of Missouri Kansas City School of Medicine
U Mo-Kansas City Sch Med

Saint Louis University School of Medicine
St Louis U

Washington University School of Medicine
Wash U, St. Louis

NEBRASKA

Creighton University School of Medicine
Creighton U

University of Nebraska College of Medicine
U Nebr Coll Med

NEVADA

University of Nevada School of Medicine
U Nevada

NEW HAMPSHIRE

Dartmouth Medical School
Dartmouth Med Sch

NEW JERSEY

University of Medicine and Dentistry of New Jersey
UMDNJ-NJ Med Sch, Newark

University of Medicine and Dentistry of New Jersey
UMDNJ-RW Johnson Med Sch

University of Medicine and Dentistry of New Jersey/School of Osteopathic Medicine
UMD-NJ Sch of Osteo Med

NEW MEXICO

University of New Mexico School of Medicine
U New Mexico

NEW YORK

Albany Medical College
Albany Med Coll

Albert Einstein College of Medicine of Yeshiva University
Albert Einstein Coll Med

State University of New York Health Science Center at Brooklyn
SUNY Health Sci Ctr, Bklyn

State University of New York at Buffalo School of Medicine & Biomedical Sciences
SUNY Buffalo

New York College of Osteopathic Medicine
NY Coll of Osteo Med

Columbia University College of Physicians and Surgeons
Columbia P&S

Cornell University Medical College
Cornell U

Mt. Sinai School of Medicine of the City University of New York
Mt Sinai Sch Med

New York University School of Medicine
NYU Sch Med

University of Rochester School of Medicine and Dentistry
U Rochester

State University of New York at Stony Brook Health Sciences Center
SUNY Hlth Sci Ctr, Stony Brook

State University of New York Health Science Center at Syracuse
SUNY Hlth Sci Ctr, Syracuse

New York Medical College
NY Med Coll

NORTH CAROLINA

University of North Carolina at Chapel Hill School of Medicine
U NC Sch Med

Duke University School of Medicine
Duke U

East Carolina University School of Medicine
E Carolina U

Bowman Gray School of Medicine
Bowman Gray

NORTH DAKOTA

University of North Dakota School of Medicine
U ND Sch Med

OHIO

University of Cincinnati College of Medicine
U Cincinnati

Case Western Reserve University School of Medicine
Case West Res U

Ohio University, College of Osteopathic Medicine
OH Coll of Osteo Med

Ohio State University College of Medicine
Ohio State U

Wright State University School of Medicine
Wright State U Sch Med

Northeastern Ohio University College of Medicine
NE Ohio U

Medical College of Ohio
MC Ohio, Toledo

OKLAHOMA

University of Oklahoma College of Medicine
U Okla Coll Med

Oklahoma State University College of Osteopathic Medicine
OSU Coll of Osteo Med

OREGON

Oregon Health Science University School of Medicine
U Oreg/Hlth Sci U, Portland

PENNSYLVANIA

Lake Erie College of Osteopathic Medicine
Lake Erie Coll of Osteo Med

Pennsylvania State University College of Medicine
Penn St U-Hershey Med Ctr

Hahnemann University School of Medicine
Hahnemann U

Jefferson Medical College of Thomas Jefferson University
Jefferson Med Coll

Medical College of Pennsylvania
Med Coll Penn

Philadelphia College of Osteopathic Medicine
Philadelphia Coll of Osteo Med

Temple University School of Medicine
Temple U

University of Pennsylvania School of Medicine
U Penn

University of Pittsburgh School of Medicine
U Pittsbrgh

PUERTO RICO

Universidad Central del Caribe School of Medicine
U del Caribe Escuela Med Cayey

Ponce School of Medicine
Ponce Med Sch

University of Puerto Rico School of Medicine
U Puerto Rico

RHODE ISLAND

Brown University Program in Medicine
Brown U

SOUTH CAROLINA

Medical University of South Carolina College of Medicine
Med U SC, Charleston

University of South Carolina School of Medicine
U SC Sch Med, Columbia

SOUTH DAKOTA

University of South Dakota School of Medicine
U SD Sch Med

TENNESSEE

East Tennessee State University James H. Quillen College of Medicine
E Tenn State U

University of Tennessee Memphis College of Medicine
U Tenn Memphis Coll Med

Meharry Medical College School of Medicine
Meharry Med Coll

Vanderbilt University School of Medicine
Vanderbilt U

TEXAS

Texas A&M University Health Science Center College of Medicine
Texas A&M U

University of Texas
U Texas, Dallas

University of North Texas Health Science Center/College of Osteopathic Medicine
U of North TX Coll of Osteo Med

University of Texas Medical School at Galveston
U Texas Med Br, Galveston

Baylor College of Medicine
Baylor

University of Texas Medical School at Houston
U Texas, Houston

Texas Tech University Health Science Center School of Medicine
Tex Tech U Sch Med

University of Texas Medical School at San Antonio
U Tex San Antonio

UTAH

University of Utah School of Medicine
U Utah

VERMONT

University of Vermont College of Medicine
U Vt Coll Med

VIRGINIA

University of Virginia School of Medicine
U Va Sch Med

Eastern Virginia Medical School of the Medical College of Hampton Roads
Eastern VA Med Sch, Norfolk

Virginia Commonwealth University Medical College of Virginia School of Medicine
Med Coll Va

WASHINGTON

University of Washington School of Medicine
U Wash, Seattle

WEST VIRGINIA

Marshall University School of Medicine
Marshall U

West Virginia School of Osteopathic Medicine
WV Sch Osteo Med

Robert C. Byrd Health Sciences Center of West Virginia University School of Medicine
W Va U Sch Med

WISCONSIN

University of Wisconsin School of Medicine
U Wisc Med Sch

Medical College of Wisconsin
Med Coll Wisc

CANADA

The University of Calgary Faculty of Medicine
U Calgary

Faculty of Medicine University of Alberta
U Alberta

University of British Columbia Faculty of Medicine
U British Columbia Fac Med

University of Manitoba Faculty of Medicine
U Manitoba

Memorial University of Newfoundland Faculty of Medicine
Meml U-St Johns, Newfoundland

Dalhousie University Faculty of Medicine
Dalhousie U

McMaster University Faculty of Health Sciences
McMaster U

Queen's University Faculty of Medicine
Queens U

University of Western Ontario Faculty of Medicine
U Western Ontario

University of Ottawa Faculty of Medicine
U Ottawa

University of Toronto Faculty of Medicine
U Toronto

McGill University Faculty of Medicine
McGill U

Laval University Faculty of Medicine
Laval U, Quebec

NOTES:

APPENDIX M

HOSPITAL LISTING

Following is an alphabetical listing of hospitals noted in doctors' entries. The abbreviations as they appear in the listings are in italics below. Due to the many mergers taking place in the hospital industry these days, the names on this list periodically may change.

Alexian Brothers Medical Center
Alexian Brothers Med Ctr
800 Biesterfield Road
Elk Grove Village, IL 60007
(847) 437-5500
Cook

Bethany Hospital
Bethany Hosp
3435 W Van Buren St
Chicago, IL 60624
(773) 265-7700
Cook

BHC Streamwood Hospital
BHC Streamwood Hosp
1400 E Irving Park Road
Streamwood, IL 60107
(630) 837-9000
Cook

Central Du Page Hospital
Central Du Page Hosp
25 N Winfield Road
Winfield, IL 60190
(630) 682-1600
Du Page

Chicago Lakeshore Hospital
Chicago Lakeshore Hosp
4840 N Marine Dr
Chicago, IL 60640
(773) 878-9700
Cook

Chicago VA Health Care System--The Westside Division
Chicago VA Hlth Care System--Westside
820 S Damen Ave
Chicago, IL 60612
(773) 666-6500
Cook

Chicago-Read Mental Health Center
Chicago-Read Mental Hlth Ctr
4200 N Oak Park Ave
Chicago, IL 60634
(773) 794-4000
Cook

Institutions in bold are profiled in this edition of the Castle Connolly Guide.

Children's Memorial Medical Center
Children's Mem Med Ctr
Part of Northwestern Healthcare
2300 Children's Plaza
Chicago, IL 60614
(773) 880-4000
Cook

Christ Hospital & Medical Center
Christ Hosp & Med Ctr
Part of Advocate Health Care
4440 W 95th St
Oak Lawn, IL 60453
(708) 425-8000
Cook

Columbus Hospital
Columbus Hosp
2520 N Lakeview
Chicago, IL 60614
(773) 883-7300
Cook

Condell Medical Center
Condell Med Ctr
801 South Milwaukee Ave
Libertyville, IL 60048
(847) 362-2900
Lake

Cook County Hospital
Cook Cty Hosp
1835 W Harrison St
Chicago, IL 60612
(312) 633-6000
Cook

Delnor Community Hospital
Delnor Comm Hosp
300 Randall Road
Geneva, IL 60134
(630) 208-3000
Kane

Doctors Hospital of Hyde Park
Doctors Hosp
5800 S Stony Island Ave
Chicago, IL 60637
(773) 643-9200
Cook

Edgewater Medical Center
Edgewater Med Ctr
5700 N Ashland Ave
Chicago, IL 60660
(773) 878-6000
Cook

Edward Hines Jr VA Hospital
Hines VA Hosp
Fifth Ave & Roosevelt Road, PO Box 5000
Hines, IL 60141
(708) 202-8387
Cook

Edward Hospital
Edward Hosp
801 S Washington St
Naperville, IL 60566
(630) 355-0450
Du Page

Elgin Mental Health Center
Elgin Mental Hlth Ctr
750 S State St
Elgin, IL 60123
(847) 742-1040
Kane

Elmhurst Memorial Hospital
Elmhurst Mem Hosp
200 Berteau Ave
Elmhurst, IL 60126
(630) 833-1400
Du Page

Institutions in bold are profiled in this edition of the Castle Connolly Guide.

Evanston Hospital
Evanston Hosp
Part of Northwestern Healthcare System
2650 Ridge Ave
Evanston, IL 60201
(847) 570-2000
Cook

Forest Hospital
Forest Hosp
555 Wilson Lane
Des Plaines, IL 60016
(847) 635-4100
Cook

Glen Oaks Hospital and Medical Center
Glen Oaks Hosp and Med Ctr
Part of Adventist Health System
701 Winthrop Ave
Glendale Heights, IL 60139
(630) 545-8000
Du Page

Glenbrook Hospital
Glenbrook Hosp
2100 Pfingsten Road
Glenview, IL 60025
(847) 657-5800
Cook

Good Samaritan Hospital
Good Samaritan Hosp
Part of Advocate Health Care
3815 Highland Ave
Downers Grove, IL 60515
(630) 275-5900
Du Page

Good Shepherd Hospital
Good Shepherd Hosp
450 W Hwy 22
Barrington, IL 60010
(847) 381-9600
Lake

Gottlieb Memorial Hospital
Gottlieb Mem Hosp
701 W North Ave
Melrose Park, IL 60160
(708) 681-3200
Cook

Grant Hospital
Grant Hosp
550 W Webster Ave
Chicago, IL 60614
(773) 883-2000
Cook

Hartgrove Hospital
Hartgrove Hosp
520 N Ridgeway Ave
Chicago, IL 60624
(773) 722-3113
Cook

Havard Memorial Hospital
Havard Mem Hosp
901 Grant St, PO Box 850
Harvard, IL 60033
(815) 943-5431
McHenry

Highland Park Hospital
Highland Park Hosp
Part of Northwestern Healthcare System
718 Glenview Ave
Highland Park, IL 60035
(847) 432-8000
Lake

Hinsdale Hospital
Hinsdale Hosp
Part of Adventist Health System
120 N Oak St
Hinsdale, IL 60521
(630) 856-9000
Du Page

Institutions in bold are profiled in this edition of the Castle Connolly Guide.

Holy Cross Hospital
Holy Cross Hosp
2701 W 68th St
Chicago, IL 60629
(773) 471-8000
Cook

Holy Family Medical Center
Holy Family Med Ctr
100 N River Road
Des Plaines, IL 60016
(847) 297-1800
Cook

Illinois Masonic Medical Center
Illinois Masonic Med Ctr
836 W Wellington Ave
Chicago, IL 60657
(773) 975-1600
Cook

Ingalls Memorial Hospital
Ingalls Mem Hosp
Part of Northwestern Healthcare System
One Ingalls Drive
Harvey, IL 60426
(708) 333-2300
Cook

Jackson Park Hospital & Medical Center
Jackson Park Hosp & Med Ctr
7531 Stony Island Ave
Chicago, IL 60649
(773) 947-7500
Cook

John J Madden Mental Health Center
John J Madden Mental Hlth Ctr
1200 S First Ave
Hines, IL 60141
(708) 338-7400
Cook

La Grange Memorial Hospital
La Grange Mem Hosp
Part of Adventist Health System
5101 Willow Springs Road
La Grange, IL 60525
(708) 352-1200
Cook

La Rabida Children's Hospital
La Rabida Children's Hosp
E 65th at Lake Michigan
Chicago, IL 60649
(773) 363-6700
Cook

Lake Forest Hospital
Lake Forest Hosp
660 N Westmoreland Road
Lake Forest, IL 60045
(847) 234-5600
Lake

Linden Oaks Hospital
Linden Oaks Hosp
852 West St
Naperville, IL 60540
(630) 305-5500
Du Page

Little Company of Mary Hospital & Health Care Centers
Little Company of Mary Hosp & Hlth Care Ctrs
2800 W 95th St
Evergreen Park, IL 60805
(708) 422-6200
Cook

Loretto Hospital
Loretto Hosp
645 S Central Ave
Chicago, IL 60644
(773) 626-4300
Cook

Institutions in bold are profiled in this edition of the Castle Connolly Guide.

Louis A Weiss Memorial Hospital
Louis A Weiss Mem Hosp
4646 N Marine Sr
Chicago, IL 60640
(773) 878-8700
Cook

Lovellton Academy
Lovellton Academy
600 Villa
Elgin, IL 60120
(847) 695-0077
Kane

Loyola University Medical Center
Loyola U Med Ctr
2160 S 1st Ave
Maywood, IL 60153
(708) 216-9000
Cook

Lutheran General Hospital
Lutheran Gen Hosp
Part of Advocate Health Care
1775 Dempster St
Park Ridge, IL 60068
(847) 723-2210
Cook

Macneal Memorial Hospital
Macneal Mem Hosp
3249 S Oak Park Ave
Berwyn, IL 60402
(708) 783-9100
Cook

Marianjoy Rehabilitation Hospital
Marianjoy Rehab Hosp & Clinics
26 W 171 Roosevelt Road
Wheaton, IL 60189
(630) 462-4000
Du Page

Memorial Medical Center
Mem Med Ctr
Hwy 14 & Doty Road
Woodstock, IL 60098
(815) 338-2500
McHenry

Mercy Hospital & Medical Center
Mercy Hosp & Med Ctr
2525 South Michigan Ave
Chicago, IL 60616
(312) 567-2000
Cook

Methodist Hospital of Chicago
Methodist Hosp of Chicago
5025 N Paulina St
Chicago, IL 60640
(773) 271-9040
Cook

Michael Reese Hospital & Medical Center
Michael Reese Hosp & Med Ctr
2929 S Ellis Ave
Chicago, IL 60616
(312) 791-3545
Cook

Midwestern Regional Medical Center
Midwestern Regional Med Ctr
2520 Elisha Ave
Zion, IL 60099
(847) 872-4561
Lake

Mount Sinai Hospital Medical Center
Mount Sinai Hosp Med Ctr
California Ave at 15th St
Chicago, IL 60608
(773) 542-2000
Cook

Institutions in bold are profiled in this edition of the Castle Connolly Guide.

Naval Hospital
Naval Hosp
2705 Sheridan Road, Bldg 200-H
Great Lakes, IL 60088
(847) 688-4560
Lake

Northern Illinois Medical Center
Northern Illinois Med Ctr
4201 Medical Center Drive
McHenry, IL 60050
(815) 344-5000
McHenry

Northwest Community Healthcare
Northwest Comm Hlthcare
Part of Northwestern Healthcare System
800 W Central Road
Arlington Heights, IL 60005
(847) 618-1000
Cook

Northwestern Memorial Hospital
Northwestern Mem Hosp
Part of Northwestern Healthcare System
251 East Huron St
Chicago, IL 60611
(312) 926-2000
Cook

Norwegian-American Hospital
Norwegian-American Hosp
1044 N Francisco Ave
Chicago, IL 60622
(773) 292-8200
Cook

Oak Forest Hospital
Oak Forest Hosp
15900 S Cicero Ave
Oak Forest, IL 60452
(708) 687-7200
Cook

Oak Park Hospital
Oak Park Hosp
520 S Maple Ave
Oak Park, IL 60304
(708) 383-9300
Cook

Our Lady Of the Resurrection Medical Center
Our Lady Of the Resurrection Med Ctr
5645 W Addison St
Chicago, IL 60634
(773) 282-7000
Cook

Palos Community Hospital
Palos Comm Hosp
12251 S 80th Ave
Palos Heights, IL 60463
(708) 923-4000
Cook

Provena Mercy Center
Provena Mercy Ctr
1325 N Highland Ave
Aurora, IL 60506
(630) 859-2222
Kane

Provena St. Therese Medical Center
Provena St Therese Med Ctr
2615 W Washington St
Waukegan, IL 60085
(847) 249-3900
Lake

Provident Hospital
Provident Hosp
500 E 51st St
Chicago, IL 60615
(312) 572-2000
Cook

Institutions in bold are profiled in this edition of the Castle Connolly Guide.

Ravenswood Hospital Medical Center
Ravenswood Hosp Med Ctr
4550 N Winchester Ave
Chicago, IL 60640
(773) 878-4300
Cook

Rehabilitation Institute of Chicago
Rehab Institute of Chicago
345 E Superior St
Chicago, IL 60611
(312) 908-6000
Cook

Resurrection Medical Center
Resurrection Med Ctr
7435 W Talcott Ave
Chicago, IL 60631
(773) 774-8000
Cook

Riveredge Hospital
Riveredge Hosp
8311 W Roosevelt Road
Forest Park, IL 60130
(708) 771-7000
Cook

Rock Creek Center
Rock Creek Ctr
40 Timberline Drive
Lemont, IL 60439
(630) 257-3636
Cook

Roseland Community Hospital
Roseland Comm Hosp
45 W 111th St
Chicago, IL 60628
(773) 995-3000
Cook

Rush North Shore Medical Center
Rush North Shore Med Ctr
9600 Gross Point Road
Skokie, IL 60076
(847) 677-9600
Cook

Rush-Copley Medical Center
Rush-Copley Med Ctr
2000 Ogden Ave
Aurora, IL 60504
(630) 978-6200
Kane

Rush-Presbyterian-St. Luke's Medical Center
Rush-Presbyterian-St Luke's Med Ctr
1653 W Congress Parkway
Chicago, IL 60612
(312) 942-5000
Cook

Sacred Heart Hospital
Sacred Heart Hosp
3240 W Franklin Blvd
Chicago, IL 60624
(773) 722-3020
Cook

Schwab Rehabilitation Hospital and Care Network
Schwab Rehab Hosp and Care Network
1401 S California Blvd
Chicago, IL 60608
(773) 522-2010
Cook

Sherman Hospital
Sherman Hosp
934 Center St
Elgin, IL 60120
(847) 742-9800
Kane

Institutions in bold are profiled in this edition of the Castle Connolly Guide.

Shriners Hospital for Children
Shriners Hosp for Children
2211 N Oak Park Ave
Chicago, IL 60707
(773) 622-5400
Cook

Silver Cross Hospital
Silver Cross Hosp
Part of Northwestern Healthcare System
1200 Maple Road
Joliet, IL 60432
(815) 740-1100
Will

South Shore Hospital
South Shore Hosp
8012 S Crandon
Chicago, IL 60617
(773) 768-0810
Cook

South Suburban Hospital
South Suburban Hosp
17800 S Kedzie Ave
Hazel Crest, IL 60429
(708) 799-8000
Cook

St. Alexius Medical Center
St Alexius Med Ctr
1555 N Barrington Road
Hoffman Estates, IL 60194
(847) 843-2000
Cook

St. Anthony Hospital
St Anthony Hosp
2875 W 19th St
Chicago, IL 60623
(773) 521-1710
Cook

St Bernard Hosp
326 W 64th
Chicago, IL 60621
(773) 962-3900
Cook

St. Elizabeth's Hospital
St Elizabeth's Hosp
1431 N Claremont Ave
Chicago, IL 60622
(773) 278-2000
Cook

St. Francis Hospital
St Francis Hosp
12935 S Gregory St
Blue Island, IL 60406
(708) 597-2000
Cook

St. Francis Hospital of Evanston
St Francis Hosp of Evanston
355 Ridge Ave
Evanston, IL 60202
(847) 316-4000
Cook

St. James Hospital & Health Centers
St James Hosp & Hlth Ctrs
1423 Chicago Rd
Chicago Heights, IL 60411
(708) 756-1000
Cook

St. Joseph Hospital--Chicago
St Joseph Hosp--Chicago
2900 N Lake Shore Dr
Chicago, IL 60657
(773) 665-3000
Cook

Institutions in bold are profiled in this edition of the Castle Connolly Guide.

St. Joseph Hospital--Elgin
St Joseph Hosp--Elgin
77 N Airlite St.
Elgin, IL 60123
(847) 695-3200
Kane

St. Joseph Medical Center--Joliet
St Joseph Med Ctr--Joliet
333 N Madison St
Joliet, IL 60435
(815) 725-7133
Will

St. Mary's of Nazareth Hospital Center
St Mary's of Nazareth Hosp Ctr
2233 W Division St
Chicago, IL 60622
(312) 770-2000
Cook

Swedish Covenant Hospital
Swedish Covenant Hosp
Part of Northwestern Healthcare System
5145 N California Ave
Chicago, IL 60625
(773) 878-8200
Cook

Thorek Hospital & Medical Center
Thorek Hosp & Med Ctr
850 W Irving Park Rd
Chicago, IL 60613
(773) 525-6780
Cook

Tinley Park Mental Health Center
Tinley Park Mental Hlth Ctr
7400 W 183rd St
Tinley Park, IL 60477
(708) 614-4000
Cook

Trinity Hospital
Trinity Hosp
2320 E 93rd St
Chicago, IL 60617
(773) 978-2000
Cook

University of Chicago Hospitals
U Chicago Hosp
5841 S Maryland
Chicago, IL 60637
(773) 702-1000
Cook

University of Illinois at Chicago Eye & Ear Infirmary
Univ of Illinois at Chicago Eye & Ear
1855 W Taylor St
Chicago, IL 60612
(312) 996-6500
Cook

University of Illinois at Chicago Medical Center
Univ of Illinois at Chicago Med Ctr
1740 W Taylor St.
Chicago, IL 60612
(312) 996-7000
Cook

University of Illinois at Chicago Psychiatric Institute
Univ of Illinois at Chicago Psychiatric
1601 West Taylor St MC 912
Chicago, IL 60612
(312) 413-4500
Cook

VA Healthcare Systems-Lakeside
VA Hlthcare Systems-Lakeside
333 E Huron St
Chicago, IL 60611
(312) 943-6600
Cook

Institutions in bold are profiled in this edition of the Castle Connolly Guide.

VA Medical Center
VA Med Ctr
3001 Green Bay Road
North Chicago, IL 60064
(847) 688-1900
Lake

Vencor Hospital
Vencor Hosp
365 E North Ave
Northlake, IL 60164
(708) 345-8100
Cook

Vencor Hospital Chicago-Central
Vencor Hosp Central
4058 W Melrose St
Chicago, IL 60641
(773) 736-7000
Cook

Vencor Hospital Chicago-North
Vencor Hosp North
2544 W Montrose
Chicago, IL 60618
(773) 267-2622
Cook

Victory Memorial Hospital
Victory Mem Hosp
1324 N Sheridan Road
Waukegan, IL 60085
(847) 360-3000
Lake

Westlake Community Hospital
Westlake Comm Hosp
1225 Lake St
Melrose Park, IL 60160
(708) 681-3000
Cook

West Suburban Hospital Medical Center
West Suburban Hosp Med Ctr
Erie at Austin
Oak Park, IL 60302
(708) 383-6200
Cook

Institutions in bold are profiled in this edition of the Castle Connolly Guide.

APPENDIX N

HMO/PPO AFFILIATIONS

Listed below are the HMOs and PPOs that the doctors included in the Castle Connolly Guide designated as among their affiliations. A single HMO may offer a variety of plans and a doctor may be affiliated with only a few. We recommend you check with the doctor's office or HMO since these affiliations are subject to change.

HMO/PPO

AARP
Accord
Advocate
Aetna Hlth Plan
Aetna-US Healthcare
Affordable Hlth Plan
Americaid
American Health Plan
Anchor
AV-MED Health Plan
Bay State Health Plan
Beech Street
Blue Choice
Blue Cross
Blue Cross & Blue Choice
Blue Cross & Blue Shield
Blue Shield
Californiacare
CapCare
Caterpillar
CCN
Century Medical Health Plan
Champus
Chicago HMO
Choicecare
CIGNA
Compare Health Service

HMO/PPO

Compass
Comprecare Healthcare
Evanston NW HC
Family Med Net
FHP Inc
First Choice
First Health
Fortis
Foundation Health
Gottlieb West Towns
Greenspring
Group Health Cooperative
Guardian
Harmony
Harvard Community Health Plan
Health Alliance Plan
Health Direct
Health First
Health One
Health Options
Health Preferred
Healthamerica
Healthcare America
HealthNet
Healthpartners
Healthplus
HealthStar

APPENDIX N

HMO/PPO

Heritage National Healthplan
Highland Park IPA
HIP Network
HMO Blue
HMO Illinois
Humana Health Plan
Independent Health Plan
Intergroup Healthcare
IPA
IPG HMO
IVPA
John Deere Health Plan
John Hancock
Joliet PPO
Kaiser Foundation Health Plan
Keystone Health Plan East
La Grange IPA
Lutheran General
Magellan
Magnacare
Masonicare
Maxicare Health Plan
Mercy Health Plans
Merit Behavioral Health Plans
Metrahealth
Metropolitan
Michael Reese Phys Grp
MMS
Napierville Health Care

HMO/PPO

Northwestern POS
NYLCare
Oxford
Pacificare Health System
PHCS
PHS
Pilgrim Health Care
Preferred Plan
Principal Health Care
Prucare
Prudential
Rush Health Plans
Rush Prudential
Sanus
Select
SEMS
Share
St Mary HMO
Takecare Health Plan
Travelers
UHC
Unicare Primary Plus
Unihealth America
United Healthcare
United Mineworkers
US Hlthcre
VBH
Wellmark Health

ACKNOWLEDGMENTS

We would like to thank the following people for their hard work in the production of this book:

Director of Information Services:	*Fred Ramen*
Director of Research:	*Jean Morgan, M.D.*
Director of Communications:	*Deborah Tropp*
Vice President, Business Development:	*William Liss-Levinson, Ph.D.*
Director, Health Partners Program:	*Michael D. Wolf, Ph.D.*
Senior Advisor, Chicago Metropolitan Area:	*Harlan H. Newkirk*
Research Staff:	*Maxine Atkins, Alicia Buckley, Anita Holder, Connie Johnson, Paige Lewis, Wagner Orellona, Riedar Syvertsen*
Design:	*Lissa Milea, Harper & Case, Ltd., NYC*

SUBJECT INDEX

SPECIAL PRACTICE INTEREST INDEX

DIRECTORY OF DOCTORS

Note: When reviewing this index, please recognize that the physicians may describe a given condition in different ways (ex: AIDS, HIV) so be sure to look under a number of key words, not just one (ex: Cosmetic Surgery, Aesthetic Surgery).

Some special interests may be condensed due to space considerations.

DIRECTORY OF DOCTORS

DIRECTORY OF DOCTORS

SPECIAL INTEREST	NAME	PAGE
Hives	Langiewicz, Janusz (MD)	145
Hodgkin's Disease	Fisher, Richard (MD)	190
Holistic Health	Fischer, Tessa (MD)	172
Holistic Medicine	Blanks, Mary (MD)	203
Holistic Pain Relief-Laser	Kurland, Howard D (MD)	243
Hormone Replacement Therapy	Nye, Elizabeth (MD)	207
Huntington's Disease	Wong, Paul (MD)	189
Hydrocephalus	Tomita, Tadanori (MD)	198
Hyperactivity Disorder	Dulcan, Mina K (MD)	155
Hypercholesterolemia	Dillon, Charles (MD)	181
Hypertension	Arguello, Maria (MD)	163
Hypertension	Arteaga, Waldo (MD)	179
Hypertension	Dillon, Charles (MD)	181
Hypertension	Dodda, Lakshmi (MD)	165
Hypertension	Kuznetsky, Kenneth (MD)	195
Hypertension	Landsberg, Lewis (MD)	162
Hypertension	Miller, Albert (MD)	153
Hypertension	Miller, Kenneth (MD)	226
Hypertension	Roseman, Melvin K. (MD)	195
Hypertension	Simon, Norman (MD)	195
Hypertension	Simovic, Predrag (MD)	187
Hypertension	Tatar, Arnold M (MD)	187
Hypertension	Zikos, Demetrios (MD)	196
Hypertension, Kidney Failure	Bhorade, Maruti (MD)	179
Hypertension-Cholesterol	Kopin, Jeffrey (MD)	183
Hypogonadism	Layman, Lawrence (MD)	206
Immune Deficiency	Rich, Kenneth (MD)	222
Immune Deficiency Diseases	Gotoff, Samuel (MD)	222
Immunotherapy	Klingerman, Hans (MD)	190
In Vitro Fertilization	Kaplan, Brian (MD)	252
Inborn Errors of Metabolism	Hoganson, George E (MD)	189
Infection-Nervous System	Yogev, Ram (MD)	235
Infections Disease	Dechovitz, Arthur (MD)	230
Infectious Disease	Frank, Arthur L (MD)	230
Infectious Diseases	De Bofsky, Harvey (MD)	230
Infectious Diseases	Ismail, Mahmoud (MD)	188
Infectious Diseases	Johnson, Daniel (MD)	226
Infectious Diseases	White, G Wesley (MD)	179
Infertility	Blankstein, Josef (MD)	203
Infertility	Confino, Edmund (MD)	251
Infertility	Hoxsey, Rodney J (MD)	251
Infertility	Kaplan, Brian (MD)	252
Inflammatory Bowel Disease	Franklin, James L (MD)	168
Inflammatory Bowel Disease	Hanauer, Stephen (MD)	169
Inflammatory Bowel Disease	Kirschner, Barbara (MD)	224
Inflammatory Bowel Disease	Sales, David (MD & PhD)	170
Inflammatory Bowel Disease	Stryker, Steven J. (MD)	261
Inflammatory Bowel Diseases	Breuer, Richard (MD)	168
Intensive Care	Naidu, Shrinivas (MD)	223
Intensive Care Medicine	Rothenberg, David (MD)	149
Interstitial Lung Diseases	Sporn, Peter (MD)	248
Interventional Cardiology	Davidson, Charles J (MD)	151
Interventional Cardiology	Khadra, Suhail (MD)	152
Interventional Cardiology	Millman, William (MD)	153
Intestinal Diseases	Konicek, Frank (MD)	169
Intraocular Lens Implants	Scelzo, Frederick (MD)	213
Invasive Procedures	Chiu, Y Christopher (MD)	150
Irritable Bowel Syndrome	Markey, W S (MD)	184
Irritable Bowel Syndrome	Zarling, Edwin (MD)	171
Jehovah's Witness Patients	Blakeman, Bradford (MD)	262
Joint Replacement	Beigler, David (MD)	214
Joint Replacement	Finn, Henry A (MD)	215
Joint Replacement	Hopkinson, William J (MD)	216
Kawasaki Disease	Shulman, Stanford (MD)	234
Kidney & Bladder Cancer	Carter, Michael (MD)	265
Kidney Failure	Berns, Arnold (MD)	194
Kidney Failure Dialysis	John, Eunice (MD)	232
Kidney Stones	Albala, David Mois (MD)	265
Kidney Stones	Berns, Arnold (MD)	194
Kidney Stones	Coe, Fredric (MD)	180
Kidney Stones	Hoeksema, Jerome (MD)	266
Kidney Stones	Langman, Craig (MD)	226
Kidney Stones	Zikos, Demetrios (MD)	196
Kidney Transplant Care	Bansal, Vinod (MD)	194
Knee Injuries	Nuber, Gordon (MD)	217
Knee Injuries	Schafer, Michael F. (MD)	255
Knee Replacement	Al-Aswad, Basel (MD)	214
Knee Replacement	Meltzer, William (MD)	216
Knee Surgery	Chand, Kishan (MD)	214
Knee Surgery	Egwele, Richard (MD)	215
Knee, Ankle Injuries	Hefferon, John (MD)	215
Knees and Shoulders	Sweeney, Howard J (MD)	217
Laparoscopic Cholecystectomy	Joehl, Raymond (MD)	257
Laparoscopic Cholecystectomy	Kaplan, Gerald (MD)	258
Laparoscopic Gallbladder	Chhablani, Asha (MD)	256
Laparoscopic Procedures	Pozzi, Patrick (MD)	208
Laparoscopic Surgery	Albala, David Mois (MD)	265
Laparoscopic Surgery	Cahill, Gerald (MD)	256
Laparoscopic Surgery	Duboe, Fred (MD)	204
Laparoscopic Surgery	Hasson, Harith M (MD)	205
Laparoscopic Surgery	Krause, Lawrence (MD)	258
Laparoscopic Surgery	Mc Grail, Michael (MD)	259
Larynx Surgery	Bastian, Robert (MD)	218
Laser Bronchoscopy	Warren, William (MD)	264
Laser Corrective Surgery	Taub, Susan J (MD)	213
Laser Surgery IVF	Jacobs, Laurence (MD)	251
Laser Surgery of Eye	Jay, Walter (MD)	211
Laser Treatments	Benvenuto, Riccardo (MD)	255
LASIK	Epstein, Randy J (MD)	210
Latex Allergy	Woody, Lisa (MD)	209
Leg Amputation	Jedrychowska, Krystyna (MD)	236
Leukemia	Chediak, Juan (MD)	175
Leukemia	Stein, Robert N (MD)	176
Leukemia, Lymphoma, Myeloma	Newman, Steven (MD)	191
Leukemia/Lymphoma	Golomb, Harvey (MD)	190
Leukemia-Aplastic Anemia	Morgan, Elaine (MD)	225
Leukemias	Gregory, Stephanie (MD & PhD)	176
Leukemias & Cancers	Salvi, Sharad (MD)	225
Limb Salvage	Finn, Henry A (MD)	215
Limited To Breast Disease	Michel, Arthur (MD)	259
Liposuction	Makhlouf, Mansour V (MD)	239
Liver and Pancreas Surgery	Pickleman, Jack R (MD)	260
Liver Disease	Breuer, Richard (MD)	168
Liver Disease	Jensen, Donald (MD)	169
Liver Disease	Nagpal, Rajeev (MD)	225
Liver Disease	Shah, Nikunj (MD)	170
Liver Disease	Whitington, Peter (MD)	235
Liver Diseases	Konicek, Frank (MD)	169
Liver Transplantation	Whitington, Peter (MD)	235
Low Back Pain	Mayer, Robert Samuel (MD)	237
Low Back Pain	Press, Joel (MD)	237
Low Back Pain	Worwag, Ewelina (MD)	222
Lower Back Disorders	Miz, George (MD)	216
Lower Back Pain	Andersson, Gunnar (MD)	214
Lower Urinary Tract Syndrome	Bormes, Thomas Pat (MD)	265
Lung Cancer	Albain, Kathy (MD)	189
Lung Cancer	Bonomi, Philip (MD)	189
Lung Cancer	Evans, Richard (MD)	262

DIRECTORY OF DOCTORS

DIRECTORY OF DOCTORS

Du Page County

Kane County

Lake County

SPECIAL INTEREST	NAME	PAGE
Breast Disease	Sobinsky, Kim (MD)	322
Breast Lumps	Strohmayer, Paul (MD)	322
Breast Reduction/Augmentation	Steinwald, Osmar (MD)	320
Breast Surgery	Furman, Richard (MD)	322
Cancer treatments	Mehta, Yashbir (MD)	321
Catheter Based Treatments for Coronary Artery Disease	Mayer, Thomas (MD)	312
Chest Diseases	Mintzer, Richard (MD)	313
Child Development	O'Brien, Charles (MD)	319
Cholesterol Reduction	Monahan, James (MD)	312
Chronic Sinus Problems	Kentor, Paul (MD)	311
Colon Cancer Prevention	Kane, Mary (MD)	314
Colon Cancer Screening	Moller, Neal (MD)	314
Cosmetic Dermatology	Lazar, Andrew (MD)	313
Emphysema	Katz, Howard (MD)	321
Epilepsy	Rowley, Wilbur F (MD)	316
Fibromyalgia	Hozman, Robert (MD)	322
Gall Bladder-Thyroid	Sobinsky, Kim (MD)	322
General Dermatology	Lazar, Andrew (MD)	313
General Obstetrics	Burstein, Harry (MD)	317
Hearing Loss	Nelson, Erik George (MD)	318
Hemochromatosis	Rudy, David R (MD)	314
Hernias	Strohmayer, Paul (MD)	322
High Risk Infertility & Gynecology	Burstein, Harry (MD)	317
Infertility	Valle, Jorge (MD)	321
Inflammatory Bowel Disease	Kane, Mary (MD)	314
Inflammatory Bowel Disease	Moller, Neal (MD)	314
Laparoscopic Hernia	Ganshirt, Stephen (MD)	322
Laparoscopic Nissen	Ganshirt, Stephen (MD)	322
Laparoscopic Surgery	Furman, Richard (MD)	322
Laparoscopic Surgery	Scheer, Michael (MD)	322
Mammography	Mintzer, Richard (MD)	313
Multiple Sclerosis	Rowley, Wilbur F (MD)	316
Muscular Pain	Lanoff, Martin (MD)	320
Obstetric Anesthesia	Matthew, Edward (MD)	311
Osteo- and Rheumatoid Arthritis	Gall, Eric P (MD)	322
Osteoporosis	Capezio, Jennifer (MD)	321
Osteoporosis	Gall, Eric P (MD)	322
Otitis	Mishell, Joseph (MD)	318
Pancreatic Surgery	Scheer, Michael (MD)	322
Pediatric Dermatology	Bronson, Darryl (MD)	312
Preventative Medicine	Einfalt, Melinda (MD)	315
Preventive Medicine	Tucci, Mark (MD)	316
Prostate Cancer	Janson, Kenneth (MD)	323
Prostate Seed Implants	Mehta, Yashbir (MD)	321
Reproductive Surgery	Valle, Jorge (MD)	321
Rheumatoid Arthritis	Hozman, Robert (MD)	322
Shoulder	Brna, John (MD)	318
Sinusitis	Mishell, Joseph (MD)	318
Travel Medicine	Einfalt, Melinda (MD)	315
Travel Medicine Immunization	Semel, Jeffery (MD)	315
Treatment of Mood Disorders	Greenspan, Brad (MD)	320
Urinary Tract Infections	Kurowski, Kurt (MD)	313
Vascular Surgery	Romeiser Jr, Adam (MD)	322
Work Injuries	Sturm, Richard E (MD)	317

McHenry County

SPECIAL INTEREST	NAME	PAGE
Generalized Pain	Prunskis, John (MD)	328
Intensive Care	Dellinger, Richard (MD)	327
Spine Pain-Neck & Back	Prunskis, John (MD)	328

Will County

SPECIAL INTEREST	NAME	PAGE
Anorectal Problems	Bass, Eric (MD)	331
Assist Devices	Foy, Bryan (MD)	335
Asthma	Schubert, Robert (MD)	332
Breast Cancer	Mc Call, Anne (MD)	334
Breast Diseases	Marshall, Wendy (MD)	335
Breast Surgery	Marvin, Joy (MD)	335
Breast-Vascular Surgery	Anderson, Allan (MD)	334
Cardiac Transplantation	Foy, Bryan (MD)	335
Colonoscopy	Nicosia, Jon (MD)	331
Epilepsy	Mc Cahill, Kathleen (MD)	333
Gynecologic Cancer	Mc Call, Anne (MD)	334
Headache	Schubert, Robert (MD)	332
Hernia Surgery	Marvin, Joy (MD)	335
Incontinence	Schuster, George (MD)	335
Incontinence Therapy	Beck, Daniel Lee (MD)	333
Laparoscopic Surgery	Beck, Daniel Lee (MD)	333
Laparoscopic Surgery	Danielson, Mark (MD)	334
Laparoscopic Surgery	Natesha, Ramanathapur K. (MD)	335
Laparoscopy	Anderson, Allan (MD)	334
Low Back Pain	Deppe, Frances (MD)	334
Neurology Stroke-Adult	Analytis, Peter (MD)	332
Pain Management	Gorski, Daniel W (MD)	331
Parkinson's Disease	Mc Cahill, Kathleen (MD)	333
Prostatitis	Schuster, George (MD)	335
Rectal Cancer	Bass, Eric (MD)	331
Rectal Cancer	Nicosia, Jon (MD)	331
Sleep Medicine	Analytis, Peter (MD)	332
Stroke Rehab	Deppe, Frances (MD)	334
Thoracic Surgery	Altergott, Rudolph (MD)	335
Trauma/Critical Care	Marshall, Wendy (MD)	335
Urinary Stones	Lewis, Gregory (MD)	335
Urological Cancers	Lewis, Gregory (MD)	335
Vascular Surgery	Altergott, Rudolph (MD)	335
Vascular Surgery	Natesha, Ramanathapur K. (MD)	335

PRIMARY CARE PHYSICIAN INDEX

NAME	TOWN	HOSPITAL	PAGE

Cook County / Family Practice

NAME	TOWN	HOSPITAL	PAGE
Arguello, Maria (MD)	Chicago	St Mary's of Nazareth Hosp Ctr	163
Arya, Jai (MD)	Chicago	Roseland Comm Hosp	163
Bardwell, Jacqueline (MD)	Oak Lawn	Christ Hosp & Med Ctr	163
Becker, Bruce (MD)	Chicago	St Mary's of Nazareth Hosp Ctr	164
Beusse, Walter (DO)	Bartlett	St Alexius Med Ctr	164
Blair, Kenneth (MD)	River Forest	West Suburban Hosp Med Ctr	164
Blankemeier, Julie (MD)	Des Plaines	Lutheran Gen Hosp	164
Blumen, Edward (MD)	Evanston	Evanston Hosp	164
Brander, William (MD)	Park Ridge	Lutheran Gen Hosp	164
Burns, Elizabeth (MD)	Chicago	Univ of Illinois at Chicago Med Ctr	164
Casey, Gerald M (MD)	Palos Heights	Palos Comm Hosp	164
Cherny, Yuri (MD)	Chicago	Swedish Covenant Hosp	164
Collins, Mark (MD)	Elk Grove Village	Alexian Brothers Med Ctr	164
Cullinane, Kevin (MD)	River Forest	West Suburban Hosp Med Ctr	164
Cupic, Dragana (MD)	Oak Lawn	Christ Hosp & Med Ctr	164
Daum, Thomas (MD)	Evergreen Park	Little Company of Mary Hosp & Hlth Care Ctrs	164
Di'Pasquo, Raymond (DO)	Orland Park	St Francis Hosp	164
Dodda, Lakshmi (MD)	Chicago	Jackson Park Hosp & Med Ctr	165
Doot, Martin (MD)	Des Plaines	Lutheran Gen Hosp	165
Early, Michael (MD)	Chicago	St Mary's of Nazareth Hosp Ctr	165
Eisenstein, Steven (MD)	Northbrook	Highland Park Hosp	165
Evans-Beckman, Linda (MD)	Evergreen Park	Christ Hosp & Med Ctr	165
Fischer, Calvin (DO)	Hoffman Estates	St Alexius Med Ctr	165
Freedman, Mark (MD)	Chicago	Ravenswood Hosp Med Ctr	165
Gomez, Carlos Alberto (MD)	Chicago	St Mary's of Nazareth Hosp Ctr	165
Goyal, Arvind (MD)	Rolling Meadows	Northwest Comm Hlthcare	165
Gros, William (MD)	Westchester	La Grange Mem Hosp	165
Grosdidier, Maureen (MD)	Glenview	Lutheran Gen Hosp	165
Hannon, Margaret (MD)	La Grange	La Grange Mem Hosp	166
Hernandez, Jose (MD)	Chicago	Norwegian-American Hosp	166
Homan, Diane (MD)	Worth	Christ Hosp & Med Ctr	166
Iagmin, Peter (MD)	Olympia Fields	St James Hosp & Hlth Ctrs	166
Kelly, Derek (MD)	Chicago	Swedish Covenant Hosp	166
Levy, Howard (MD)	Chicago	Louis A Weiss Mem Hosp	166
Lipsky, Martin (MD)	Glenview	Evanston Hosp	166
Locke, Susan (MD)	River Forest	West Suburban Hosp Med Ctr	166
Lubben, Georgia (MD)	Chicago	Jackson Park Hosp & Med Ctr	166
March, Anthony (DO)	Park Ridge	Lutheran Gen Hosp	166
Marchi, Michael (MD)	Chicago	Resurrection Med Ctr	166
Mc Donough, Richard (MD)	Barrington	Good Shepherd Hosp	166
Mercado, Ramiro (MD)	Chicago	St Mary's of Nazareth Hosp Ctr	166
O'Neill, Hugh (MD)	Evergreen Park	Christ Hosp & Med Ctr	167
Patel, Kokila (MD)	Chicago	Resurrection Med Ctr	167
Pector, Steven (DO)	Elk Grove Vlg	Alexian Brothers Med Ctr	167
Perish, Cressa (MD)	Matteson	Ingalls Mem Hosp	167
Rothschild, Steven (MD)	Chicago	Rush-Presbyterian-St Luke's Med Ctr	167
Sadowski, Joseph (MD)	Chicago	Resurrection Med Ctr	167
Sage, John (MD)	Glenview	Lutheran Gen Hosp	167
Schwer, William (MD)	Worth	Rush-Presbyterian-St Luke's Med Ctr	167
Slusinski, Bernard (DO)	Chicago	Holy Cross Hosp	167
Spishakoff, Leonard (MD)	Chicago	St Elizabeth's Hosp	167
Sproul, Stephen (MD)	Arlington Hts	Lutheran Gen Hosp	167
Veldman, Marie Ann (DO)	Tinley Park	Christ Hosp & Med Ctr	167
Walsh, Katherine (MD)	River	West Suburban Hosp Med Ctr	167
Wollner, Timothy (DO)	Evergreen Park	Little Company of Mary Hosp & Hlth Care Ctrs	168
Zalski, Andrew (MD)	Chicago	Illinois Masonic Med Ctr	168

NAME	TOWN	HOSPITAL	PAGE

Cook County / Internal Medicine (Geriatrics)

NAME	TOWN	HOSPITAL	PAGE
Birhanu, Kidanu (MD)	Burbank	Little Company of Mary Hosp & Hlth Care Ctrs	172
Grant, Mark (MD)	River Forest	West Suburban Hosp Med Ctr	172
Sier, Herbert (MD)	Park Ridge	Lutheran Gen Hosp	172

Cook County / Internal Medicine

NAME	TOWN	HOSPITAL	PAGE
Adelson, Bernard (MD)	Winnetka	Evanston Hosp	179
Altkorn, Diane (MD)	Chicago	U Chicago Hosp	179
Aronson, Alan (MD)	Skokie	Rush North Shore Med Ctr	179
Arteaga, Waldo (MD)	Chicago	Holy Cross Hosp	179
Barrocas, Salvador (MD)	Elk Grove Vlg	Alexian Brothers Med Ctr	179
Berlin, Gabriel (MD)	Glenview	Evanston Hosp	179
Bogacz, Kathleen (MD)	Skokie	Evanston Hosp	180
Brill, John (MD)	Chicago	Rush-Presbyterian-St Luke's Med Ctr	180
Brongiel, Alan (MD)	Streamwood	St Alexius Med Ctr	180
Bulmash, Jack (MD)	Chicago	Illinois Masonic Med Ctr	180
Burton, Wayne N (MD)	Chicago	Northwestern Mem Hosp	180
Candocia, Santiago (MD)	Buffalo Grove	Evanston Hosp	180
Carlson, Bruce (MD)	Barrington	Good Shepherd Hosp	180
Clarke, John (MD)	Chicago	Northwestern Mem Hosp	180
Cole, James (MD)	Arlington Hts	Northwest Comm Hlthcare	180
Curry, Raymond (MD)	Chicago	Northwestern Mem Hosp	181
Danon, Joseph (MD)	Chicago	St Mary's of Nazareth Hosp Ctr	181
Deano, Danilo (MD)	Chicago	St Mary's of Nazareth Hosp Ctr	181
Dillon, Charles (MD)	Chicago	Rush-Presbyterian-St Luke's Med Ctr	181
Fainman, Zachary (MD)	Des Plaines	Lutheran Gen Hosp	181
Farrell, Richard (MD)	Oak Lawn	Little Company of Mary Hosp & Hlth Care Ctrs	181
Foody, James (MD)	Chicago	U Chicago Hosp	181
Furey, Warren (MD)	Chicago	Mercy Hosp & Med Ctr	181
Gardner, Allen (MD)	Glenview	Evanston Hosp	181
Ginsburg, David Lee (MD)	Hoffman Estates	St Alexius Med Ctr	181
Grendon, Michael Todd (MD)	Chicago	St Joseph Hosp-Elgin	182
Gupta, Ashutosh (MD)	Chicago	Jackson Park Hosp & Med Ctr	182
Havey, Robert (MD)	Chicago	St Joseph Hosp-Chicago	182
Hering, Paul (MD)	Maywood	Loyola U Med Ctr	182
Horowitz, Kenneth (MD)	Arlington Heights	Northwest Comm Hlthcare	182
Hoyer, Danuta (MD)	Chicago	Rush-Presbyterian-St Luke's Med Ctr	182
Jaffe, Harry (MD)	Evanston	Evanston Hosp	182
Katz, Richard (MD)	Northbrook	Highland Park Hosp	182
Kehoe, William (MD)	Skokie	Rush-Presbyterian-St Luke's Med Ctr	182
Kerchberger, Vern (MD)	Arlington Hts	Northwest Comm Hlthcare	183
Kirby, Joanne (MD)	Chicago	Columbus Hosp	183
Kogan, Edward (MD)	Hoffman Estates	St Alexius Med Ctr	183
Kopin, Jeffrey (MD)	Chicago	Northwestern Mem Hosp	183
Kreamer, Jeffry (MD)	Palatine	Good Shepherd Hosp	183
Krishnan, Meera (MD)	Oak Lawn	Christ Hosp & Med Ctr	183
Kroger, Elliott (MD)	River Forest	West Suburban Hosp Med Ctr	183
Lewis, Gerald (MD)	Des Plaines	Lutheran Gen Hosp	183
Logan, Patrick (MD)	Winnetka	Evanston Hosp	183
Madhav, Gopal (MD)	Evergreen Park	Christ Hosp & Med Ctr	183
Meyers, Kim (MD)	Evanston	Evanston Hosp	184
Michael, Magdy (MD)	Chicago	St Mary's of Nazareth Hosp Ctr	184
Miller, James (MD)	Oak Park	Mount Sinai Hosp Med Ctr	184
Milner, Larry (MD)	Northbrook	Highland Park Hosp	184
Morgan, Herman (MD)	Chicago	Trinity Hosp	184

NAME	TOWN	HOSPITAL	PAGE
Mozwecz, Jeffrey (MD)	Oak Lawn	Christ Hosp & Med Ctr	184
Murphy, Joseph Leroy (MD)	Chicago	St Joseph Hosp-Elgin	184
Mutterperl, Robert (DO)	Chicago	Resurrection Med Ctr	184
Newberger, Todd (MD)	Evanston	Evanston Hosp	184
Nora, Maryannette (MD)	Lincolnwood	Columbus Hosp	184
Ohri, Arun (MD)	Chicago	Resurrection Med Ctr	185
Palmer, Scott Bradley (MD)	Chicago	Rush North Shore Med Ctr	185
Patel, Jayant (MD)	Chicago	Holy Cross Hosp	185
Patel, Natubhai (MD)	Chicago	St Mary's of Nazareth Hosp Ctr	185
Paul, Tarak (Dharam) (MD)	Chicago	Grant Hosp	185
Pearson, Marilyn (MD)	Chicago	Illinois Masonic Med Ctr	185
Perez, Andrew (MD)	Evergreen Park	Little Company of Mary Hosp & Hlth Care Ctrs	185
Pierce, Warren (MD)	Hoffman Estates	St Alexius Med Ctr	185
Pieri, Italo D. (MD)	Chicago	Resurrection Med Ctr	185
Polychronopoulos, Soterios G (MD)	Chicago	Little Company of Mary Hosp & Hlth Care Ctrs	185
Principe, John R (MD)	Chicago	Christ Hosp & Med Ctr	185
Raines, Robert (MD)	Oak Lawn	Christ Hosp & Med Ctr	185
Ramsey, Michael (MD)	Chicago	Rush-Presbyterian-St Luke's Med Ctr	186
Reddy, Rajagopal (MD)	Chicago	St Elizabeth's Hosp	186
Rehusch, Steven (MD)	Streamwood	St Alexius Med Ctr	186
Ringel, Paul (MD)	Chicago	Illinois Masonic Med Ctr	186
Rotenberg, Morry (MD)	Arlington Hts	Holy Family Med Ctr	186
Rowley, Guy (MD)	Chicago	St Joseph Hosp-Elgin	186
Sabbagh, Haissam (MD)	Berwyn	Macneal Mem Hosp	186
Saheb, Farid (MD)	Norridge	Our Lady Of the Resurrection Med Ctr	186
Sattar, Abdul (MD)	Chicago	Ravenswood Hosp Med Ctr	186
Shah, Ashok (MD)	Chicago	Ravenswood Hosp Med Ctr	186
Siegler, Mark (MD)	Chicago	U Chicago Hosp	187
Siglin, Martin (MD)	Chicago	Louis A Weiss Mem Hosp	187
Simovic, Predrag (MD)	Chicago	St Joseph Hosp-Chicago	187
Skul, Vesna (MD)	Chicago	Rush-Presbyterian-St Luke's Med Ctr	187
Sokol, Norton (MD)	Chicago	Mount Sinai Hosp Med Ctr	187
Starr, Byron (MD)	Chicago	Northwestern Mem Hosp	187
Tatar, Arnold M (MD)	Chicago	Northwestern Mem Hosp	187
Tatar, Audrey (MD)	Chicago	Northwestern Mem Hosp	187
Thomas, Michael (DO)	Evergreen Park	Little Company of Mary Hosp & Hlth Care Ctrs	187
Tosetti, Patrick (MD)	Hickory Hills	Loyola U Med Ctr	187
Tulley, John E. (MD)	Chicago	Michael Reese Hosp & Med Ctr	187
Twaddle, Martha (MD)	Skokie	Evanston Hosp	188
Wechter, David T (MD)	Chicago	Michael Reese Hosp & Med Ctr	188
Wistenberg, Lexy (MD)	Morton Grove	Rush North Shore Med Ctr	188
Wyse, Joseph (MD)	Skokie	Evanston Hosp	188
Yegelwel, Eric (MD)	Arlington Hts	Lutheran Gen Hosp	188
Zimmanck Jr, Robert D (MD)	Park Ridge	Lutheran Gen Hosp	188

Cook County / Obstetrics & Gynecology

NAME	TOWN	HOSPITAL	PAGE
Acharya, Vasant (MD)	Oak Park	West Suburban Hosp Med Ctr	202
Archie, Julian (MD)	Oak Park	Rush-Presbyterian-St Luke's Med Ctr	203
Beck, Herbert (MD)	Evanston	Evanston Hosp	203
Boatwright, Patricia (MD)	Chicago	Rush-Presbyterian-St Luke's Med Ctr	203
Charles, Allan (MD)	Chicago	Michael Reese Hosp & Med Ctr	204
Chiranand, Pinit (MD)	Chicago	St Bernard Hosp	204
Cislak, Carol (MD)	Evanston	Evanston Hosp	204
Cromer, David (MD)	Evanston	Evanston Hosp	204
Dooley, Sharon L (MD)	Chicago	Northwestern Mem Hosp	204
Duboe, Fred (MD)	Hoffman Estates	St Alexius Med Ctr	204

NAME	TOWN	HOSPITAL	PAGE
Frederiksen, Marilynn (MD)	Chicago	Northwestern Mem Hosp	205
Hayes, Ernest (MD)	Chicago	Bethany Hosp	205
Hussey, Michael J. (MD)	Chicago	Rush-Presbyterian-St Luke's Med Ctr	206
Kim, Kee Chong (MD)	Melrose Park	Westlake Comm Hosp	206
Koduri, Anur (MD)	Chicago	Ravenswood Hosp Med Ctr	206
O'Connor, Therese Marie (MD)	Park Ridge	Lutheran Gen Hosp	207
Olsen, Norman (MD)	Chicago	Swedish Covenant Hosp	207
Pozzi, Patrick (MD)	Elk Grove Vlg	Alexian Brothers Med Ctr	208
Thomas, Joseph (MD)	Chicago	Little Company of Mary Hosp & Hlth Care Ctrs	209
Tyler, Lamarr (DO)	Vernon Hills	Highland Park Hosp	209

Cook County / Pediatrics

NAME	TOWN	HOSPITAL	PAGE
Barrows, William (MD)	Chicago	Michael Reese Hosp & Med Ctr	228
Benuck, Irwin (MD)	Evanston	Children's Mem Med Ctr	228
Boblick, John (MD)	Oak Park	Elmhurst Mem Hosp	228
Brown, Donald (MD)	Chicago	Children's Mem Med Ctr	229
Burnet, Deborah (MD)	Chicago	U Chicago Hosp	229
Burnstine, Richard (MD)	Buffalo Grove	Evanston Hosp	229
Cabrera, Bertha (MD)	Chicago	St Mary's of Nazareth Hosp Ctr	229
Chande, Sumitra (MD)	Oak Lawn	Christ Hosp & Med Ctr	229
Chaudhary, Mohammad Y (MD)	Chicago	Bethany Hosp	229
Ciskoski, Ronald (MD)	Evanston	St Francis Hosp	229
Clark, Aleta (MD)	Chicago	Northwestern Mem Hosp	229
Cohn, Richard (MD)	Chicago	Children's Mem Med Ctr	229
Collins, Mary Ann (MD)	Evergreen Park	Christ Hosp & Med Ctr	229
Cueva, John Paul (MD)	Chicago	Christ Hosp & Med Ctr	229
Cupeles, Angela B (MD)	Chicago	St Mary's of Nazareth Hosp Ctr	230
De Bofsky, Harvey (MD)	Chicago	Trinity Hosp	230
De Paul, Virginia (MD)	Evanston	Evanston Hosp	230
De Stefani, Thomas (MD)	Maywood	Loyola U Med Ctr	230
Dechovitz, Arthur (MD)	Evanston	Evanston Hosp	230
Delach, Anthony (MD)	Palos Park	Christ Hosp & Med Ctr	230
Diamond, Sean (MD)	Orland Park	Loyola U Med Ctr	230
Downey, James (MD)	Evanston	Evanston Hosp	230
Espinosa, Roberto (MD)	Chicago	Swedish Covenant Hosp	230
Esposito, Patrick (MD)	Streamwood	St Alexius Med Ctr	230
Freed, Marc (DO)	Berwyn	Macneal Mem Hosp	230
Gruszka, Mary (MD)	Berwyn	Macneal Mem Hosp	231
Hankin, Bernard (MD)	Skokie	Evanston Hosp	231
Hanna, Wafaa (MD)	Richton Park	South Suburban Hosp	231
Harris, George (MD)	Palos Park	Christ Hosp & Med Ctr	231
Hoess, Cynthia (MD)	Chicago	Rush-Presbyterian-St Luke's Med Ctr	231
Holland, Julie (MD)	Evanston	Evanston Hosp	231
Hrycelak, Maria (MD)	Park Ridge	Lutheran Gen Hosp	231
Jacob, Molly (MD)	Chicago	Illinois Masonic Med Ctr	231
Jaudes, Paula (MD)	Chicago	La Rabida Children's Hosp	231
John, Eunice (MD)	Chicago	Univ of Illinois at Chicago Med Ctr	232
Kaufman, Jonathan (MD)	Barrington	Good Shepherd Hosp	232
Kaye, Bennett (MD)	Chicago	Children's Mem Med Ctr	232
Kramer, Jane (MD)	Chicago	Rush-Presbyterian-St Luke's Med Ctr	232
Lantos, John David (MD)	Chicago	U Chicago Hosp	232
Linares, Oscar (MD)	Cicero	St Anthony Hosp	232
Lotsu, Solace (MD)	Glencoe	Columbus Hosp	232
Matray, Mark (MD)	Western Springs	La Grange Mem Hosp	232
Narayan, M S Laxmi (MD)	Chicago	Rush-Presbyterian-St Luke's Med Ctr	233
Noah, Zehava (MD)	Chicago	Children's Mem Med Ctr	233

NAME	TOWN	HOSPITAL	PAGE
Paterek, Malgorzata (MD)	Chicago	Columbus Hosp	233
Pervos, Richard (MD)	Park Ridge	Lutheran Gen Hosp	233
Polin, Kenneth (MD)	Northbrook	Children's Mem Med Ctr	233
Qamar, Izhar Ui (MD)	Chicago	La Rabida Children's Hosp	233
Radfar, Baroukh (MD)	South Holland	St Francis Hosp	233
Rangsithienchai, Pisit (MD)	Chicago	Little Company of Mary Hosp & Hlth Care Ctrs	233
Rauen, Mary (MD)	Chicago	Children's Mem Med Ctr	233
Reifman, Cathy (MD)	Bridgeview	Macneal Mem Hosp	233
Roth, Susan (MD)	Chicago	Children's Mem Med Ctr	233
Salafsky, Ira (MD)	Evanston	Evanston Hosp	234
Saleh, Nabil (MD)	Westchester	Gottlieb Mem Hosp	234
Saul, Richard (MD)	Northbrook	Highland Park Hosp	234
Simpson, Elda (MD)	Glenwood	Ingalls Mem Hosp	234
Skarpathiotis, Georgios I (MD)	Palos Heights	Christ Hosp & Med Ctr	234
Slavik, Charles (MD)	Buffalo Grove	Northwest Comm Hlthcare	234
Slivnick, Barbara Yates (MD)	Chicago	Children's Mem Med Ctr	234
Sud, Madhupa (MD)	Homewood	Ingalls Mem Hosp	234
Surati, Natverlal B (MD)	Chicago	Ravenswood Hosp Med Ctr	235
Traisman, Edward (MD)	Evanston	Children's Mem Med Ctr	235
Typlin, Bonnie (MD)	Chicago	Northwestern Mem Hosp	235
Wheeler, Wendell (MD)	Chicago	Trinity Hosp	235
Whitington, Peter (MD)	Chicago	Northwestern Mem Hosp	235
Yanong, Procopio U (MD)	Chicago	Ravenswood Hosp Med Ctr	235
Yao, Tito (MD)	Chicago	Loretto Hosp	235
Yogev, Ram (MD)	Chicago	Children's Mem Med Ctr	235
Zieserl, Edward (MD)	Evanston	Evanston Hosp	235
Zollar, Lowell (MD)	Chicago	Provena Mercy Ctr	236

Du Page County / Family Practice

NAME	TOWN	HOSPITAL	PAGE
Balodis, Anita (MD)	Elmhurst	Elmhurst Mem Hosp	280
Bednar, Patrick (MD)	Winfield	Central DuPage Hosp	280
Fortman, Lisa (MD)	Hinsdale	Hinsdale Hosp	280
Frigo, Judith (MD)	Hinsdale	Hinsdale Hosp	280
Hubbard, Robert (MD)	Naperville	Edward Hosp	281
Johnson, Robert (MD)	Carol Stream	Glen Oaks Hosp and Med Ctr	281
Lis, Linda (MD)	Burr Ridge	Hinsdale Hosp	281
Morris, Thomas (DO)	Burr Ridge	Hinsdale Hosp	281
Neumann, Charles (DO)	Downers Grove	Good Samaritan Hosp	281
Siebert, Joseph (MD)	Downers Grove	Good Samaritan Hosp	281

Du Page County / Internal Medicine

NAME	TOWN	HOSPITAL	PAGE
Allen, James E (MD & PhD)	Hinsdale	Hinsdale Hosp	283
Arain, Azizur (MD)	Downers Grove	Hinsdale Hosp	283
Carbone, Robert (MD)	Hinsdale	Hinsdale Hosp	283
Collins, James J (MD)	Naperville	Edward Hosp	283
Dunphy, James V (MD)	Naperville	Edward Hosp	283
Fearon, Maureen (MD)	Oak Brook Terrace	Loyola U Med Ctr	283
Gallagher, Thomas J (MD)	Hinsdale	Hinsdale Hosp	283
Klickman, Howard (MD)	Downers Grove	Good Samaritan Hosp	283
Kolbaba, Scott (MD)	Wheaton	Central DuPage Hosp	283
Krouse, Richard (MD)	Downers Grove	Elmhurst Mem Hosp	284
Kulczycki, Ted (MD)	Aurora	Rush-Copley Med Ctr	284
Loeb, Barbara (MD)	Downers Grove	Good Samaritan Hosp	284
O'Leary, Brian (MD)	Naperville	Edward Hosp	284
Zimmerman, Richard (MD)	Downers Grove	Good Samaritan Hosp	284

NAME	TOWN	HOSPITAL	PAGE

Du Page County / Obstetrics & Gynecology

NAME	TOWN	HOSPITAL	PAGE
Barbour, Christopher (MD)	Downers Grove	Good Samaritan Hosp	287
Carver, Thomas Richard (MD)	Oak Brook	Edward Hosp	287
Chen, Thomas (MD)	Oakbrook Terrace	Edward Hosp	287
Fitzmaurice, William (MD)	Elmhurst	Elmhurst Mem Hosp	287
Gulling, Edward (MD)	Glen Ellyn	Central DuPage Hosp	288
Shangle, Elizabeth (MD)	Lombard	Elmhurst Mem Hosp	288
Yu, Mario (MD)	Oak Brook	Hinsdale Hosp	288

Du Page County / Pediatrics

NAME	TOWN	HOSPITAL	PAGE
Campbell, Daniel (MD)	Hinsdale	Hinsdale Hosp	291
Coufal, Stanislava (MD)	Downers Grove	Good Samaritan Hosp	291
Coyer, William (MD)	Naperville	Central DuPage Hosp	291
Eckberg, Lorene (MD)	Aurora	Rush-Copley Med Ctr	291
Grunenwald, Christienne (MD)	Wheaton	Central DuPage Hosp	291
Han, Sang Jo (MD)	Bloomingdale	St Alexius Med Ctr	291
Huang, Pamela Claire (MD)	Darien	Good Samaritan Hosp	292
Liber, Peter (MD)	Wheaton	Central DuPage Hosp	292
Moosabhoy, Nafeesa (MD)	Hinsdale	Hinsdale Hosp	292
Morris, David (MD)	Naperville	Central DuPage Hosp	292
Veselik, Keith (MD)	Darien	Loyola U Med Ctr	292

Kane County / Family Practice

NAME	TOWN	HOSPITAL	PAGE
Neubauer, Joseph (MD)	Geneva	Delnor Comm Hosp	301
Poulos, Dorothea (MD)	Elgin	Sherman Hosp	301

Kane County / Internal Medicine (Geriatrics)

NAME	TOWN	HOSPITAL	PAGE
Susarla, Visi (MD)	Elgin	St Joseph Hosp-Elgin	302

Kane County / Internal Medicine

NAME	TOWN	HOSPITAL	PAGE
Baley, Richard (MD)	Elgin	Sherman Hosp	302
Kerpe, Algimantas Steponas (MD)	Geneva	Delnor Comm Hosp	302
Shah, Devendra (MD)	Elgin	Sherman Hosp	302

Kane County / Obstetrics & Gynecology

NAME	TOWN	HOSPITAL	PAGE
Epstein, Brad (MD)	Elgin	Sherman Hosp	303
Schleifer, Donald (MD)	Elgin	Sherman Hosp	303

Kane County / Pediatrics

NAME	TOWN	HOSPITAL	PAGE
Hao, Crispin (MD)	Aurora	Provena Mercy Ctr	305

Lake County / Family Practice

NAME	TOWN	HOSPITAL	PAGE
Kurowski, Kurt (MD)	North Chicago	Highland Park Hosp	313
Rudy, David R (MD)	North Chicago	Highland Park Hosp	314

NAME	TOWN	HOSPITAL	PAGE
Salazar, Luis (MD)	Grayslake	Condell Med Ctr	314
Szyman, Edward (MD)	Deerfield	Highland Park Hosp	314
Tanney, Robert (DO)	Long Grove	Highland Park Hosp	314
Uhler, Jeffrey (MD)	Lake Zurich	Good Shepherd Hosp	314

Lake County / Internal Medicine (Geriatrics)

Goldberg, Barry (MD)	Highland Park	Highland Park Hosp	314

Lake County / Internal Medicine

Braunlich, Scott (MD)	Lake Forest	Lake Forest Hosp	315
Einfalt, Melinda (MD)	Barrington	Good Shepherd Hosp	315
Frazin, Bruce (MD)	Waukegan	Victory Mem Hosp	315
Goldberg, Barry (MD)	Highland Park	Highland Park Hosp	315
Hadesman, Robert (MD)	Libertyville	Condell Med Ctr	315
Osher, Gerald (MD)	Lake Forest	Lake Forest Hosp	315
Pickard, Maurice (MD)	Highland Park	Lake Forest Hosp	315
Polyak, Valentina (MD)	Gurnee	Victory Mem Hosp	315
Sultan, John (MD)	Highland Park	Highland Park Hosp	315
Tucci, Mark (MD)	Fox Lake	Provena St Therese Med Ctr	316

Lake County / Obstetrics & Gynecology

Logan, Scott (MD)	Lake Forest	Lake Forest Hosp	317

Lake County / Pediatrics

Bismonte, Albino (MD)	Gurnee	Victory Mem Hosp	319
Fondriest, Diane (MD)	Lake Forest	Good Shepherd Hosp	319
Goldman, Barry (MD)	Lake Villa	Provena St Therese Med Ctr	319
Goldstein, Arnold (MD)	Highland Park	Highland Park Hosp	319
Lasin, Gerald (MD)	Lake Forest	Lake Forest Hosp	319
Levy, Barbara (MD)	Deerfield	Highland Park Hosp	319
Levy, Robert L (MD)	Deerfield	Highland Park Hosp	319
O'Brien, Charles (MD)	Deerfield	Evanston Hosp	319
Zwirn, Marilyn (DO)	Libertyville	Highland Park Hosp	320

McHenry County / Family Practice

Bruah, David (MD)	Woodstock	Mem Med Ctr	327

McHenry County / Internal Medicine

Hernandez, Michael (MD)	Elgin	Sherman Hosp	327
Lipov, Sergei (MD)	Lake in the Hills	St Joseph Hosp-Elgin	327

McHenry County / Obstetrics & Gynecology

Warren, Ann (MD)	Barrington	Good Shepherd Hosp	327

ALPHABETICAL DOCTOR LISTING

DIRECTORY OF DOCTORS

NAME	SPECIALTY	PAGE
A		
Aaronson, Donald W (MD)	A&I	145
Abbasy, Iftikharul (MD)	S	295
Abcarian, Herand (MD)	CRS	156
Abraham, Edward (MD)	OrS	214
Abreu, Jose (MD)	Anes	146
Acharya, Vasant (MD)	ObG	202
Acino, Shawn (MD)	U	264
Adair, Roy (MD)	PMR	236
Adams, Elaine (MD)	Rhu	252
Adelson, Bernard (MD)	IM	179
Adler, Solomon (MD)	Hem	175
Agarwal, Mahesh (MD)	Pul	321
Agarwal, Suresh (MD)	Anes	277
Agarwala, Brojendra N (MD)	PCd	222
Agnoli, Francis (MD)	EDM	280
Agrawal, Rekha (MD)	Nep	193
Ahmad, Nasir (MD)	Nep	302
Ahmad, Shahida (MD)	N	199
Ahmad, Zubair (MD)	Pul	246
Ahmed, Vasia (MD)	Onc	189
Ahuja, Satya (MD)	Nep	194
Airan, Mohan (MD)	S	295
Ajmani, Harpinder (MD)	Rhu	252
Akhtar, Riaz (MD)	Cv	278
Akhter, Iqbal (MD)	Cv	150
Akhter, Javeed (MD)	Pul	246
Al-Aswad, Basel (MD)	OrS	214
Albain, Kathy (MD)	Onc	189
Albala, David Mois (MD)	U	265
Albert, Brian (MD)	Cv	150
Albion, Timothy (MD)	ObG	202
Albrecht, Ronald (MD)	Anes	146
Alcala, Gilda (MD)	Ped	334
Alderman, Sarah (MD)	Pul	246
Alexander, Bonita (MD)	PMR	236
Alexander, Frederick S (MD)	Inf	332
Alexander, Jay (MD)	Cv	312
Ali, Fatima (MD)	Psyc	293
Al-Khudari, Mohammad A (MD)	ObG	333
Allen, Albert (MD & PhD)	Psyc	241
Allen, James E (MD & PhD)	IM	283
Allen, Neil (MD)	N	199
Alleva, Joseph (MD)	SM	255
Alshabkhoun, Shakeab (MD)	TS	262
Altergott, Rudolph (MD)	TS	335
Altimari, Anthony (MD)	S	295
Altkorn, Diane (MD)	IM	179
Altman, David (MD)	Psyc	241
Ambrose, Steven (MD)	MF	188
Ampel, Leon Louis (MD)	Anes	146
Analytis, Peter (MD)	N	332
Anderson, Allan (MD)	S	334
Anderson, Douglas E (MD)	NS	196
Anderson, Kenneth (MD)	S	255
Andersson, Gunnar (MD)	OrS	214
Andreoni, John (MD)	Inf	177
Andrews, Robert (MD)	CRS	312
Andrews, Thomas (MD)	D	279
Angres, Dan (MD)	AdP	277
Ankin, Michael (MD)	Pul	321
Anstadt, Brad (MD)	Oph	209
Anwar, Syed (MD)	Psyc	305
Anzia, Daniel (MD)	Psyc	241
Applebaum, Edward (MD)	Oto	218
Arain, Azizur (MD)	IM	283
Aranha, Gerard (MD)	S	255
Archie, Julian (MD)	ObG	203
Arensman, Robert (MD)	PdS	227
Argaez, Juvenal (MD)	IM	179
Arguello, Maria (MD)	FP	163
Ariano, Moira (MD)	D	279
Arias, Ada (MD)	Pul	246
Aron, Raul (MD)	S	305
Aronson, Alan (MD)	IM	179
Aronson, Solomon (MD)	Anes	146
Arteaga, Waldo (MD)	IM	179
Arya, Jai (MD)	FP	163
Astrachan, Boris (MD)	Psyc	241
Atzeff, Luben (MD)	PlS	320
Augustinsky, James (MD)	Inf	282
Ausman, James (MD)	NS	196
Awan, Azhar (MD)	RadRO	249
Axelrod, Edward (MD)	ObG	203
Azizi, Freidoon (MD)	GO	173
Azuma, Dennis (MD)	Onc	284
B		
Baba, Walten (MD)	EDM	161
Bach, Bernard (MD)	OrS	214
Backer, Carl (MD)	PdS	227
Bailey, Larry (MD)	Oto	218
Baim, Howard (MD)	Oto	218
Baker, Dennis (MD)	DR	280
Baker, William (MD)	GVS	268
Baker, William (MD)	GVS	268
Bakhos, Mamdouh (MD)	TS	262
Balandrin, Jorge (MD)	IM	179
Baldwin, David (MD)	EDM	161
Balesteri, Anthony (MD)	Cv	150
Baley, Richard (MD)	IM	302
Balk, Robert (MD)	Pul	246
Ball, John T (MD)	Nep	194
Ballester, Oscar (MD)	Hem	314
Balling, David (MD)	Inf	177

NAME	SPECIALTY	PAGE
Balodis, Anita (MD)	FP	280
Banerji, Manatosh (MD)	Hem	175
Banich, Francis (MD)	S	296
Bansal, Vinod (MD)	Nep	194
Banti, Gustavo (MD)	U	306
Barbour, Christopher (MD)	ObG	287
Bardwell, Jacqueline (MD)	FP	163
Barhamand, Fariborze B (MD)	Onc	284
Barnes, Robert J (MD)	Oph	288
Barnett, Arden (MD)	Psyc	293
Barnett, Morton (MD)	D	331
Baron, Joseph M. (MD)	Hem	175
Barr, Lewis (MD)	Pul	246
Barrera Jr, Ermilo (MD)	S	255
Barriuso, Eduardo (MD)	ObG	203
Barrocas, Salvador (MD)	IM	179
Barrows, William (MD)	Ped	228
Barsanti, Carl (MD)	Pul	294
Bartizal, John (MD)	CRS	156
Barton, John (MD)	ObG	203
Bass, Eric (MD)	CRS	331
Bassuk, Angel (MD)	PdS	228
Bastian, Robert (MD)	Oto	218
Batjer, Hunt (MD)	NS	196
Battista, Robert (MD)	Oto	290
Bauer, Bruce (MD)	PlS	237
Bauer, Jerry (MD)	NS	196
Baughman, Verna (MD)	Anes	146
Bawani, Mohammad (MD)	Ge	314
Bayer, William (MD)	EDM	280
Bayly Jr, Melvyn (MD)	ObG	203
Beatty, Robert (MD)	NS	286
Beck, Daniel Lee (MD)	ObG	333
Beck, Herbert (MD)	ObG	203
Becker, Bruce (MD)	FP	164
Becker, Thomas Ray (MD)	OrS	318
Bednar, Michael S (MD)	HS	174
Bednar, Patrick (MD)	FP	280
Behal, Rajan (MD)	NuM	303
Behinfar, Mehdi (MD)	Rad	250
Beigler, David (MD)	OrS	214
Bekele, Alemaychu (MD)	S	255
Bekerman, Carlos (MD)	NuM	202
Belavic, Andrew (MD)	PM	291
Belizario, Evangelina (MD)	ChAP	279
Bell, Anthony (MD)	NP	285
Bello, John (MD)	Oph	209
Belmonte, John (MD)	S	296
Benawara, Raghbir (MD)	NP	192
Bennett, David A (MD)	N	199
Benson, Leon (MD)	HS	174
Benuck, Irwin (MD)	Ped	228
Benvenuto, Riccardo (MD)	S	255
Benzon, Honorio (MD)	Anes	146
Berent, Philip (MD)	Psyc	241
Berger, David (MD)	S	322
Berger, Scott (MD)	Ge	281
Berk, Richard (MD)	S	255
Berkelhammer, Charles (MD)	Ge	168
Berkowitz, Gerald (MD)	IM	179
Berkowitz, Richard A (MD)	Anes	146
Berkson, Michael (MD)	OrS	304
Berlin, Gabriel (MD)	IM	179
Berlin, Leonard (MD)	DR	159
Berlinger, Frederick (MD)	EDM	161
Berman, Andrew (MD)	Oph	210
Berman, James (MD)	PGe	224
Bernardino, Elizabeth (MD)	Psyc	293
Berns, Arnold (MD)	Nep	194
Bernstein, Ira (MD)	Cv	150
Bernstein, Joel R (MD)	DR	159
Bernstein, Lawrence (MD)	N	199
Bernstein, Sidney (MD)	Oph	303
Bethke, Kevin (MD)	S	256
Beusse, Walter (DO)	FP	164
Bhalla, Suresh (MD)	Ge	332
Bharani, Sakina N. (MD)	A&I	277
Bhatt, Anjali (MD)	Oph	303
Bhatt, Nikhil (MD)	Oto	304
Bhorade, Maruti (MD)	IM	179
Bielinski, Roger (MD)	U	328
Bielski, Steven (MD)	EDM	301
Bikshorn, Barry (MD)	N	199
Birhanu, Kidanu (MD)	Ger	172
Bismonte, Albino (MD)	Ped	319
Bitran, Jacob (MD)	Hem	175
Bittar, Sami (MD)	PlS	238
Black, Henry (MD)	Nep	194
Black, Preston (MD)	PdS	291
Blackwell, Mable (MD)	Ped	228
Blair, Kenneth (MD)	FP	164
Blakeman, Bradford (MD)	TS	262
Blankemeier, Julie (MD)	FP	164
Blanks, Mary (MD)	ObG	203
Blankstein, Josef (MD)	ObG	203
Blasco, Thomas (MD)	Anes	146
Blitstein, Mark D. (MD)	Ge	314
Bloch, Steven (MD)	PlS	320
Block, Leslie (MD)	Oto	318
Bloom, Allen (MD)	S	296
Bloom, Robert (MD)	Psyc	241
Bloomer, William (MD)	RadRO	249
Blumen, Edward (MD)	FP	164
Boarden, Wilfred (MD)	Anes	146
Boatwright, Patricia (MD)	ObG	203
Boblick, John (MD)	Ped	228
Bockrath, John M. (MD)	U	297
Bogacz, Kathleen (MD)	IM	180

NAME	SPECIALTY	PAGE
Bonomi, Philip (MD)	Onc	189
Bonow, Robert O (MD)	Cv	150
Booth, Carol (MD)	MG	189
Bormes, Thomas Pat (MD)	U	265
Boury, Harb (MD)	NS	286
Boyer, Kenneth (MD)	Ped	228
Boyer, Martin (DO)	RadRO	249
Bradley, Craig (MD)	PlS	238
Brander, William (MD)	FP	164
Brandman, James (MD)	Onc	285
Brash, Richard (MD)	OrS	289
Braund, Victoria (MD)	Ger	172
Braunlich, Scott (MD)	IM	315
Braverman, Charles (MD)	Ped	328
Braxton, Jeffrey (MD)	S	296
Bray, James (MD)	ObG	203
Bregman, Andrew (MD)	Ge	281
Brendler, Charles B (MD)	U	265
Bresler, Michael E. (MD)	DR	159
Bresnahan, Joseph (MD)	Ge	168
Breuer, Richard (MD)	Ge	168
Brey, Steven (MD)	Anes	146
Breyer, Robert (MD)	TS	262
Brill, John (MD)	IM	180
Briller, Joan (MD)	Cv	150
Briner, William (MD)	SM	255
Brna, John (MD)	OrS	318
Broido, Peter (MD)	S	296
Brongiel, Alan (MD)	IM	180
Bronner, Abraham Jay (MD)	DR	159
Bronson, Darryl (MD)	D	312
Brosnan, Joseph (MD)	S	256
Brown, Calvin (MD)	Rhu	252
Brown, Charles Marshal (MD)	TS	262
Brown, Donald (MD)	Ped	229
Brown, Douglas V (MD)	Anes	147
Brown, Frederick (MD)	NS	196
Brown, James Louis (MD)	U	265
Brown, Steven (MD)	Oph	210
Brown, Susan (MD)	Hem	175
Broy, Susan (MD)	Rhu	252
Bruah, David (MD)	FP	327
Brubaker, Linda (MD)	ObG	203
Bruno, Edward (MD)	DR	332
Bubala, Paul (MD)	ObG	203
Buch, Piyush (MD)	GerPsy	173
Budinger, G R Scott (MD)	Pul	246
Bufalino, Vincent (MD)	Cv	278
Bulger, Richard (MD)	Oto	290
Bulmash, Jack (MD)	IM	180
Bumstead, Robert (MD)	Oto	290
Burget, Gary C. (MD)	PlS	238
Burke, Allan (MD)	N	199
Burnet, Deborah (MD)	Ped	229
Burns, Elizabeth (MD)	FP	164
Burnstine, Richard (MD)	Ped	229
Burnstine, Thomas (MD)	N	199
Burstein, Harry (MD)	ObG	317
Burt, Richard K. (MD)	Onc	189
Burton, Barbara (MD)	MG	189
Burton, Robert (MD)	Psyc	241
Burton, Wayne N (MD)	IM	180
Bush-Joseph, Charles (MD)	OrS	214
Byrne, Mitchel (MD)	S	256

C

NAME	SPECIALTY	PAGE
Cabana, Emilio C (MD)	PNep	333
Cabrera, Bertha (MD)	Ped	229
Cacioppo, Phillip (MD)	S	256
Cahill, Gerald (MD)	S	256
Cahill, John (MD)	Cv	278
Calandra, David (MD)	TS	297
Caldarelli, David (MD)	Oto	218
Calvin, James E (MD)	Cv	150
Camba, Noel (MD)	Cv	150
Campbell, Daniel (MD)	Ped	291
Campbell, David (MD)	Cv	312
Campo, Adalberto (MD)	Cv	150
Camras, Louis E (MD)	Ped	304
Canaday, Lucy (MD)	FP	332
Candocia, Santiago (MD)	IM	180
Canelas, Elizabeth W (MD)	Psyc	241
Cann, Stephen R (MD)	AdP	311
Cannon, Mary Jean (MD)	ObG	287
Capezio, Jennifer (MD)	Rhu	321
Caplan, Michael (MD)	NP	192
Carbone, Robert (MD)	IM	283
Caridi, Robert (MD)	PlS	238
Carlson, Bruce (MD)	IM	180
Caro, William (MD)	D	157
Carobene, Holly (MD)	PM	221
Carroll, Charles (MD)	OrS	214
Carroll, Gregory (MD)	Anes	277
Carroll, John (MD)	ObG	287
Carson, Maureen (MD)	ObG	203
Carter, Michael (MD)	U	265
Carver, Thomas Richard (MD)	ObG	287
Casas, Laurie (MD)	PlS	238
Casey, Gerald M (MD)	FP	164
Castillo, Samuel (MD)	Ge	168
Cavallino, Robert (MD)	DR	159
Cavallo, Charles A. (MD)	TS	306
Cavanaugh, James (MD)	Psyc	241
Cavanaugh, Jean A (MD)	PMR	236
Cerullo, Leonard (MD)	NS	196
Chand, Kishan (MD)	OrS	214

NAME	SPECIALTY	PAGE
Chande, Sumitra (MD)	Ped	229
Chang, Rowland (MD)	Rhu	252
Chapman, Lawrence (MD)	Oph	210
Charles, Allan (MD)	ObG	204
Charnogursky, Gerald (MD)	EDM	161
Chaudhary, Mohammad Y (MD)	Ped	229
Chaudhry, Naseem (MD)	Psyc	293
Chaudhry, Urmila (MD)	NP	192
Chaudhuri, Gouri (MD)	PMR	292
Chawla, Bhuvan (MD)	Nep	332
Chawla, Manjeet S (MD)	Onc	189
Chediak, Juan (MD)	Hem	175
Chen, David (MD)	PMR	236
Chen, Thomas (MD)	ObG	287
Cheng, Elaine (MD)	ObG	287
Cherala, Sundaraj (MD)	Anes	301
Cherny, Yuri (MD)	FP	164
Chhablani, Asha (MD)	S	256
Childers, Sara Jean (MD)	Anes	147
Chiranand, Pinit (MD)	ObG	204
Chiu, Y Christopher (MD)	Cv	150
Chodak, Gerald (MD)	U	265
Chor, Philip (MD)	Psyc	241
Chua, David (MD)	Ge	281
Chua-Apolinario, Susan (MD)	A&I	277
Chwals, Walter (MD)	PdS	228
Chyu, Juliana (MD)	D	327
Ciric, Ivan (MD)	NS	197
Ciskoski, Ronald (MD)	Ped	229
Cislak, Carol (MD)	ObG	204
Citronberg, Robert (MD)	Inf	177
Clardy, Christopher (MD)	PNep	226
Clark, Aleta (MD)	Ped	229
Clark, Elizabeth (MD)	GVS	268
Clark, James (MD)	Cv	278
Clarke, John (MD)	IM	180
Clemis, Jack (MD)	Oto	219
Co, Richard (MD)	Cv	151
Cobleigh, Melody (MD)	IM	180
Cochran, Michael (MD)	Onc	316
Coe, Fredric (MD)	IM	180
Cohen, Bruce (MD)	N	199
Cohen, Edward (MD)	Nep	194
Cohen, Issac (MD)	Onc	285
Cohen, Lewis (MD)	Rhu	253
Cohen, Mark (MD)	OrS	214
Cohen, Mimis (MD)	PlS	238
Cohn, Arnold (MD)	OrS	318
Cohn, Richard (MD)	Ped	229
Cohn, Susan (MD)	PHO	225
Cole, James (MD)	IM	180
Cole, Roger (MD)	PCd	222
Collins, James J (MD)	IM	283
Collins, John (MD)	N	286
Collins, Karen L. (MD)	ObG	204
Collins, Mark (MD)	FP	164
Collins, Mary Ann (MD)	Ped	229
Collins, Merry (MD)	Ped	328
Collins, Michael (MD)	OrS	289
Collins, Roger (MD)	OrS	318
Collins, Sharon (MD)	Oto	290
Confino, Edmund (MD)	RE	251
Connolly, Mark (MD)	S	256
Consiglio, Angelo (MD)	Oto	304
Conterato, Dean (MD)	RadRO	249
Conway, James (MD)	NuM	202
Cook, Francis (MD)	Inf	177
Cook, John Q (MD)	PlS	238
Cooke, David (MD)	Cv	151
Costas, Chris (MD)	Inf	177
Coufal, Stanislava (MD)	Ped	291
Coupet, Edouard (MD)	ObG	204
Covert, Robert (MD)	NP	285
Coyer, William (MD)	Ped	291
Coyle, John (MD)	S	256
Cozzens, Jeffrey (MD)	NS	197
Cozzi, Laura (MD)	Oto	219
Craig, Nona (MD)	D	157
Craig, Robert (MD)	Ge	168
Crandall, David (MD)	ObG	204
Crane, Kenneth (MD)	Rhu	253
Crawford, Karen (MD)	ChAP	155
Crawford, Paul (MD)	Nep	194
Creticos, Catherine (MD)	Inf	177
Cromer, David (MD)	ObG	204
Cromydas, George (MD)	Pul	246
Cruz, Sidney (MD)	IM	180
Cuasay, Nestor (MD)	DR	159
Cueva, John Paul (MD)	Ped	229
Cullinane, Kevin (MD)	FP	164
Cunningham, Myles (MD)	S	256
Cupeles, Angela B (MD)	Ped	230
Cupic, Dragana (MD)	FP	164
Cupic, Milorad (MD)	PM	221
Curnyn, Arnold D (MD)	Oph	210
Currie, James (MD)	Inf	177
Curry, Raymond (MD)	IM	181
Cybulski Jr., George R. (MD)	NS	197

D

NAME	SPECIALTY	PAGE
Daddono, Anthony (MD)	A&I	311
D'Agostino, Anthony M (MD)	ChAP	155
Dahlinghaus, Daniel (MD)	S	256
Dahodwala, Mohamed (MD)	Cv	151
Daily, Mark (MD)	Oph	288
Daniels, John (MD)	SM	328

DIRECTORY OF DOCTORS

NAME	SPECIALTY	PAGE
Danielson, Mark (MD)	S	334
Danon, Joseph (MD)	IM	181
Darrell, Brenda A (MD)	ObG	204
Das Gupta, Tapas (MD)	S	256
Daum, Robert S (MD)	Ped Inf	226
Daum, Thomas (MD)	FP	164
Davidson, Charles J (MD)	Cv	151
Davis, Floyd (MD)	N	199
Davis, Gilla (MD)	Psyc	241
Davis, James (MD)	D	279
Davis, Lloyd S (MD)	N	199
Davis-Fourte, Felicia (MD)	Anes	147
Davison, Richard (MD)	Cv	151
Deam, Malcolm (MD)	Inf	177
Deano, Danilo (MD)	IM	181
De Backer, Noel (MD)	IM	181
De Bartolo Jr, Hansel M (MD)	Oto	304
De Bofsky, Harvey (MD)	Ped	230
De Bruin, Ronald E. (MD)	NuM	317
De Bustros, Andree C (MD)	EDM	161
Dechovitz, Arthur (MD)	Ped	230
Deddish, Ruth B (MD)	NP	192
De Geest, Koen (MD)	GO	173
De Girolami, Daniele (MD)	Cv	331
De Groot, Leslie (MD)	EDM	161
Delach, Anthony (MD)	Ped	230
Del Busto, Paul (MD)	Rhu	253
DeLeon, Antonio (MD)	Oto	219
Delicata, Dino S (MD)	Oto	290
Dellinger, Richard (MD)	CCM	327
De Marco, Carl (MD)	U	265
Demos, Terrence (MD)	DR	159
De Paul, Virginia (MD)	Ped	230
Deppe, Frances (MD)	PMR	334
Derman, Gordon (MD)	HS	174
Desai, Kirtiben P (MD)	Anes	147
Desai, Narendra (MD)	Oto	219
De Stefani, Thomas (MD)	Ped	230
Detjen, Paul (MD)	A&I	145
Deutsch, Stephen (MD)	Ge	168
Deutsch, Thomas (MD)	Oph	210
Dhiman, Surender (MD)	OrS	333
Diamond, Merle (MD)	IM	181
Diamond, Sean (MD)	Ped	230
Diamond, Terrence (MD)	Pul	246
Dias, Luciano (MD)	OrS	215
Dieter, Raymond (MD)	TS	297
Diettrich, Nancy (MD)	S	256
DiGianflippo, Anthony (MD)	NS	286
Dillehay, Gary (MD)	NuM	202
Dillon, Bruce C (MD)	S	296
Dillon, Charles (MD)	IM	181
Dini, Morteza (MD)	GO	173
Dinwiddie, Stephen H (MD)	FPsy	302

NAME	SPECIALTY	PAGE
Di'Pasquo, Raymond (DO)	FP	164
Dixon, Donald (MD)	Cv	151
Dodda, Lakshmi (MD)	FP	165
Dolan, James R (MD)	GO	173
Dold, Henry (MD)	PA&I	222
Dolezal, Rudolph (MD)	PlS	238
Donahue, Philip E (MD)	S	257
Donaldson, James S (MD)	DR	159
Dongas, John F (MD)	Cv	331
Doolas, Alexander (MD)	S	257
Dooley, Sharon L (MD)	ObG	204
Doot, Martin (MD)	FP	165
Doud, Debra (MD)	Cv	278
Dougal, Mary (MD)	Oph	210
Douglas, Daniel (MD)	S	296
Douglas, Zachariah (MD)	Psyc	241
Downey, James (MD)	Ped	230
Drachler, A Michael (MD)	ObG	204
Drazkiewicz, Maciej K. (MD)	Hem	176
Druzak, Karen (MD)	ObG	287
Duboe, Fred (MD)	ObG	204
Dubrow, Ira (MD)	PCd	222
Duck, Stephen C (MD)	PEn	224
Duda, Eugene (MD)	NRad	201
Duerinck, Mark (MD)	Cv	278
Dugan, Robert (MD)	OrS	318
Dulcan, Mina K (MD)	ChAP	155
Dumitru, Rodica (MD)	Inf	282
Dunham, Michael E (MD)	POto	226
Dunkas, Nicholas (MD)	Psyc	242
Dunphy, James V (MD)	IM	283
Durburg, John R (MD)	Psyc	242
Dwarakanathan, Arcot A (MD)	EDM	161
Dworin, Aaron (MD)	D	313

E

NAME	SPECIALTY	PAGE
Earley, Willie R (MD)	Psyc	242
Early, Michael (MD)	FP	165
Ebenhoeh, Patrick (MD)	Psyc	242
Echiverri, Henry C (MD)	N	287
Eckberg, Lorene (MD)	Ped	291
Edger, Robert (MD)	Psyc	242
Edidin, Deborah V (MD)	PEn	224
Egan, William (MD)	Psyc	242
Egel, Robert Terrell (MD)	ChiN	156
Egwele, Richard (MD)	OrS	215
Eilers, Robert (MD)	PMR	292
Einfalt, Melinda (MD)	IM	315
Eisenstein, Richard (MD)	Psyc	242
Eisenstein, Steven (MD)	FP	165
Eller, Theodore (MD)	NS	197
Ellman, Michael H (MD)	Rhu	253

NAME	SPECIALTY	PAGE
Emanuele, Mary Ann (MD)	EDM	161
Emanuele, Nicholas (MD)	EDM	161
Engel, Geoffery (MD)	U	265
Enzmann, Dieter (MD)	DR	159
Epstein, Brad (MD)	ObG	303
Epstein, Paul A. (MD)	EDM	162
Epstein, Randy J (MD)	Oph	210
Ertle, James O (MD)	D	279
Espinosa, Gustavo (MD)	Rad	250
Espinosa, Roberto (MD)	Ped	230
Esposito, Patrick (MD)	Ped	230
Evans, Richard (MD)	PA&I	222
Evans, Richard (MD)	TS	262
Evans-Beckman, Linda (MD)	FP	165
Evrard, Marilyn (MD)	Onc	285

F

NAME	SPECIALTY	PAGE
Faber, L Penfield (MD)	TS	262
Fahey, Patrick J (MD)	Pul	247
Fainman, Zachary (MD)	IM	181
Falkowski, Walter (MD)	U	265
Fantus, Richard J. (MD)	SCC	262
Faraci, Philip (MD)	TS	262
Farbota, Leo (MD)	S	305
Farrell, Richard (MD)	IM	181
Faulk, David (MD)	Ge	302
Fawcett, Jan A. (MD)	Psyc	242
Fearon, Maureen (MD)	IM	283
Feinberg, James (MD)	D	157
Feingold, Michael (MD)	ObG	204
Feinstein, Jeffrey M (MD)	RadRO	294
Feldman, Joseph (MD)	PMR	236
Feldman, Ted (MD)	Cv	151
Ferguson, Mark (MD)	TS	262
Ferguson, R Lawrence (MD)	NS	197
Ferlmann, James (MD)	PlS	293
Fermin, Ramone E (MD)	Anes	147
Fernbach, Sandra (MD)	PR	227
Fiakpui, E Z (MD)	ObG	204
Finkel, Sanford (MD)	Psyc	242
Finley, Robert (MD)	Cv	278
Finn, Henry A (MD)	OrS	215
Firlit, Casimir (MD)	U	265
Fischer, Calvin (DO)	FP	165
Fischer, Tessa (MD)	Ger	172
Fischer, William (MD)	RadRO	294
Fisher, Elizabeth (MD)	PCd	222
Fisher, Raymond (MD)	Cv	151
Fisher, Richard (MD)	Onc	190
Fishman, David (MD)	Cv	151
Fishman, David A (MD)	GO	173
Fishman, Gerald (MD)	Oph	210
Fitzgerald, Michael (MD)	NP	285
Fitzmaurice, William (MD)	ObG	287
Flaherty, Joseph (MD)	Psyc	242
Fogelfeld, Leon (MD)	EDM	162
Fondriest, Diane (MD)	Ped	319
Foody, James (MD)	IM	181
Foody, Robert (MD)	Oph	303
Fortman, Lisa (MD)	FP	280
Fox, Jacob H (MD)	N	200
Foy, Bryan (MD)	TS	335
Franco, Joseph Anthony (MD)	S	257
Frank, Angela R (MD)	S	257
Frank, Arthur L (MD)	Ped	230
Frank, Helge (MD)	N	287
Frank, Judith (MD)	Rhu	253
Frank, Lawrence W (MD)	SM	255
Frank, Stasia (MD)	NuM	202
Franklin, James L (MD)	Ge	168
Frazin, Bruce (MD)	IM	315
Frederiksen, Marilynn (MD)	ObG	205
Freebeck, Peter (MD)	Pul	294
Freed, Marc (DO)	Ped	230
Freedberg, Howard (MD)	OrS	215
Freedman, Mark (MD)	FP	165
Freier, Paul (MD)	Cv	278
Freint, Alan (MD)	Oto	318
Fretzin, David (MD)	D	157
Friedman, Michael (MD)	Oto	219
Friedman, Neil R (MD)	U	323
Frigo, Judith (MD)	FP	280
Froelich, Christopher (MD)	Rhu	253
Fronczak, Stanley (MD)	NS	286
Fry, Willard (MD)	TS	263
Fuentes, Henry (MD)	OrS	215
Fuld, Irving (MD)	DR	159
Fullerton, David (MD)	TS	263
Furey, Warren (MD)	IM	181
Furman, Richard (MD)	S	322

G

NAME	SPECIALTY	PAGE
Gagnon, James D (MD)	Rad	334
Gaiha, Vishnu (MD)	Cv	151
Galal, Hatem (MD)	PlS	238
Galante, Jorge O (MD)	OrS	215
Galinsky, Dennis (MD)	RadRO	295
Gall, Eric P (MD)	Rhu	322
Gallagher, Thomas J (MD)	IM	283
Gallo, Martin (MD)	ObG	288
Galston, Stephen Al (MD)	Psyc	320
Galvez, Angel Galvez (MD & PhD)	Hem	176
Gamelli, Richard Louis (MD)	S	257
Gamez, Ramon (MD)	NS	316

DIRECTORY OF DOCTORS

NAME	SPECIALTY	PAGE
Gandhi, Vikram (MD)	OrS	289
Ganshirt, Stephen (MD)	S	322
Garcia-Buder, Sofia A (MD)	EDM	162
Gardner, Allen (MD)	IM	181
Gardner, Thomas (MD)	NP	192
Gartlan, Michael (MD)	Oto	333
Garvey, Daniel (MD)	U	266
Gavino, Wayne (MD)	N	303
Gaviria, Moises (MD)	Psyc	242
Gehlhoff, David A (MD)	Psyc	242
Geisler, Fred (MD)	NS	197
Gekas, Paul (MD)	Ge	302
Geldner, Peter (MD)	PlS	239
Gelfand, Richard (MD)	Anes	147
Geller, Robert (MD)	S	257
Gendleman, Mark (MD)	D	157
George, Jeffrey (DO)	NP	192
Geppert, Eugene (MD)	Pul	247
Gerard, David (MD)	Ge	281
Gerbie, Melvin (MD)	ObG	205
Gerding, Dale Nicholas (MD)	Inf	177
Gerolimatos, Spiridon G (MD)	DR	327
Gersack, John (MD)	U	266
Ghahremani, Gary (MD)	DR	159
Ghai, Vivek (MD)	NP	193
Ghazanfari, K (MD)	Ge	168
Gianopoulos, John (MD)	ObG	205
Giardina, John Joseph (MD)	Cv	278
Gidding, Samuel (MD)	PCd	223
Giese, Todd (MD)	Ped	328
Gilden, Janice Laurie (MD)	EDM	313
Gill, Santosh (MD)	Cv	301
Gill, Sukhjit (MD)	Cv	151
Gilligan, William (MD)	OrS	289
Gilman, Alan (MD)	Hem	176
Gilmer, William (MD)	Psyc	243
Ginde, Jay (MD)	Rad	250
Ginsburg, David Lee (MD)	IM	181
Ginsburg, David S (MD)	Nep	316
Girgis, Samuel (MD)	Oto	219
Giroux, John (MD)	Ped	334
Girzadas, Daniel (MD)	OrS	215
Gitelis, Michael (MD)	OrS	304
Gitelis, Steven (MD)	OrS	215
Gittler, Michelle (MD)	PMR	236
Glaser, Scott (MD)	Anes	277
Glazer, Scott (MD)	D	157
Glick, Ellen (MD)	Inf	315
Glickman, Paul (MD)	Rhu	253
Glista, Glen (MD)	N	287
Gluckman, Gordon (MD)	U	266
Gluskin, Lawrence (MD)	Ge	168
Go, Margaret (MD)	NP	285
Gojkovich, Dusan (MD)	Psyc	243
Golan, John (MD)	GVS	268
Golbus, Glenn (MD)	Cv	151
Golbus, Joseph (MD)	Rhu	253
Goldberg, Barry (MD)	Ger	314
Goldberg, Barry (MD)	IM	315
Goldberg, Salmon (MD)	A&I	145
Goldflies, Mitchell (MD)	OrS	215
Goldin, Marshall D (MD)	TS	263
Goldman, Barry (MD)	Ped	319
Goldman, Michael (MD)	Oto	219
Goldrath, David (MD)	U	266
Goldstein, Arnold (MD)	Ped	319
Goldstein, Wayne (MD)	OrS	215
Golomb, Harvey (MD)	Onc	190
Gomez, Carlos Alberto (MD)	FP	165
Gonzalez, Mark Henry (MD)	HS	174
Goodell, William (MD)	PHO	319
Goodman, Allan L (MD)	DR	313
Goodman, Larry J (MD)	Inf	178
Goodwin, James (MD)	N	200
Gordon, Leo I (MD)	Hem	176
Gore, Richard M (MD)	DR	160
Gorelick, Philip (MD & PhD)	N	200
Gorski, Daniel W (MD)	Anes	331
Gotoff, Samuel (MD)	PA&I	222
Gott, Laurence (MD)	U	266
Gottlieb, Lawrence (MD)	PlS	239
Govostis, Dean (MD)	GVS	298
Goyal, Arvind (MD)	FP	165
Grad, Gary I. (MD)	Onc	190
Graham, Lee D (MD)	Rhu	295
Grammer III, Leslie C (MD)	A&I	145
Granger, Sylvia (MD)	Ped	304
Grant, Evalyn N (MD)	A&I	145
Grant, Mark (MD)	Ger	172
Grant, Thomas H (DO)	DR	160
Grayhack, John (MD)	U	266
Green, Daniel (MD & PhD)	Oph	317
Green, David (MD)	Hem	176
Green, Thomas P (MD)	PCCM	223
Greenberg, Mark (MD)	Rad	321
Greenberg, Sheldon (MD)	Psyc	243
Greenberger, Paul (MD)	A&I	145
Greendale, Robert (MD)	Psyc	320
Greene, Scott (MD)	Anes	147
Greenland, Philip (MD)	Cv	151
Greenspahn, Bruce (MD)	Cv	152
Greenspan, Brad (MD)	Psyc	320
Gregory, Stephanie (MD & PhD)	Hem	176
Grendon, Michael Todd (MD)	IM	182
Gress, Damian (MD)	PlS	239
Grieco, John (MD)	TS	297
Griem, Katherine (MD)	RadRO	249
Griffin, Andrew (MD)	PCd	223

NAME	SPECIALTY	PAGE
Grill, Stephen (MD)	Ge	281
Grober, James (MD)	Rhu	253
Gros, William (MD)	FP	165
Grosdidier, Maureen (MD)	FP	165
Grossman, Bruce (MD)	Oto	219
Grunenwald, Christienne (MD)	Ped	291
Gruszka, Mary (MD)	Ped	231
Guastella, Frank (MD)	Oph	210
Guay-Bhatia, Lise Anne (MD)	Oph	304
Gulati, Surendra (MD)	N	333
Gulling, Edward (MD)	ObG	288
Gunasekaran, T S (MD)	PGe	224
Gunderson, Holly (MD)	S	334
Gunn, Larry (MD)	S	296
Gunnar, William (MD)	TS	297
Gupta, Ashutosh (MD)	IM	182
Gupta, Raj G (MD)	Pul	247
Gutman, Arnold (MD)	A&I	311
Gutta, Gandhi (MD)	S	296

H

NAME	SPECIALTY	PAGE
Haag, Jeffery (MD)	Oph	288
Haag, Mary (MD)	ObG	205
Hadesman, Robert (MD)	IM	315
Hadesman, William (MD)	OrS	289
Hagan, Colleen (MD)	S	257
Hahn, June (MD)	Anes	147
Hahn, Yoon (MD)	NS	197
Haid, Max (MD)	Hem	314
Halderman, John (MD)	Psyc	243
Hale, David (MD)	Cv	152
Hall, Steven (MD)	Anes	147
Halstead, R David (MD)	PCd	328
Halstuk, Kevin (MD)	GVS	268
Hambrick, Ernestine (MD)	CRS	156
Hamburger, Ronald (MD)	Nep	194
Hamming, Bruce (MD)	OrS	318
Han, Sang Jo (MD)	Ped	291
Hanan, Ira (MD)	Ge	168
Hanauer, Stephen (MD)	Ge	169
Hankin, Bernard (MD)	Ped	231
Hanlon, John P (MD)	Oph	210
Hann, Sang (MD)	S	257
Hanna, Wafaa (MD)	Ped	231
Hanna, Wafik (MD)	Oto	290
Hannigan, James (MD)	Onc	190
Hannon, Margaret (MD)	FP	166
Hansen, Jack (MD)	DR	160
Hansfield, Scott (MD)	ObG	317
Hanson, David (MD)	Oto	219
Hantel, Alexander (MD)	Onc	285
Hanus, Steven (MD)	ChAP	155
Hao, Crispin (MD)	Ped	305
Haraf, Daniel (MD)	RadRO	249
Harden, R. Norman (MD)	PM	221
Harford, Francis (MD)	S	257
Harris, George (MD)	Ped	231
Harris, Gerald D (MD)	HS	174
Harris, Max (MD)	Rhu	253
Hart, Robert W (MD)	Pul	247
Hartman, Edith (MD)	Psyc	305
Hartmann, Joseph (MD)	Cv	278
Hartz, Wilson (MD)	S	257
Harvey, Richard (MD)	PMR	236
Hass, Marsie (MD)	ObG	205
Hasson, Harith M (MD)	ObG	205
Havalad, Suresh (MD)	Ped	231
Havey, Robert (MD)	IM	182
Hayek, Richard (MD)	OrS	215
Hayes, Ernest (MD)	ObG	205
Hedberg, Carl Anderson (MD)	IM	182
Hedger, Robert (MD)	Nep	194
Hefferon, John (MD)	OrS	215
Heim, Stephen (MD)	OrS	289
Heiser, William (MD)	DR	160
Hekmatpanah, Javad (MD)	NS	197
Helgason, Cathy (MD)	N	200
Herbst, Arthur (MD)	ObG	205
Herena, Juan (MD)	Pul	247
Hering, Paul (MD)	IM	182
Hernandez, Jose (MD)	FP	166
Hernandez, Michael (MD)	IM	327
Herndon, Karyn (MD)	ObG	205
Hewell, Charles (MD)	Anes	301
Hickey, Michael (MD)	RE	295
Hier, Daniel (MD)	N	200
Hill, James (MD)	OrS	215
Hillman, David (MD)	Oph	210
Hines, Jerome (MD)	Cv	278
Hirsch, Sheldon (MD)	Nep	194
Ho, Sam (MD)	N	200
Ho, Sherwin (MD)	SM	255
Hoag, Emily (MD)	Psyc	243
Hoag, J M (MD)	D	157
Hoard, Donald (MD)	U	266
Hobart, John (MD)	ObG	205
Hobbs, John (MD)	ObG	205
Hoeksema, Jerome (MD)	U	266
Hoeltgen, Thomas (MD)	Onc	190
Hoess, Cynthia (MD)	Ped	231
Hogan, George (MD)	Rad	250
Hoganson, George E (MD)	MG	189
Holden, John (MD)	Ge	281
Holinger, Lauren (MD)	Oto	219
Holland, Julie (MD)	Ped	231
Holt, Linda (MD)	ObG	205

DIRECTORY OF DOCTORS

NAME	SPECIALTY	PAGE
Homan, Diane (MD)	FP	166
Homer, Daniel (MD)	N	200
Hong, Dennis (MD)	CCM	156
Honig, George (MD)	Ped	231
Hopkins, Gail (MD)	OrS	333
Hopkins, William (MD)	S	257
Hopkinson, William J (MD)	OrS	216
Horan, Daniel (MD)	Rad	328
Horowitz, Kenneth (MD)	IM	182
Horowitz, Steven (MD)	Oto	219
Hossain, Zahur (MD)	Ge	302
Hosseinian, Abdol (MD)	ObG	206
Hotaling, Andrew J (MD)	Oto	219
Hoxsey, Rodney J (MD)	RE	251
Hoyer, Danuta (MD)	IM	182
Hoyme, K Dan (MD)	U	266
Hozman, Robert (MD)	Rhu	322
Hrycelak, Maria (MD)	Ped	231
Huang, Pamela Claire (MD)	Ped	292
Hubbard, Robert (MD)	FP	281
Hueter, David C (MD)	Cv	152
Hui, Peter (MD)	S	296
Huq, Zahurul (MD)	S	257
Husayni, Tarek Saad (MD)	PCd	223
Hussain, Ahmed (MD)	Psyc	294
Hussein, Jaafar (MD)	Cv	152
Hussey, Michael (MD)	MF	284
Hussey, Michael J. (MD)	ObG	206
Hutchinson Jr, James C (MD)	Oto	219
Huttenlocher, Peter (MD)	ChiN	156
Hutter, Loren (MD)	ObG	206
Hwang, Kwang-Ko (MD)	PM	291

I

NAME	SPECIALTY	PAGE
Iagmin, Peter (MD)	FP	166
Iammartino, Albert (MD)	Rhu	295
Ibrahim, Kamal (MD)	OrS	289
Ignatoff, Jeffrey M (MD)	U	266
Indiraraj, Chenni (MD)	S	296
Ingall, David (MD)	Ped	231
Ismail, Mahmoud (MD)	MF	188
Israel, Jeannette (MD)	MG	189
Issleib, Stuart (MD)	Ge	282
Itkonen, Jerry (MD)	Pul	247
Ivankovich, Anthony (MD)	Anes	147
Ivanovic, Lou (MD)	Cv	152
Ivanovich, Peter (MD)	Nep	194

J

NAME	SPECIALTY	PAGE
Jabamoni, Reena (MD)	ObG	206
Jablon, Michael (MD)	HS	174
Jacob, Abraham (MD)	S	257
Jacob, Molly (MD)	Ped	231
Jacobs, Jeffrey (MD)	Ge	169
Jacobs, Laurence (MD)	RE	251
Jacobs, Leo (MD)	Psyc	243
Jaffe, Harry (MD)	IM	182
Jain, Bhagwan (MD)	Cv	152
Jain, Dinesh (MD)	Ge	282
Jain, Neeraj (MD)	Anes	277
Jajeh, Fahd (MD)	Cv	312
Jameson, James Larry (MD & PhD)	EDM	162
Jampol, Lee (MD)	Oph	211
Janevicius, Raymond V (MD)	PlS	293
Janson, Kenneth (MD)	U	323
Jaudes, Paula (MD)	Ped	231
Javaheri, Ghodrat (MD)	GO	173
Jay, Mary Susan (MD)	Ped	231
Jay, Walter (MD)	Oph	211
Jedrychowska, Krystyna (MD)	PMR	236
Jellish, Walter Scott (MD & PhD)	Anes	147
Jenks, James (MD)	ObG	288
Jensen, Donald (MD)	Ge	169
Joehl, Raymond (MD)	S	257
John, Eunice (MD)	Ped	232
Johnson, Daniel (MD)	Ped Inf	226
Johnson, Maryl (MD)	Cv	152
Johnson, Peter (MD)	PlS	239
Johnson, Robert (MD)	FP	281
Johnstone, Helen (MD)	Ped	232
Jones, George (MD)	U	335
Jones, Lynwood A (MD)	Inf	178
Jones, Paul (MD)	Cv	152
Jones, Paul John (MD)	Oto	220
Joob, Axel (MD)	TS	263
Josephson, Michelle (MD)	Nep	194
Joshi, Nalinaksha (MD)	N	200
Julka, Naresh (MD)	Nep	286

K

NAME	SPECIALTY	PAGE
Kadish, Alan (MD)	Cv	152
Kagan, Robert (MD)	HS	174
Kahrilas, Peter (MD)	Ge	169
Kalichman, Miriam (MD)	Ped	232
Kalimuthu, Ramasamy (MD)	PlS	239
Kaminer, Lynne (MD)	Hem	176
Kane, Mary (MD)	Ge	314
Kane Jr, James M (MD)	S	258
Kao, Cheng Fu (MD)	Anes	331
Kapadia, Naren (MD)	Onc	316
Kaplan, Brian (MD)	RE	252
Kaplan, Bruce (MD)	Oph	211
Kaplan, Gerald (MD)	S	258

NAME	SPECIALTY	PAGE
Kaplan, Richard (MD)	PNep	226
Kapoor, Deepak (MD)	Psyc	243
Karasick, Jeffrey (MD)	NS	197
Kashian, Stephen M (MD)	IM	182
Kathpalia, Satish (MD)	Nep	332
Katz, Howard (MD)	Pul	321
Katz, Jeffrey (MD)	PM	221
Katz, Richard (MD)	IM	182
Katz, Robert (MD)	Rhu	253
Kaufman, Jonathan (MD)	Ped	232
Kaye, Bennett (MD)	Ped	232
Kaymakcalan, Orhan (MD)	S	258
Kayton, Lawrence (MD)	Psyc	243
Kazan, Robert (MD)	NS	286
Kazer, Ralph (MD)	RE	252
Kazmar, Raymond E (MD)	Rhu	254
Keane, Dennis (MD)	PMR	292
Keane, John (MD)	D	157
Kearns, William (MD)	Oph	211
Keeler, Thomas (MD)	U	266
Keen, Mary (MD)	PMR	292
Kehoe, Thomas (MD)	Pul	247
Kehoe, William (MD)	IM	182
Kelly, Derek (MD)	FP	166
Kelly, James (MD)	N	200
Kelly, Jonathan (MD)	Psyc	243
Kelly, Joseph Francis (MD)	A&I	277
Kemel, Alexander (MD)	NuM	317
Kennard, Donald R (MD)	DR	301
Kennedy, Lofton (MD)	ObG	206
Kennedy, Michael (MD)	S	258
Kent, Vernon (MD)	ObG	333
Kentor, Paul (MD)	A&I	311
Kerchberger, Vern (MD)	IM	183
Kern, Richard (MD)	Pul	247
Kerpe, Algimantas Steponas (MD)	IM	302
Kerr, William (MD)	IM	183
Kessler, Harold (MD)	Inf	178
Kessler, Robert (MD)	S	328
Ketterling, Kevan (MD)	OrS	304
Keuer, Edward J. (MD)	D	157
Khadra, Suhail (MD)	Cv	152
Khan, A Haye (MD)	S	258
Khan, Hamid (MD)	OrS	289
Khandekar, Janardan (MD)	Onc	190
Khandeparker, Vilas (MD)	U	266
Khorsand, Joubin (MD)	S	258
Khurana, Anil (MD)	Pul	321
Khurana, Deepak (MD)	Ge	327
Kiel, Krystyna D (MD)	RadRO	249
Kies, Merrill (MD)	Onc	190
Killian, Dennis (MD)	Cv	331
Kim, Chang (MD)	S	305
Kim, Jinsup (MD)	IM	183

NAME	SPECIALTY	PAGE
Kim, Kee Chong (MD)	ObG	206
Kim, Moon (MD)	NP	193
Kim, Taek (MD)	ObG	288
Kinney, Michael R (MD)	S	258
Kirby, Joanne (MD)	IM	183
Kirch, E P (MD)	Ge	314
Kirschner, Barbara (MD)	PGe	224
Kirschner, Kristi (MD)	PMR	236
Kismartoni, Karoly R (MD)	ObG	206
Klamut, Michael (MD)	Ge	169
Klein, Joel (MD)	A&I	311
Klein-Gitelman, Marisa (MD)	Ped Rhu	227
Klickman, Howard (MD)	IM	283
Klingerman, Hans (MD)	Onc	190
Klowden, Arthur (MD)	Anes	147
Klugman, Vanessa (MD)	EDM	162
Klygis, Linas (MD)	Ge	169
Knepper, Paul (MD)	Oph	211
Koch, Donald F (MD)	Rad	250
Koduri, Anur (MD)	ObG	206
Koenigsberg, David (MD)	Cv	152
Kogan, Edward (MD)	IM	183
Kohn, Arthur (MD)	Oph	211
Koht, Antoun (MD)	Anes	148
Kolb, Louis (MD)	OrS	216
Kolbaba, Scott (MD)	IM	283
Kolbusz, Robert (MD)	D	279
Koltun, Douglas (MD)	PMR	236
Konicek, Frank (MD)	Ge	169
Kontrick, Andrew (MD)	PlS	320
Kopin, Jeffrey (MD)	IM	183
Kornmesser, Thomas (MD)	GVS	268
Koshy, Mabel (MD)	IM	183
Kosova, Leonard (MD)	Hem	176
Kozeny, Keith (MD)	D	158
Kozney, Gregory (MD)	Nep	286
Kozuh, Gerald (MD)	Onc	285
Kraft, Avram R (MD)	S	322
Kraft, Bertram (MD)	Oph	211
Kramer, Jane (MD)	Ped	232
Krantz, Heather (MD)	ObG	317
Kranzler, Leonard (MD)	NS	197
Kraus, Helen (MD)	PlS	239
Kraus, Louis (MD)	Psyc	243
Krause, Lawrence (MD)	S	258
Krause, Philip (MD)	Cv	152
Krauss, Stuart (MD)	Onc	190
Krawczyk, Mitchell (MD)	ObG	206
Kreamer, Jeffry (MD)	IM	183
Krieger, Richard (MD)	PMR	292
Krinski, Roseanne (MD)	S	258
Krishnan, Meera (MD)	IM	183
Kritsas, John (MD)	U	297
Kroczek, Bohdan (MD)	S	258

NAME	SPECIALTY	PAGE
Kroger, Elliott (MD)	IM	183
Krouse, Richard (MD)	IM	284
Krueger, Barbara (MD)	S	258
Kucich, Vincent (MD)	TS	263
Kuderna, James (MD)	OrS	216
Kuhs, Leon (MD)	Psyc	243
Kulczycki, Ted (MD)	IM	284
Kumar, Sanath (MD)	S	258
Kumar, Vijay P (MD)	Cv	278
Kuppuswami, Narmadha (MD)	ObG	288
Kurland, Howard D (MD)	Psyc	243
Kurowski, Kurt (MD)	FP	313
Kurtzman, Daniel (MD)	Oto	220
Kuznetsky, Kenneth (MD)	Nep	195

L

NAME	SPECIALTY	PAGE
Lalmalani, Gopal (MD)	Cv	153
Lalyre, Yolanda (MD)	Ge	169
Landsberg, Lewis (MD)	EDM	162
Langiewicz, Janusz (MD)	A&I	145
Langman, Craig (MD)	PNep	226
Lanoff, Martin (MD)	PMR	320
Lantos, John David (MD)	Ped	232
La Palio, Lawrence (MD)	Ger	172
La Pata, Robert (MD)	ObG	206
Larson, Bruce (MD)	Oph	289
Larson, Paul (MD)	ObG	206
Lasin, Gerald (MD)	Ped	319
Lavoll, Gunnbjorg (MD)	Psyc	243
La Voo, Elizabeth (MD)	D	158
Lawson, Thomas (MD)	DR	160
Layden, Thomas (MD)	Ge	169
Layman, Lawrence (MD)	ObG	206
Lazar, Andrew (MD)	D	313
Lease, John (MD)	PlS	239
Lebbin, Dennis (MD)	EDM	280
Lebel, Robert (MD)	MG	284
Le Compte, Benjamin (MD)	NS	197
Lee, Kwang-Sun (MD)	NP	193
Lee, Seung Soo (MD)	ObG	206
Lee-Chuy, Ismael (MD & PhD)	GerPsy	173
Leff, Joel (MD)	Psyc	243
Leibach, Steven J (MD)	Onc	190
Leonetti, John (MD)	Oto	220
Lerner, Ira (MD)	PMR	236
Lertsburapa, Yukhol (MD)	TS	263
Lester, Lucy (MD)	Pul	247
Leventhal, Bennett (MD)	Psyc	244
Levin, Jay (MD)	OrS	216
Levin, Murray (MD)	Nep	195
Levin, Stuart (MD)	Inf	178
Levine, Elliot (MD)	ObG	207
Levine, Laurence (MD)	U	266
Levine, Toni (MD)	Oto	304
Levinson, Monte (MD)	Ger	172
Levit, Fred (MD)	D	158
Levitan, Ruven (MD)	Ge	169
Levitt, Leonard (MD)	D	158
Levy, Barbara (MD)	Ped	319
Levy, Howard (MD)	FP	166
Levy, Richard (MD)	PEn	224
Levy, Robert L (MD)	Ped	319
Lewicky, Andrew O (MD)	Oph	211
Lewis, Edmund (MD)	Nep	195
Lewis, Gerald (MD)	IM	183
Lewis, Gregory (MD)	Cv	153
Lewis, Gregory (MD)	U	335
Lewis, Steven (MD)	Ger	302
Lewis, Victor (MD)	PlS	239
Lewy, Peter (MD)	PNep	226
Liao, Thomas E (MD)	Pul	247
Liber, Peter (MD)	Ped	292
Libit, Sherwood (MD)	PNep	319
Licameli, Greg (MD)	Oto	220
Lichon, Francis (MD)	Rhu	295
Lichtenberg, Lee (MD)	Rhu	305
Lieberman, Howard (MD)	Oph	211
Lieblich, Jeffrey (MD)	EDM	313
Liebovitz, Susan (MD)	D	158
Lifchez, Aaron (MD)	ObG	207
Light, Terry (MD)	HS	174
Linares, Oscar (MD)	Ped	232
Lind, Richard (MD)	S	328
Lind, Stuart E (MD)	Hem	176
Lindberg, C Ronald (MD)	Oph	211
Lindquist, John (MD)	EDM	162
Linn, Edward S (MD)	ObG	207
Lipinski, Casimir (MD)	Cv	153
Lipov, Eugene G (MD)	Anes	148
Lipov, Sergei (MD)	IM	327
Lipsky, Martin (MD)	FP	166
Liptay, Michael (MD)	TS	263
Lis, Linda (MD)	FP	281
Lisberg, Edward E (MD)	A&I	145
Liske, Thomas (MD)	Pul	305
Listernick, Robert (MD)	Ped	232
Litvin, Julia (MD)	EDM	162
Locher, Frederick G (MD)	OrS	216
Locher, Stephen (MD)	ObG	207
Locke, Susan (MD)	FP	166
Locker, Gershon (MD)	Onc	190
Locker, Gershon (MD)	Onc	191
Loeb, Barbara (MD)	IM	284
Loeff, Deborah (MD)	PdS	228
Logan, Patrick (MD)	IM	183
Logan, Scott (MD)	ObG	317

NAME	SPECIALTY	PAGE
Lopata, Randee (MD)	ObG	207
Lopez, Eugene (MD)	OrS	216
Lopez, Osvaldo (MD)	Oph	211
Lopez, Ramon (MD)	ObG	333
Lotsu, Solace (MD)	Ped	232
Lowenthal, Mark (MD)	IM	315
Lubben, Georgia (MD)	FP	166
Lubeck, David (MD)	Oph	211
Lubicky, John (MD)	OrS	216
Lubienski, Mark (MD)	S	259
Luchins, Daniel (MD)	GerPsy	173
Luck, Susan (MD)	S	259
Luger, Gerald (MD)	CCM	157
Luken, Martin (MD)	NS	197
Lurain, John (MD)	GO	173
Luskin-Hawk, Roberta (MD)	Inf	178
Lygizos, Nicholas (MD)	Oto	220
Lyon, Alice (MD)	Oph	212
Lyon, Susan (MD)	Oto	220

M

NAME	SPECIALTY	PAGE
Madamala, Thakshaka Mani (MD)	ChAP	327
Madda, Frank (MD)	PlS	239
Madej, Patricia (MD)	Onc	285
Madhav, Gopal (MD)	IM	183
Madison, Laird (MD)	EDM	162
Mael, David (MD)	Rhu	254
Mafee, Mahmood (MD)	DR	160
Mahoney, Eileen (MD)	Oto	290
Majumdar, Sanjoy (MD)	IM	184
Maker, Vijay (MD)	S	259
Makhlouf, Mansour V (MD)	PlS	239
Malhotra, Rabindra (MD)	Cv	278
Maltezos, Stavros (MD)	NS	198
Malvar, Thomas (MD)	U	267
Manam, Bob (MD)	Inf	283
Mandrea, Eugene (MD)	D	158
Mangurten, Henry (MD)	MF	188
Mann, Stewart (MD)	Pul	247
Mansfield, James (MD)	NS	303
Manus, Dean (MD)	PlS	305
March, Anthony (DO)	FP	166
Marchi, Michael (MD)	FP	166
Marciniak, Christina (MD)	PMR	237
Marcus, Elizabeth (MD)	S	259
Margolis, Benjamin (MD)	Pul	247
Marinberg, Boris (MD)	DR	160
Marinelli, Anthony (MD)	Pul	248
Markey, W S (MD)	IM	184
Markovitz, David (MD)	N	200
Markus, Norman (MD)	PlS	320
Marschall, Michael (MD)	PlS	293
Marshall, Wendy (MD)	S	335
Martell, John (MD)	OrS	216
Martinez, Charles J. (MD)	NuM	202
Martini, D Richard (MD)	Psyc	244
Martini, Seif (MD)	Cv	331
Martonffy, Denes (MD)	NS	286
Martorana, Andrew (MD)	Psyc	244
Martucci, John (MD)	Anes	277
Marut, Edward (MD)	RE	321
Marvin, Joy (MD)	S	335
Marwah, Birinder (MD)	IM	184
Marymont, Jesse (MD)	Anes	148
Matalon, Terrence (MD)	DR	160
Mategrano, Victor (MD)	DR	280
Mathew, Moly (MD)	Anes	331
Matray, Mark (MD)	Ped	232
Matthew, Edward (MD)	Anes	311
Matz, Gregory (MD)	Oto	220
Maximovich, Stanley (MD)	PlS	293
Mayer, John (MD)	OrS	318
Mayer, Robert Samuel (MD)	PMR	237
Mayer, Thomas (MD)	Cv	312
Mazur, John (MD)	NS	303
Mazzone, Theodore (MD)	EDM	162
Mc Cahill, Kathleen (MD)	N	333
Mc Call, Anne (MD)	RadRO	334
McCarthy III, Walter J (MD)	GVS	269
Mc Coyd, Kevin (MD)	N	287
Mc Donough, Richard (MD)	FP	166
McFadden, John (MD)	Rad	250
McGee, John (MD)	Anes	148
Mc Grail, Michael (MD)	S	259
McGrath, Kris (MD)	A&I	145
McIlree, Nina (MD)	PMR	237
McKeever, Louis (MD)	Cv	279
Mc Kenna, Kathleen (MD)	Psyc	244
Mc Kenna, Michael E (MD)	Ge	282
Mc Kinney, Peter (MD)	PlS	239
Mc Kinney, William (MD)	Psyc	244
Mc Laughlin, Desmond (MD)	Anes	148
Mc Leod, Evan (MD)	Pul	248
McLeod, Rima (MD)	Inf	178
McLone, David (MD)	NS	198
McLone, David (MD)	NS	198
Mc Nally, Randall (MD)	PlS	239
Mehta, Harshad M (MD)	Psyc	244
Mehta, Yashbir (MD)	RadRO	321
Meiselman, Mick (MD)	IM	184
Meisles, Jeffrey (MD)	OrS	216
Melam, Howard (MD)	A&I	145
Meltzer, William (MD)	OrS	216
Menezes, Ralph (MD)	Psyc	244
Mercado, Ramiro (MD)	FP	166
Meredith, Heidi (MD)	Psyc	244

DIRECTORY OF DOCTORS

NAME	SPECIALTY	PAGE
Merkel, Douglas (MD)	Onc	191
Merlotti, Gary J (MD)	SCC	262
Merrick, Frank (MD)	ObG	207
Merrick, Paul (MD)	U	297
Merrill, Timothy (MD)	DR	160
Merrin, Claude (MD)	U	267
Mershon, Stephen (MD)	GerPsy	173
Mesleh, George (MD)	S	259
Messer, Joseph V. (MD)	Cv	153
Messersmith, Richard (MD)	Rad	250
Metrick, Scott (MD)	N	316
Mets, Marilyn (MD)	Oph	212
Metzger, Boyd (MD)	EDM	162
Meyer, James (MD)	Psyc	244
Meyer, Joel (MD)	Rad	251
Meyers, Kim (MD)	IM	184
Michael, Magdy (MD)	IM	184
Michalska, Margaret (MD)	Rhu	254
Michel, Arthur (MD)	S	259
Michelotti, Joseph (MD)	S	305
Miller, Alan (MD)	Psyc	320
Miller, Albert (MD)	Cv	153
Miller, Frank (MD)	DR	160
Miller, Frederick E (MD)	Psyc	244
Miller, James (MD)	IM	184
Miller, Kenneth (MD)	PNep	226
Miller, Laura Jo (MD)	Psyc	244
Miller, Marilyn T (MD)	Oph	212
Miller, Paul E. (MD)	Anes	148
Miller, Robert (MD)	Oto	220
Miller, Ronald W (MD)	ObG	207
Miller, Scott (MD)	Cv	153
Miller, Sheldon (MD)	Psyc	245
Millman, Leonard (MD)	Oph	212
Millman, William (MD)	Cv	153
Milner, Larry (MD)	IM	184
Mintzer, Richard (MD)	DR	313
Mishell, Joseph (MD)	Oto	318
Mittal, Bharat (MD)	RadRO	249
Miz, George (MD)	OrS	216
Moawad, Atef (MD)	ObG	207
Mohan, Jagan (MD)	N	200
Mokarry, Victor Peter (MD)	Oto	220
Molitch, Mark (MD)	EDM	162
Moller, Neal (MD)	Ge	314
Molloy Jr, Robert E (MD)	Anes	148
Monahan, James (MD)	Cv	312
Monasterio, Jack (MD)	PlS	293
Montana, Louis (MD)	S	296
Mooney, Gabriel (MD)	PlS	240
Moore, Dennis (MD)	Oto	220
Moore, Thomas (MD)	Ped	334
Moosabhoy, Nafeesa (MD)	Ped	292
Moran, Brian (MD)	RadRO	249

NAME	SPECIALTY	PAGE
Moran, Michael (MD)	OrS	217
Morgan, David (MD)	RadRO	250
Morgan, Elaine (MD)	PHO	225
Morgan, George (MD)	Ge	282
Morgan, Herman (MD)	IM	184
Morgan, Nathaniel (MD)	D	158
Morimoto, David (MD)	Oph	333
Morimoto, Paul (MD)	Oph	333
Morris, David (MD)	Ped	292
Morris, Thomas (DO)	FP	281
Morrow, Monica (MD)	S	259
Moscoso, Eloy (MD)	S	259
Moser, Richard P (MD)	NS	198
Moss, Jonathan (MD)	Anes	148
Motto, George S (MD)	EDM	163
Mozwecz, Jeffrey (MD)	IM	184
Muasher, Issa E (MD)	TS	263
Mukherjee, Ashish (MD)	Cv	153
Mullane, Michael (MD)	Onc	191
Mullin, Kimberly Anne (MD)	ObG	207
Munoz, Maria (MD)	ObG	207
Muraskas, Jonathon (MD)	NP	193
Murphy, Joseph Leroy (MD)	IM	184
Murphy, Sharon (MD)	PHO	225
Murthy, Anantha (MD)	RadRO	295
Murthy, Vemuri (MD)	Anes	148
Muscarello, Vincent (MD)	Ge	170
Mustoe, Thomas (MD)	PlS	240
Mutchnik, David (MD)	U	323
Muthuswamy, Petham (MD)	Pul	248
Mutterperl, Robert (DO)	IM	184
Myers, Phil (MD)	Anes	331
Myers, William (MD)	Oph	212

N

NAME	SPECIALTY	PAGE
Nadimpalli, Chitra (MD)	Oph	212
Nadimpalli, Surya P R (MD)	Rad	251
Nagle, Daniel J. (MD)	HS	175
Nagpal, Krishan (MD)	Oph	289
Nagpal, Rajeev (MD)	PGe	225
Naidu, Shrinivas (MD)	PCCM	223
Narayan, M S Laxmi (MD)	Ped	233
Nash, Donald (MD)	S	259
Natesha, Ramanathapur K. (MD)	S	335
Nayden, John (MD)	Rad	251
Nelson, Erik George (MD)	Oto	318
Nelson, Suzanne P (MD)	PGe	225
Nemickas, Rimgaudas (MD)	Cv	153
Neubauer, Joseph (MD)	FP	301
Neumann, Charles (DO)	FP	281
Newberger, Todd (MD)	IM	184
Newman, Daniel (MD)	OrS	217

NAME	SPECIALTY	PAGE
Newman, Steven (MD)	Onc	191
Newmark, Jay (MD)	U	267
Nicosia, Jon (MD)	CRS	331
Nierman, Peter (MD)	ChAP	155
Nighswander, J Richard (MD)	IM	284
Nigro, Salvatore (MD)	TS	297
Noah, Zehava (MD)	Ped	233
Nold, Stephen (MD)	U	267
Nootens, Raymond (MD)	Oph	212
Nora, Maryannette (MD)	IM	184
Nora, Nancy (MD)	Nep	316
Norman, Douglas (MD)	TS	263
Noskin, Gary (MD)	Inf	178
Nour, Fred (MD)	N	287
Nuber, Gordon (MD)	OrS	217
Nuzzarello, Joseph (MD)	U	297
Nye, Elizabeth (MD)	ObG	207

O

NAME	SPECIALTY	PAGE
Obasi, Ejikeme (MD)	Nep	195
O'Brien, Charles (MD)	Ped	319
O'Connor, Scott (MD)	OrS	304
O'Connor, Therese Marie (MD)	ObG	207
O'Donoghue, Marianne Nelson (MD)	D	279
O'Donoghue, Michael (MD)	S	259
Ogata, Edward (MD)	NP	193
O'Grady, Richard (MD)	Oph	212
Ohri, Arun (MD)	IM	185
O'Keefe, James Paul (MD)	Inf	178
Oken, Jeffrey Edward (MD)	PMR	292
Olak, Jemi (MD)	TS	263
O'Leary, Brian (MD)	IM	284
Olinger, Edward (MD)	Ge	170
Olsen, Norman (MD)	ObG	207
O'Neill, Hugh (MD)	FP	167
O'Reilly, William (MD)	Onc	191
Orlowski, Janis (MD)	Nep	195
Orth, David (MD)	Oph	212
Osher, Gerald (MD)	IM	315
Overton, Margaret Eileen (MD)	Anes	148
Ow, Earl Phillip (MD)	PCd	223
Oyama, Joseph (MD)	Nep	195
Ozog, Diane Louise (MD)	A&I	277

P

NAME	SPECIALTY	PAGE
Pachman, Lauren (MD)	Rhu	254
Pahl, Elfriede (MD)	PCd	223
Painter, Thomas (MD)	GVS	269
Palella, Thomas Daniel (MD)	Rhu	254
Paller, Amy Susan (MD)	D	158
Palmer, David (MD)	Oph	212
Palmer, Scott Bradley (MD)	IM	185
Panchal, Kanu (MD)	NS	198
Pandit, Jay (MD)	S	259
Panje, William (MD)	Oto	220
Park, C Lucy (MD)	PA&I	222
Parnass, Samuel (MD)	Anes	148
Parrillo, Joseph E (MD)	CCM	157
Parvathaneni, K (MD)	TS	263
Pasternak, Joseph F (MD)	ChiN	156
Patek, Robert (MD)	OrS	217
Patel, Ambalal K (MD)	S	259
Patel, Jayant (MD)	IM	185
Patel, Kaushik (MD)	Onc	285
Patel, Kokila (MD)	FP	167
Patel, Natubhai (MD)	IM	185
Paterek, Malgorzata (MD)	Ped	233
Paton, John (MD)	NP	193
Paul, Tarak (Dharam) (MD)	IM	185
Pavel, Dan (MD)	NuM	202
Pavese, Joseph (MD)	ObG	208
Pavlatos, Christ (MD)	SM	322
Pawlikowski, James (MD)	S	260
Payne, Deming (MD)	PlS	293
Payne, Timothy (MD)	OrS	290
Pearce, William (MD)	GVS	269
Pearson, Marilyn (MD)	IM	185
Peckler, M Scott (MD)	S	260
Pector, Steven (DO)	FP	167
Pedemonte, Walter (MD)	Psyc	245
Peller, Patrick (MD)	NuM	202
Pelletiere, Vincent (MD)	PlS	240
Pensler, Jay Michael (MD)	PlS	240
Perez, Andrew (MD)	IM	185
Perez-Tamayo, Alejandra (MD)	S	260
Pergament, Eugene (MD)	CG	156
Perish, Cressa (MD)	FP	167
Perlman, Reid (MD)	NuM	202
Perri, John (MD)	Psyc	245
Pervos, Richard (MD)	Ped	233
Pesavento, Daniel (MD)	ObG	317
Pessis, Dennis (MD)	U	323
Petasnick, Jerry (MD)	Rad	251
Petchenik, Lon (MD)	Oto	221
Peterson, Carol (MD)	Onc	332
Phillips, Richard (MD)	Rad	251
Pickard, Maurice (MD)	IM	315
Pickleman, Jack R (MD)	S	260
Piel, Ira (MD)	Onc	191
Pielet, Bruce (MD)	ObG	208
Pierce, Karen (MD)	ChAP	155
Pierce, Scott (MD)	ObG	208
Pierce, Warren (MD)	IM	185
Pieri, Italo D. (MD)	IM	185

NAME	SPECIALTY	PAGE
Pillsbury, Lisa (MD)	Nep	195
Pineless, Gary (MD)	Cv	312
Plotnick, Bennett (MD)	Ge	170
Polin, Kenneth (MD)	Ped	233
Polin, Stanton (MD)	TS	264
Polk, Dan (MD)	NP	193
Pollock, James (MD)	A&I	145
Polyak, Valentina (MD)	IM	315
Polychronopoulos, Soterios G (MD)	IM	185
Poma, Pedro A (MD)	ObG	208
Pomerantz, Rhoda (MD)	Ger	172
Pope, Richard Mitchell (MD)	Rhu	254
Porter, Gregory Anthony (MD)	Anes	148
Portugal, Louis (MD)	Oto	221
Pottenger, Lawrence (MD)	OrS	217
Poulos, Dorothea (MD)	FP	301
Poznanski, Andrew (MD)	PR	227
Poznanski, Elva (MD)	ChAP	155
Pozzi, Patrick (MD)	ObG	208
Prajka, Valerie (DO)	FP	332
Preisler, Harvey (MD)	Onc	191
Press, Joel (MD)	PMR	237
Principe, John R (MD)	IM	185
Prinz, Richard (MD)	S	260
Prunskis, John (MD)	PM	328
Przypyszny, John (MD)	S	260
Pucci, Rita (MD)	S	260
Pundaleeka, Sarode (MD)	Hem	332
Pupillo, Louis (MD)	NS	198

Q

NAME	SPECIALTY	PAGE
Qamar, Izhar Ui (MD)	Ped	233
Quigg, Rebecca Jayne (MD)	Cv	153
Quinn, Thomas (MD)	Cv	153

R

NAME	SPECIALTY	PAGE
Rabin, David (MD)	DR	313
Radfar, Baroukh (MD)	Ped	233
Radhakrishnan, Jayant (MD)	PdS	228
Radwanska, Eva (MD)	RE	295
Raine, Talmage (MD)	PlS	293
Raines, Robert (MD)	IM	185
Ramakrishna, Bhagavatula (MD)	Inf	178
Ramilo, Jose (MD)	PR	227
Ramsey, Michael (MD)	IM	186
Ramsey, Ruth Godwin (MD)	Rad	251
Randolph, David (MD)	PlS	240
Rangsithienchai, Pisit (MD)	Ped	233
Rao, Noel (MD)	PMR	292
Rathi, Manohar (MD)	NP	193
Rattner, Zachary (MD)	DR	160
Rauen, Mary (MD)	Ped	233
Rauh, R Andrew (MD)	Cv	279
Razma, Antanas (MD)	Pul	248
Reddy, Chandra (MD)	Anes	148
Reddy, Rajagopal (MD)	IM	186
Reddy, Ravindranath (MD)	NP	285
Redondo, Luis J (MD)	OrS	217
Reeves, Robert (MD)	Psyc	245
Regan, Michael (MD)	ObG	208
Rehusch, Steven (MD)	IM	186
Reider, Bruce (MD)	OrS	217
Reifman, Cathy (MD)	Ped	233
Rejowski, James (MD)	Oto	290
Renshaw, Domeena (MD)	Psyc	245
Repasy, Andrew Bela (MD)	Ger	172
Resnick, Alan (MD)	A&I	311
Resnick, Kenneth (MD)	Oph	212
Reyes, Hernan M (MD)	PdS	228
Rezak, Michael (MD)	N	200
Rhee, Chang (MD)	Rad	251
Riaz, Muhamad Khalid (MD)	Cv	301
Rich, Barry H (MD)	PEn	291
Rich, Kenneth (MD)	PA&I	222
Rich, Stuart (MD)	Cv	153
Ries, Michael (MD)	Pul	248
Rinehart, John (MD)	RE	252
Ringel, Paul (MD)	IM	186
Ripeckyj, Andrew (MD)	Psyc	245
Roberts, Jack (MD)	TS	264
Robin, Arnold (MD)	S	260
Robinson, Barbara (MD)	ObG	208
Robinson, June (MD)	D	158
Rodenas, Jesus (MD)	Anes	149
Rodts, Thomas (MD)	OrS	290
Rogers, B H Gerald (MD)	Ge	170
Rogin, Alan (MD)	U	267
Romeiser Jr, Adam (MD)	S	322
Rosanova, Albert (MD)	S	260
Rosanova, Mark (MD)	Oph	212
Roseman, Melvin K. (MD)	Nep	195
Rosen, Barry (MD)	S	260
Rosen, Jeffrey (MD)	S	260
Rosen, Steven (MD)	Onc	191
Rosenberg, Aaron (MD)	OrS	217
Rosenberg, James (MD)	Ge	170
Rosenberg, Michael (MD)	A&I	146
Rosenberg, Neil (MD)	Pul	248
Rosenblum, Leigh (MD)	NuM	202
Rosenbush, Stuart (MD)	Cv	154
Rosenfield, Robert (MD)	PEn	224
Rosenow, Mary (MD & PhD)	S	261
Rosenthal, Gayle (MD)	Ge	170
Rosi, David (MD)	Onc	191

NAME	SPECIALTY	PAGE
Ross, Lawrence (MD)	U	267
Ross, Matthew (MD)	NS	286
Rotenberg, Morry (MD)	IM	186
Roth, Andrew G (MD)	Anes	149
Roth, David (MD)	Anes	149
Roth, Elliot (MD)	PMR	237
Roth, Susan (MD)	Ped	233
Rothenberg, David (MD)	Anes	149
Rothschild, Steven (MD)	FP	167
Rotmensch, Jacob (MD)	ObG	208
Rowan, Daniel (DO)	Cv	154
Rowley, Guy (MD)	IM	186
Rowley, Stephen (MD)	Cv	279
Rowley, Wilbur F (MD)	N	316
Rozental, Jack M. (MD & PhD)	N	200
Rubach, Bryan (MD)	Oto	291
Rubin, Gary (MD)	Oph	213
Rubin, Michael (MD)	ObG	208
Rubin, Susan (MD)	N	201
Rubinstein, Wayne (MD)	N	201
Ruchim, Michael (MD)	Ge	170
Ruder, Henry (MD)	EDM	163
Rudy, David R (MD)	FP	314
Ruff, Bradley (MD)	Oph	318
Ruge, John (MD)	NS	198
Russ, Joseph (MD)	S	306
Rydel, James (MD)	Nep	195

S

NAME	SPECIALTY	PAGE
Sabbagh, Haissam (MD)	IM	186
Sabesin, Seymour M (MD)	Ge	170
Saclarides, Theodore John (MD)	CRS	156
Sacy, George (MD)	DR	161
Sadauskas, J Linas (MD)	Psyc	294
Sadowski, Joseph (MD)	FP	167
Sage, John (MD)	FP	167
Saheb, Farid (MD)	IM	186
Salafsky, Ira (MD)	Ped	234
Salazar, Jose (MD)	NS	198
Salazar, Luis (MD)	FP	314
Saleh, Nabil (MD)	Ped	234
Salem, Mohamed (MD)	Nep	195
Sales, David (MD & PhD)	Ge	170
Salinger, Michael H (MD)	Cv	154
Salvi, Sharad (MD)	PHO	225
Samuels, Brian (MD)	Onc	191
Sandage, Scott (DO)	ChAP	155
Sandler, Richard (MD)	PGe	225
Santos, Rene (MD)	Inf	178
Sarin, Pramila (MD)	RadRO	250
Sarwark, John (MD)	PdS	228
Sastri, Suriya (MD)	IM	284
Sattar, Abdul (MD)	IM	186
Saul, Richard (MD)	Ped	234
Saxena, S V Amod (MD)	RadRO	250
Scafuri, Ralph (MD)	OrS	217
Scanlon, Patrick (MD)	Cv	154
Scelzo, Frederick (MD)	Oph	213
Schaeffer, Anthony (MD)	U	267
Schafer, Michael F. (MD)	SM	255
Schanbacher, Paul (MD)	Anes	149
Scheer, Michael (MD)	S	322
Schenck, Robert (MD)	HS	175
Schewitz, David (MD)	ObG	317
Schickler, Renee (MD)	EDM	163
Schiffman, Kenneth (MD)	OrS	290
Schleifer, Donald (MD)	ObG	303
Schlenker, James (MD)	PlS	240
Schmidt, Greg (MD)	CCM	157
Schneider, Joseph (MD)	GVS	269
Schreiber, Ronald (MD)	Cv	154
Schroeder, James (MD)	Rhu	254
Schroeder, Keith E (MD)	OrS	217
Schubert, Robert (MD)	IM	332
Schuette, Patrick (MD)	Rhu	254
Schuler, James (MD)	GVS	269
Schulte, Edward (DO)	Anes	149
Schupp, Elizabeth (MD)	Pul	294
Schuster, George (MD)	U	335
Schwartz, Janice (MD)	Ger	172
Schwartz, Jerrold (MD)	Ge	170
Schwartz, Lee (MD)	Psyc	245
Schwartz, Michael (MD)	N	201
Schwartz, Michael (MD)	DR	301
Schwer, William (MD)	FP	167
Schy, Susan (MD)	ObG	208
Sciarra, John (MD)	ObG	208
Seed, Randolph (MD)	S	261
Seeler, Ruth A (MD)	PHO	225
Seidenberg, Henry (MD)	Psyc	245
Semel, Jeffery (MD)	Inf	315
Semel, Jeffrey (MD)	Inf	178
Sener, Stephen (MD)	S	261
Septon, Robert (MD)	D	313
Serushan, Majid (MD)	IM	186
Sethi, Manjeet (MD)	Cv	154
Sethna, Jehangir (MD)	S	261
Shadel, Robert F (MD)	OM	288
Shafer, Jeff (MD)	RadRO	305
Shah, Ashok (MD)	IM	186
Shah, Devendra (MD)	IM	302
Shah, Nikunj (MD)	Ge	170
Shah, Prabodh (MD)	Onc	191
Shah, Rajendra (MD)	PlS	240
Shah, Ranchhodlal (MD)	IM	186
Shah, Shirish (MD)	Cv	154

NAME	SPECIALTY	PAGE
Shah, Upendra (MD)	EDM	163
Shahani, Bhagwan (MD)	PMR	237
Shangle, Elizabeth (MD)	ObG	288
Shapiro, Barry (MD)	Anes	149
Shapiro, Daniel (MD)	Psyc	245
Sharifi, Roohollah (MD)	U	267
Sharma, Madie M. (MD)	RadRO	250
Shashoua, Abe (MD)	ObG	208
Shaw, Geoffrey (MD)	Psyc	245
Shaw, James C (MD)	D	158
Shaw, John M (MD)	Onc	191
Shayani, Vafa (MD)	S	296
Shea, John (MD)	NS	198
Sheaff, Charles (MD)	S	261
Sheftel, David (MD)	Ped	234
Sherman, Edward (MD)	Inf	283
Sherman, Richard (MD)	OrS	318
Shirazi, S Javed (MD)	RadRO	250
Shkolnik, Arnold (MD)	PR	227
Shoults, David (MD)	Anes	311
Shulman, Stanford (MD)	Ped	234
Siddique, Teepu (MD)	N	201
Sidrys, Jonas (MD)	RadRO	295
Siebert, Joseph (MD)	FP	281
Siegler, Mark (MD)	IM	187
Sier, Herbert (MD)	Ger	172
Siglin, Martin (MD)	IM	187
Silver, Michael (MD)	Pul	248
Silver, Richard (MD)	ObG	208
Silverman, Bernard (MD)	PEn	224
Silverman, Irwin (MD)	Cv	154
Simon, Norman (MD)	Nep	195
Simovic, Predrag (MD)	IM	187
Simpson, Elda (MD)	Ped	234
Simpson, Kevin (MD)	Pul	248
Sinibaldi, Mark (MD)	Psyc	334
Sinsheimer, Erica (MD)	EDM	163
Sison, Jose (MD)	Anes	301
Sisung, Charles (MD)	PMR	237
Sittler, Stephen (MD)	Ge	171
Sizemore, Glen (MD)	EDM	163
Skarpathiotis, Georgios I (MD)	Ped	234
Skosey, John (MD)	Rhu	254
Skul, Vesna (MD)	IM	187
Slavik, Charles (MD)	Ped	234
Slivnick, Barbara Yates (MD)	Ped	234
Sliwa, James A (DO)	PMR	237
Sloane, Herman (MD)	Oph	213
Slogoff, Stephen (MD)	Anes	149
Slusinski, Bernard (DO)	FP	167
Smith, Joanne C (MD)	PMR	293
Smith, Lewis (MD)	Pul	248
Smith, Matthew (MD)	Ge	171
Sobinsky, Kim (MD)	S	322
Socol, Michael (MD)	ObG	209
Sodt, Peter (MD)	PCd	223
Soifer, Neil (MD)	Nep	196
Sokol, Norton (MD)	IM	187
Solomon, Samuel (MD)	D	313
Soltes, Barbara (MD)	RE	252
Soltes, Steven (MD)	Oto	221
Somers, Jonathon (MD)	TS	264
Sosenko, George (MD)	U	298
Sosenko, Maria (MD)	Rhu	334
Sowray, Paul (MD)	Onc	192
Sparberg, Marshall (MD)	Ge	171
Spencer, Charles (MD)	Ped Rhu	227
Sperling, Richard (MD)	PlS	240
Spero, Neal (MD)	D	158
Spies, Stewart (MD)	NuM	202
Spishakoff, Leonard (MD)	FP	167
Sporn, Peter (MD)	Pul	248
Sprague, Stuart (MD)	Nep	196
Springer, David (MD)	Oph	213
Springer, Harry (MD)	PlS	240
Sproul, Stephen (MD)	FP	167
Srinivasan, Chida (MD)	Anes	149
Stankiewicz, James (MD)	Oto	291
Starr, Byron (MD)	IM	187
Steimle, Cynthia (MD)	TS	306
Stein, Robert N (MD)	Hem	176
Steiner, Monica (MD)	PMR	293
Steinwald, Osmar (MD)	PlS	320
Stephenson, Richard E (MD)	Anes	149
Stern, Mark (MD)	Cv	312
Stipisic, Ana (MD)	Rad	321
Stobnicki, Aleksandra (MD)	N	201
Stock, E Lee (MD)	Oph	213
Stoller, Walter A (MD)	EDM	280
Stone, Neil (MD)	Cv	154
Strassner, Howard T (MD)	MF	188
Streicher, Lauren F (MD)	ObG	209
Strohmayer, Eileen T (MD)	ObG	317
Strohmayer, Paul (MD)	S	322
Stryker, Steven J. (MD)	S	261
Sturm, Richard E (MD)	OM	317
Sublette, Gerard (MD)	Ge	282
Sud, Madhupa (MD)	Ped	234
Sugar, Joel (MD)	Oph	213
Suk, Churl-Soo (MD)	OrS	217
Sulayman, Rabi F (MD)	Ped	234
Suleiman, Khair A (MD)	NP	286
Sullivan, Daniel J (MD)	DR	280
Sullivan, Henry (MD)	TS	264
Sultan, John (MD)	IM	315
Sumida, Colin (MD)	Cv	331
Sunbulli, Talal (MD)	Ge	171
Sundar, Balakrishna (MD)	U	267

NAME	SPECIALTY	PAGE
Wander, John (MD)	S	297
Warpeha, Raymond L (MD)	PlS	240
Warren, Ann (MD)	ObG	327
Warren, William (MD)	TS	264
Wassef, Samir Y (MD)	NP	193
Wasserman, David (MD)	DR	161
Wasserman, Michael (MD)	N	201
Waters, William Bedford (MD)	U	267
Watt, Cathleen M (MD)	Anes	150
Wayne, Audrey (MD)	Oph	289
Wayne, Ralph W. (MD)	DR	280
Wechter, David T (MD)	IM	188
Wehner, Julie (MD)	OrS	218
Weigel, Thomas (MD)	PCd	223
Weiner, Glenn (MD)	Rhu	254
Weingarten, Charles (MD)	Oto	221
Weinstein, Robert Alan (MD)	Inf	178
Weir, Bryce (MD)	NS	198
Weise, Roger A (MD)	Ger	172
Weisman, Robert (MD)	CRS	156
Weiss, Regis (MD)	GO	174
Weiss, Robert (MD)	Oph	213
Wenzel, Dave (MD)	Anes	277
Werner, Phillip Ladd (MD)	EDM	163
West, Ann (MD)	ObG	303
West, James (MD)	Pul	249
Wheeler, John (MD)	U	268
Wheeler, Wendell (MD)	Ped	235
Whisler, Walter (MD)	NS	199
White, G Wesley (MD)	Inf	179
White, John (MD)	S	306
Whitington, Peter (MD)	Ped	235
Wichter, Melvin (MD)	N	201
Wickman, Doris (MD)	ObG	288
Wicks, Mark (MD)	Pul	294
Wiedrich, Thomas (MD)	HS	175
Wieland, John (MD)	Ge	171
Wiener, Pauline K (MD)	GerPsy	282
Wiggins, Henry W Jr (MD)	Rad	251
Wilber, David (MD)	Cv	155
Wilczynski, Michael (MD)	Rad	251
Wilensky, Jacob (MD)	Oph	213
Wilner, Gary (MD)	Cv	155
Winans, Charles (MD)	Ge	171
Winnie, Alon (MD)	Anes	150
Winter, Christine (MD)	Onc	285
Wise, Ronald (MD)	D	158
Wistenberg, Lexy (MD)	IM	188
Witt, Paul (MD)	OrS	304
Witt, Thomas (MD)	S	261
Wiznitzer, Israel (MD)	Onc	316
Wiznitzer, Israel (MD)	Onc	316
Wohlberg, Frederick (MD)	U	268
Wollner, Timothy (DO)	FP	168
Wolpert, Edward (MD)	Psyc	246
Wolter, Janet (MD)	Onc	192
Wong, Alton (MD)	Hem	177
Wong, Paul (MD)	MG	189
Woodley, David T (MD)	D	159
Wood-Molo, Mary (MD)	RE	252
Woods, William (MD)	ObG	317
Woody, Lisa (MD)	OM	209
Worwag, Ewelina (MD)	PM	222
Wright, Robert (MD)	N	201
Wrona, Leo A (MD)	ObG	333
Wuertz, Peter M. (DO)	Anes	311
Wurtz, Rebecca (MD)	Inf	179
Wyma, Daniel (MD)	Psyc	294
Wyse, Joseph (MD)	IM	188

Y

NAME	SPECIALTY	PAGE
Yanong, Procopio U (MD)	Ped	235
Yao, James (MD)	GVS	269
Yao, Tito (MD)	Ped	235
Yapor, Wesley (MD)	NS	199
Yapp, Rockford (MD)	Ge	282
Yario, Robert (MD)	TS	264
Yee, Martin J (MD)	PMR	237
Yegelwel, Eric (MD)	IM	188
Yeh, Stephen (MD)	Oto	221
Yellen, Steven (MD)	Cv	155
Yogev, Ram (MD)	Ped	235
Yohay, Daniel (MD)	Nep	196
Yordan, Edgardo (MD)	GO	174
Young, I James (MD)	N	201
Young, Michael (MD)	U	268
Young, Nancy (MD)	Oto	221
Yu, Mario (MD)	ObG	288
Yuk, Antonio (MD)	NS	327

Z

NAME	SPECIALTY	PAGE
Zachary, Lawrence (MD)	PlS	241
Zahid, Mohammad (MD)	Nep	302
Zahrebelski, George (MD)	Ge	171
Zaino, Ricca Yao (MD)	ObG	328
Zajecka, John (MD)	Psyc	246
Zalski, Andrew (MD)	FP	168
Zanetti, Claude (MD)	Pul	249
Zaret, Cheryl Riva (MD)	Oph	214
Zarian, Lawrence P (MD)	DR	313
Zarling, Edwin (MD)	Ge	171
Ziai, Fuad (MD)	PEn	224
Zieserl, Edward (MD)	Ped	235
Zikos, Demetrios (MD)	Nep	196

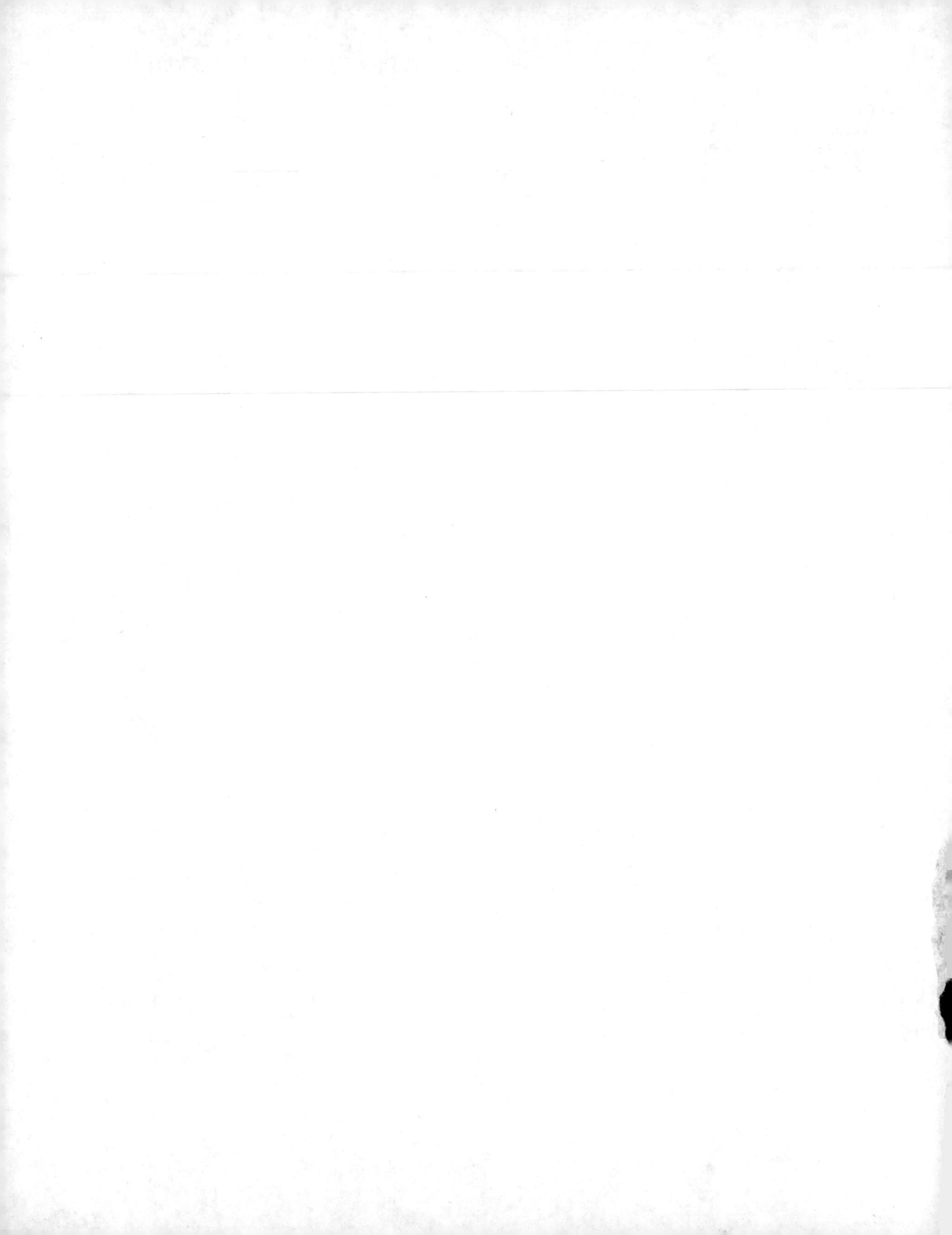